Pediatric Atlas of Ultrasound- and Nerve Stimulation-Guided Regional Anesthesia

Ban C.H. Tsui • Santhanam Suresh
Editors

Pediatric Atlas of Ultrasound- and Nerve Stimulation-Guided Regional Anesthesia

Springer

Editors
Ban C.H. Tsui, Dip Eng, BSc (Math), B Pharm, MSc, MD, FRCPC
Professor and Director of Clinical Research
Department of Anesthesiology and Pain Medicine
University of Alberta
Edmonton, Alberta
Canada

Pediatric and Adult Anesthesiologist
Stollery Children's Hospital/University of Alberta Hospital
Site Chief, Anesthesia, Cross Cancer Institute
Edmonton, Alberta
Canada

Santhanam Suresh, MD
Arthur C. King Professor and Chair of Pediatric Anesthesiology
Department of Pediatric Anesthesiology
Ann and Robert H. Lurie Children's Hospital of Chicago
Chicago, IL
USA

Professor of Anesthesiology and Pediatrics
Feinberg School of Medicine
Northwestern University
Chicago, IL
USA

ISBN 978-0-387-79963-6 ISBN 978-0-387-79964-3 (eBook)
DOI 10.1007/978-0-387-79964-3

Library of Congress Control Number: 2015949112

Springer New York Heidelberg Dordrecht London

Printed on acid-free paper

Springer Science+Business Media LLC New York is part of Springer Science+Business Media (www.springer.com)

We would like to dedicate this edition of the book to our patients, our teachers, our students, and our families. In addition, Dr. Tsui would especially like to express his deepest appreciation of the great encouragement provided to him during his academic career by his father, Woon-Tak Tsui, who he lost suddenly during the preparation of this edition.

Ban C.H. Tsui, MD
Santhanam Suresh, MD

To my wife, Eliza, and my children, Jenkin and Jeremy—the real loves of my life. Without their support and understanding, I could not have completed this demanding project. I would also like to dedicate this opus to my parents, Woon-Tak and Kau-Wan, for their love and guidance throughout my life.

Ban C.H. Tsui, MD

I would like to dedicate this book to my family; my wife, Nina, and my children, Aneesha, Sunitha, and Madhav, who have been my greatest inspiration and love in my life; my mother Chandra Santhanam who has been my avid supporter; and to the memory of my late father R. Santhanam whose extraordinary love and dedication to our family fostered my growth. I want to thank all the members of the Department of Pediatric Anesthesiology at the Ann & Robert H. Lurie Children's Hospital of Chicago, whose support was imperative in getting this book off the ground. Finally to my colleague and friend Ban Tsui whose dedication and commitment is what evolved into this atlas.

Santhanam Suresh, MD

Foreword

Over the past 30 years, pediatric regional anesthesia has come of age. There is now a large and rapidly growing body of information regarding the impact of development on pain responses, local anesthetic pharmacology, and the adaptation of a full range of regional anesthetic techniques for infants and children. There is also a quickly expanding literature on safety and efficacy from registries and clinical trials. Thirty years ago, in most pediatric centers worldwide, regional anesthesia was used for only a small fraction of surgeries. Today, it is an essential part of pediatric anesthetic and analgesic management throughout the world. For children in tertiary centers in highly developed countries, regional anesthesia is recognized as an essential component of multimodal analgesic regimens that seek to provide pain relief with movement; diminish opioid use, with a corresponding reduction in opioid side-effects; and facilitate early mobilization, early enteral feeding, and early hospital discharge. Some preliminary studies in infant humans and infant animals suggest that regional anesthesia may have an impact on preventing prolonged changes in central nervous system responses to surgical trauma. In lower resource settings, pediatric regional anesthesia is more often used as a primary anesthetic approach, based on considerations of cost, safety, and reduced need for postoperative intensive care. In the face of ongoing controversy over the impact of general anesthetics on the developing brain, regional anesthesia has a growing role for neonates, infants, and toddlers as an approach to limiting general anesthetic dosing and overall exposure.

Ban Tsui and Santhanam Suresh have been pioneers in this effort, and it is fitting that they are co-editing this wonderful textbook. Both editors have made fundamental innovations in the field over the past 20 years, and both continue to innovate and to mentor to a new generation of investigators and clinicians.

This book is superb in every way. As an atlas, it is first-rate. Anatomic drawings, diagrams, photos, and ultrasound images are combined in ways that masterfully guide the reader. The introductory sections outline the physics behind nerve stimulation and ultrasound in a way that is both sophisticated and highly practical for the clinician. The chapter entitled "Clinical and Practical Aspects of Ultrasound Use" codifies a set of clinical pearls in a clear and useful manner. The chapters that discuss pain assessment, pharmacology, and complications are practical and up-to-date. Part III covers the clinical anatomy of the various regions of the body with relevance to the conduct of regional anesthesia. Throughout these sections, the illustrations are outstanding, with just the right level of detail and the right points of emphasis. Parts IV, V, VI, VII, VIII, IX, and X build on these foundations to elucidate the "how-to" for the full range of regional anesthetic blocks. No other textbook, adult or pediatric, gives such clear guidance on how to perform a block, how to troubleshoot, how to avoid pitfalls, and how to analyze and solve clinical problems. Throughout these sections, there is a great balance between the science and the art of regional anesthesia. In every chapter, there is an authoritative reference list.

I am left with only one criticism, namely the title. This book is a magnificent atlas, but it is really much more than that: it is by far the definitive textbook on pediatric regional anesthesia.

Charles Berde, MD, PhD
Professor of Anesthesia (Pediatrics), Harvard Medical School,
Children's Hospital Boston, Boston, MA, USA

Preface

In 2007, Tsui, with Springer, published the first textbook and atlas devoted entirely to ultrasound-guided regional blockade in adults, entitled *Atlas of Ultrasound and Nerve Stimulation-Guided Regional Anesthesia*. Since then, many textbooks and atlases with a similar focus have been written, albeit for the adult population only. Despite the extensive progress made in regional anesthesia over the past decades, there still exists no textbook and/or atlas dedicated to both ultrasound- and nerve stimulation-guided regional blockades for the pediatric population.

In preparing this, the first textbook focused on ultrasound and nerve stimulation for pediatric regional anesthesia; we had the privilege of gathering friends and colleagues as contributing authors. Similar to the situation for the adult population, pediatric regional anesthesia has long been regarded as an "art," and success with these techniques is perceived widely to be the domain of a few skilled pediatric anesthesiologists. Around 30 years ago, the introduction of nerve stimulation technology began to nudge regional anesthesia closer toward a "science." However, nerve stimulation has its limitations; the technique relies on electrical impulses to elicit a physiological response from nerves, and considerable variation exists among individuals with respect to this phenomenon. Nerve stimulation guidance is also limited by a number of other factors, including the properties of injectates, physiological fluids (e.g., blood), and disease. Nevertheless, it proved to be a useful and objective method to place, with some reliability, the needle tip close to a target nerve. Surprisingly, the introduction of nerve stimulation did not spark a renewed interest in regional anesthesia, although it proved quite a benefit to those of us who were performing nerve blocks on a regular basis. This is particularly true in the case of pediatric patients, who are usually unable to provide feedback since their blocks are administered under heavy sedation and/or general anesthesia.

Ultrasound imaging is one of the most exciting technological advancements to be applied to regional anesthesia. For the first time in over 100 years, we can visualize the nerve which we intend to block. Unlike nerve stimulation, we foresee ultrasound being a catalyst to draw anesthesiologists toward devoting more of their practice to regional anesthesia. We must remember, however, that the images ultrasound provides us are indirect and open to individual interpretation, depending on the user's experience level, training, and where they received that experience and training. While some practitioners have a natural gift for interpreting ultrasound images, this is not the case with the majority. There is a significant learning curve that goes with mastering ultrasound-guided regional anesthesia. What is more, it has been shown that combining ultrasound and nerve stimulation can improve block success, meaning that two techniques must be learned and mastered to be used to achieve a common goal. This was the main reason for describing and covering the advantages of both technologies in the adult atlas.

It is our hope that the adult atlas spurred readers to incorporate ultrasound (and nerve stimulation) technology into their practice and become better regional anesthesiologists. As with that book, the main objective of this one is to shorten the learning curve associated with regional anesthesia—this time for use in pediatric patients. For those practitioners who are already adept and experienced with pediatric regional anesthesia, this book may serve to increase their knowledge and provide new insights into this field. The ultimate goal of this book is to continue to develop and uncover new knowledge by amalgamating landmark, nerve stimulation, and ultrasound guidance techniques in regional anesthesia, thereby improving patient care.

This atlas follows a layout similar to the one in the adult atlas. The book begins with several chapters providing information on both ultrasound and nerve stimulation. Equipment and setup, with a focus on needs for pediatric regional anesthesia, are also discussed. Chapter 4 provides perhaps the most important information, including many practical ideas and approaches for using ultrasound during pediatric regional blockade. As with the adult book, we have also included a chapter discussing the fundamental ideas and physical tenets underlying electrical stimulation for regional blockade. In the clinical chapters, the reader will find helpful tables and flowcharts which describe step-by-step procedures for finding a nerve using electrical stimulation as well as troubleshooting tips in case of unexpected or unwanted responses during nerve stimulation. This atlas also includes a chapter on the use of ultrasound for placement of perineural catheters for continuous nerve blocks; many readers will find this chapter applicable to blocks in adults as well.

In the same way that a sound knowledge of anatomy forms the basis of success in regional anesthesia, anatomy forms the core of this book. As Gaston Labat, the father of modern regional anesthesia, stated, "Anatomy is the foundation upon which the entire concept of regional anesthesia is built. Anyone who wishes to be an expert in the art of regional anesthesia must be thoroughly grounded in anatomy." This advice remains as true today as when it was given a century ago. Thus, there are six consecutive chapters discussing pediatric anatomy with relevance to regional anesthesia, each supplemented with diagrams and illustrations to provide the reader with a comprehensive rendering of the anatomy associated with blocks in a particular region of the body. In the clinical chapters, there is a brief description of relevant anatomy with illustrations. In the absence of a readily available pediatric cadaver, we utilized an adult cadaver software program to obtain cross-sectional images showing gross anatomy, and we have used MRI and ultrasound, in pediatric subjects where possible, to capture detailed images of the corresponding block location. This is followed by a clinical description of how to perform ultrasound imaging during regional blockade. These sections describe and illustrate the positioning of the probe, the specific needling technique used, how to use nerve stimulation, and pre- and post-local anesthetic application. This sequential format gives the reader a realistic simulation of the management of each clinical situation.

The images used in this book are those from our everyday practice and are achievable by any newcomer using ultrasound for regional anesthesia. We have been mindful not to concentrate on anatomically perfect ultrasound images—which can be obtained occasionally—but instead show images that are representative of those encountered on an average day. As with the adult atlas, MRI images were captured from consenting patients to further illustrate the neuroanatomy and relationship to surrounding anatomical structures. Where possible, we have also provided schematic drawings to show the relationship between nerves, vessels, bone, muscle, and other structures that one must contend with when using ultrasound to guide nerve blocks. For the ultrasound images, we have again provided unlabeled and labeled images along with a diagram showing the location of the ultrasound probe footprint. The unlabeled image allows the reader to familiarize themselves with a realistic clinical image without the distraction of labels. In our experience, the side-by-side presentation of unlabeled and labeled ultrasound images acts as a helpful learning tool for novice users.

Since ultrasound-guided regional anesthesia is still an emerging field, the literature is constantly being updated with new ideas about how to best apply this technology. In this book, we focus on the most common approaches used and supplement these by including, in clinical pearls and notes, alternative approaches as described in the literature or by the chapter authors. This allows the reader to attempt and select the most suitable approach for his/her own needs. Throughout the book, dynamic and systematic scanning techniques are emphasized. As with adults, ultrasound-guided visualization of obvious nearby landmarks (i.e., blood vessels) is recommended as a first step in identifying target nerves in pediatric patients. From there, shifting the view to the associated neural structures and "tracing back" to the desired block site is, in our experience, a more user-friendly method than "hunting" for the target nerve and block site without the guidance of any familiar subcutaneous landmarks. In this way, the dynamic method reemphasizes the importance of anatomical knowledge as the foundation for successful regional anesthesia.

It is almost certain that when they are first beginning to use ultrasound for regional blockade, anesthesiologists will encounter difficulty in learning how to use the technology to identify neural structures and place the needle tip accurately. In many cases, this will result in frustration and failure, which likely deters many anesthesiologists from persisting in improving their technique and adopting the technology for their practice. This is especially pertinent to pediatric regional anesthesia since the patients are, in general, uncooperative and the anatomy is that much smaller and, in some cases, underdeveloped compared to adults. We anticipate that the concepts and methods described in this textbook will ease the learning curve for pediatric anesthesiologists wishing to incorporate regional blockade into their repertoire. Finally, the contents of this book provide a useful refresher and resource for all regional anesthesiologists wishing to hone their skills and adapt cutting-edge techniques into their practice.

Edmonton, Alberta, Canada
Chicago, IL, USA

Ban C.H. Tsui, MSc, MD, FRCPC
Santhanam Suresh, MD

Acknowledgments

We wish to acknowledge the following individuals for their support, hard work, and contributions in preparing this book. Dr. Tsui's research manager, Dr. Gareth Corry, spent many extra hours and worked diligently to contribute toward and assemble the material contained in this book. His continual assistance with editing helped organize and expedite our and our colleagues' writing and editing process. We also wish to thank a group of students, medical students, fellows, and research assistants over the past 5 years, including Natalie Chua, Kim Cochrane, Jason Ha, Sarah Henschke, Alex Kwan, Danika Leung, Paul Li, Jennifer Pillay, and Jenkin Tsui from the University of Alberta, and Dr. Amod Sawardekar from Northwestern University, who assisted in organizing chapter drafts, labeling of the images, and contribution of the written material. The Chair of the University of Alberta Department of Anesthesiology and Pain Medicine, Dr. Mike Murphy, provides ongoing support and encouragement. Dr. Michelle Noga, of the University of Alberta Department of Diagnostic Imaging and Radiology, facilitated access to the institution's MRI technology and operators. We also acknowledge the work done by Teresa Liang, now a radiology resident at the University of British Columbia, who diligently collected the MRI images used in this book. We acknowledge the Ecole Polytechnique Fédérale de Lausanne, Switzerland, Visible Human Web Server (http://visiblehuman.epfl.ch) as the data source for the anatomical slices used throughout the book. Staff members from the University of Alberta Hospital, the Stollery Children's Hospital, and Northwestern University/Lurie Children's Hospital Chicago always provide an excellent environment for patient care, teaching, and research that has directly facilitated the advancement of clinical regional anesthesia practice. A Clinical Scholar Award from the Alberta Heritage Foundation for Medical Research allowed Dr. Tsui to pursue this project by helping to support his academic work. The unrestricted grant from Springer to start this project was a financial help and support, and Shelley Reinhardt and Michael D. Sova from Springer are greatly appreciated for providing their expertise and assistance for this project.

Edmonton, Alberta, Canada
Chicago, IL, USA

Ban C.H. Tsui, MSc, MD, FRCPC
Santhanam Suresh, MD

Contents

Part VI Nerve Blocks Below the Clavicle

Contributors

Alex Baloukov, MPH Faculty of Health Sciences, Simon Fraser University, Burnaby, BC, Canada

Karen R. Boretsky, MD Department of Anesthesia, Perioperative and Pain Medicine, Harvard Medical School, Boston Children's Hospital, Boston, MA, USA

Kelly P.A. Byrne, MB ChB, FANZCA Department of Anesthesia, Waikato Hospital, Hamilton, New Zealand

Bruce D. Dick, PhD, R Psych Division of Pain Medicine, Department of Anesthesiology and Pain Medicine, Stollery Children's Hospital, University of Alberta, Edmonton, AB, Canada

Bryan J. Dicken, MSc, MD, FRCSC Division of Pediatric Surgery, Department of Surgery, University of Alberta Hospital, Edmonton, AB, Canada

Derek Dillane, MB, BCh, BAO, MMedSci, FFARCSI Department of Anesthesiology and Pain Medicine, University of Alberta Hospital, Edmonton, AB, Canada

Adam M. Dryden, MD Department of Anesthesiology and Pain Medicine, University of Alberta Hospital, Edmonton, AB, Canada

Vivian H.Y. Ip, MB ChB, MRCP, FRCA Department of Anesthesiology and Pain Medicine, University of Alberta Hospital, Edmonton, AB, Canada

Glenn Merritt, MD Department of Anesthesiology, University of Colorado Hospital and Children's Hospital Colorado, Aurora, CO, USA

Peter D. Metcalfe, MD, MSc, FRCSC Division of Pediatric Surgery, Division of Urology, Department of Surgery, Stollery Children's Hospital, University of Alberta Hospital, Edmonton, AB, Canada

Michelle L. Noga, MD, FRCPC Department of Radiology and Diagnostic Imaging, University of Alberta, Edmonton, AB, Canada

Kathy Reid, RN, MN, NP Pediatric Anesthesia, Stollery Children's Hospital, Edmonton, AB, Canada

Adam O. Spencer, MSc, MD, FRCPC Vi Riddell Complex Pain and Rehabilitation Centre, Alberta Children's Hospital, Calgary, AB, Canada

Santhanam Suresh, MD Department of Pediatric Anesthesiology, Ann & Robert Lurie Children's Hospital of Chicago, Chicago, IL, USA

Heather Yizhen Z. Ting, MD, FRCPC Department of Anesthesiology and Pain Medicine, University of Alberta Hospital, Edmonton, AB, Canada

Ban C.H. Tsui, Dip Eng, BSc (Math), B Pharm, MSc, MD, FRCPC Department of Anesthesiology and Pain Medicine, Stollery Children's Hospital/University of Alberta Hospital, Edmonton, AB, Canada

Michelle J. Verrier, BA Department of Anesthesiology and Pain Medicine, University of Alberta, Edmonton, AB, Canada

Anil H. Walji, MD, PhD Division of Anatomy, Department of Surgery, Faculty of Medicine and Dentistry, University of Alberta, Edmonton, AB, Canada

Part I

Equipment and Technique for Nerve Stimulation and Ultrasound Guidance in Regional Anesthesia

1 Regional Block Area Setup, Equipment, and Monitoring

Vivian H.Y. Ip and Ban C.H. Tsui

Contents

V.H.Y. Ip, MB ChB, MRCP, FRCA
Department of Anesthesiology and Pain Medicine,
University of Alberta Hospital, 2-150 Clinical Sciences Building,
Edmonton, AB T6G 2G3, Canada
e-mail: hip@ualberta.ca

B.C.H. Tsui, Dip Eng, BSc (Math), B Pharm, MSc, MD, FRCPC (✉)
Department of Anesthesiology and Pain Medicine,
Stollery Children's Hospital/University of Alberta Hospital,
2-150 Clinical Sciences Building, Edmonton, AB T6G 2G3, Canada
e-mail: btsui@ualberta.ca

B.C.H. Tsui, S. Suresh (eds.), *Pediatric Atlas of Ultrasound- and Nerve Stimulation-Guided Regional Anesthesia*,
DOI 10.1007/978-0-387-79964-3_1

1.1 Differences Between the Pediatric and Adult Populations That Affect Regional Blocks

It is important to recognize that there are distinct differences between the pediatric and adult populations that can affect regional block technique. In order to understand the setup and equipment used for children in regional anesthesia, one must appreciate that:

- Children do not understand the importance of lying still for a procedure.
- Children are not able to communicate or differentiate paresthesia, pain, or pressure on injection.
- Anatomical structures are smaller and are situated more closely to each other and to the adjacent vessels.
- Target nerves are more superficial to the skin.
- There is a lower concentration of plasma protein binding, especially in young children.

To overcome these differences, regional anesthesia is usually performed in children under deep sedation or general anesthesia. There is ongoing debate regarding performing regional anesthesia in anesthetized adults, but such practice is well accepted in pediatric patients, primarily due to the differences outlined above. This encourages development of other techniques to minimize the incidence of nerve damage, namely, nerve stimulators, ultrasonography, and injection pressure monitoring.

When performing a regional block, the equipment should be appropriate for the size of the patient. In particular, the size of the needle must be adapted to the size of the child. This allows for improved control of the needle while performing the blocks, which are often superficial. The SLA "hockey stick" (25 mm, 13–6 MHz) is a good example of an ultrasound transducer that provides good resolution for superficial structures and has a small footprint. These are essential characteristics when using ultrasound to guide regional blocks in the pediatric population.

1.2 Block Area and Monitoring

Performing regional anesthesia in children requires meticulous attention to detail and concentration. Having a quiet environment with all of the drugs and equipment needed to perform regional anesthesia and resuscitation on hand is of paramount importance. An induction room is an ideal place where the patient can be sedated or anesthetized away from surgical staff and where the regional block could be performed before entering into the operating room. Available space and setups will, however, vary between hospitals. In adults, a designated block area can be used to provide the ideal environment while speeding up turnover time; however, this type of area may be unnecessary for pediatric patients, as the majority will receive a general anesthetic before regional anesthesia is performed. Also, since the regional block is for analgesia, the time for the block to take effect is not as essential as compared to its application for surgical anesthesia.

An assistant trained in regional anesthesia, with experience in monitoring pediatric patients under sedation or general anesthesia, should be present. This is important not only for monitoring the child during the procedure but also to handle the nerve stimulator and to help with the injectate.

Regardless of the area, it is critical to have all equipment, drugs, and monitoring available in the room where the block is to be performed. The best way to gather all the necessary equipment and drugs is to use a well-labeled storage cart (Fig. 1.1) where the supplies are organized and easily identifiable.

The following outlines the contents of this cart:

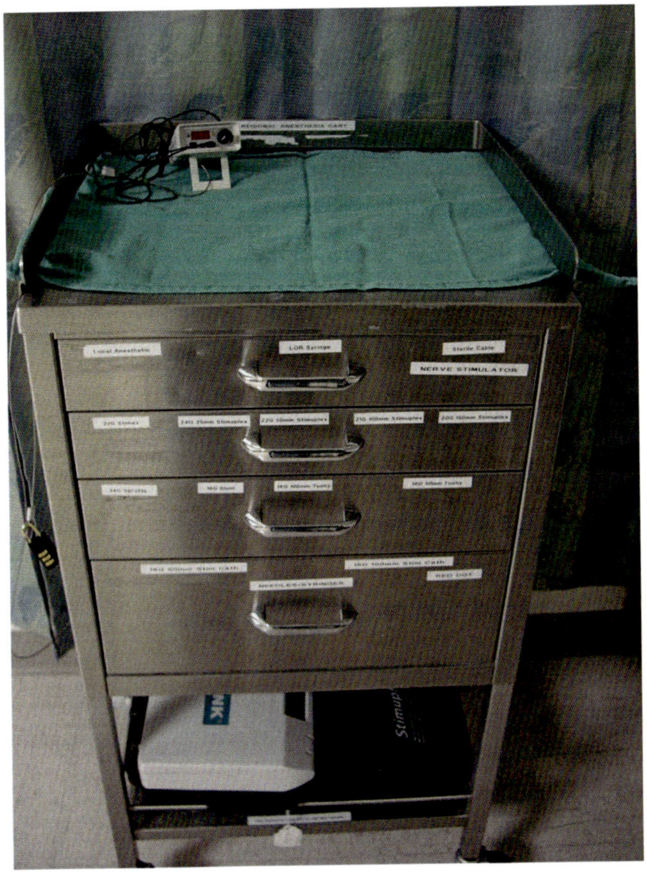

Fig. 1.1 Equipment storage cart with clear identification of equipment, supplies, and medication

1.2.1 General Equipment

- Sterile skin preparation solution.
- Sponges/gauze.
- Drape.
- Marking pen and ruler for landmark identification.
- Selection of different sizes of syringes.
- A variety of needles with a selection of gauges for skin infiltration, drawing up 5 % dextrose, local anesthetics, sedation, or induction of general anesthetic.
- In pediatric patients, most regional blocks are performed under general anesthesia without a muscle relaxant. However, selections of sedatives and hypnotics can be used for cooperative mature pediatric patients as follows:
  - Midazolam (IM/IV: 0.1–0.15 mg/kg up to 0.5 mg/kg, IV infusion with loading dose of 0.05–0.2 mg/kg over 2–3 min. Continuous infusion initiated at a rate of 0.06–0.12 mg/kg/h)
  - Propofol (IV: 1–2 mg/kg for sedation, then 100–150 μg/kg/min infusion)
  - Short-acting opioids:
    - Fentanyl (IV sedation: 1–2 μg/kg, then 0.5–1 μg/kg/h IV infusion).
    - Remifentanil (IV: 2–18 years: 1 μg/kg over 30–60 s, then 0.05–0.1 μg/kg/min IV infusion). All sedation medication should be titrated to response.
  - Several commonly used local anesthetics with different concentrations, as well as 50 mL bags or ampules of normal saline for drug dilution if necessary.
  - *All local anesthetics should be stored separately from the intravenous drugs.*

1.2.2 Emergency Drugs and Resuscitating Equipment

- Although the use of ultrasound allows reduced volumes of local anesthetic to accomplish a successful nerve block, it is pertinent to have resuscitation equipment and drugs available.
- Children have a higher tolerance to local anesthetic on a weight-dependent basis owing to a greater volume of distribution; this increases the threshold in reaching the toxic dose. However, in newborns less than 6 months, the threshold in reaching the toxic dose is reduced due to the lower concentration of serum protein for local anesthetic binding, namely, alpha-1 acid glycoprotein. This results in a higher plasma concentration of unbound local anesthetic.

1.2.3 Resuscitation Equipment

- Oxygen supply, nasal prongs, and face masks.
- A selection of different sizes of Guedel airways, face masks, laryngeal masks, and endotracheal tubes.
- Laryngoscopes (Macintosh and Miller blades) and gum elastic bougie.
- Ambu® bag (bagger).
- Suction.
- Selections of various sizes of intravenous cannulae.
- Defibrillator should also be accessible.

1.2.4 Resuscitation Drugs (Intravenous Doses)

- Atropine (0.02 mg/kg)
- Epinephrine (0.01 mg/kg)
- Suxamethonium (2 mg/kg)
- Ephedrine (1–12 years: 0.2–0.3 mg/kg; 12–18 years: 2.5–5 mg)
- Glycopyrrolate (5–10 μg/kg)
- Intralipid® 20 % (1.5 mL/kg bolus over 1 min followed by 0.25 mL/kg/min infusion; bolus dose can be repeated at 5-min intervals if there is no return of spontaneous circulation) (see Chaps. 7 and 8).

1.2.5 Monitoring

- Routine monitoring should be applied before sedation or general anesthetic is induced. This includes:
  - Electrocardiogram
  - Noninvasive blood pressure
  - Pulse oximetry
  - Capnography
  - End-tidal gas monitoring

1.2.6 Nerve Block and Catheter Equipment

There is a variety of different needles for single-shot nerve blocks and Tuohy needles for peripheral nerve catheter insertion. The needles for single-shot nerve blocks usually have a female attachment for the nerve stimulator and another extension to facilitate aspiration and injection of 5 % dextrose or local anesthetics. Extension tubing is also available to facilitate flexible attachment of a syringe to the Tuohy needle for catheter insertions.

1.2.7 Needles

1.2.7.1 Needle Tip Design

A blunt needle (Fig. 1.2) reduces the risk of nerve damage and provides a better feel for the "pop" of puncturing through the fascia. However, if the needle is too blunt, the user may have to apply extra pressure to perforate the fascia, which can result in "overshooting" the nerve.

Long-beveled needles increase the risk of damage to nerves and vascular structures in the case of intraneural puncture.

- For continuous peripheral nerve blocks, the commonly used needles are:
  - Tuohy needles (Fig. 1.3), 18G (20G catheter) or 20G (22–24G catheter). These are the same needles as used for epidural anesthesia.
  - Special Sprotte® cannulas (Fig. 1.4) have a lateral "eye" with smooth edges to prevent shearing of the catheter. They also have an atraumatic tip.
  - Facet tip needles (Fig. 1.5) are used when the catheter is to be positioned parallel to the nerve.

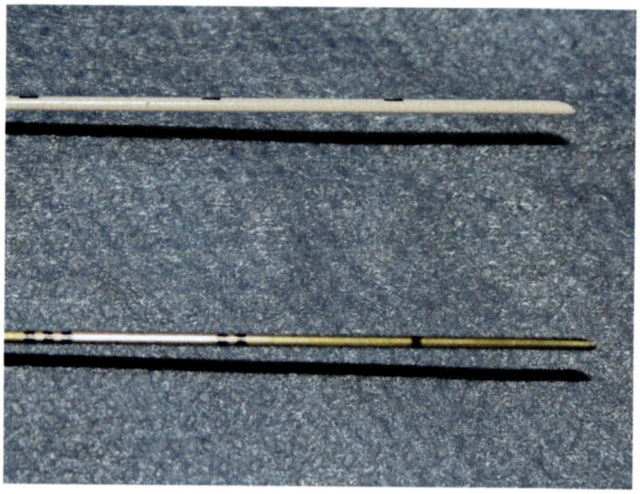

Fig. 1.2 Blunt needles for single-shot nerve blocks

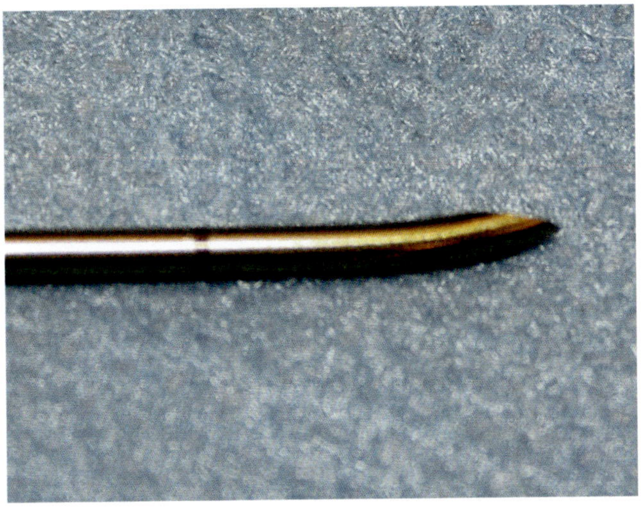

Fig. 1.3 Tuohy needle for continuous peripheral nerve blocks

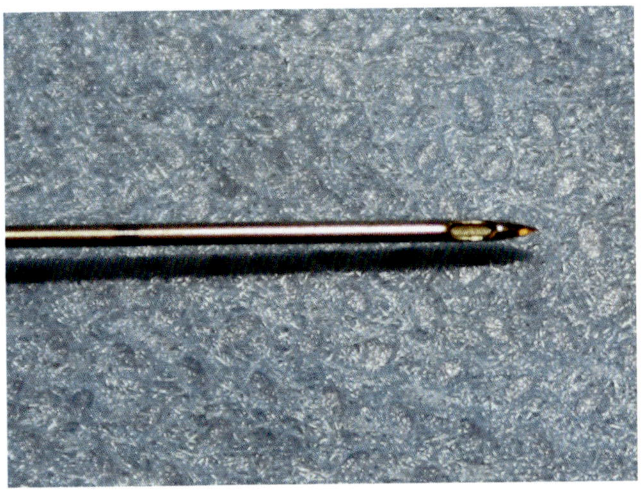

Fig. 1.4 Special Sprotte® cannula with a lateral "eye" with smooth edges and an atraumatic tip

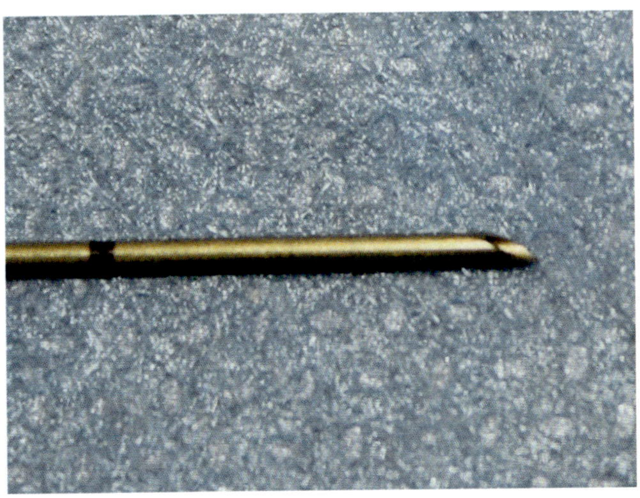

Fig. 1.5 Facet tip needle. To be used when the catheter is to be positioned parallel to the nerve

1.2.7.2 Needle Lengths

The choice of the needle length depends on the specific block and the size of the child. The use of ultrasound can help determine the depth to the target nerve. Some needles have centimeter markings (Fig. 1.6) which indicate the depth of penetration into the tissue. The use of the shortest possible needle for the required block allows for better handling and manipulation. The range of needles available is given by the following examples:

- 25 mm (ProBloc SC® by Life-Tech INC., Texas, USA; Arrow, Reading, PA)
- 30 mm (Life-Tech INC., Texas, USA; Pajunk, Geisingen, Germany; B Braun, Melsungen, Germany)
- 40 mm (ProBloc SC® by Life-Tech INC., Texas, USA)
- 50 mm (Life-Tech INC., Texas, USA; Pajunk, Geisingen, Germany; Arrow, Reading, PA)

1.2.7.3 Needle Gauges

- Generally, a 22G insulated needle is used for single-shot peripheral nerve blocks, although 25G insulated needles are also available.
- For catheter insertion, 20–21G and 24G catheters are inserted with 18G and 20G Tuohy needles, respectively.

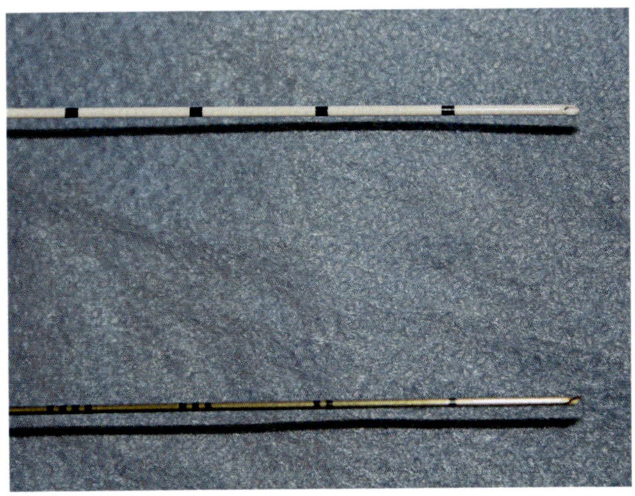

Fig. 1.6 Centimeter markings along the entire length of needles are useful for measuring depth of penetration

1.2.7.4 Other Needle Designs

Other needles are echogenic (e.g., Stimuplex®, B Braun, Melsungen, Germany) or have echogenic "dots" made by "Cornerstone" reflectors (e.g., SonoPlex®, Pajunk, Geisingen, Germany) (Fig. 1.7) to facilitate better imaging of the needle under ultrasound.

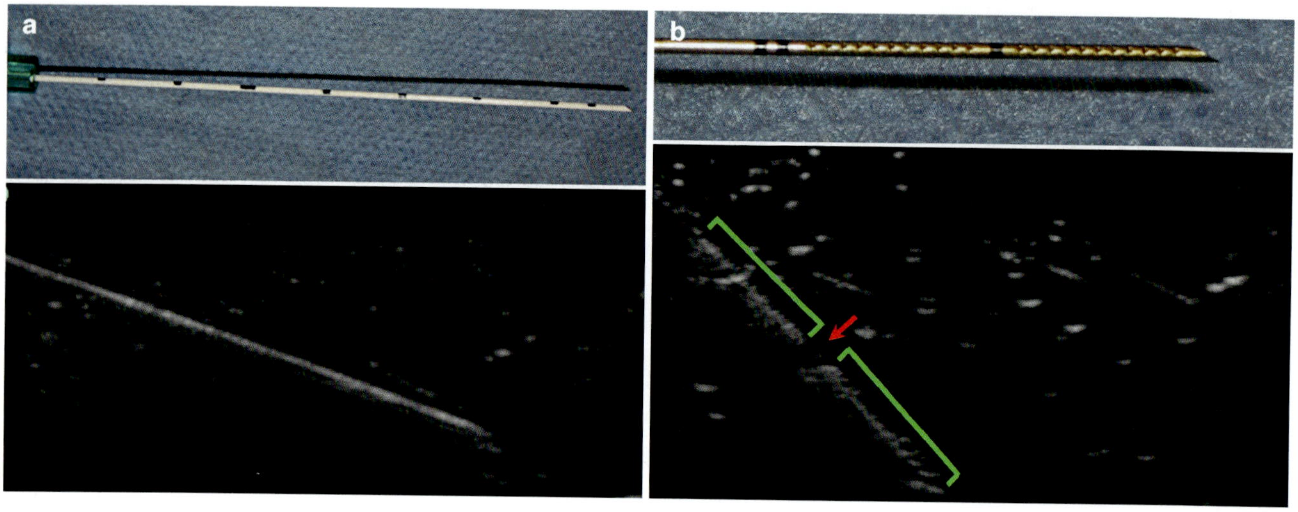

Fig. 1.7 (**a**) Echogenic needles or (**b**) needles with echogenic "dots" made by "Cornerstone" reflectors facilitate better imaging of the needle under ultrasound

1.2.8 Peripheral Nerve Catheters

Approaches (see Chap. 5)

1. Catheter through needle
   There are two broad types of catheters: stimulating catheters and non-stimulating catheters. The advancement and course of stimulating catheters are guided by the motor response achieved by nerve stimulation.
2. Catheter over needle
   The approach has just recently been introduced into the market. Ultrasound guidance is critical when using the catheter-over-needle approach. The introducing needle can be stimulating or non-stimulating, whereas the catheter itself is only available in non-stimulating format. Detailed discussion is presented in Chap. 5.

1.2.9 Neuraxial Nerve Blocks/Catheters

There are ready-made packs with various needles, syringes, drapes, gauze/sponges, aseptic solutions, and catheters (if appropriate) for caudal, spinal, and epidural anesthesia. These should also be available in the storage cart. Details of epidural catheter placement are presented in Chaps. 5 and 33.

1.2.10 Additional Equipment

When performing a regional block, patient feedback and communication are often used as one of the indicators of neural damage. As children are more often than not anesthetized when performing a regional block, it is important to have other tools to increase success rate while minimizing adverse effects. These include:

1.2.10.1 Nerve Stimulator

A functioning, high-quality nerve stimulator with digital display of the current amplitude between 0 and 5 mA and short pulse width is adequate for peripheral nerve blocks. When performing nerve stimulation, the negative electrode is attached to the needle, and the positive electrode is attached to the patient. Higher current (1–15 mA) is required for electrical stimulation via the epidural catheter (the Tsui test). A smooth, gradual increment and decrement of current is important for fine adjustment of the block needle or catheter.

1.2.10.2 Ultrasound Machine

A detailed discussion about the principles of ultrasound machines and related equipment is discussed in Chap. 3, and the practical aspects of ultrasound-guided anesthesia are discussed in Chap. 4.

To ensure a good-quality image, selecting an appropriate transducer and a high-resolution machine is essential. Good needling technique needle and visualization are also crucial when performing blocks in children since anatomical structures are close together.

1.2.10.3 Injection Pressure Monitoring

Monitoring of injection pressure is important when performing peripheral nerve blocks. High-pressure injections may indicate intraneural injection, which can cause persistent neurological deficit. There are commercially available, single-use, in-line pressure monitors (Fig. 1.8), as well as the use of a column of air in the syringe and the compressed air injection technique (CAIT) (Fig. 1.9) to prevent high injection pressure. A compressed air injection technique involves withdrawing a set amount of air above a volume of injectate in a syringe, with the subsequent compression and maintenance of this volume during injection to maintain the pressure at a chosen level. The compression of the air volume in the syringe during injection at 50 % or less will ensure an injection pressure below 760 mmHg. This is substantially lower than the threshold associated with increased risk for clinical neurological deficit (1,293 mmHg); however, there are no data for injection pressure limits associated with neurological injury in the pediatric population.

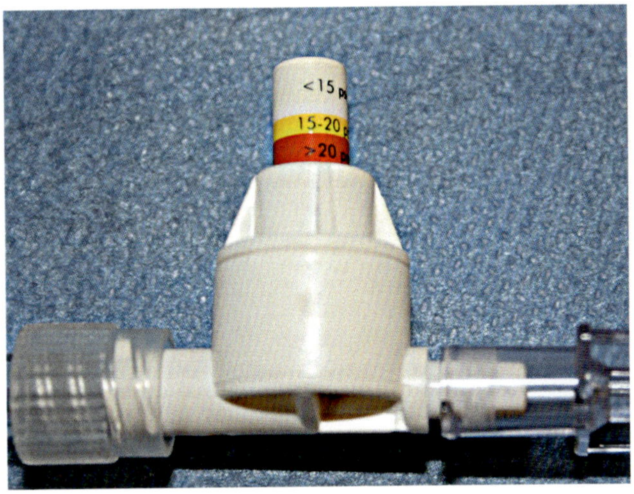

Fig. 1.8 Commercially available single-use, in-line pressure monitor for monitoring injection pressure during peripheral nerve blockade

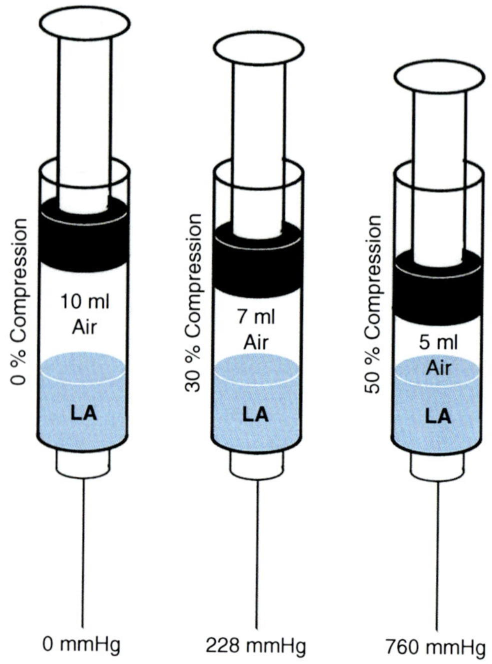

Fig. 1.9 Compressed air injection technique (CAIT) to prevent high injection pressure. 50 % compression of air volume in the syringe corresponds to an injection pressure of 760 mmHg. *LA* local anesthetic (Adapted from Tsui BC, Li LX, Pillay JJ. Compressed air injection technique to standardize block injection pressures. Can J Anesth. 2006;53:1098–102. With permission from Springer Verlag)

1.2.10.4 Syringe/Infusion Pumps

Syringe pumps are devices which enable continuous infusion (with or without boluses of local anesthetic) to be administered during the postoperative period, thereby increasing the duration of the peripheral/neuraxial nerve block(s). There is a range of commercially available pumps that are most often classified as mechanical, electrical spring driven, or elastic balloon driven.

Quality of life can be improved with disposable infusion pumps for ambulatory continuous peripheral blocks. The use of these pumps has been reported in children as young as 8 years of age, although it requires vigilant patient selection, education, and follow-up. The flow of local anesthetic through the catheter should be confirmed before discharge.

Suggested Reading

Cave G, Harvey M. Intravenous lipid emulsion as antidote beyond local anesthetic toxicity: a systematic review. Acad Emerg Med. 2009;16:815–24.

Gadsden J, McCally C, Hadzic A. Monitoring during peripheral nerve blockade. Curr Opin Anaesthesiol. 2010;23:656–61.

Hadzic A, Dilberovic F, Shah S, et al. Combination of intraneural injection and high injection pressure leads to fascicular injury and neurologic deficits in dogs. Reg Anesth Pain Med. 2004;29:417–23.

Ilfeld BM, Smith DW, Enneking FK. Continuous regional analgesia following ambulatory pediatric orthopedic surgery. Am J Orthop. 2004;33:405–8.

Kapur E, Vuckovic I, Dilberovic F, et al. Neurologic and histologic outcome after intraneural injections of Lidocaine in canine sciatic nerves. Acta Anaesthesiol Scand. 2007;51:101–7.

Pitcher CE, Raj PP, Ford DJ. The use of peripheral nerve stimulators for regional anaesthesia: a review of experimental characteristics, technique, and clinical applications. Reg Anesth. 1985;10:49–58.

Tsui BC. Equipment for regional anesthesia in children. Tech Reg Anesth Pain Manag. 2007a;11:235–46.

Tsui BC. Regional block room setup and equipment. In: Tsui BC, editor. Atlas of ultrasound and nerve stimulation-guided regional anesthesia. New York: Springer; 2007b. p. 1–7.

Tsui BC, Li LX, Pillay JJ. Compressed air injection technique to standardize block injection pressures. Can J Anesth. 2006;53:1098–102.

Weinberg G, Ripper R, Feinstein DL, Hoffman W. Lipid emulsion infusion rescues dogs from bupivacaine-induced cardiac toxicity. Reg Anesth Pain Med. 2003;28:198–202.

Pediatric Electrical Nerve Stimulation

2

Kelly P.A. Byrne and Ban C.H. Tsui

Contents

K.P.A. Byrne, MB ChB, FANZCA
Department of Anesthesia, Waikato Hospital,
Pembroke Street, Hamilton 3204, New Zealand
e-mail: Kelly.Byrne@waikatodhb.health.nz

B.C.H. Tsui, Dip Eng, BSc (Math), B Pharm, MSc, MD, FRCPC (✉)
Department of Anesthesiology and Pain Medicine,
Stollery Children's Hospital/University of Alberta Hospital,
2-150 Clinical Sciences Building,
Edmonton, AB T6G 2G3, Canada
e-mail: btsui@ualberta.ca

B.C.H. Tsui, S. Suresh (eds.), *Pediatric Atlas of Ultrasound- and Nerve Stimulation-Guided Regional Anesthesia*,
DOI 10.1007/978-0-387-79964-3_2

2.1 Nerve Stimulation Procedure

The general procedure for nerve stimulation with peripheral nerve blocks is as follows:

1. The patient is anesthetized or sedated without the use of muscle relaxants and positioned appropriately for the desired block.
2. The stimulating needle is connected to the cathode.
3. After the patient has been draped and the skin has been prepared, the needle is advanced toward the nerve with a current of 1–2 mA and pulse width of 0.1–0.2 ms.
4. At this high current, the nerve will depolarize and muscle twitches will be seen when the needle tip is between 1 and 2 cm from the nerve.
5. The current intensity is then decreased as the needle is advanced further toward the nerve. The aim is to obtain nerve depolarization and a resulting muscle twitch at a current of 0.4–0.5 mA. The muscle twitch should disappear at currents below this (i.e., the threshold current is 0.4–0.5 mA).
6. Attempting to observe a twitch at lower current levels (<0.4 mA) may result in inadvertent intraneural injection and is not necessary to increase success.
7. When attempting to place perineural catheters, a higher current is generally required for stimulation of the nerve. This is true especially if normal saline is used for hydrodissection since the ionic conduction of normal saline will disperse the electrical stimulus.
8. Once an acceptable threshold current is reached, aspiration for potential intravascular placement is performed. If this is negative, then the Raj test is preformed, where 1–2 mL of injectate, either local anesthetic or normal saline, is given. With the administration of the injectate, the muscle twitch should diminish. This phenomenon was initially attributed to the displacement of the nerve by the injectate, where the distance between nerve and needle tip increases such that the current is no longer sufficient to stimulate the nerve; however, more recent work by Tsui et al. [1], suggests that the underlying cause is dispersion of the electrical current by injection of ionic solutions (i.e., normal saline or local anesthetic). The use of nonionic solutions, such as 5 % dextrose in water (D5W), leads to preservation of the muscle twitch and improved accuracy of placement of blocks and perineural catheters.

Other applications of electrical stimulation include the use of percutaneous electrodes to guide the initial needle puncture site. This is particularly useful in children, where the distance from skin to nerve is small. Electrical stimulation can also be used to place epidural catheters; a description of this technique will be given later in this chapter.

2.2 Electrophysiology

The characteristics of the electrical impulse will determine its ability to stimulate a nerve, and the quality of stimulation will be affected by the polarity and type of the electrode, by the distance between the needle and the nerve, and by potential interactions at the tissue-needle interface.

2.2.1 Characteristics of Electrical Impulses

Spinal nerves are comprised of fascicles containing neurons and small blood vessels held together by endoneurium (Fig. 2.1). The current intensity required to stimulate a nerve is determined by the nerve fiber type and diameter. Larger, myelinated fibers are more easily stimulated than smaller, unmyelinated ones. It is important to choose the current judiciously as higher currents becomes less specific for stimulation of motor nerves. Thus, when the correct current is used, one can theoretically produce a motor response without stimulating the pain fibers, allowing the patient to remain awake for the procedure.

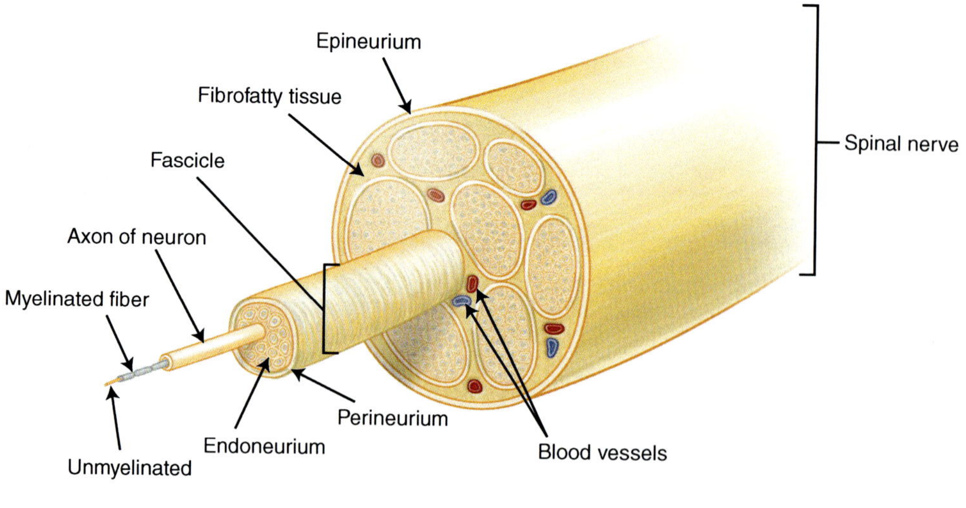

Fig. 2.1 Schematic of cross section of a spinal nerve

2.2.2 Current Intensity and Duration

Whether or not a nerve is stimulated depends on a combination of both the strength and duration of the stimulus and the polarity of the electrode. All modern nerve stimulators produce a square wave pulse of current. The total energy (or charge) applied to the nerve (Q) is a product of the current intensity (I) and the duration of the stimulus (t): $Q = (I)(t)$. The relationship between the characteristics of the nerve, its excitability, and the current required to stimulate it is described by the formula $I = \mathrm{Ir}(1 + C/t)$ (Fig. 2.2), where I is current required, Ir is the rheobase, C is the chronaxie, and t is the duration of the stimulus. Rheobase is the minimum current (in mA) required to stimulate a nerve using a long pulse duration or pulse width. As seen in Fig. 2.2, the current required to stimulate the nerve is at a minimum once the pulse duration exceeds 0.3 ms. The chronaxie is determined from the strength-duration curve and is defined as the duration of stimulus (in ms) required to stimulate the nerve at twice the rheobase; in other words, the stimulus applied is twice the strength of the minimum strength required to stimulate the nerve. As Raj et al. [2] stated, "The chronaxie can be used as a measure of the threshold for any particular nerve and is useful when comparing different nerves or nerve fiber types." The pulse width can therefore be varied in order to target different fiber types. In mammalian peripheral nerves, the respective chronaxies are Aα fibers, 0.05–0.1 ms; Aδ fibers, 0.17 ms; and C fibers, 0.4 ms.

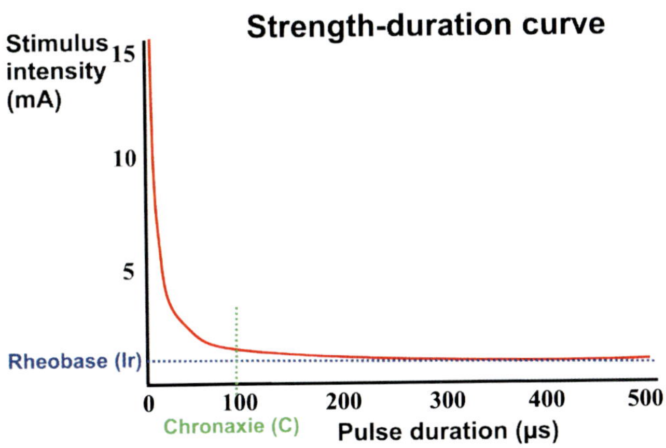

Fig. 2.2 Stimulation curve plotting current intensity and pulse duration

2.2.3 Rate of Current Change

- Regardless of the stimulus intensity, a rate of current change that is too low will reduce nerve excitability.
- Low subthreshold intensity or slowly increasing rates will inactivate sodium conductance and prevent depolarization – this is termed accommodation.

2.2.4 Polarity of Stimulating and Returning Electrodes

The polarity of the needle will affect its ability to stimulate the nerve at a given current. If the needle is connected to the anode, the current required to stimulate the nerve will be up to four times greater than if the needle is attached to the cathode. The flow of current within the needle when it is attached to the cathode produces an area of depolarization around the needle tip. This reduces the resting membrane potential of the neuronal cell membrane, causing depolarization and an action potential. When the needle is connected to the anode, the flow of current produces hyperpolarization in the area around the needle tip and leads to a higher current being required for stimulation. This phenomenon is known as preferential cathodal stimulation (Fig. 2.3) and refers to the significantly reduced current that is required to elicit a motor response when the cathode is used as the stimulating electrode. Hence, it is normal practice to attach the cathode to the needle. The anode is then attached to the patient's skin and acts as a returning electrode to complete the circuit. It was previously thought that the distance between the needle and the returning electrode was an important contributor to the resistance of the entire circuit; however, it is now known that the overall resistance remains much the same regardless of where the returning electrode is positioned.

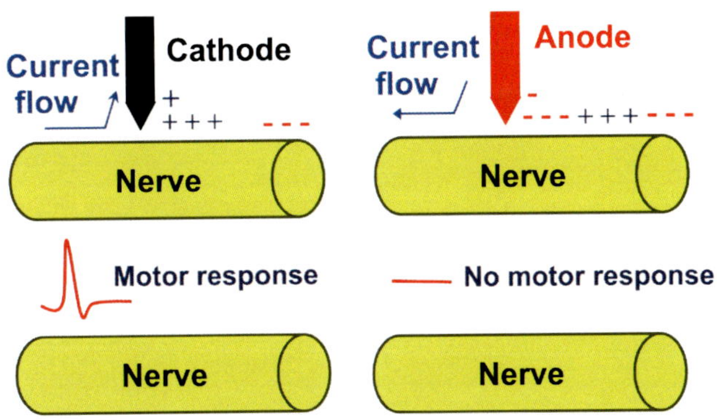

Fig. 2.3 Preferential cathodal stimulation. The flow of current within the needle when attached to the cathode causes depolarization around the needle tip. This reduces the resting membrane potential of the neuronal cell membrane, resulting in an action potential

2.2.5 Distance-Current Relationship

As one would expect, the further the distance between the stimulating electrode and the nerve, the greater the current that is required to stimulate the nerve (Fig. 2.4). This relates to the current intensity at a given distance from the stimulating electrode and is described by Coulomb's law, $I = k(i/r^2)$, where I = current required, k is Coulomb's constant, i = minimal current, and r = distance from nerve. From this equation it can be seen that the current required is inversely proportional to the square of the distance from the nerve. Hence, small changes in the distance from the nerve greatly affect the current required. The current required to stimulate the nerve at 2 cm away can be 400 times greater than that required to stimulate the nerve when the electrode is in direct contact with the nerve.

Another factor in determining whether or not the nerve will be stimulated at a particular distance and current is the pulse width of the stimulus. As shown by the pulse width-current curve, short pulse widths (i.e., 0.04 ms) are a better indicator of the distance between the nerve stimulator and the nerve, based on changes in current (Fig. 2.5). With long pulse widths (i.e., 1 ms), there is little difference in the current required to stimulate the nerve, regardless of whether the stimulating needle is in direct contact with the nerve or 1 cm away. In contrast, at a pulse width of 0.04 ms, there is a large difference in the stimulating current required when comparing direct contact with the nerve versus a distance of 1 cm away.

When undertaking a peripheral nerve block, an initial current of between 1 and 2 mA (pulse width of 0.1–0.2 ms) is used to elicit a response superficially. Accurate placement of the needle is indicated when a response is still generated once the current is reduced to between 0.2 and 0.5 mA. If stimulation of the nerve continues at a current below 0.2 mA, then intraneural injection is possible and the needle should be repositioned. Thus, nerve stimulation below 0.2 mA has a high positive predictive value for intraneural placement of the needle.

Several recent studies have raised concerns that intraneural injection can occur in the absence of nerve stimulation within a range that is normally considered a risk for intraneural injection. Bigeleisen et al. [3] examined supraclavicular blocks and found that in 54 % of patients intraneural needle placement was associated with a motor response in the 0.2–0.5 mA range. These results contradicted the previously established guidelines which stated that a motor response below 0.2 mA indicated intraneural needle placement. Robards et al. [4] combined ultrasound and nerve stimulation for localization of the sciatic nerve at the popliteal fossa and found that, in 20 of 24 patients, a motor response was not obtained until the needle tip was advanced into an intraneural location. Given these findings, other methods of determining intraneural placement of the needle, such as changes in electrical impedance, have been explored.

Percutaneous electrode guidance can be used to determine the optimal site for needle insertion. The negative electrode of the nerve stimulator connects to a commercially available surface electrode (0.5 cm diameter) (Fig. 2.6). The initial current used is generally 5 mA with a 0.2 ms pulse width. The current is then reduced to a minimum using the technique explained above. The widespread use of ultrasound has led to a significant reduction in the use of percutaneous guidance systems.

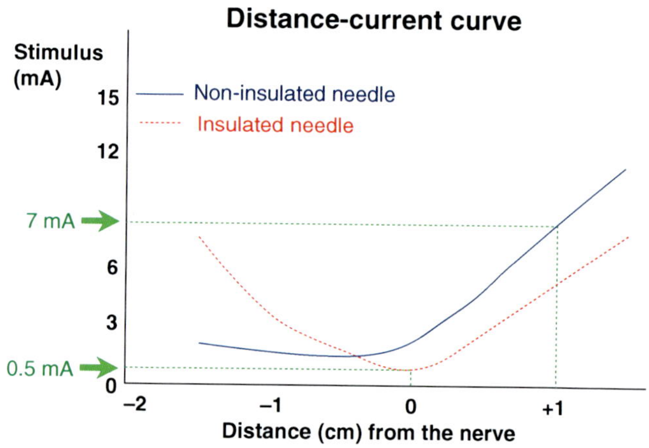

Fig. 2.4 Distance-current curve. Noninsulated needles require more current than insulated needles at the same distance from the nerve and have less discrimination of distances as the needle approaches the nerve. The current threshold is minimal (0.5 mA) for insulated needles when the needle is on the nerve

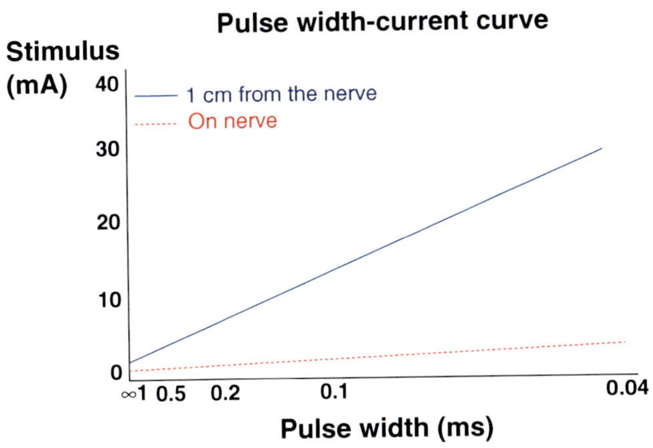

Fig. 2.5 Current intensity at different pulse widths. A shorter pulse width requires more current with greater nerve-needle distances but is a good discriminator

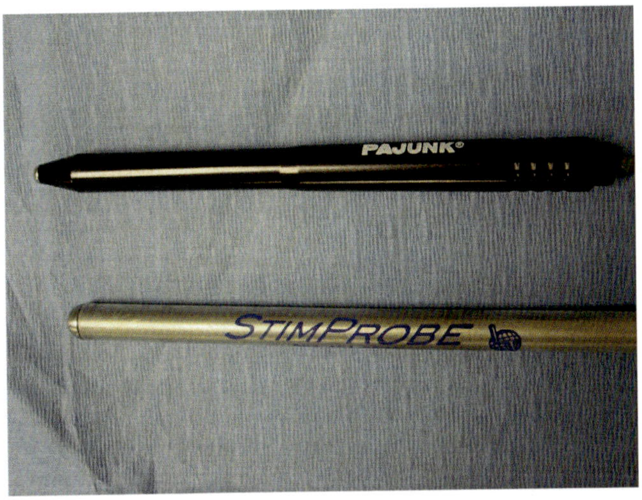

Fig. 2.6 Surface electrodes for percutaneous electrode guidance. The large diameter (0.5 cm) electrodes attach to the negative electrode of the nerve stimulator

2.2.6 Current Density of Electrodes and Injectates

At the needle tip, the conductive area for current flow will modify the current density and response threshold. Small conductive areas will condense the current and reduce the threshold current needed for motor responses. The needle/catheter-tissue interface can also affect the density of the current, as the area of conductance can change with different injectates and with different tissue compositions. Whether the injectate has conducting properties or not will significantly affect the current at the needle tip.

2.2.7 Electrodes

Types of electrodes include insulated and noninsulated needles and stimulating catheters. Insulated needles have nonconducting shafts (e.g., Teflon) that direct the current density to a sphere around the uncoated needle tip – the smaller the conducting area, the higher the density of current. This means that a lower stimulating current can be used to elicit a motor response. Noninsulated needles are bare metal and transmit current throughout their entire shaft. The current density at the tip is therefore much lower as compared to insulated needles, meaning that noninsulated needles often require more than 1 mA of current for nerve stimulation. Stimulating catheters are similar to insulated needles, although when normal saline is used as a priming solution or a dilating medium, a much higher threshold current is often required to determine correct placement due to the dispersion of current by the ionic solution.

2.2.8 Injectates

- Injection of ionic solutions such as local anesthetic or normal saline results in an increase in the conductive area at the needle tip and an increase in the threshold requirement for stimulation of the nerve (Fig. 2.7). This effect, rather than the displacement of the nerve from the needle tip, is responsible for the abolition of motor response with test dose of local or normal saline (the Raj test).
- The use of nonelectrolyte/nonconducting injectates, such as D5W, reduces the conductive area and increases the current density at the needle tip, resulting in maintenance or augmentation of the motor response at a low current (<0.5 mA).
- Nerve stimulation is clearly sensitive to changes at the tissue-needle/catheter interface. In a physiological context, the electrical field surrounding the needle tip and the conductive area generated by the needle tip are nonuniform, occasionally leading to an unstable electrical stimulation response.

- During advancement of a stimulating catheter, it may be beneficial to use nonconducting solutions to dilate the perineural space, because as long as the tip of the stimulating catheter stays in proximity to the nerve, the use of nonconducting solutions will reduce the current leakage and promote continued motor response during advancement of the catheter.

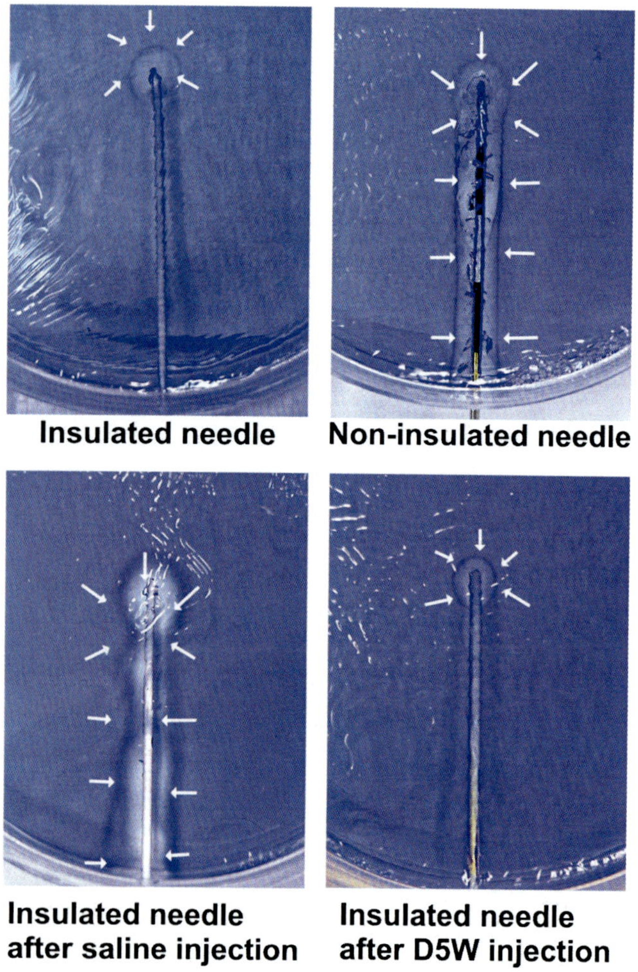

Fig. 2.7 Conductive properties of electrodes and injectates. *Top row*, insulated needles have a small conducting area, allowing low threshold current stimulation, while noninsulated needles transmit current through their entire length and have a lower current density at the tip. *Bottom row*, conducting solutions (e.g., saline or local anesthetic) increase the conductive area at the needle tip and increase the threshold current requirement. Nonconducting (nonelectrolyte) solutions (e.g., D5W) reduce the conductive area at the tip and increase the current density. The motor response from nerve stimulation after D5W injection remains the same (or is augmented) during needle/catheter placement

2.2.9 Electrical Impedance

At the most basic level, impedance is defined as resistance in an AC circuit. It is calculated as the voltage-current ratio for a single complex exponential at a particular frequency. Impedance is highly sensitive to tissue composition and has been shown to vary depending on the water content of the tissue. A significant difference between extraneural and intraneural impedance, resulting from differences in the physical composition of tissue components, has been demonstrated in the porcine sciatic nerve [5]. This difference in electrical impedance may be explained by variation in water and lipid content between the intraneural and extraneural space (Fig. 2.8): the intraneural compartment contains considerably greater amounts of nonconducting lipid and lower water content (5–20 % by weight) compared to the surrounding muscle (73–78 % water by weight).

The highly variable response to nerve stimulation as observed during ultrasound-guided regional anesthesia may be explained in part by the significant difference between intraneural and extraneural tissue impedance at different sites along the same nerve. An inverse relationship between electrical impedance and current threshold was demonstrated for the median nerve [6]; stimulation of the nerve in the axilla required significantly higher current thresholds than at the elbow. The lower impedance of the axillary muscle tissue may have produced a region of highly conductive tissue around the needle tip, dispersing current away from the nerve. Higher current settings may be required when a stimulating needle is advanced through low-impedance muscle tissue. On the other hand, lower current settings may be needed for nerves located in high-impedance fat or connective tissue.

A recent study assessing accidental nerve puncture during ultrasound-guided blocks in adult patients demonstrated the utility of electrical impedance in clinical scenarios [7]. It was shown that a >4.3 % increase in impedance may indicate intraneural needle placement. To date, an investigation of the use of electrical impedance in guiding needle placement in pediatric regional blocks has yet to be performed.

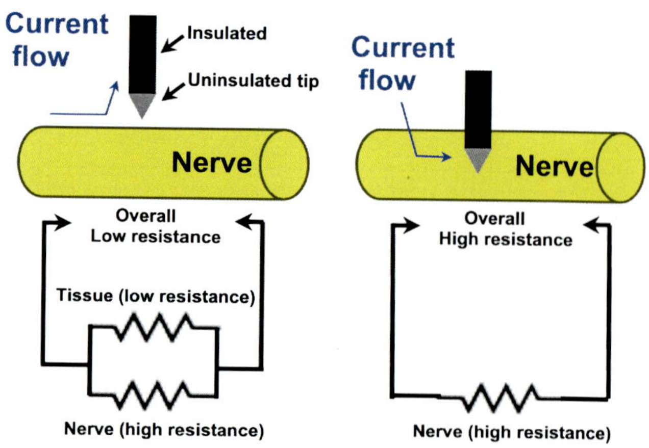

Fig. 2.8 Differences in intra- and extraneural impedance. This may be explained by variation in water and lipid content between the two spaces

2.3 Electrical Epidural Stimulation

Electrical stimulation of an epidural catheter can confirm epidural placement and can be used to determine the optimal position to deliver postoperative analgesia. This technique is particularly relevant in children where small distances can significantly alter the nerve distribution blocked by the epidural.

The epidural stimulation test (aka the Tsui test) [8] applies similar principles to those of peripheral nerve blockade, that is, using electrical pulses and the current versus nerve-distance relationship. This test possesses between 80 and 100 % positive predictive value for epidural placement and has been effective in guiding catheters within two segmental levels of the target level, as confirmed by radiological imaging. This can facilitate appropriate placement and allow adjustments in the event of catheter migration, kinking, or coiling. In addition to confirming and guiding epidural catheter placement, this test has the potential to detect intrathecal, subdural, or intravascular catheter placement. The principles of this test can be applied to both catheter and single-shot techniques with both epidural and caudal approaches.

2.3.1 Test Equipment and Procedure

There are specialized kits available for use in electrical epidural stimulation (Tsui epidural kit, Pajunk, Geisingen, Germany). A conventional epidural kit can also be modified for electrical stimulation. This test is designed to be used in addition to the traditional loss-of-resistance technique:

1. Anesthetize or sedate the patient without the use of muscle relaxants, and position them appropriately. Insert the epidural via the traditional loss-of-resistance technique, and advance the catheter into the epidural space. The epidural catheter must contain a metal coil to enable electrical stimulation.
2. After sterile preparation, connect a nerve stimulator to the epidural catheter using an electrode adaptor (e.g., Arrow-Johans ECG adaptor, Arrow International Inc., Reading, PA, USA) (Fig. 2.9).
3. Prime the catheter and adaptor with sterile normal saline.
4. Attach the cathode lead of the nerve stimulator to the metal hub of the adaptor. Attach the grounding anode lead to an electrode on the patient's body surface.
5. Set the nerve stimulator to low frequency and pulse width (1 Hz, 0.2 ms).
6. Carefully and slowly increase the current intensity until motor activity begins.
7. Depending on the characteristics of the response, as described in Table 2.1, the catheter location can be indentified and appropriate adjustments can be made.
8. If a single-shot epidural is planned, a similar technique can be used to confirm needle placement. The only exception is that the nerve stimulator is attached to an insulated needle (e.g., 18–24 G insulated needles) rather than to the already positioned catheter.
9. The threshold current for determining correct needle placement is similar for the lumbar and caudal routes, but the upper limit of 10 mA may be extended for thoracic epidural placement (up to 17 mA).
10. The stimulator should be versatile enough to allow the current to be increased by small increments and applied for short intervals.

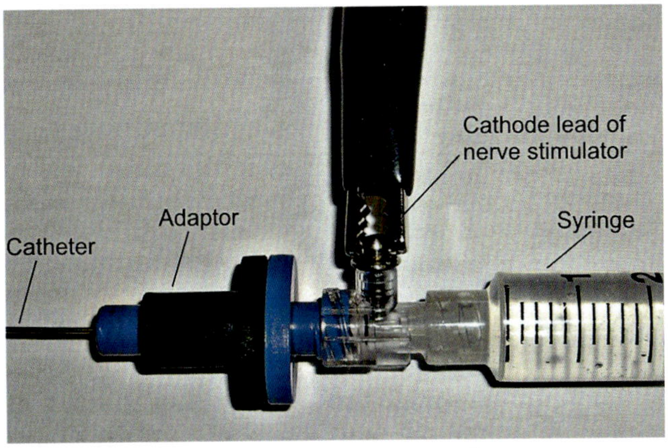

Fig. 2.9 An adaptor (Arrow-Johans ECG Adaptor) is attached to the connector of the epidural catheter (19 G Arrow FlexTip Plus); the adaptor and catheter are filled with normal saline, and the cathode lead of the nerve stimulator is attached to the metal hub of the adapter

Table 2.1 Test dose with dextrose 5 % in water (D5W) prior to local anesthetic injection

- A test dose of a nonconducting solution (e.g., D5W) is beneficial prior to local anesthetic injection during peripheral nerve blockade
- The solution can be visualized easily with ultrasound, especially with color Doppler, and can indicate the approximate spread of local anesthetic.
- Carefully observing the spread of D5W will help confirm extravascular and extraneural needle placement, especially when the threshold current during nerve stimulation is <0.4 mA
- When used with nerve stimulation, D5W will confirm needle placement near the nerve if the motor response is maintained or augmented

2.4 Mechanisms of the Epidural Stimulation Test

Catheter placement is confirmed by stimulating the spinal nerve roots (not the spinal cord) with a catheter that conducts a low-amplitude electrical current through normal saline. A correct motor response (1–10 mA) confirms accurate placement of the epidural catheter tip (Table 2.2). Correct placement is defined as 1–2 cm from the nerve roots (Fig. 2.4). Responses observed with a significantly lower threshold current (<1 mA), especially if substantially diffuse or bilateral, may warn of incorrect catheter placement, either in proximity to a nerve root or in the subarachnoid or subdural space, where the catheter contacts the highly conductive cerebrospinal fluid (CSF). Previous studies have used insulated needles to elicit a motor response in the epidural space (11.1 ± 3.1 mA [9] and 3.84 ± 0.99 mA) [10] and showed that these currents are higher than that required in the intrathecal space (0.77 ± 0.32 mA and 0.6 ± 0.3 mA) [11]. The segmental level of the catheter tip may be predicted based on the progressive nature of the motor twitches (i.e., from lower limbs and back to intercostals and upper limb) as the catheter is advanced.

A local anesthetic test dose helps confirm epidural versus intravascular location. If the catheter is placed correctly, the motor threshold current should increase after the local anesthetic application. This is due to the dispersion of the current by the ionic solution. If the catheter is in an intravascular position, then the local anesthetic will be removed from the area into the systemic circulation resulting in no change in the current required for motor stimulation. To further confirm placement of the catheter, administering an epinephrine test dose (0.5 μg/kg) and observing the subsequent ECG changes, in particular >25 % increase in T wave or ST segment changes irrespective of chosen lead, is recommended.

The electrical resistance and threshold currents differ between stimulating needles and catheters. Insulated needles will provide a lower electrical resistance and should therefore be used for stimulation. When using a needle to stimulate, the upper limit of the threshold current indicating a positive test is similar to catheter placement at the caudal space (mean = 3.7 mA); however, at the thoracic level, the threshold current becomes higher (up to 17 mA). The lower limit of >1 mA applies to all segmental levels. The higher threshold currents that may be seen with direct insertion at the thoracic level may be related to the minimal depth of needle penetration that is normally used for precautionary measures at this level.

Table 2.2 Epidural catheter location determined by standard test dose (lidocaine with 1:200,000 epinephrine) versus the epidural stimulation test

Catheter location	Test dose	Epidural stimulation test
Subarachnoid	Hypotension/total spinal response (<1 mA)	Positive unilateral/bilateral motor
Subdural	? (<1 mA)	Diffuse motor response in many segments
Epidural space		
Close to nerve	?	Unilateral motor response (<1 mA)
Against nerve root	?	Positive motor response (1–10 mA); threshold current increase after local anesthetic injection
Non-intravascular	Heart rate increase	Remains or returns to baseline positive motor response (1–10 mA) even after local anesthetic injection
Intravascular	Blood pressure increase	ECG changes
Subcutaneous	?	Negative response

2.4.1 Stimulating Epidural Catheter Requirements

There are two major areas where the requirements for stimulating epidural catheters vary from that of conventional epidural kits: (1) the need for effective conduction of electrical current and (2) the ability to advance the catheter significant distances.

2.4.2 Effective Conduction of Electrical Current

In order to induce electrical pulses, the catheter's electrical resistance must remain low. Any highly conductive ionic solution (e.g., normal saline) can be used to prime the catheter. A metal coil in the lumen is required because of the catheter length and the risk of air trapping, both of which can increase the resistance to current flow. A soft, metal-containing epidural catheter (Fig. 2.10a) (e.g., Flextip Plus from Arrow International, Reading, PA, USA; Perifix from B. Braun, Bethlehem, PA, USA; Spirol from Sims, Portex, Markham, ON, Canada) is effective for epidural stimulation testing. Peripheral stimulating catheters (e.g., StimuLong Plus from Pajunk, Geisingen, Germany, or StimuCath, Arrow International, Reading, PA, USA) contain an internal fixed wire that extends beyond the distal lumen tip (Fig. 2.10b); these have been used for the epidural stimulation test without the requirement for priming with normal saline. However, there is limited experience with these catheters, and they may not have any benefit over the conventional metal-coil-containing catheters.

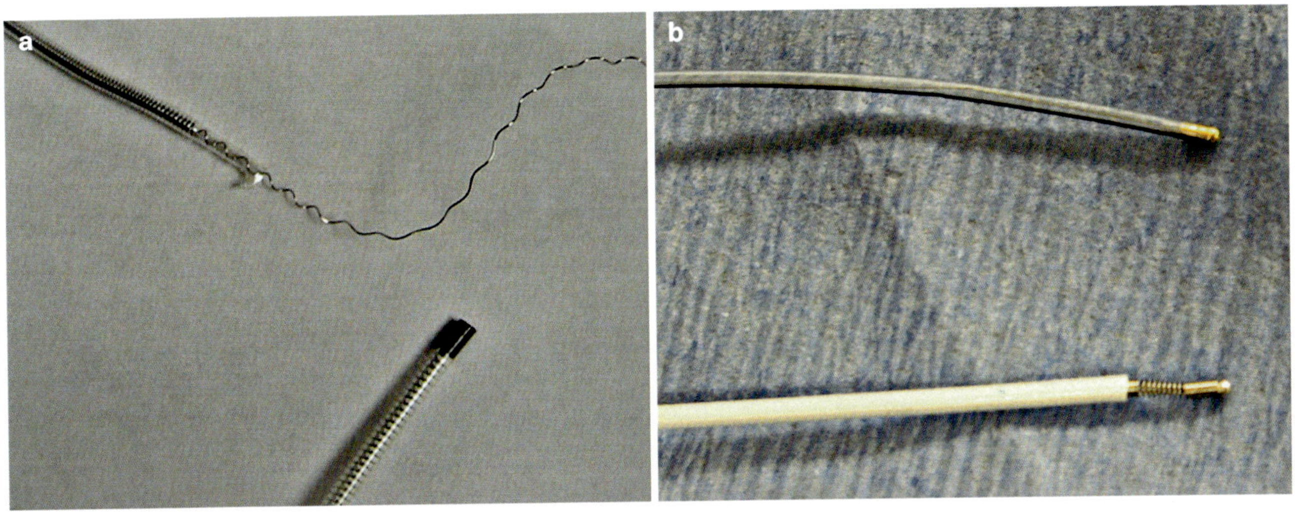

Fig. 2.10 (**a**) Soft, metal-containing epidural catheters can be used for the epidural stimulation test (metal wire has been exposed and unwound in the top catheter); (**b**) other peripheral stimulating catheters, with a wire extension beyond the distal tip, have been used for epidural catheter insertion using electrical stimulation

2.4.3 Advancement of the Catheter

Conventional metal-coil-containing catheters are soft and pliable in nature, and as a result, when threading them, they either require modification with a metal stylet or substitution with a specialized styletted catheter setup (Fig. 2.11; StimuLong Tsui, Pajunk, Geisingen, Germany) that includes an injection port system. When advancing the catheter, minor resistance to the passage of the catheter can be overcome by injecting normal saline through the catheter or by flexion or extension of the patient's vertebral column. The ejected fluid may reduce the friction between the catheter and surrounding tissues, and this may be more effective when a multiport catheter is used. Clinicians must remain vigilant as epidural catheter placement has the potential for neurological injury. Therefore, under no circumstances should any force be used to advance the catheter.

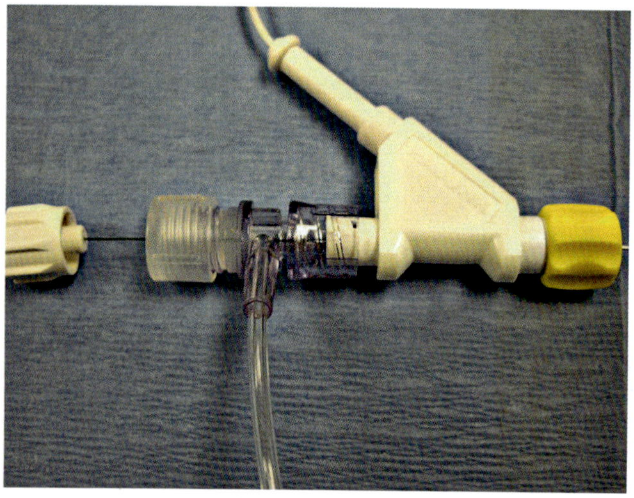

Fig. 2.11 A specialized styletted catheter setup (StimuLong Tsui, Pajunk, Geisingen, Germany) that includes an injection port system

2.4.4 Considerations for Test Performance and Interpretation

Because local muscle contraction in the trunk region can be confused with epidural stimulation, it is recommended that an anode be placed on the upper extremity for lumbar epidurals and the lower extremity for thoracic epidurals. The 1–10 mA range for epidural stimulation should be used only as a guideline, as epidural stimulation may occur outside this range. Some cases will require stimulation of greater than 17 mA, for example, when using insulated needles in the thoracic region. We recommend this range for several reasons: it is easy to remember, and stimulation below 1 mA is suggestive of intrathecal placement or placement in close proximity to a nerve root.

The best predictor of correct epidural placement is a combination of threshold current level and distribution of elicited motor responses (i.e., correlation with approximate segmental location) since subcutaneous placement would not elicit such predictive and segmental responses.

Although no known complications of epidural electrical stimulation have been described, it is recommended that the current remain fairly low (<15–20 mA) and that the period of stimulation last only a few minutes. This helps to confirm the safety of epidural electrical stimulation. Other studies of spinal cord stimulators in chronic pain settings and intraoperative spinal cord monitoring during spinal surgery have used stimulation in the 2–40 mA range.

2.4.5 Limitations of Epidural Stimulation

- Significant clinical neuromuscular blockade or local anesthetics in the epidural space limit the use of this test. An alternative technique to the epidural stimulation test uses an ECG to monitor catheter location. When the catheter tip is at or near the target level, the ECG complex recorded from the epidural catheter should match the ECG measured from a surface electrode. Unlike the epidural stimulation test, the ECG technique cannot warn of intrathecal or intravascular position of the catheter nor can it guide catheter placement when the threading distance is short (see Fig. 33.7).
- Ultrasound imaging is an alternative method for catheter guidance and placement in young children.
- Limitations of electrical stimulation are minor and include the need for and cost of a "specialized" stimulating catheter. This, however, is offset by the more accurate postoperative analgesia and avoidance of intrathecal or intravascular placement of the catheter.

2.5 Useful Equipment Features in Nerve Stimulation

In 1985, Pither et al. [12] described essential features of a nerve stimulator, and there have been few alterations to these criteria since then. There are multiple different makes and models of nerve stimulators, many of which share similar features. Anesthesiologists should familiarize themselves with the equipment that is commonly used at their institution.

2.5.1 Constant Current Output and Display

Historically, nerve stimulators produced a constant voltage, although most modern nerve stimulators now produce a constant current (Fig. 2.12). This means that the resistance of the circuit is monitored and the voltage adjusted accordingly to provide a constant current. Most nerve stimulators have an adjustable frequency, pulse width, and current strength (Fig. 2.13). Additionally, clear digital displays show the current delivered to the patient, the target current setting, and impedance. Some stimulators have low (<6 mA) and high (<80 mA) ranges for increased accuracy during localization of peripheral nerves and monitoring neuromuscular blockade, respectively. The current requirements for epidural stimulation (1–17 mA) often fall outside the usual working range for peripheral nerve stimulators. Other makes and models of nerve stimulators may be required for this technique.

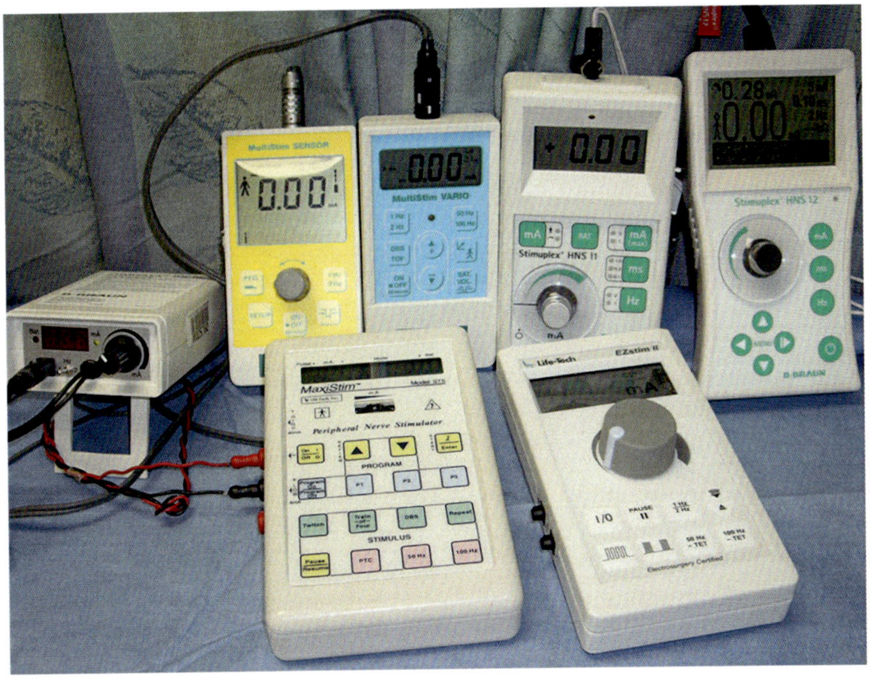

Fig. 2.12 Many constant current nerve stimulators are on the market and will vary in their current output ranges

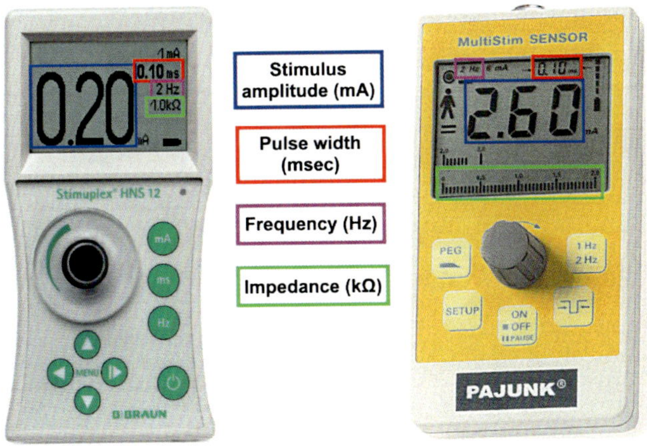

Fig. 2.13 Peripheral nerve stimulators showing display of stimulus amplitude, pulse width, frequency, and impedance

2.5.2 Variable Pulse Width and Frequency

Pulse width determines the amount of charge delivered to the patient and may enable selective stimulation of different types of nerve fibers. For example, sensory fibers are more effectively stimulated at longer pulse widths (0.4 ms), whereas shorter pulse widths (0.05–0.15 ms) are sufficient for motor fibers. Some devices allow width ranges from 0.05 to 1 ms for high variation and selectivity, depending on specific nerve location. The frequency of stimulation will affect the needle advancement rate, as low frequencies (<1 Hz) may result in the target nerve being missed, and high frequencies can cause twitches which are similar to involuntary fasciculations. Most practitioners use 2 Hz as a compromise between these two extremes.

2.5.3 Other Features

A specialized male connector designed to fit into the female conducting portion of the stimulating needle is a useful addition. Indicators displaying the battery status and warning of an incomplete circuit or pulse delivery failure are important components of the nerve stimulator. Foot pedal or handheld remote controls to adjust current output (Fig. 2.14) may improve the operator's ability to undertake the procedure without assistance.

Probes may be available for surface mapping during percutaneous electrode guidance procedures (Fig. 2.6).

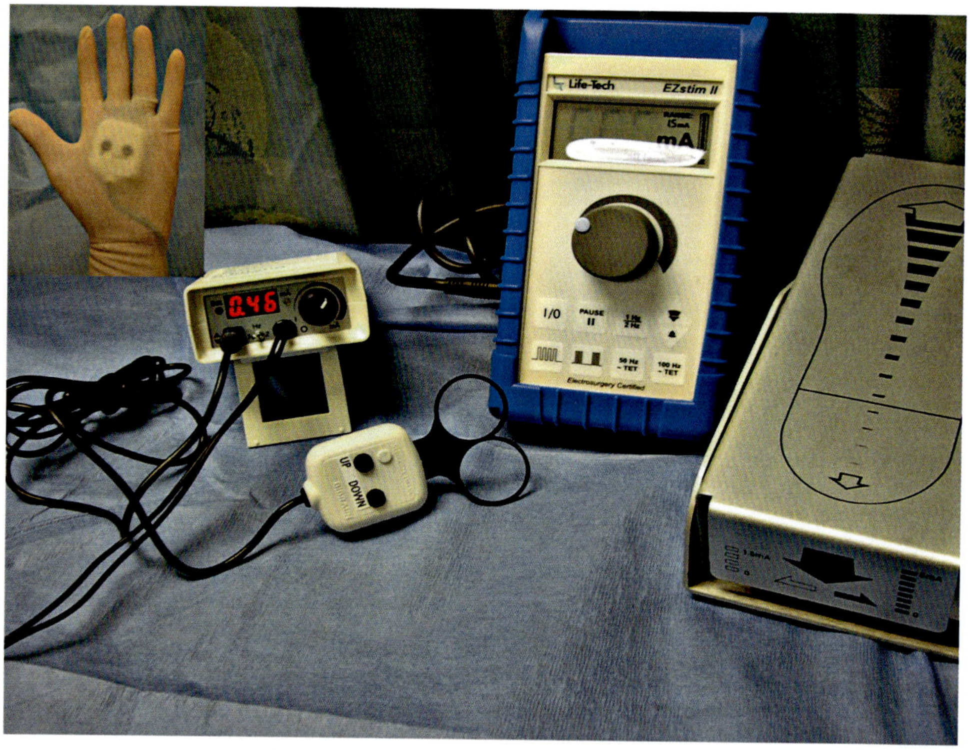

Fig. 2.14 Foot pedal or handheld remote control adjusters of current output

2.6 Practical Considerations

2.6.1 Documentation

Documentation of the procedure and performance of the nerve block is a critical part of the procedure, both for quality assurance and medicolegal reasons. It is important to document the block procedure, the specific current at which the muscle twitch is present and at which it disappears, and the presence or absence of any pain or paresthesia.

2.6.2 Population Considerations

Specific groups of patients may require increased current intensity levels (e.g., diabetics, obese, nerve conduction disorders, and under anesthesia [13]); however, this is not as relevant in the pediatric population.

2.6.3 Does Nerve Stimulation Make a Difference?

Current research has evaluated the success and side effects of nerve stimulator-based blocks compared to ultrasound-guided blocks. There is emerging evidence to show that ultrasound-guided blocks may have an earlier onset time, a reduced local anesthetic dose, and possibly an increased success rate in certain settings. Does this mean that nerve stimulation is a relic of the past? We argue strongly that this is not the case. While ultrasound is rapidly becoming the standard of care in many parts of the world, nerve stimulation should at least be considered the minimum standard of safety when performing a nerve block. In the pediatric setting, nerve stimulation has been vital in providing an objective method of identifying nerves in anesthetized patients and provides a complementary role to ultrasound in performing nerve blocks. Currently ultrasound is limited, as it cannot reliably detect intraneural injection while nerve blockade is performed. Intraneural injection may be avoided if ultrasound is used in conjunction with nerve stimulation. The development of new approaches, such as the measurement of electrical impedance and the epidural stimulation test, may provide other advantages to the use of nerve stimulation in regional anesthesia.

Clinical Pearls

- In children, since the regional block is typically performed under general anesthesia, it is critical to not use muscle relaxant if one is planning to utilize nerve stimulation.
- Peripheral nerve blocks:
  - There is no clear evidence to prove the benefits of nerve stimulation, but it can help to make the block safer; the authors use nerve stimulation at 0.2 mA to warn if the needle tip is too close to the nerve.
  - In addition, a recent report suggests that threshold currents used for motor response from nerve stimulation under general anesthesia might be higher than those used for awake patients [13].
- Central neuraxial blocks:
  - The authors find it useful and practical to monitor and guide epidural catheter advancement when threading the catheter from the caudal space.

References

1. Tsui BCH, Kropelin B, Ganapathy S, Finucane B. Dextrose 5% in water: fluid medium for maintaining electrical stimulation of peripheral nerves during stimulating catheter placement. Acta Anaesthesiol Scand. 2005;49:1562–5.
2. Raj PP, Rosenblatt R, Montgomery SJ. Use of the nerve stimulator for peripheral blocks. Reg Anesth. 1980;5:14–21.
3. Bigeleisen PE, Moayeri N, Groen GJ. Extraneural versus intraneural stimulation thresholds during ultrasound-guided supraclavicular block. Anesthesiology. 2009;110:1235–43.
4. Robards C, Hadzic A, Somasundaram L, Iwata T, Gadsden J, Xu D, Sala-Blanch X. Intraneural injection with low-current stimulation during popliteal sciatic nerve block. Anesth Analg. 2009;109: 673–7.
5. Tsui BC, Pillay J, Tsung C, Dillane D. Electrical impedance to distinguish intraneural from extraneural needle placement in porcine nerves under direct exposure and ultrasound guidance. Anesthesiology. 2008;109:479–83.
6. Sauter AR, Dodgson MS, Kalvøy H, Grimnes S, Stubhaug A, Klaastad O. Current threshold for nerve stimulation depends on electrical impedance of the tissue: a study of ultrasound-guided electrical nerve stimulation of the median nerve. Anesth Analg. 2009;108:1338–43.
7. Bardou P, Merle JC, Woillard JB, Nathan-Denizot N, Beaulieu P. Electrical impedance to detect accidental nerve puncture during ultrasound-guided peripheral nerve blocks. Can J Anesth. 2013;60: 253–8.
8. Tsui BC, Gupta S, Finucane B. Confirmation of epidural catheter placement using nerve stimulation. Can J Anesth. 1998;45:640–4.
9. Tsui BC, Wagner A, Cave D, Seal R. Threshold current for an insulated epidural needle in pediatric patients. Anesth Analg. 2004;99:694–6.
10. Tsui BC, Wagner AM, Cunningham K, Perry S, Desai S, Seal R. Can continuous low current electrical stimulation distinguish insulated needle position in the epidural and intrathecal spaces in pediatric patients? Paediatr Anaesth. 2005;15:959–63.
11. Tsui BCH, Wagner AM, Cunningham K, et al. Threshold current of an insulated needle in the intrathecal space in pediatric patients. Anesth Analg. 2005;100:662–5.
12. Pither CE, Raj PP, Ford DJ. The use of peripheral nerve stimulators for regional anaesthesia: a review of experimental characteristics, technique, and clinical applications. Reg Anesth. 1985;10:49–58.
13. Tsui BC. The effects of general anaesthesia on nerve-motor response characteristics (rheobase and chronaxie) to peripheral nerve stimulation. Anaesthesia 2014;69:374–9.

Suggested Reading

Baranoswki AP, Pither CE. A comparison of three methods of axillary brachial plexus anaesthesia. Anaesthesia. 1990;45:362–5.

Bosenberg AT, Raw R, Boezaart AP. Surface mapping of peripheral nerves in children with a nerve stimulator. Pediatr Anesth. 2002;12: 398–403.

Bouaziz H, Narchi P, Mercier FJ, Labaille T, Zerrouk N, Girod J, Benhamou D. Comparison between conventional axillary block and a new approach at the midhumeral level. Anesth Analg. 1997;84: 1058–62.

Capdevila X, Lopez S, Bernard N, Dadure C, Motais F, Biboulet P, Choquet O. Percutaneous electrode guidance using the insulated needle for prelocation of peripheral nerves during axillary plexus blocks. Reg Anesth Pain Med. 2004;29:206–11.

de Medicis E, Tetrault JP, Martin R, Robichaud R, Laroche L. A prospective comparison study of two indirect methods for confirming the localization of an epidural catheter for postoperative analgesia. Anesth Analg. 2005;101:1830–3.

Dillane D, Tsui BC. Is there still a place for the use of nerve stimulation? Pediatr Anesth. 2012;22:102–8.

Ganta R, Cajee RA, Henthorn RW. Use of transcutaneous nerve stimulation to assist interscalene block. Anesth Analg. 1993;76:914–5.

Goldberg ME, Gregg C, Larijani GE, Norris MC, Marr AT, Seltzer JL. A comparison of three methods of axillary approach to brachial plexus blockade for upper extremity surgery. Anesthesiology. 1987; 66:814–6.

Guyton AC, Hall JE. Textbook of medical physiology. 9th ed. Philadelphia: WB Saunders; 1995. p. 57–71.

Hadzic A, Vloka JD, Claudio RE, Hadzic N, Thys DM, Santos AC. Electrical nerve localization: effects of cutaneous electrode placement and duration of the stimulus on motor response. Anesthesiology. 2004;100:1526–30.

Kimura J. Electrodiagnosis in diseases of nerve and muscle: principles and practice. 3rd ed. Oxford: Oxford University Press; 2001. p. 178–214.

Lena P, Martin R. Subdural placement of an epidural catheter detected by nerve stimulation. Can J Anesth. 2005;52:618–21.

Magora F, Rozin R, Ben-Menachem Y, Magora A. Obturator nerve block: an evaluation of technique. Br J Anaesth. 1969;41:695–8.

Marhofer P, Schrogendorfer K, Koinig H, Kapral S, Weinstabl C, Mayer N. Ultrasonographic guidance improves sensory block and onset time of three-in-one blocks. Anesth Analg. 1997;85:854–7.

Shannon J, Lang SA, Yip RW, Gerard M. Lateral femoral cutaneous nerve block revisited. A nerve stimulator technique. Reg Anesth. 1995;20:100–4.

Sia S, Bartoli M, Lepri A, Marchini O, Ponsecchi P. Multiple-injection axillary brachial plexus block: a comparison of two methods of nerve localization-nerve stimulation versus paresthesia. Anesth Analg. 2000;91:647–51.

Tamai H, Sawamura S, Kanamori Y, Takeda K, Chinzei M, Hanaoka K. Thoracic epidural catheter insertion using the caudal approach assisted with an electrical nerve stimulator in young children. Reg Anesth Pain Med. 2005;29:92–5.

Tsui BC, Tarkkila P, Gupta S, Kearney R. Confirmation of caudal needle placement using nerve stimulation. Anesthesiology. 1999;91: 374–8.

Tsui BC, Gupta S, Finucane B. Detection of subarachnoid and intravascular epidural catheter placement. Can J Anesth. 1999;46: 675–8.

Tsui BC, Seal R, Koller J, Entwistle L, Haugen R, Kearney R. Thoracic epidural analgesia via the caudal approach in pediatric patients undergoing fundoplication using nerve stimulation guidance. Anesth Analg. 2001;93:1152–5.

Tsui BC, Wagner A, Finucane B. Electrophysiologic effect of injectates on peripheral nerve stimulation. Reg Anesth Pain Med. 2004;29: 189–93.

Tsui BC, Wagner A, Cave D, Kearney R. Thoracic and lumbar epidurals via the caudal approach using electrical stimulation guidance in pediatric patients: a review of 289 patients. Anesthesiology. 2004; 100:683–9.

Tsui BC, Hopkins D. Electrical stimulation for regional anesthesia. In: Boezaart AP, editor. Anesthesia and orthopaedic surgery. New York: McGraw-Hill; 2006. p. 249–56.

Tsui BC. Electrical nerve stimulation. In: Tsui BC, editor. Atlas of ultrasound and nerve stimulation-guided regional anesthesia. New York: Springer; 2007. p. 9–18.

Urmey WF, Stanton J. Inability to consistently elicit a motor response following sensory paresthesia during interscalene block. Anesthesiology. 2002;96:552–4.

Urmey WF, Grossi P. Percutaneous electrode guidance: a noninvasive technique for prelocation of peripheral nerves to facilitate peripheral plexus or nerve block. Reg Anesth Pain Med. 2002;27: 261–7.

Urmey WF, Grossi P. Use of sequential electrical nerve stimulation (SENS) for location of the sciatic nerve and lumbar plexus. Reg Anesth Pain Med. 2006;31:463–9.

Williams R, Saha B. Ultrasound placement of needle in three-in-one nerve block. Emerg Med J. 2006;23:401–3.

Ultrasound Basics

3

Michelle L. Noga, Vivian H.Y. Ip, and Ban C.H. Tsui

Contents

M.L. Noga, MD, FRCPC
Department of Radiology and Diagnostic Imaging,
University of Alberta, 2A2.41 Walter Mackenzie
Centre 8440-112 Street, Edmonton, AB T6G 2B7, Canada
e-mail: mnoga@ualberta.ca

V.H.Y. Ip, MB ChB, MRCP, FRCA
Department of Anesthesia and Pain Medicine,
University of Alberta Hospital,
2-150 Clinical Sciences Building,
Edmonton, AB T6G 2G3, Canada
e-mail: hip@ualberta.ca

B.C.H. Tsui, Dip Eng, BSc (Math), B Pharm, MSc, MD, FRCPC (✉)
Department of Anesthesiology and Pain Medicine,
Stollery Children's Hospital/University of Alberta Hospital,
2-150 Clinical Sciences Building,
Edmonton, AB T6G 2G3, Canada
e-mail: btsui@ualberta.ca

B.C.H. Tsui, S. Suresh (eds.), *Pediatric Atlas of Ultrasound- and Nerve Stimulation-Guided Regional Anesthesia*,
DOI 10.1007/978-0-387-79964-3_3

3.1 Basic Ultrasound Physics and Technology

3.1.1 Basic Principles

- Ultrasound waves are oscillating sound pressure waves with frequencies that typically exceed 20,000 cycles per second (Hertz; Hz).
- An image is acquired by sending a pulse of ultrasound waves which propagates through a medium (such as liquid or soft tissue) until it encounters an interface with a different medium; at this point, an echo is produced. Returning echoes are processed and an image is created.
- Ultrasound waves are created by converting electrical energy into sound waves or mechanical energy through vibrating objects known as piezoelectric crystals such as barium titanate or lead zirconate.
- A transducer houses the piezoelectric crystals which temporarily deform when an alternating voltage is applied.
- The sound wave generated travels in a well-defined beam and direction.
- These crystals also detect ultrasound that is reflected back (echo) and convert the pressure change into electrical energy.
- The receiver amplifies the signals and displays them in the following ways:
  - A-mode: echo information as amplitude signals
  - B-mode: brightness information as an image slices down the beam (most commonly used in regional anesthesia)
  - M-mode: motion with respect to time

3.2 Transducers

- These are the most important part of the ultrasound machine, as they affect the quality of the image in scanning a patient. Higher frequencies result in higher spatial resolution, but penetrate less depth of tissue.
- They emit ultrasound waves in pulses.
- A typical ultrasound pulse contains two to five cycles of the same frequency.
- Pulse length is the duration of each pulse.
- Pulse repetition frequency is the number of pulse emitted by the transducer and is measured in pulses per second. The pulse repetition frequency must be set such that all the echoes from the target have returned before the next pulse is generated.

3.2.1 Types of Ultrasound Transducers

The transducers are named after the geometric arrangement of their piezoelectric elements. There are many different transducers available commercially (Fig. 3.1). In general, there are three array types:

Linear Array

- Piezoelectric elements are arranged in parallel, forming a row of rectangular elements that produces a rectangular image.
- High frequency with good resolution but shallow depth penetration.
- There is a one-to-one ratio of coupling between the contact (footing) area and the image size (i.e., large coupling area) which can be a disadvantage of these transducers.
- This array is widely used in the pediatric population owing to its good imaging quality in superficial structures of 3–4 cm in depth.

Convex (or Curved) Arrays

- These are curved linear transducers with linear arrays shaped into convex curves, covering a large surface field of view.
- The advantage is the larger image field produced with less coupling to the contact (footing) area.
- The main disadvantage is the nonlinear line density in the image, which can make it slightly more difficult for the beginner to comprehend the image.
- The C60 probe is a low-frequency transducer (5–2 MHz), giving good penetration but poor resolution in superficial structures. Therefore, it is seldom used in children.
- The C11 probe is a medium-frequency (7–4 MHz) transducer which can be used for abdominal imaging in children for ilioinguinal/iliohypogastric nerve blocks.

Phased Array (12–2 MHz)

- These transducers are similar to the linear array in that they contain a row of rectangular elements, but there are fewer elements in this transducer, and the elements are smaller.
- The advantage with this transducer is the large field of view produced despite the small coupling area.
- The disadvantages are the small near field (see below) and the nonlinear line density.
- This transducer is generally dedicated to cardiac imaging or pediatric abdominal imaging.

Broadband Transducers

- These transducers cover a range of bandwidths, such as 10–5 MHz or 14–8 MHz.
- They have shorter pulse length, giving higher axial resolution and a wide bandwidth, which is important for harmonic imaging (at the expense of axial resolution).
- They offer an excellent resolution of superficial structures in the upper limbs and good penetration depths in the lower limbs without having to change the transducer.

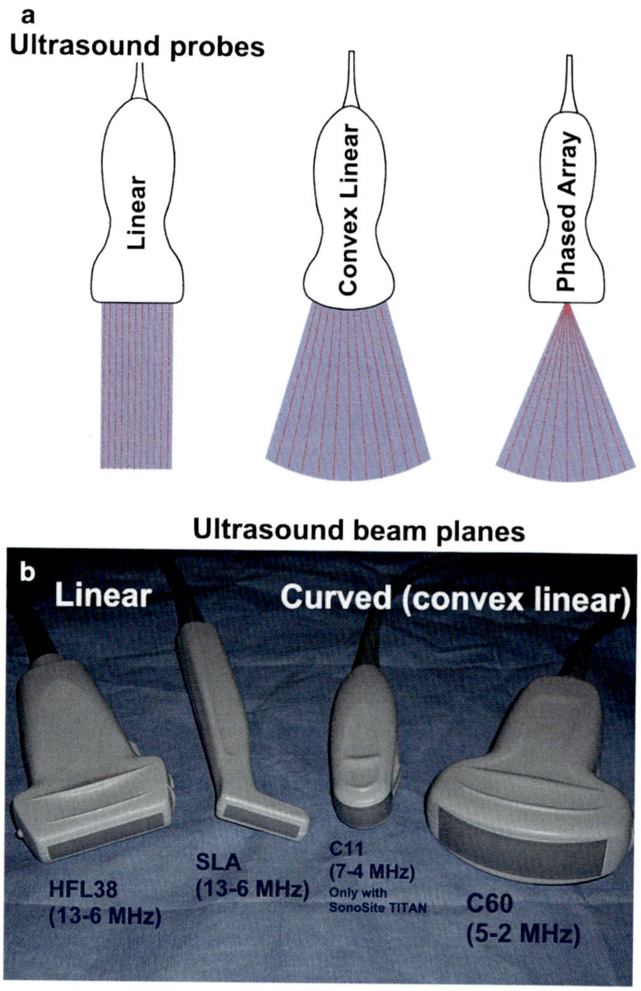

Fig. 3.1 (**a**) Schematic of ultrasound transducer types: linear array, convex linear array, and phased array. (**b**) Linear and curved (convex linear) transducers (e.g., SonoSite MicroMaxx) are the most common types used for regional anesthesia. Each has different beam frequencies

3.3 Sound Wave Properties in Tissue

In order to understand and interpret the image obtained by ultrasound scanning, it is important to grasp the basic principle of the propagation of ultrasound through tissues. Table 3.1 shows the summary of the practical aspects of ultrasound imaging.

Table 3.1 Practical aspects of ultrasound wave characteristics

Frequency (Hz)
Number of periods per second
High frequency provides high spatial resolution for superficial structures, but poor penetration; lower frequencies are required for deeper structures
Wavelength (mm)
Length of one cycle in one direction of propagation of the wave
Velocity (m/s)
Displacement of the wave per unit of time
Different acoustic impedances (densities) of tissue determine the velocity of ultrasound waves
Period (s)
Time for one complete wave cycle
Amplitude
Strength of the wave, calculated by the square root of the wave energy
Amplifier gain function adjusts the strength of weak echoes to improve the signal-to-noise ratio
Attenuation
Ultrasound wave amplitude decreases with time as it travels through tissue
Time gain compensation (TGC) compensates for the attenuation of the wave by increasing the amplification factor of the signal as a function of time after the initial pulse; all interfaces are then uniform in signal regardless of their depth
Field
Characterizes the propagation of ultrasound energy within a medium
Near field (Fresnel region) is the non-diverging portion of the beam adjacent to the transducer face; the length is a function of transducer frequency and diameter
Far field (Fraunhofer region) is the diverging portion of the ultrasound beam with diminishing energy causing decreases in lateral resolution (or sharpness); less divergence occurs with high-frequency, large-diameter transducers
Focused transducers can change the field interface, i.e., focal zone, being the area of greatest image resolution
Reflection
Each interface (from various acoustic impedances) within the tissue reflects sound waves back to the emitting transducer; good contour definition thus results between different tissues
Fluids allow perfect sound transmission, with no echoes, and result in a black image; tissues attenuate and disperse sound waves, resulting in homogeneous or heterogeneous appearances

3.3.1 Speed of Sound

- The speed of ultrasound through tissue depends on the properties of the tissue.
- Gases have the slowest propagation speed (e.g., air=330 m/s); liquids have an intermediate speed (e.g., water=1,480 m/s); solids have a high propagation speed (e.g., bone=3,400 m/s).

3.3.2 Reflection

- When an ultrasound wave arrives at the interface between two different types of tissue, it is partially reflected and partially transmitted.
- The intensity of the echo depends on the acoustic impedance of the two tissues. Acoustic impedance is determined by the density and stiffness of the tissue.
- The acoustic impedance of soft tissues ranges between 1.3 and 1.7×10^{6} kg · m/s; air=430 kg · m/s; bone=6.47×10^{6} kg · m/s. The greater the difference in the acoustic impedance of two tissues, the more the reflection there is (e.g., soft tissue-air interface or soft tissue-bone interface). There will be little transmission beyond these boundaries; therefore, imaging beyond these boundaries is usually impossible.
- The subsequent subsection of this chapter will cover the ultrasonographic appearance of different tissues in more detail.

3.3.3 Scattering

- For interfaces whose dimensions are very small, such as blood vessels, reflections are known as scattering.
- Scattered waves spread in all directions and distort the resulting image.
- Different types of tissues cause different degrees of scattering; hence, it is more important as a diagnostic tool.

3.3.4 Resolution

- Spatial resolution describes the ability to discriminate two adjacent objects on the display.
  There are two types:
  - Axial resolution: the ability to distinguish objects that are located parallel to each other along the beam axis or at different depths. This depends on the pulse length, which is a function of the wavelength and the number of cycles in the pulse. The higher the frequency or shorter the pulse length, the better the axial resolution is produced. This is particularly important for the pediatric population, as their structures are smaller than in adults.
  - Lateral resolution: the ability to distinguish objects located beside each other. This depends on the beam width and the number of transducer elements per centimeter (line density).

3.3.5 Refraction

- A sound wave meeting a boundary layer at an angle will change direction as it enters the next medium; this depends on the change of velocity of propagation.
- If the velocity is greater in the first medium, refraction occurs toward the perpendicular and vice versa.

3.3.6 Absorption

- Absorption is the main cause of energy loss as ultrasound propagates through the tissue.
- When sound waves enter a body, friction causes kinetic energy to be converted to heat energy, and the energy lost cannot be used to construct an image.
- Absorption depends on the tissue and the frequencies employed. High absorption occurs in the bone; hence, an acoustic shadow is cast. The higher the frequency, the greater the damping and the less the maximum depth of penetration.

3.4 Optimization of Image Quality: Knobology

3.4.1 Frequency

- Selection of a transducer with a frequency appropriate to the depth of the target nerve being examined is the first step in obtaining a good ultrasound image.
- With each transducer, there is a range of frequency, and a more precise frequency can be selected by choosing the type of examination to be performed, for example, the Resolution (or nerve examination), General, or Penetration (or abdomen examination) buttons on the ultrasound machine.

3.4.2 Depth

- It is important to select the appropriate depth since too much depth results in a smaller target and too shallow produces an inadequate image which may exclude important neighboring structures necessary to perform a nerve block safely.

3.4.3 Gain

- By increasing the gain, the amplitude of the echoes is increased, and the image will appear brighter.
- This function serves to improve the signal-to-noise ratio such that weak echoes can be detected (Fig. 3.2).

3.4.4 Time Gain Compensation

- This function offers adjustment of gain in various image depths.
- This is important since the amplitude of ultrasound decreases as it propagates the tissue; therefore, by adjusting gain at different depths of the image enables a uniform display of the signal throughout the image.

3.4.5 Focal Zone

- There are three parts to the ultrasound energy as it propagates the tissue:
  - *Near field* (*Fresnel region*)
    This is adjacent to the transducer surface and is a nondiverging portion of the ultrasound beam.
    Its width is the same as that of the transducer.
    Its length is a function of the transducer frequency and width.
  - *Focal zone*
    At this point, the sound cone is at its narrowest and is at the end of the near field and before the far field.
    This area has the best lateral resolution.
    Some ultrasound machines allow the focal zone to be selected, and it should lie where the target nerve is.
  - *Far field* (*Fraunhofer region*)
    This is where the ultrasound beam begins to diverge and diminish in energy since it is absorbed by the tissue.
    Lateral resolution decreases as this diverging beam progresses.

3.4.6 Doppler Ultrasound

- Doppler ultrasound uses continuous (rather than pulsed) ultrasound beams to detect the presence and measure the velocity of moving interfaces.
- It detects frequency shift in echoes from moving subjects. As a moving object approaches, the received frequency is higher than the emitted frequency and is lower as it moves away. This change in frequency is known as Doppler shift.
- It is useful since it can detect the presence of vessels which can be landmarks to aid identification of the targeted nerve.
- It also highlights the location of vessels adjacent to the targeted nerve such that the trajectory of the needle can be planned to avoid the vessels. This is particularly important in the supraclavicular region since aberrant vessels such as transverse cervical artery and suprascapular artery can be present in the field of the needle trajectory.

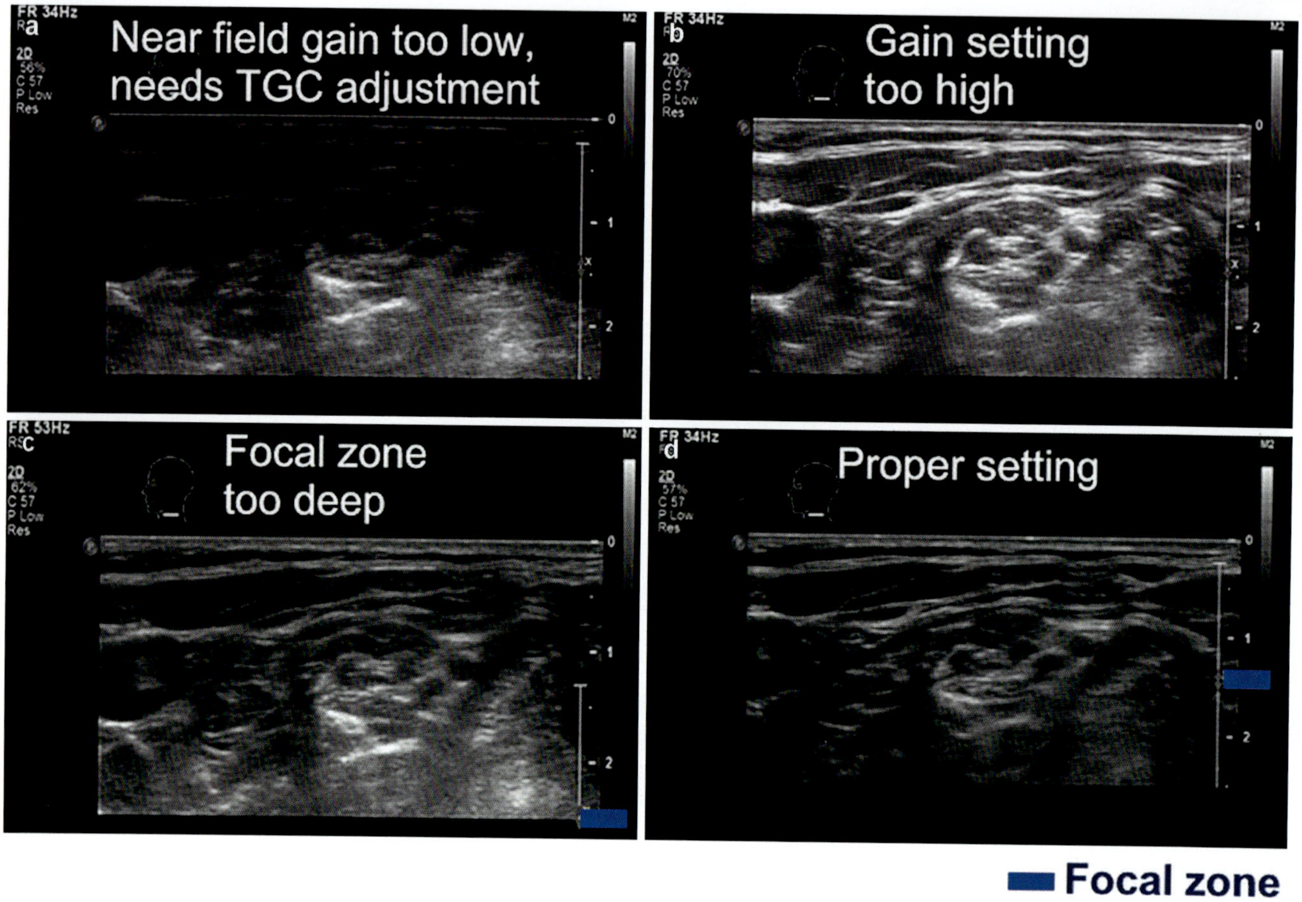

Fig. 3.2 Gain adjustments and focal zone depth. Increasing the gain will increase the amplitude of echoes and improve the signal-to-noise ratio. Gain settings that are either too high (**a**) or too low (**b**) will result in artifactual images and poor resolution between structures. The focal zone (area of greatest image resolution) is adjusted by effectively reducing the beam diameter (compare **c** and **d**)

3.5 Anisotropy and Artifacts

3.5.1 Anisotropy

- Anisotropy is the property of tendons, nerves, and muscles to vary in their ultrasound appearance depending on the angle of incidence between the ultrasound beam and the structure.
- This is important since these three structures are our landmarks or objects to be differentiated when performing a nerve block. This becomes more challenging when the structures are small, as in children.
- The loss of a 90° angle of incidence between the transducer and the structure being imaged can produce a peculiar image in nerves, for example, in the supraclavicular region when the contact between the transducer and the skin is lost. This can be overcome by using an SLA "hockey stick" probe in small children or C11 curved array probe for older children when the brachial plexus is not too superficial.
- This effect is also commonly seen when imaging the femoral nerve in the inguinal region.

3.5.2 Artifacts

An artifact is an image attribute which does not reflect the original structures being scanned. This can be a result of the operator or the interaction of ultrasound with the adjacent tissue.

There are various forms of artifacts:

Acoustic shadowing

- Any structure with a high attenuation coefficient (e.g., bone) diminishes the penetration of the ultrasound beam resulting in minimal or no transmission through the structure (Fig. 3.3).
- Some artifacts may form important landmarks in identifying the target nerve (e.g., the radial nerve "rolling" on the humerus).

Acoustic enhancement

- When the ultrasound beam propagates from a tissue with low attenuation to that with a high attenuation, a hyperechoic area may be seen just below the interface (Fig. 3.4).
- This can be minimized by reducing the overall gain or decreasing the far gain.

Reverberation artifact

- This is caused by ultrasound passing through two adjacent structures with markedly different acoustic properties (Fig. 3.5).

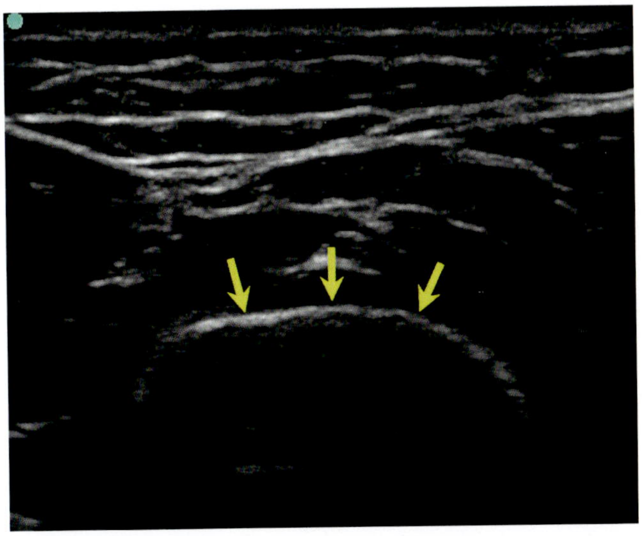

Fig. 3.3 Example of acoustic shadowing. Bone (*arrows*) prevents penetration of the ultrasound beam, leading to reflection of the beam and shadowing underneath

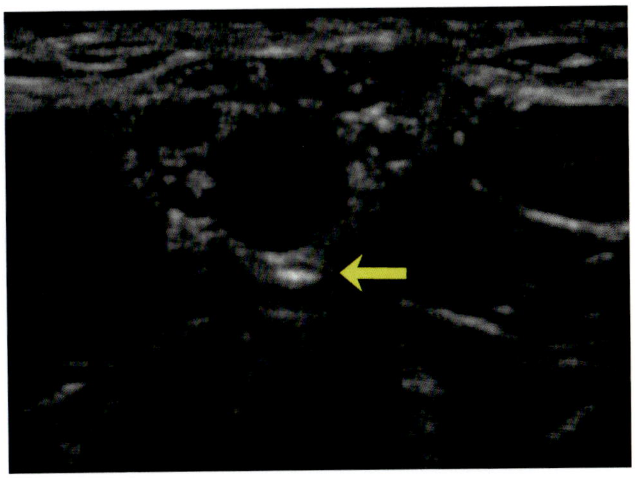

Fig. 3.4 Example of acoustic enhancement. The bright white area indicated by the *arrow* is acoustic enhancement which is reflected onto the tissue

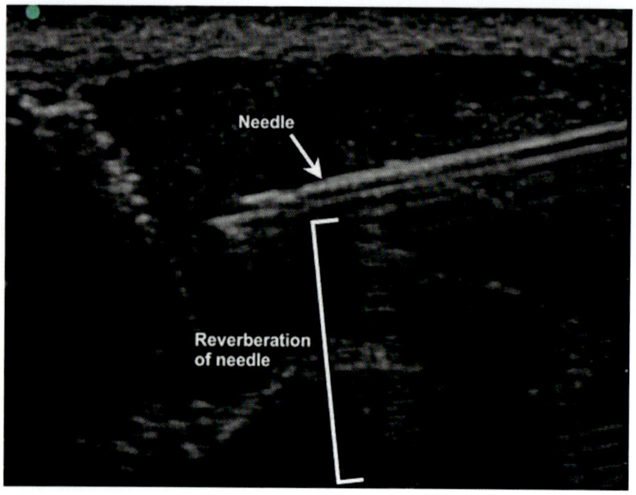

Fig. 3.5 Example of reverberation artifact (multiple hyperechoic lines deep to the needle).

3.6 Echogenic Appearance of Various Tissues

Different tissues have their own ultrasonographic appearance (Table 3.2). Transducers with a high frequency and bandwidth are necessary to differentiate between the fascicular appearance of the nerves and the fibrillar characteristics of tendons. This is particularly challenging in areas where the nerves and tendons are close together, such as those at the wrist or ankle.

There are two common views for ultrasound tissue imaging in regional anesthesia:

- Cross-sectional view when the ultrasound image gives a view of a "cut across the structure." This is also known as the short axis or transverse view.
- Longitudinal view is when the ultrasound images the structure by following its course. This is otherwise called the long axis view.

Table 3.2 Ultrasonographic characteristics of various tissues

Tissue/cavity	Sonographic appearance
Nerves	*Fascicular* appearance
Long axis	Hyperechoic (bright) tubular connective tissue with dispersed elongated hyperechoic fascicles
Short axis	Round/elliptical hypoechoic (dark) fascicles in hyperechoic homogeneous background
Plexus level	Long axis view more hypoechoic than in the periphery
Tendons	*Fibrillar* appearance
Long axis	Fine, highly linear parallel hyperechoic lines separated by fine hypoechoic lines
Short axis	Alternating hyper- and hypoechoic longitudinal areas; no round fascicular appearance
Muscle	
Long axis	Pennate or feather-like
Short axis	"Starry night" with uniform hypoechoic pattern; more hypoechoic than nerves and tendons
Bone	Linear hyperechoic bone density with hypoechoic shadow
Blood vessels	Hypo- or anechoic circular structures on short axis viewing. Arteries can be distinguished from veins by their darker, more defined circular structure, as well as their lack of easy compressibility
Fat	Generally hypoechoic, may contain pathological hyperechoic connective tissue
Fascia	Hyperechoic marking well-defined boundary
Pleura and air	Pleura appears hyperechoic with either anechoic fluid-filled cavity or diffuse hyperechoic air cavity (e.g., aerated lung)

Nerves and tendons

- Long axis view of the nerves in the peripheral appears as hyperechoic (bright) tubular structures from the connective tissues with elongated and well-defined hypoechoic (dark) spaces within this tubule, which are neuronal fascicles (Fig. 3.6).
- Short axis view of a nerve in the periphery shows small elliptical or round hypoechoic structures which are fascicles, each surrounded by a homogeneous hyperechoic connective tissue, giving a honeycomb appearance to the nerve. The nerve can also be "traced back" using the traceback approach (see Sect. 4.4.2) since it is a continuous structure and is usually adjacent to the vessel(s) (Fig. 3.7).
- Nerve roots, such as those seen in the cervical region during interscalene blocks, appear monofascicular. The trunks and cords of the brachial plexus have an even better defined fascicular pattern owing to the hyperechoic thick epineurium. This fascicular pattern is more difficult to appreciate at the cord level since it is deeper.
- With a longitudinal view, the brachial plexus is hypoechoic compared to the nerves in the periphery due to the increased amount of connective tissues accompanying the nerves in the periphery.
- It may be difficult to differentiate between a nerve and a tendon with ultrasound although there are certain differences, as shown in Table 3.3.

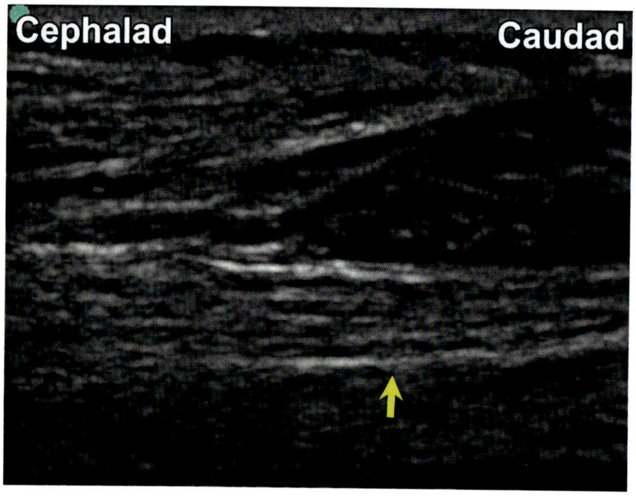

Fig. 3.6 Long axis view of peripheral nerves shows hyperechoic tubular structures (*yellow arrow*). Elongated and well-defined hypoechoic spaces within this tubule are neuronal fascicles

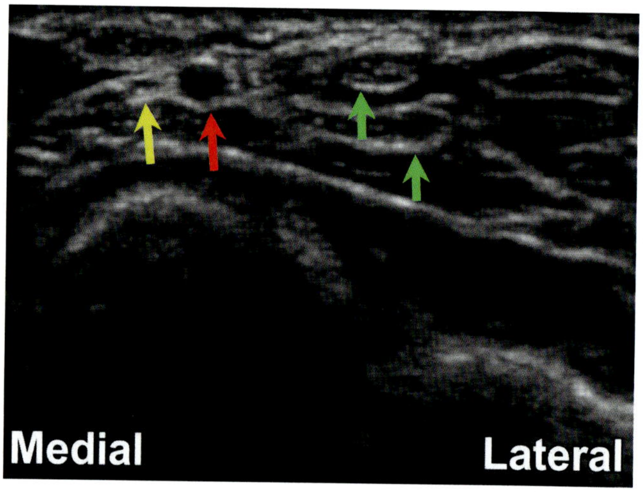

Fig. 3.7 Short axis view of a peripheral nerve (*yellow arrow*) shows small elliptical or round hypoechoic structures which are fascicles, each surrounded by a homogeneous hyperechoic connective tissue, giving a honeycomb-like appearance to the nerve. *Red arrow* indicates artery; *green arrows* indicate tendon

Table 3.3 Differences in ultrasonographic appearance of nerves and tendons

	Nerves	Tendons
General appearance	Fascicular	Fibrillar
Long axis view (at 90° incidence angle)	Less pronounced and fewer hyperechoic lines, but these lines are thicker	Numerous fine, parallel, hyperechoic lines (fibrillar pattern) separated by hypoechoic lines
Transverse view	No specific patterns to hyper- or hypoechoic areas	Alternating hyper-, hypoechoic longitudinal areas
	Honeycomb-like appearance, especially the periphery	
Consistency in shape	Fairly consistent in shape	Profile changes abruptly
Longitudinal view with active or passive movement	Stationary among the surrounding mobile tissue	Mobile

Muscle

- In a short axis (cross-sectional) view, there is a uniform, hypoechoic "starry night" pattern; on longitudinal scanning (long axis view), there is a typical pennate or feather-like appearance (Fig. 3.8).
- The hyperechoic lines within the muscle are separated by wider spaces of hypoechoicity compared to the nerves.

Bone

- The bone has a linear, hyperechoic appearance which casts a hypoechoic shadow beneath (acoustic shadowing) (Fig. 3.3).
- This striking appearance is ideal for providing landmarks for nerve blocks, such as the greater trochanter of the femur as a landmark for subgluteal approach to the sciatic nerve or the radial groove/deltoid tuberosity, medial epicondyle, and lateral epicondyle for radial, median, and ulnar nerve locations, respectively.

Vascular structure

- Blood vessels appear as anechoic structures on cross-sectional view.
- Arteries are typically circular and pulsatile; the latter characteristic is enhanced upon external compression by the transducer on the skin.
- Veins are compressible, so care must be taken when performing nerve blocks since pressure exerted on the transducer during scanning may occlude the veins, making them invisible on the image. This is particularly true when the vessels are small, such as those in children.

Fat

- Fatty tissue is slightly hypoechoic relative to the skin, although abnormalities such as tumors may result in hyperechoic reflection.

Fascial tissue

- The fascia appears as a well-defined hyperechoic line.

Pleura and air

- The pleura has a hyperechoic linear appearance, and, beyond the pleura, the reverberation artifact creates specular reflectors which "move" on breathing (Fig. 3.5).
- The air within the lung forms a "comet tail" acoustic shadow deep from the pleura.

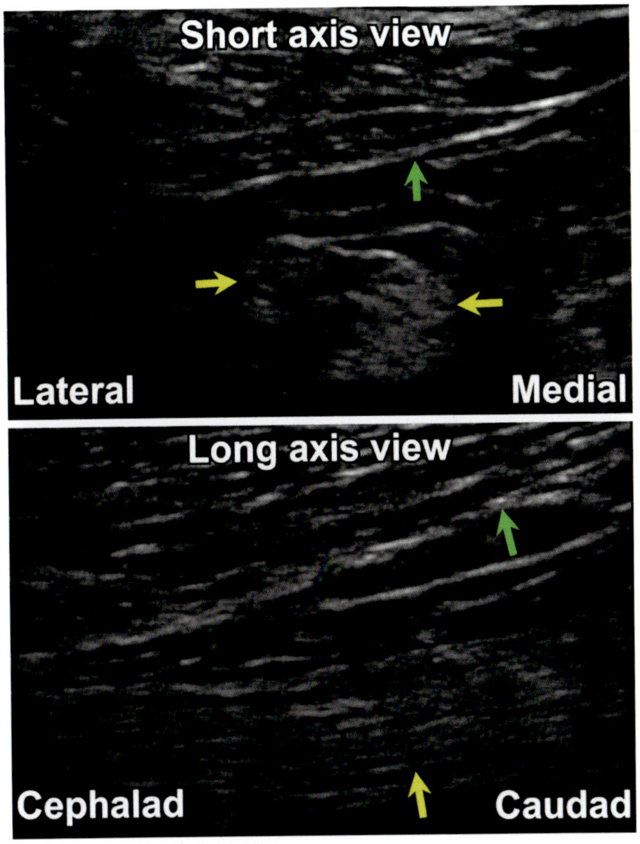

Fig. 3.8 Short (*top*) and long (*bottom*) axis view of muscle. Note the uniform, hypoechoic "starry night" pattern in the short axis view and the pennate or feather-like appearance in the long axis view. *Yellow arrows* indicate nerve; *green arrows* indicate muscle

3.7 Equipment Selection

- The necessary equipment allowing performance of ultrasound-guided regional anesthesia is, of course, an ultrasound machine. The portable laptop machines currently available offer a good-quality, high-resolution image, comparable to those of the larger, more cumbersome (and more expensive) cart-based systems. Portable machines are more practical and allow ultrasound-guided nerve blocks to be performed at the bedside.
- The machine should have the basic functions for optimizing image quality, such as gain control, color flow Doppler, and zoom.
- The machine should allow images and short video clips to be captured and stored. There should be a hard disk with high capacity for storage of the images and film sequence as well as an ability to export these to a Universal Serial Bus (USB) memory stick or compact disc (CD). The images in this book were captured with the SonoSite M-Turbo (Bothell, WA, USA), unless stated otherwise.
- A good machine should be simple to use and with the commonly used function buttons clearly visible.
- Ultrasound machines are almost like cameras. Portable units are analogous to current automatic, "point-and-click" cameras, which are simple to use and can capture reasonably good pictures. In contrast, the larger, cart-based systems are akin to complex manual cameras favored by the professional photographer.
- For most blocks performed in children, a SonoSite M-Turbo machine is adequate. However, for imaging neuraxial structures, the large, cart-based systems are superior due to higher resolution and sensitivity, which produce remarkable images and enable greater precision.
- The most crucial piece of equipment is the transducer. As mentioned previously in this chapter, high-frequency linear transducers (13–6 MHz) that allow high spatial resolution are ideal for superficial structures in children during both peripheral nerve blocks and neuraxial blocks.
- A smaller footprint, as with the SLA "hockey stick" transducer (25 mm), is practical for performing nerve blocks in small children. Transducers with a larger surface area footprint (38 mm) are more suitable for older children and provide an increased overview.
- For neuraxial blocks, a 38 mm footprint high-frequency probe (13–6 MHz) is usually used.

Preferred needle and probe options for various block locations are listed in Table 3.4.

Table 3.4 Needle and probe selection for peripheral block locations

Block location	Needle[a]	Probe[a]
Upper extremity		
Interscalene	3–5 cm, 22G	HFL38, C11
Supraclavicular	3.75 cm, 22G	SLA, C11
Infraclavicular	10 cm, 22G	HFL38, C11
Axillary	1.25–2 cm, 22G	HFL38
Radial (spiral groove)	1.25–2 cm, 22G	HFL38
Musculocutaneous (coracobrachialis)	1.25–2 cm, 22G	HFL38
Median (antecubital)	3.75 cm, 22G	HFL38
Ulnar (mid-forearm)	3.75 cm, 22G	SLA, HFL38
Lower extremity		
Lumbar plexus	15 cm, 22G	C60
Femoral	3–4 cm, 22G	HFL38
Sciatic – anterior/posterior	10 cm, 22G	C60
Popliteal – posterior	5–6 cm, 22G	HFL38
Popliteal – lateral	10 cm, 20G	HFL38
Ankle	2.5 cm, 24G	SLA, HFL38
Trunk		
Intercostal	3.75 cm, 22G	HFL38
Paravertebral	8.75 cm, 22G	HFL38, C60

[a]Selection based on commonly available needle length and SonoSite probes (see Fig. 3.1b)

3.8 Current Advances for Future Developments

Advancements in technology enable constant improvement of the quality of ultrasound images. The areas of important development are:

3.8.1 Compound Imaging

Speckle is a 2D noise in ultrasonographic images resulting from scattering media. To overcome speckle, multiple image planes are captured from different beam angles and broad bandwidth frequencies simultaneously and are then averaged to construct a speckle-reduced single image. This process is known as compounding.

3.8.2 Single-Crystal Transducers

These are sizable monocrystals produced by techniques that are similar to those employed in growing silicon. They may produce increased bandwidth, sensitivity, and high energy density for remarkable performance.

3.8.3 Capacitive Micromachined Ultrasound Transducers (CMUT)

The conversion from acoustic to electrical energy and vice versa is obtained through an electric field stored in a multitude of microscopic capacitors obtained from a silicon wafer by means of micromachining. These transducers have excellent bandwidth and impedance matching to the human body. These properties produce higher-resolution images and enable optimal tissue harmonic imaging which captures the higher-frequency echoes with less scatter and artifacts. This application is important for real-time 3D imaging.

3.8.4 Sonix GPS (Ultrasonix Medical Corp, Richmond, BC, Canada)

Sonix GPS is an electromagnetic needle tracking system with a sensor housed within the needle for real-time ultrasound-guided needle insertion. The current and predicted needle positions are displayed on the ultrasound screen, and, as the needle is advanced, the needle trajectory and ultrasound beam are aligned in real time, allowing the user to aim the needle accurately toward the final target location.

3.8.5 Power Doppler

This technique can detect lower flow vessels which would not show up in normal color Doppler, such as those with a low diastolic velocity from a perpendicular Doppler angle. Instead of estimating the frequency shift in Doppler signals, power Doppler estimates the integral of the power spectrum. The color in the power Doppler image indicates that blood flow is present but does not provide any information on flow velocity.

3.8.6 Robot-Assisted Regional Anesthesia

Recently, the multipurpose da Vinci Surgical System Type S (DVS) (Intuitive Surgical, Sunnyvale, CA) was demonstrated to place a single-injection nerve block and perineural catheter into an ultrasound phantom under real-time ultrasound guidance. The limitation with this technique is, first and foremost, the cost, and there is a need for increased manpower (two engineers, an anesthesiologist, and a urologist, in this simulation) to perform this procedure using this equipment. This is, however, an exciting experiment that proves the benefits of the twenty-first-century technology.

Suggested Reading

Bhargava R, Noga M, Lou L. Ultrasound basics. In: Tsui BC, editor. Atlas of ultrasound and nerve stimulation-guided regional anesthesia. New York: Springer; 2007. p. 19–33.

Connolly DJA, Berman L, McNally EG. The use of beam angulation to overcome anisotropy when viewing human tendon with high frequency linear array ultrasound. Br J Radiol. 2001;7(4):183–5.

Gray AT. Ultrasound-guided regional anesthesia. Anesthesiology. 2006;104:368–73.

Hemmerling TM, Taddei R, Wehbe M, et al. First robotic ultrasound-guided nerve blocks in humans using the Magellan system. Anesth Analg. 2013;116:491–4.

Karmakar MK, Kwok WH. Ultrasound-guided regional anesthesia. In: Cote CJ, Lerman J, Todres ID, editors. A practice of anesthesia for infants and children. 4th ed. Philadelphia: WB Saunders; 2009. p. 911–24.

Kelsey CA. Essentials of radiology physics. St. Louis: Warren H. Green; 1985.

Lemoigne Y, Caner A, Rahal G, editors. Physics for medical imaging applications. Dordrecht: Springer; 2007.

Marhofer P, Frickey N. Ultrasonographic guidance in pediatric regional anesthesia. Part 1: theoretical background. Pediatr Anesth. 2006;16: 1008–18.

Oakley CG, Zipparo MJ. Single-crystal piezoelectrics: a revolutionary development for transducers. Ultrason Symp 2000 IEEE. 2000;2: 1157–67.

Oralkan O, Ergun S, Johnson JA, et al. Capacitive micromachined ultrasonic transducers: next-generation arrays for acoustic imaging. IEEE Trans Ultrason Ferroelectr Freq Control. 2002;49: 1596–610.

Park SE, Hackenberger W. High performance single crystal piezoelectrics: applications and issues. Curr Opin Solid State Mater Sci. 2002;6:11–8.

Polaner DM, Suresh S, Cote CJ. Regional anesthesia. In: Cote CJ, Lerman J, Todres ID, editors. A practice of anesthesia for infants and children. 4th ed. Philadelphia: WB Saunders; 2009. p. 873–4.

Rapp H, Folger A, Grau T. Ultrasound-guided epidural catheter insertion in children. Anesth Analg. 2005;101:333–9.

Rubin K, Sullivan D, Sadhasivam S. Are peripheral and neuraxial blocks with ultrasound guidance more effective and safe in children? Pediatr Anesth. 2009;19:92–6.

Sites BD, Brull R, Chan VW, et al. Artifacts and pitfall errors associated with ultrasound-guided regional anesthesia. Part I: understanding the basic principles of ultrasound physics and machine operations. Reg Anesth Pain Med. 2007;32:412–8.

Tighe PJ, Badiyan SJ, Luria I, et al. Robot-assisted regional anesthesia: a simulated demonstration. Anesth Analg. 2010;111(3):813–6.

4 Clinical and Practical Aspects of Ultrasound Use

Michelle L. Noga, Vivian H.Y. Ip, and Ban C.H. Tsui

Contents

M.L. Noga, MD, FRCPC (✉)
Department of Radiology and Diagnostic Imaging,
University of Alberta, 2A2.41 Walter Mackenzie Centre,
8440-112 Street, Edmonton, AB T6G 2B7, Canada
e-mail: mnoga@ualberta.ca

V.H.Y. Ip, MB ChB, MRCP, FRCA
Department of Anesthesiology and Pain Medicine,
University of Alberta Hospital, 2-150 Clinical Sciences Building,
Edmonton, AB T6G 2G3, Canada
e-mail: hip@ualberta.ca

B.C.H. Tsui, Dip Eng, BSc (Math), B Pharm, MSc, MD, FRCPC
Department of Anesthesiology and Pain Medicine,
Stollery Children's Hospital/University of Alberta Hospital,
2-150 Clinical Sciences Building,
Edmonton, AB T6G 2G3, Canada
e-mail: btsui@ualberta.ca

B.C.H. Tsui, S. Suresh (eds.), *Pediatric Atlas of Ultrasound- and Nerve Stimulation-Guided Regional Anesthesia*,
DOI 10.1007/978-0-387-79964-3_4

4.1 Image Acquisition

Basic Concepts

- It is advisable to perform the block in a stress-free environment with minimal time restraints.
- The target area should be surveyed (scanned) using a generous amount of ultrasound gel prior to sterile preparation. One of the most common reasons for poor visualization is lack of sufficient gel for skin-probe contact.
- Upon location of a suitable puncture site, the probe position is marked on the skin with a sterile marker.
- The images used in this book are those from our everyday practice and are achievable by any newcomer to ultrasound-guided regional anesthesia. We have been mindful not to concentrate on presenting anatomically perfect ultrasound images, which are obtained occasionally; shown are images that are representative of what you will encounter in an average day.
- In order to facilitate learning in identification of the sonoanatomy, unlabelled ultrasound images are placed next to identical but well-labeled images. Our colleagues have found this layout to be the most effective for familiarizing themselves with realistic clinical images as there is no distraction from multiple labels, yet at the same time, they benefit from side-by-side reference to the same image that has been labeled.
- More importantly, the labeling system indicates what structures are normally visualized as well as the expected locations of any clinically relevant and important structures which may not be immediately obvious. Hopefully, this will reduce frustration and failure from unrealistic expectation in an attempt to visualize every structure.

4.2 Probe Preparation

- Both the probe and the patient's skin should be prepared for maximum sterility and optimal imaging.
- Water-soluble conductivity gel is always used to remove the air-skin interface and to allow good reflection of ultrasound waves.
- Probe sterility is paramount in performing real-time, or dynamic, ultrasound-guided nerve block. This can be maintained by standard sleeve covers, although these can be expensive and cumbersome.
- When using a probe with the standard long covers, it is important to avoid air tracking between the probe and cover, as well as between the cover and the skin, which can obscure the ultrasound image.
- For single-shot blocks, we find it practical to use a transparent dressing without the full cover of a sterile sleeve:
  - A sterile transparent dressing (Tegaderm™; 3M Health Care, St. Paul, MN, USA) can be used effectively, but to maintain a smooth surface, it must be stretched before it is adhered to the surface of the probe. The IV3000 dressing (Smith & Nephew Medical Limited, Hull, UK) is marketed for this purpose, but we have observed that, when placed over the probe surface, multiple small adhesive wells trap air underneath the dressing, leading to poor imaging and a limited ability to use the Doppler effect (Fig. 4.1) [1].
  - We also use individual sterile packs of gel.
- For continuous blocks:
  - Complete sterile preparation is required; a complete sterile cover is used for the ultrasound probe. A mask, sterile gown, and gloves should be worn by the operator.
- After completion of the procedure, the probe and related equipment (including all surfaces and cables) should be thoroughly cleaned.

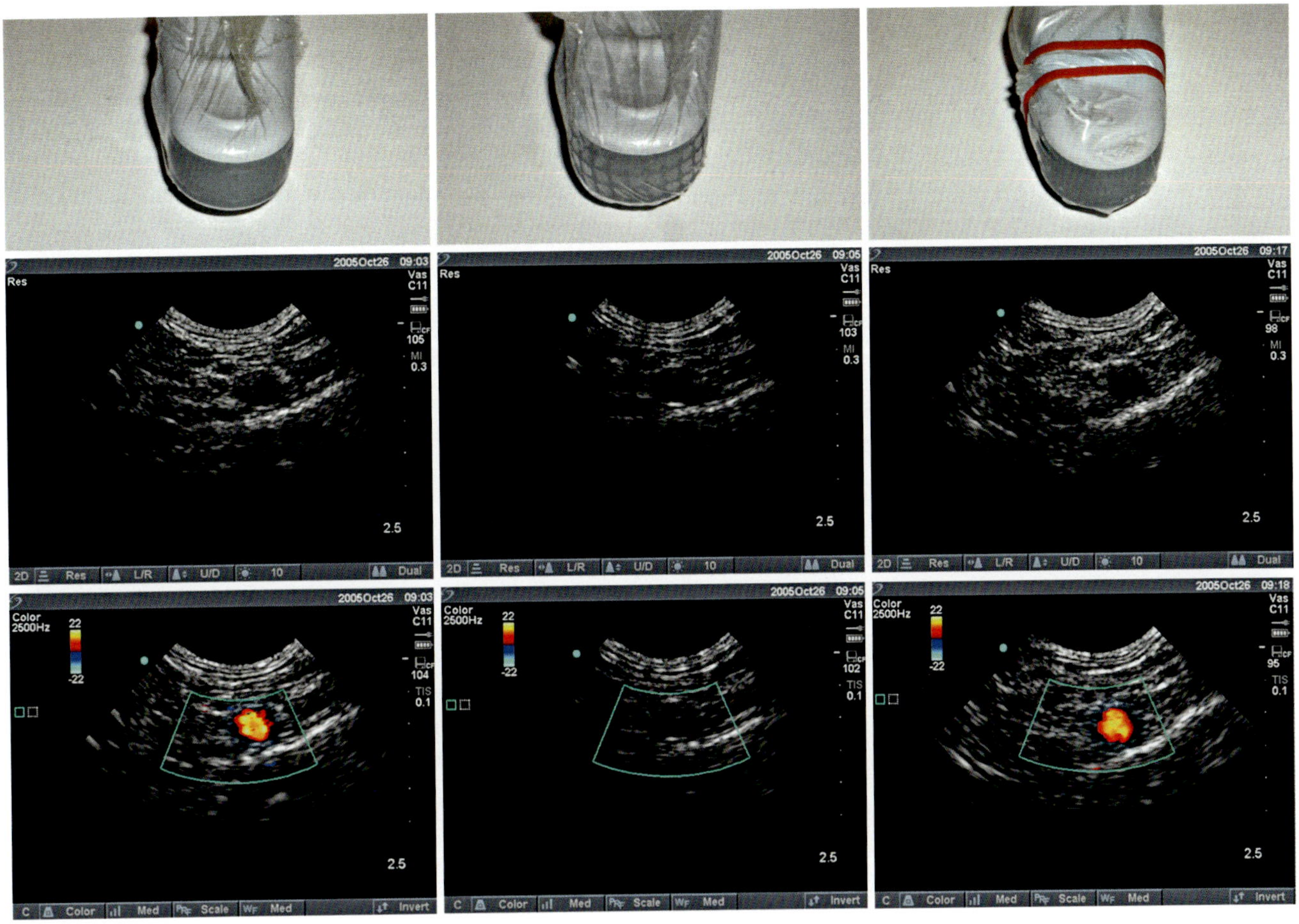

Fig. 4.1 Effects of sterile transparent dressing on image quality and ability to use Doppler ultrasound with curved probes. The Tegaderm dressing maintains image quality and ability to use Doppler as long as it is stretched (*left*). The IV3000 dressing can be used (*middle*), but multiple small adhesive wells containing air may form under the dressing, leading to poor imaging and limited ability to use Doppler. A complete commercial sterile cover (*right*) would be necessary if performing catheter insertion for continuous anesthesia/analgesia (Adapted from Tsui et al. [1]. With permission from Wolters Kluwer Health)

4.3 Image Optimization

- One of the most important factors in ultrasound-guided localization is patient positioning. The patient should be placed in a position such that the target area is well exposed. In the subsequent clinical chapters, patient positioning will be described for each individual block prior to discussing the ultrasound imaging technique.
- The operator position should be optimized to enable both a good view of the ultrasound screen and comfortable hand positioning for needle insertion.
- The reader is referred to Chap. 3 to choose the appropriate frequency of transducer at each peripheral block location; the frequency will partly determine the type of array (linear versus curved) that will be suitable. Often, a high-frequency linear array transducer (10 MHz or more) is the most appropriate for the pediatric population. If the area of interest is relatively deep, such as the gluteal region in teenagers, a lower-frequency transducer (5–7 MHz) may be advantageous with greater penetration. Whether the probe array is curved or linear depends on the region and field of view required (e.g., blocks in the lumbar region benefit from larger fields of view and lower frequencies, which curved array probes offer).

4.3.1 Probe Alignment

- The probe will have a marker or groove to show which way is "up." The marker corresponds to the top of the ultrasound image, and if you slide the probe toward the marker, the image will move in the direction that the probe is moved. Similarly, if you slide the probe away from the marker side, the image will move in the direction opposite the marker.
- In most circumstances, and particularly with transverse planes of viewing, the plane of the transducer beam should intersect the axis of the nerve structures at a perpendicular position. The lateral resolution will be optimal in this situation, and artifacts such as anisotropy (Chap. 3, Sect. 3.6) will be minimized.
- To obtain the best short-axis view in a coronal plane, such as scanning the supraclavicular region, follow these important steps for probe handling (Fig. 4.2):
  - Scan across the relevant area to obtain a transverse view of the vascular structure (e.g., subclavian artery) or nerve since it is easier to capture these structures with an ultrasound beam "transecting" in a short axis rather than obtaining a longitudinal view.
  - The image can be refined by rotating the probe (turn slightly clockwise or anticlockwise) or tilting the probe forward and backward to achieve a perpendicular beam through the target structure in order to sharpen the image.
- Adjust the time gain compensation (TGC) so that the visualized area is of uniform echotexture. Always adjust the TGC to the center when changing transducers during a study.
- Appropriate depth should be adjusted such that the target nerve is in the center of the screen with other relevant structures in view (e.g., in supraclavicular block, one should be able to visualize the subclavian artery, the first rib, and the pleura).
- The focal point should be adjusted to the where the target nerve is.
- A systematic approach allows the best image to be obtained in a timely fashion, increasing the success rate of ultrasound-guided peripheral nerve blocks.
- Most neural structures are accompanied by blood vessels (pulsatile arteries or compressible veins) or bony landmarks, which are readily identifiable using ultrasound. Color Doppler is useful in this situation to identify blood vessels. The color convention is for red to represent blood flowing toward the transducer and blue to represent blood flowing away from the transducer. Therefore, the knowledge of anatomy is always important to identify nerves around these landmarks.
- The "traceback" approach (see below) also aids the identification of a nerve, especially when differentiating between similar-looking structures such as tendons or artifacts.

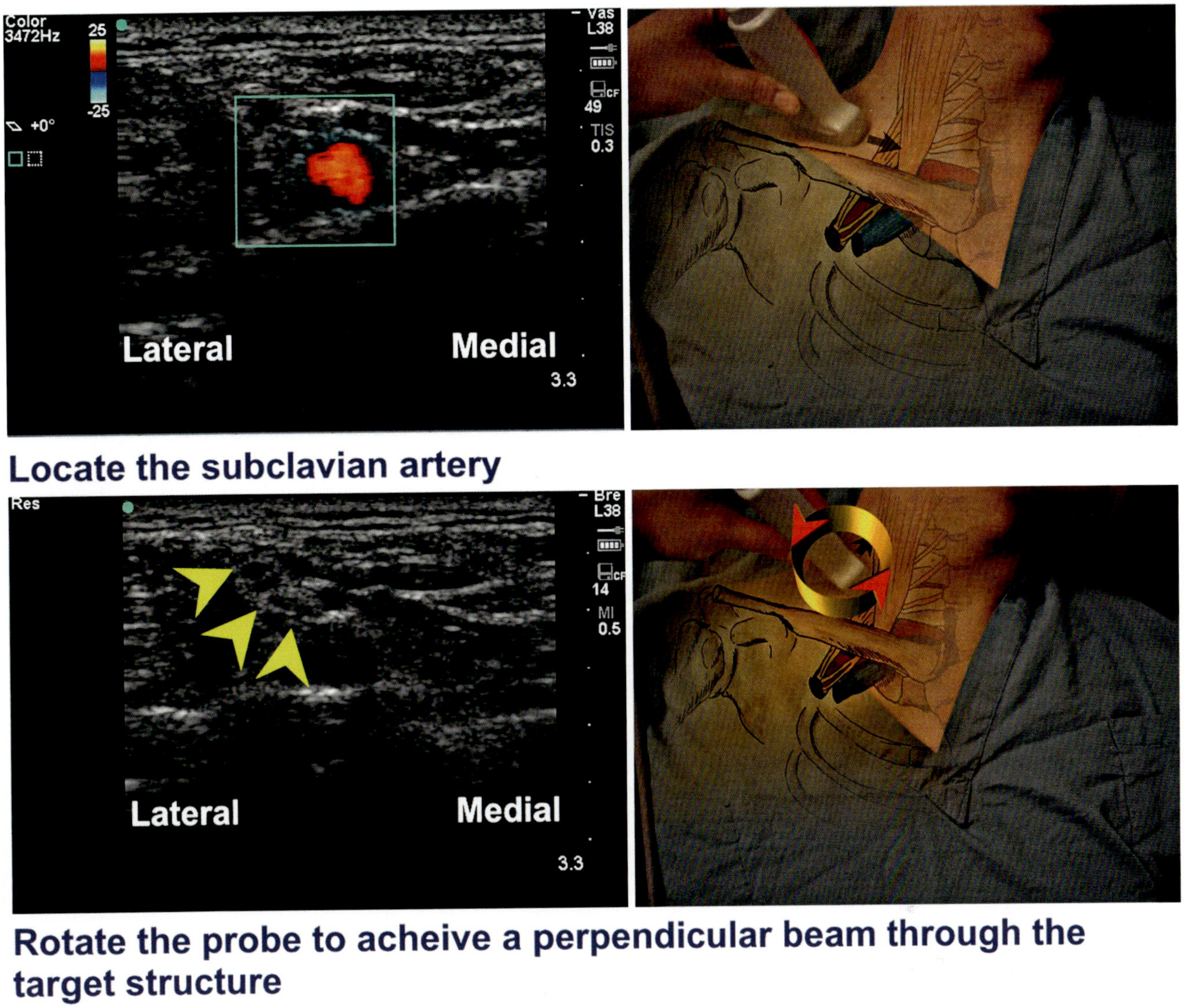

Fig. 4.2 Probe handling during supraclavicular blockade with landmark identification of the subclavian artery. Scan across the relevant area to obtain a transverse view of the vascular structure (in this case the subclavian artery; *top*). To sharpen the image, rotate the probe (*clockwise* or *anticlockwise*) or tilt the probe forward and backward to achieve a perpendicular beam through the target structure (*bottom*)

4.3.2 Practical Approach: Traceback Method

As with the conventional "blind" approach, knowledge of anatomy is of upmost importance when performing peripheral nerve blocks under ultrasound guidance. The spatial appreciation in relation to the surrounding structures is also relevant. In our experience, neural structures are not always easy to identify under ultrasound; they can appear hyper- or hypoechoic and are sometimes confused with artifacts. Nerves are continuous structures, which lend themselves to be "traced" proximally and distally. This enables the differentiation from structures with similar appearance (e.g., tendons). In this section, we will describe a systematic "traceback" approach [2] to help identify the target nerves (within various regions) of commonly used nerve blocks.

- Instead of immediately focusing on locating the target nerve at the commonly used block site, the goal of this exercise is to obtain a clear image of an obvious anatomic landmark (i.e., a blood vessel or bony landmark) not too far removed from one point along the target nerve's path.
- If suitable, it is generally preferred to perform the block at this location due to the dependable anatomical relations.
- Otherwise, the operator focuses on the nerve (often in short axis by adjusting the transducer as described above in probe alignment) and "traces" it toward the block target area by moving the ultrasound probe in a proximal or distal direction along the nerve.
- The appearance of surrounding structures (e.g., muscle and other soft tissues) changes consistently as the probe moves, whereas the appearance of the target nerve does not change in any significant manner and is traceable.
- In this way, we can more easily and reliably identify the corresponding nerve or plexus.

For illustration purposes, see Fig. 4.3, which describes a traceback practice for facilitating identification of the sciatic nerve at the popliteal fossa (using vascular landmark identification). This approach allows the operator to gain confidence in their ability to recognize and locate the nerves. During the training process, we found that the traceback approach is an easy and reliable way to become proficient at identifying neural structures prior to performing regional anesthesia. However, the traceback approach may not be necessary in some locations where the larger nerves are more easily identifiable, for example, the median nerve in the axilla and antecubital fossa and the femoral nerve in the inguinal region.

We strongly recommend that the initial step in performing ultrasound-assisted regional anesthesia is identification of obvious landmarks (usually blood vessels or bony landmarks) in the vicinity of the target nerve. Table 4.1 lists the numerous nerve blocks that can benefit from identification of highly visible and dependable structures (i.e., blood vessels (especially with color Doppler) and bone) for accurate nerve identification. Nonetheless, the traceback technique is useful for popliteal nerve for identification of the bifurcation, identifying the brachial plexus at the interscalene region, or for revealing anatomic anomalies.

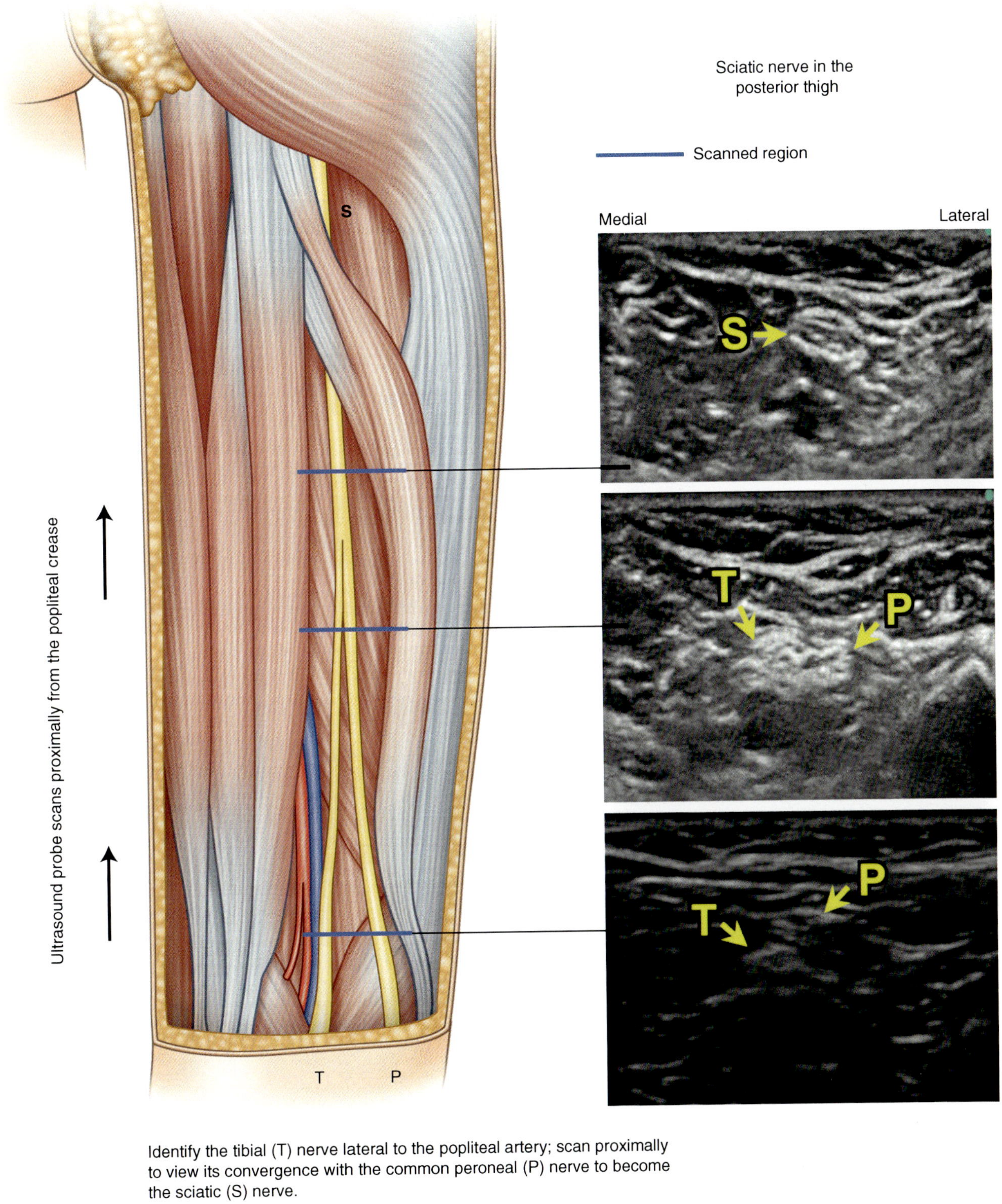

Fig. 4.3 Traceback approach in the posterior thigh for identification of the sciatic nerve at the popliteal fossa (Adapted from Tsui and Finucane [2]. With permission from Wolters Kluwer Health)

Table 4.1 Useful landmarks for identification of nerves using ultrasound; many can be used in "traceback" approaches

Block	Ultrasound landmark	Comments
Interscalene	Subclavian artery	Trace nerve proximally from the distal supraclavicular location where the artery lies medial to the nerve
Supraclavicular	Subclavian artery	Brachial plexus lies lateral and often superior to the artery
Infraclavicular	Subclavian artery and vein	Brachial plexus cords surround the artery
Axillary	Axillary artery	Terminal nerves surround the artery
Peripheral nerves		
Median at antecubital fossa	Brachial artery	Nerve lies immediately medial to the artery
Radial at posterior elbow	Humerus at spiral groove	Groove is found on posterolateral surface of humerus inferior to the deltoid insertion, and the nerve can be located (also adjacent to the deep brachial artery) and traced to the anterior elbow
Ulnar at medial forearm	Ulnar artery	The nerve lies medial and adjacent to the artery at the midpoint of the forearm
Lumbar plexus	Transverse process	Lies between and just deep to the lateral tips of the processes
Femoral	Femoral artery	Nerve lies lateral to artery (vein most medial). Insert needle above the bifurcation of the deep femoral artery
Sciatic		
Labat	Ischial bone	Nerve lies lateral to the ischial bone
Subgluteal	Greater trochanter and ischial tuberosity	Nerve lies between the two bone structures
Popliteal	Popliteal artery	Trace back from the popliteal crease where the tibial nerve is adjacent to the artery. Scanning proximally to the sciatic bifurcation, the artery becomes deeper and at a greater distance from the tibial nerve where it is joined by the peroneal nerve
Ankle		
Tibial (posterior tibial)	Posterior tibial artery	Nerve lies posterior to the artery
Deep peroneal	Anterior tibial artery	Nerve lies lateral to the artery

4.4 Control of Needle Trajectory

4.4.1 Visibility of Needles

- Common small-bore, 22G insulated block needles are adequate to perform ultrasound-guided blocks in children.
- Since neural structures are superficial in children, there is generally good needle visibility since the increased angles of penetration tend to reduce visibility.
- A larger-gauge needle, such as the 17G–20G Tuohy needles used in peripheral nerve block catheterization, can also improve visibility.
- Manufacturers are constantly improving needles for visibility, and echogenic needles are commercially available (Chap. 1).
- It is important to be able to visualize the tip of the needle. Tilting (Fig. 4.4a), rotating (Fig. 4.4b), and manipulating the transducer alignment (Fig. 4.4c) is necessary to ensure that the image of the needle includes the tip. This is particularly important for the out-of-plane approach, since the image of the needle is a hyperechoic dot which could be interpreted as either the shaft or the tip of the needle on the screen (see below).

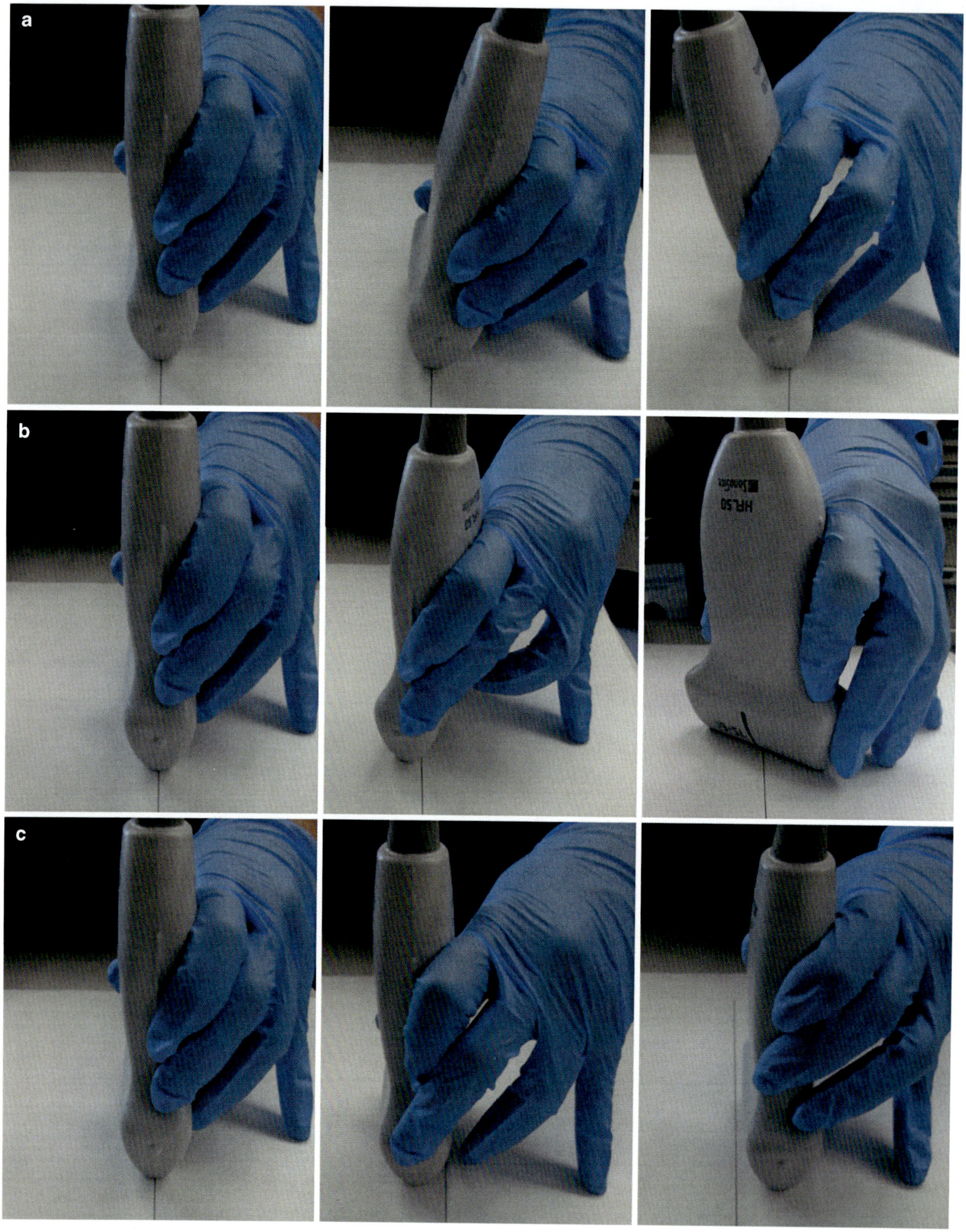

Fig. 4.4 Tilting (**a**), rotating (**b**), and manipulating (**c**) the alignment of the ultrasound probe is necessary to visualize the tip of the needle. The *line* on the paper indicates the original axis of the probe

4.4.2 Hand-Eye Coordination

One of the most common errors of the beginner learning ultrasound-guided regional anesthesia is to focus their attention on the needle in their hand, instead of observing the needle position changes on the screen. This is a cardinal error, as important information relating to the needle position and the corresponding image will be missed by concentrating on the actual needle. Today's teenage population illustrates this point by focusing on the onscreen action rather than on the controller when playing a video game (Fig. 4.5). Similarly, an experienced laparoscopic surgeon may look directly at their instruments upon initial insertion but will transfer their focus to the screen for all subsequent instrument manipulation. Although it sounds trivial to stress good hand-eye coordination, mastering it has been extremely helpful for staff at our institution.

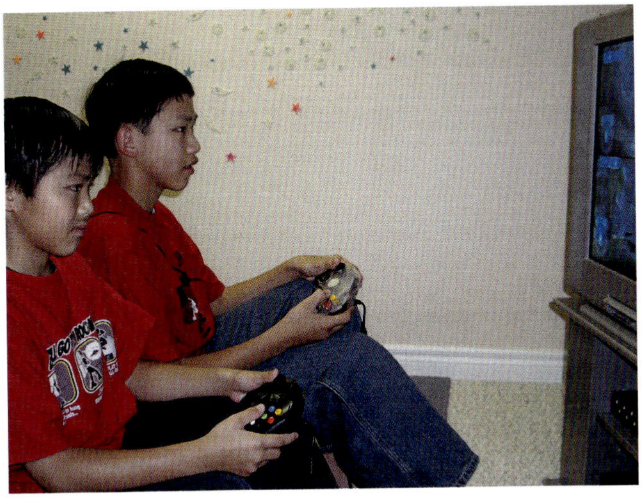

Fig. 4.5 Children demonstrating hand-eye coordination focusing on the video game screen rather than their hand movements on the controller (Reprinted from Tsui BC, Dillane D. Practical and clinical aspects of ultrasound and nerve stimulation-guided peripheral nerve blocks. In: Tsui BC, editor. Atlas of ultrasound and nerve stimulation-guided regional anesthesia. New York: Springer; 2007. p. 35–48. With permission from Springer Verlag)

4.4.3 Needling Technique

4.4.3.1 In-Plane Technique (Fig. 4.6)

- Aligning the needle to the ultrasound plane is an important concept to grasp and practice.
- In-plane (IP, long-axis, longitudinal, or axial) needling approaches with the needle parallel to the ultrasound scanning plane have the advantage of allowing continuous control of the needle trajectory due to clear visualization of both needle tip and shaft.
- The nerve structure is often placed at the edge of the ultrasound screen to ensure shallow insertion angle of the needle and, therefore, a better visualization.
- Good alignment of the needle shaft and scanning plane is required and can be attained by paying close attention when viewing the needle and probe from above or in an axial view.
- For practical reasons, it is often advisable to use a small footprint linear (e.g., hockey stick) probe or curved array probe (e.g., C11) in compact areas, such as the supraclavicular fossa. It is critical to use in-plane technique at this location (to adequately view the needle to prevent pleural puncture), and smaller probes will be beneficial for more space to maneuver the needle.
- Most commercial needle-guiding tools involve physical fixation of the needle aligned in-plane with respect to the ultrasound beam; such an apparatus is not only expensive and cumbersome to use but often limits fine adjustment of needle placement and requires extra long needles (Fig. 4.7).
- A GPS needle tracking device is available which provides real-time information of where the needle should be maneuvered for the target area (Chap. 3).
- In contrast, the freehand technique requires excellent coordination to align and maintain the needle in plane to the ultrasound beam in order to visually track the advancement of the needle toward the target in real time; accordingly, the freehand technique often requires a steep learning curve.
- Tsui [3] developed a method of needle-probe alignment using a laser attachment for the probe (Fig. 4.8); the laser line will project onto both the needle shaft and the midline of the probe, indicating an in-plane position. Alternatively, a commercially available laser attachment for the needle (SonoGuide, Pajunk, Geisingen, Germany) is also available and operates with a similar concept (Fig. 4.9).
- It should be noted that the in-plane approach can be performed as a single shot or catheter insertion when the target nerve is scanned both in a short-axis (cross-sectional view) or a long-axis (longitudinal view).

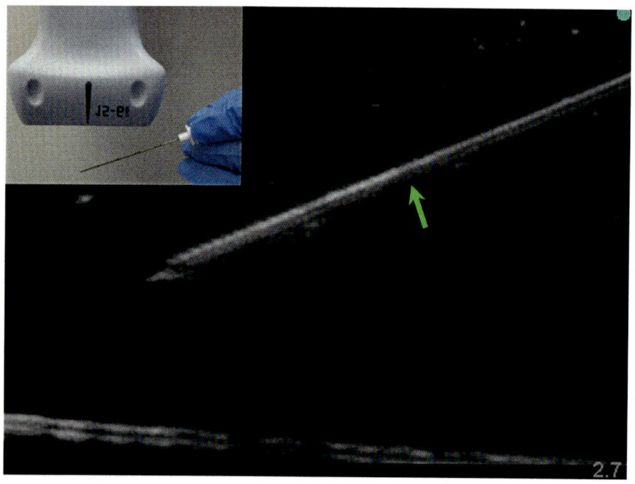

Fig. 4.6 Needle (*green arrow*), including tip and shaft during an in-plane approach

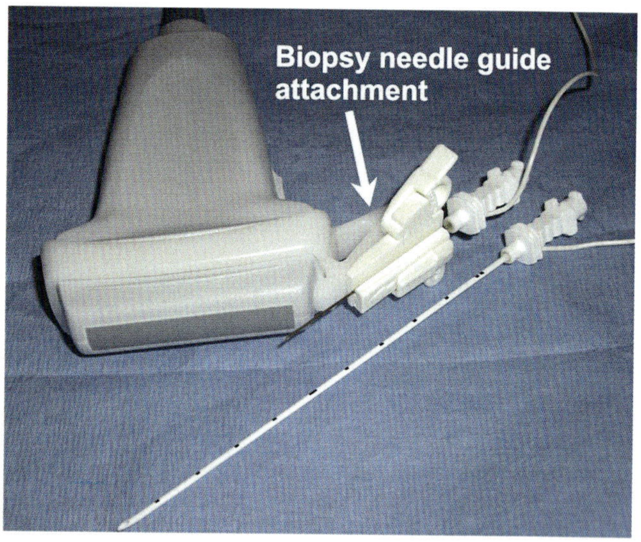

Fig. 4.7 Commercial biopsy needle attachment. The fixed needle has a limited trajectory and has to be extra long (Reprinted from Tsui BC, Dillane D. Practical and clinical aspects of ultrasound and nerve stimulation-guided peripheral nerve blocks. In: Tsui BC, editor. Atlas of ultrasound and nerve stimulation-guided regional anesthesia. New York: Springer; 2007. p. 35–48. With permission from Springer Verlag)

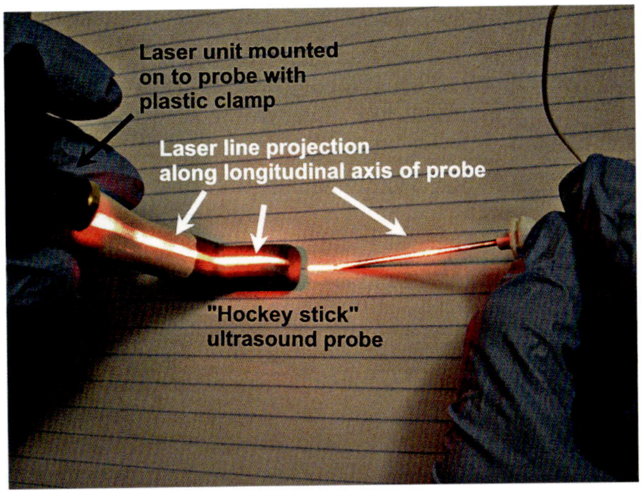

Fig. 4.8 Alignment of the block needle and ultrasound beam using a laser line (Reprinted from Tsui [3]. With permission from Wolters Kluwer Health)

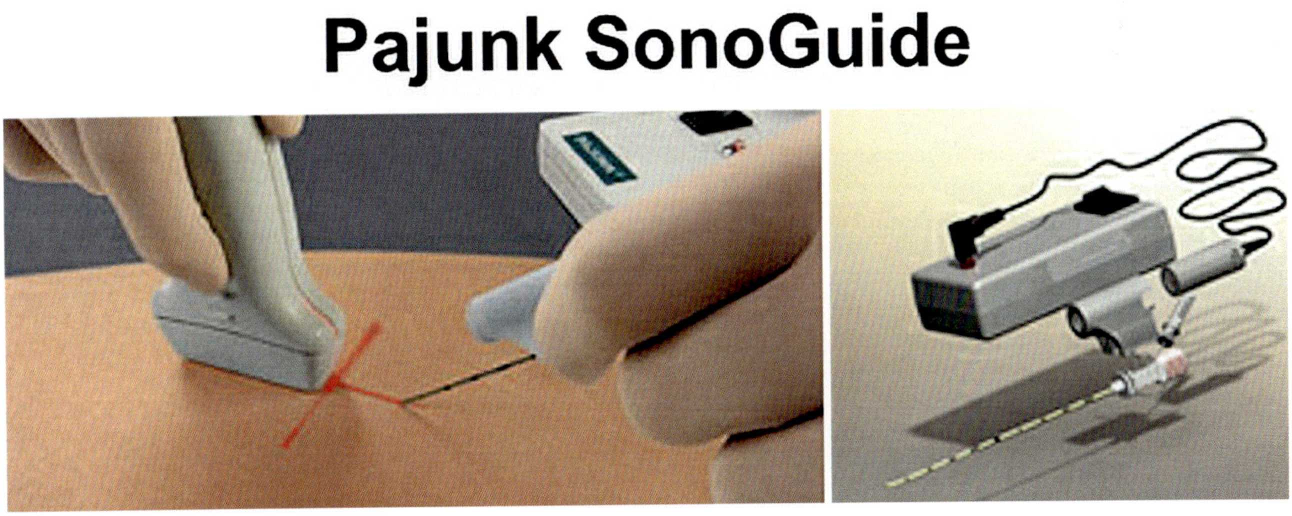

Fig. 4.9 Commercially available laser attachment for block needle

4.4.3.2 Out-of-Plane Technique: Walkdown Approach

- Out-of-plane (OOP; tangential, short-axis) alignment of the needle to the scanning plane can be useful in several block locations (e.g., popliteal, terminal nerves of the forearm, ankle blocks), but the separation between the needle tip and proximal shaft can be poorly defined.
- OOP needling can be difficult since the needle shaft can easily be mistaken for the needle tip (Fig. 4.10).
- Needle tip imaging can be improved by using shallow initial puncture angles since the tip appears as a bright dot at these angles.
- An approach that can improve needle tip visibility when using OOP approaches with linear probes involves calculating the required depth of puncture (with measurement to the related neural structure recorded using ultrasound prior to the block) and using trigonometry with the shaft angle and length to calculate a "reasonable" distance to place the initial needle puncture site (Fig. 4.11) [4].
- The initial shallow puncture will be easily seen, and the needle tip can be followed as it is *walked down* to the final calculated depth. For example, if the final depth of penetration for the block is 2 cm, the needle will ultimately obtain a 45° angle if the initial puncture site is 2 cm from the probe and the needle is incrementally angled to this level [5]. This approach works best for structures that are ≤2 cm deep.
- For target nerves deeper than 2 cm, a long needle is required. It is impractical to have the needle insertion site greater than 2 cm away from the probe since there will be a relatively large "blind" needling area. In this situation, the needle should be inserted almost perpendicularly (i.e., the needle placed just adjacent to the probe which means that in reality, it will be 0.5 cm away from the ultrasound beam). Again, applying the principles of trigonometry, a distance ≤1 cm between the needle and the ultrasound beam becomes negligible as the target depth increases, and the needle insertion depth becomes comparable to the target depth (Fig. 4.12). For instance, the difference between the depth of needle insertion and the actual depth of the target is minimal when the needle is directly adjacent to the transducer with a maximum distance of 1 cm away from the ultrasound beam:

$$\sqrt{\left((2\text{cm target depth})^2 + (1\text{cm insertion distance})^2\right)} = 2.2\text{cm needle length required}$$

Therefore, this approach helps clinicians to determine if the hyperechoic dot on the ultrasound image is the needle tip by correlating it to the length of the needle inserted.

- The nerve structure is often placed in the center of the screen to guarantee that aligning the needle puncture with the center of the probe will ensure close needle tip-nerve alignment.
- The choice of probe, whether linear or curved, can be altered depending on the anatomical situation.
- The OOP approach usually works well when the target nerve is scanned in a short-axis (cross-sectional view) for both single shot and catheter insertion.

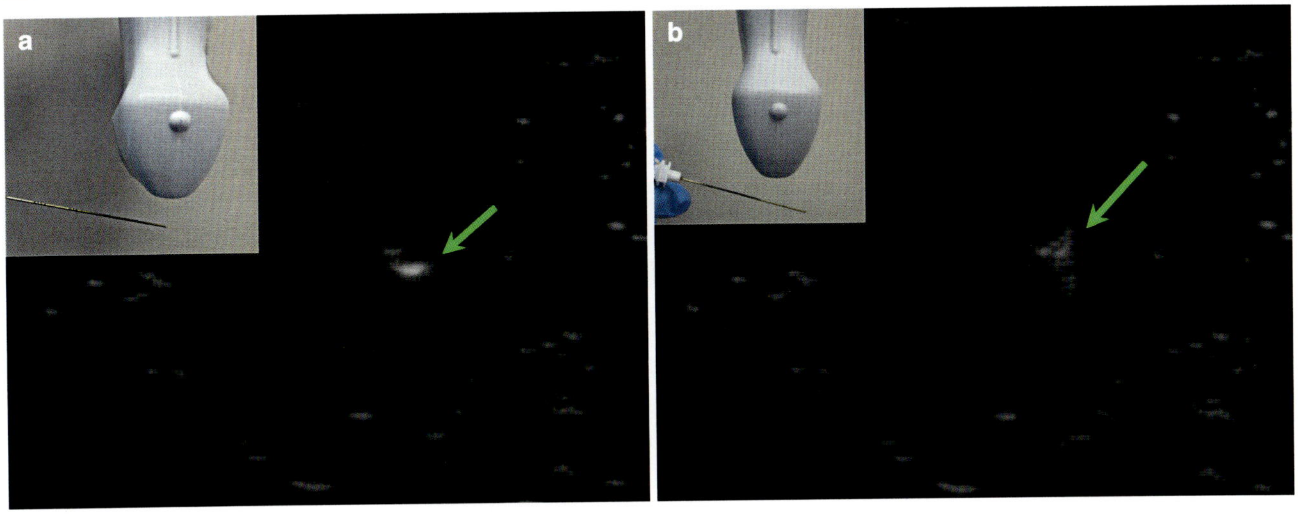

Fig. 4.10 Needle tip (**a**) and shaft (**b**) in an out-of-plane approach. *Green arrows* indicate needle position

Fig. 4.11 Walkdown approach to optimize out-of-plane needle visibility and tracking. The steep angles (*left*) often used limit the visibility of needle tips, while shallower angles (*right*) improve visibility. Incremental needle angulation (with two to three insertion angles from shallow to final 45°) can improve needle tracking. The trigonometric relationship, using an ultrasound-measured target depth, will allow an estimate of the target needle insertion site, directing the needle to the target location at a final angle of 45° (Adapted from Tsui and Dillane [4]. With permission from Wolters Kluwer Health)

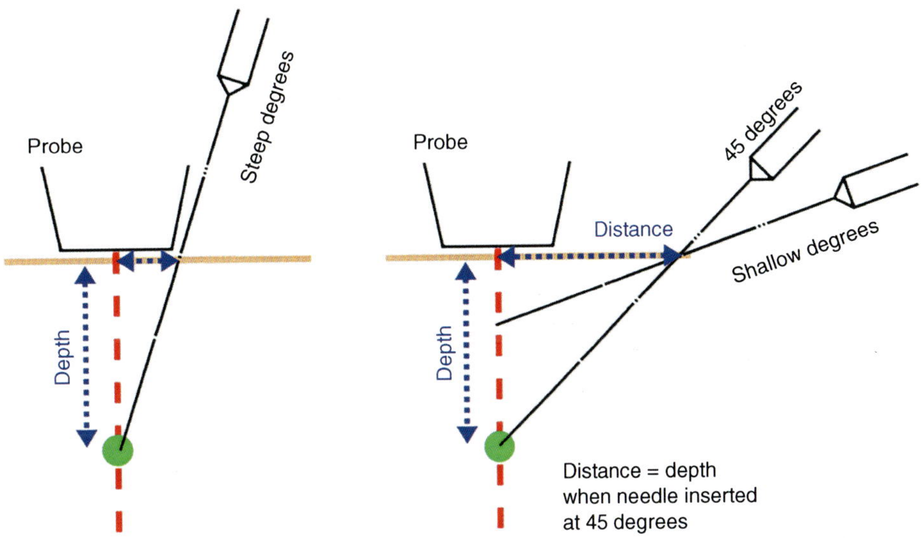

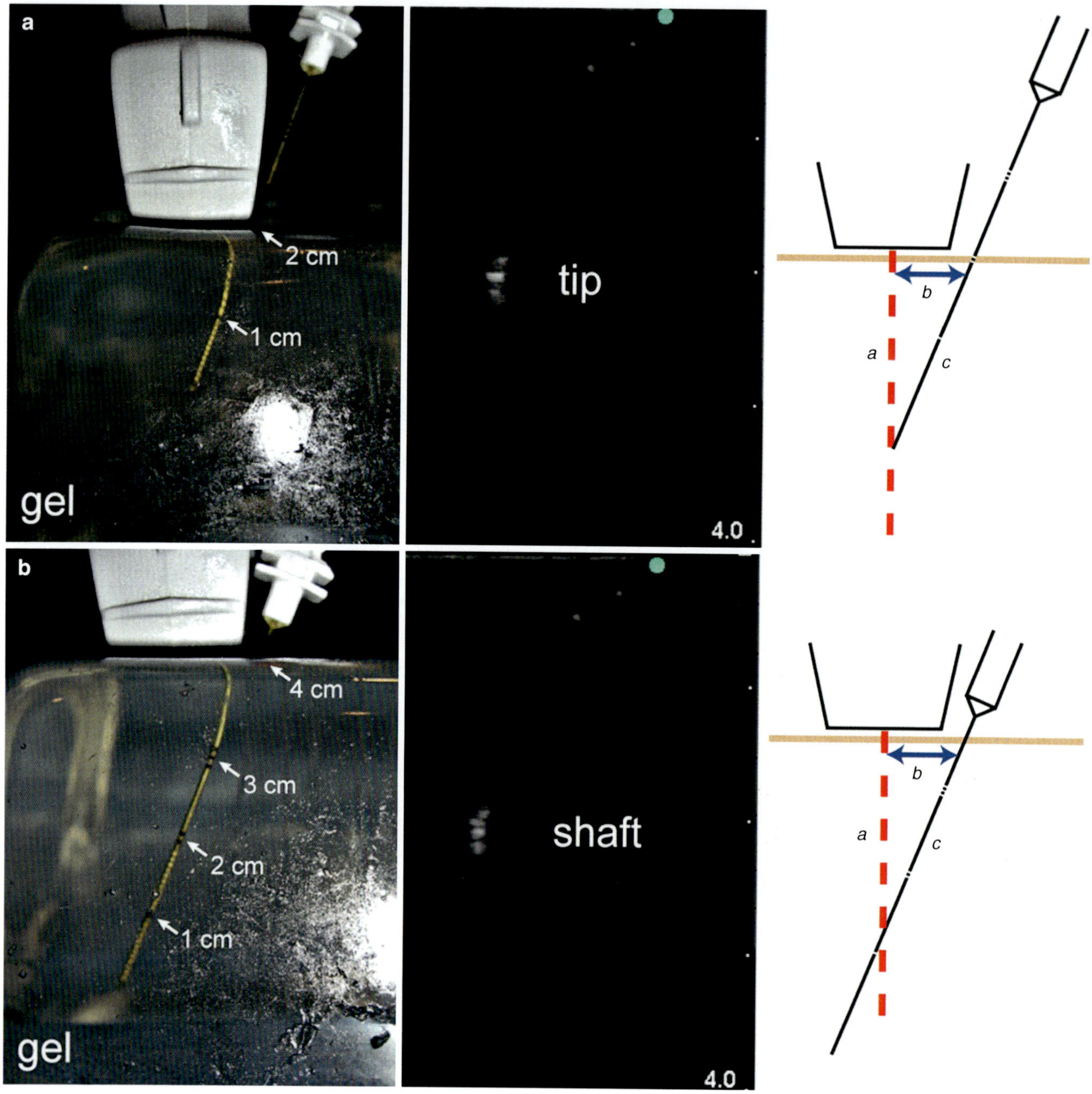

Fig. 4.12 Method to determine needle tip location by correlating it to the length of the needle inserted for target nerves deeper than 2 cm with an out-of-plane approach. The needle is placed just adjacent to the probe and inserted almost perpendicularly. According to principles of trigonometry, a distance ≤1 cm between the needle and the ultrasound beam becomes negligible as the target depth increases. The needle insertion depth therefore becomes comparable to the target depth. The hyperechoic dot on the ultrasound image can be distinguished as the needle tip (**a**) or the shaft (**b**) (Adapted from Tsui [5]. With permission from Springer Verlag)

References

1. Tsui BC, Twomey C, Finucane BT. Visualization of the brachial plexus in the supraclavicular region using a curved ultrasound probe with a sterile transparent dressing. Reg Anesth Pain Med. 2006;31:182–4.
2. Tsui BC, Finucane BT. The importance of ultrasound landmarks: a "traceback" approach using the popliteal blood vessels for identification of the sciatic nerve. Reg Anesth Pain Med. 2006;31:481–2.
3. Tsui BC. Facilitating needle alignment in-plane to an ultrasound beam using a portable laser unit. Reg Anesth Pain Med. 2007; 32(1):84–8.
4. Tsui BC, Dillane D. Needle puncture site and a "walkdown" approach for short-axis alignment during ultrasound-guided blocks. Reg Anesth Pain Med. 2006;31(6):586–7.
5. Tsui B. A trigonometric method to confirm needle tip position during out-of-plane ultrasound-guided regional blockade. Can J Anesth. 2012;59:501–2.

Suggested Reading

Chan VW. The use of ultrasound for peripheral nerve block. In: Boezaart AP, editor. Anesthesia and orthopaedic surgery. New York: McGraw-Hill; 2006. p. 283–90.

Grau T. Ultrasound in the current practice of regional anesthesia. Best Pract Res Clin Anaesth. 2005;19:175–200.

Gray AT. Ultrasound-guided regional anesthesia. Current state of the art. Anesthesiology. 2006;104:368–73.

Karmakar MK, Kwok WH. Ultrasound-guided regional anesthesia. In: Cote CJ, Lerman J, Todres ID, editors. A practice of anesthesia for infants and children. 4th ed. Philadelphia: WB Saunders; 2009. p. 911–8.

Marhofer P, Greher M, Kapral S. Ultrasound guidance in regional anesthesia. Br J Anaesth. 2005;94:7–17.

Schafhalter-Zoppoth I, McColluch CE, Gray AT. Ultrasound visibility of needles used for regional nerve block: an in vitro study. Reg Anesth Pain Med. 2004;29:480–8.

Tsui BC, Dillane D. Practical and clinical aspects of ultrasound and nerve stimulation-guided peripheral nerve blocks. In: Tsui BC, editor. Atlas of ultrasound and nerve stimulation-guided regional anesthesia. New York: Springer; 2007. p. 35–48.

Tsui BC, Finucane BT. Practical recommendations for improving needle-tip visibility under ultrasound guidance? Reg Anesth Pain Med. 2005;30:596–7.

Regional Block Catheter Insertion Using Ultrasonography and Stimulating Catheters

5

Vivian H.Y. Ip and Ban C.H. Tsui

Contents

V.H.Y. Ip, MB ChB, MRCP, FRCA (✉)
Department of Anesthesia and Pain Medicine,
University of Alberta Hospital,
2-150 Clinical Sciences Building,
Edmonton, AB T6G 2G3, Canada
e-mail: hip@ualberta.ca

B.C.H. Tsui, Dip Eng, BSc (Math), B Pharm, MSc, MD, FRCPC
Department of Anesthesiology and Pain Medicine,
Stollery Children's Hospital/University of Alberta Hospital,
2-150 Clinical Sciences Building,
Edmonton, AB T6G 2G3, Canada
e-mail: btsui@ualberta.ca

B.C.H. Tsui, S. Suresh (eds.), *Pediatric Atlas of Ultrasound- and Nerve Stimulation-Guided Regional Anesthesia*,
DOI 10.1007/978-0-387-79964-3_5

5.1 Indications, Contraindications, and Safety of Peripheral Nerve Catheter Placement

Prior to performing any procedure, the risk should be balanced against the benefit. This is particularly true in the pediatric population, where data on the efficacy and safety of peripheral nerve catheters is scarce. In general, peripheral catheters are used in children undergoing procedures that are associated with significant and prolonged postoperative pain, such as major orthopedic procedures, traction of femoral fractures, operations on congenital malformations of upper or lower limbs, and amputation, or to facilitate postoperative physiotherapy. Peripheral catheters can also be used in children to improve peripheral perfusion following microvascular surgery and to help manage chronic pain conditions.

One of the main considerations of peripheral nerve catheter placement is when there is a high risk of neurovascular injury from either the injury or surgery, for example, condylar or supracondylar fractures of the elbow. Physicians should exercise caution since there is a lack of safety data with regard to regional anesthesia in patients with preexisting neurological disorders. Another consideration is that there is continued debate regarding performing regional anesthesia in anesthetized adults. Such practice is well accepted in pediatric patients as it reduces the risk of a "moving target" and because children are often unable to communicate and differentiate between paresthesia, pain at injection site, or pressure from the injectate.

5.2 Equipment and Injectates

5.2.1 Equipment Required

5.2.1.1 Types of Catheters

1. *Non-stimulating Catheters*

The principle behind these types of catheters is the catheter-through-needle technique, in which the catheter is introduced *within* the larger-bore Tuohy needle which has been placed in proximity to the nerve. The Tuohy needle will be removed at the end of the procedure leaving the catheter in situ. Despite the concurrent use of ultrasound, catheter threading is performed essentially blind due to its small diameter. The catheter tip position is often difficult to ascertain since needle withdrawal is inevitably accompanied by simultaneous compensating advancement of the catheter. In order to facilitate threading of the catheter into the perineural space, Pajunk has designed a peripheral continuous catheter (SonoLong Curl Continuous kit, Pajunk, Geisingen, Germany) which curls immediately after exiting the needle (Fig. 5.1), allowing the tip to remain near the position of the needle tip.

2. *Stimulating Catheters*

Although it is still unclear as to whether stimulating catheters are more effective than non-stimulating catheters at positioning the catheter tip in proximity to the nerve, stimulating catheters can aid in the verification of catheter tip localization. When motor response is present at a reasonable threshold (0.5 mA), this usually signifies the correct placement of a stimulating catheter. Some stimulating needle and catheter sets, for example, the StimuCath® (Arrow International, Reading, PA, USA) with a 5 mm bare tip, may need a higher stimulation current, such as 1 mA; it should also be noted that nerve stimulation is not sensitive enough to detect intraneural placement of the catheter. Therefore, it is our recommendation that the spread of local anesthetic through the catheter tip be observed with ultrasound. Ultrasound-guided perineural catheter insertion can be technically challenging and requires a sound knowledge of sonoanatomy, good hand-eye coordination, and a competent assistant. High success rates can be obtained once these skills are acquired.

Catheters that are used in continuous peripheral nerve blocks in children are similar to those used in adults. There are four commercial varieties of catheters available with different lengths of needles required for various blocks and to accommodate the child's habitus/size. Several manufacturers now provide Tuohy needle/catheter sets specifically tailored for pediatric use.

Arrow® StimuCath (Arrow International, Reading, PA, USA)

- The insulated needle is 17G and 18G Tuohy-tipped with centimeter markings available in 4 and 8 cm (Fig. 5.2).
- The 60-cm-long catheter comes in 19G and 20G which is made more rigid by a steel stylet.
- The catheter has a female adaptor to accommodate the stimulating cable from the nerve stimulator.
- The catheter has a SnapLock™ adaptor.
- The hub of the catheter is a stimulating cable that stimulates the catheter
- The stylet has to be removed before liquid can be injected through the catheter as it is advanced for hydrodissection (see below).
- The catheter can kink if resistance is encountered during insertion.

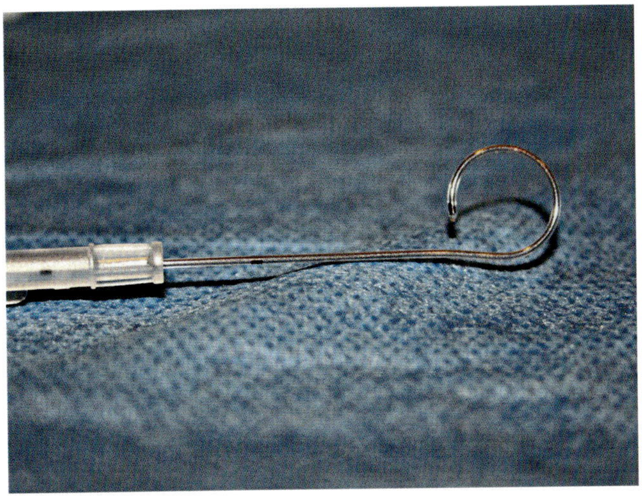

Fig. 5.1 Pajunk® SonoLong Curl

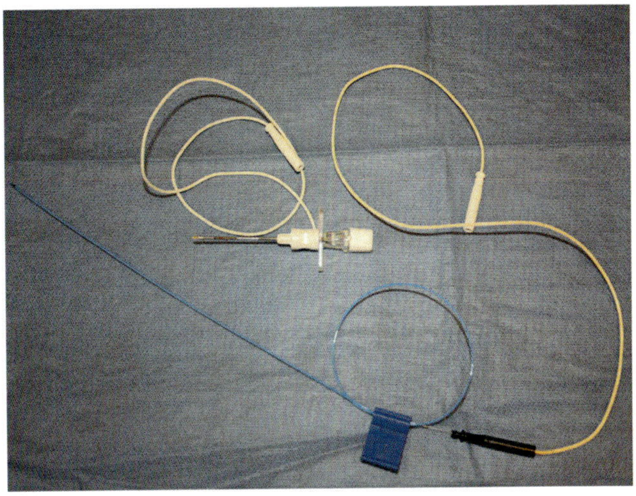

Fig. 5.2 Arrow® StimuCath

Pajunk® StimuLong Sono (Pajunk, Geisingen, Germany)

- The insulated Tuohy needles are available in 50, 100, and 110 mm lengths.
- The stimulating catheter has a gold-plated, atraumatic rounded tip with a high conductivity (Fig. 5.3).
- The catheter does not have a stylet, enabling fluid to be injected as the catheter is advanced.
- The metal coil of the catheter provides radiopacity and prevents kinking of the catheter as it meets resistance.

Pajunk® StimuLong Sono-Tsui Set (Pajunk, Geisingen, Germany)

- The insulated Tuohy needles have lengths of 50 and 100 mm (Fig. 5.4).
- The catheter design incorporates the characteristics of the StimuLong Sono catheter with two distinct features:
  - The stiffness of the catheter tip can be regulated by pushing the steel stylet forward and backward and can be locked in place by tightening or loosening a valve. This ensures atraumatic manipulation of the catheter tip.
  - Similar to the StimuLong Sono catheters, fluid can be injected through the catheter during advancement for hydrodissection.

ContiStim® Catheters (B.Braun, Melsungen, Germany)

- Life-Tech has incorporated smaller catheters (21G–24G; Prolong Micro) for pediatric use.
- The 18G, 19G, and 20G insulated Tuohy needles are available in variable lengths of 50, 100, and 150 mm.
- It has an atraumatic ball tip to reduce tissue damage and create a 360° outflow pattern.
- The catheters are said to be kink resistant.
- The fluid path/giving set connector is attached to a port for stimulation of the catheter.
- It features an EzTwist™ closure for the fluid path connector which indicates that the catheter has been securely connected.

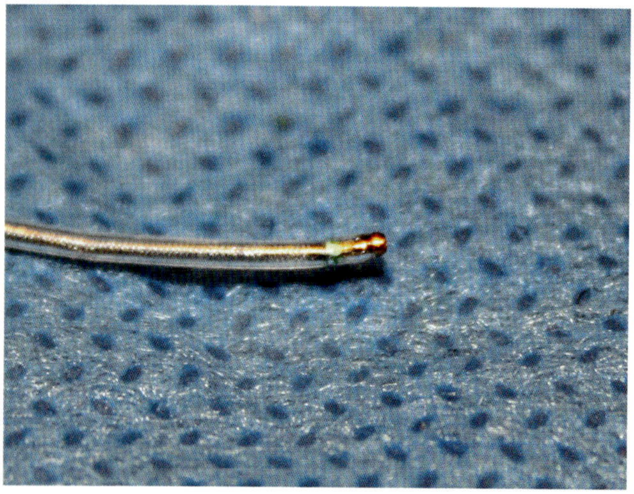

Fig. 5.3 Stimulating catheter (Pajunk® StimuLong Sono) featuring a gold-plated, atraumatic rounded tip with a high conductivity

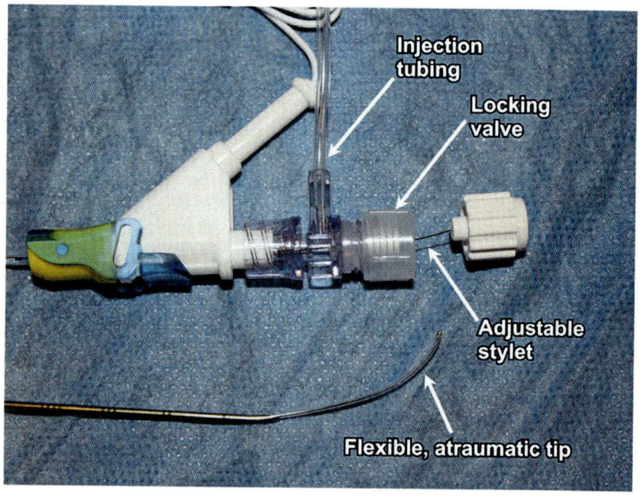

Fig. 5.4 Pajunk® StimuLong Sono-Tsui Set. Catheter tip with steel stylet to adjust stiffness. Stylet can be pushed forward or backward and can be locked in place with a valve

3. *Catheter-over-needle assembly*

- There are a few variations on this design marketed by different brands:
  - Pajunk, whose feature design is its two components, the outer catheter sheath and the flexible, non-kinkable inner catheter (Figs. 5.5 and 5.6). This assembly was initially designed and modified by Dr. Ban Tsui. The inner catheter is introduced within the outer catheter and is Luer-locked in place for injection (Fig. 5.7).
  - B.Braun, with the catheter-over-needle as a sole component (Fig. 5.8)
  - Arrow, with a catheter-over-needle with a blunt needle and a sharp injection needle for the initial puncture of the skin (Fig. 5.9).
- To position the distal end of the outer catheter in proximity to the target nerve, a 21G needle is inserted *within* the outer catheter with its distal end protruding for its electrically conductive property.
- The insertion of this catheter/needle unit is under real-time ultrasound guidance and nerve stimulation. The latter is used mainly to monitor for the absence of motor response to prevent intraneural injection.
- The distal end of the outer catheter is tapered and thin for smooth advancement within the tissue. The second component of the inner catheter is inserted *into* the outer catheter after the needle has been withdrawn.
- The main difference between this catheter-over-needle assembly and the traditional catheter-through-needle assembly is the position of the needle in relation to the catheter. In the traditional assembly, the catheter is introduced within the Tuohy needle; therefore, upon removal of the Tuohy needle, a gap is left between the skin and the catheter. In contrast, the needle in the catheter-over-needle assembly is within the outer catheter which remains in situ at the end of the procedure. This enables a tight fit between the skin and the catheter. Moreover, the inner catheter literally replaces the needle, which was initially placed in proximity to the nerve before its withdrawal. This enables the tip of the inner catheter to be in proximity to the nerve.

Several advantages of this design include:

- Simple to use with the insertion technique comparable to that of a single-shot nerve block
- Less risk of leakage from the catheter insertion site, which is particularly important in shoulder surgery where the patient is in a sitting position with a potential for surgical field contamination
- Less risk of dressing adhesive disruption
- Less risk of dislodgement
- Less cumbersome steps
- Easy visualization of the catheter, especially the catheter tip

A preassembled peripheral catheter pack is an efficient way of bringing together all the essential equipment to perform a peripheral nerve catheter. If such a pack is not available, a cart/trolley with all the necessary equipment should be prepared. The equipment required includes:

- Sterilizing solution.
- Sponges/gauze.
- Drapes.
- Lidocaine in a small syringe and 23G hypodermic needle for skin infiltration if necessary.
- Sterile ultrasound transducer cover, sterile gel, and elastic bands for transducer preparation (see below).
- Appropriately sized (gauge and length) Tuohy needle and extension tubing, nerve block catheter, or catheter-over-needle.
- 5 % dextrose in water (D5W) and appropriate syringes for hydrodissection.
- Micro-filter or giving set attachment for the injecting into the catheter.
- Appropriate dressings.
- Sterile gowns and gloves (it is recommended that full sterile procedure should be observed for peripheral catheter insertion, including a face mask, hat, sterile gown, and gloves).
- Ultrasound machine with appropriate settings.
- The nerve stimulator should be set up and ready to use for the initial placement of the needle and/or if a stimulating catheter is to be used.

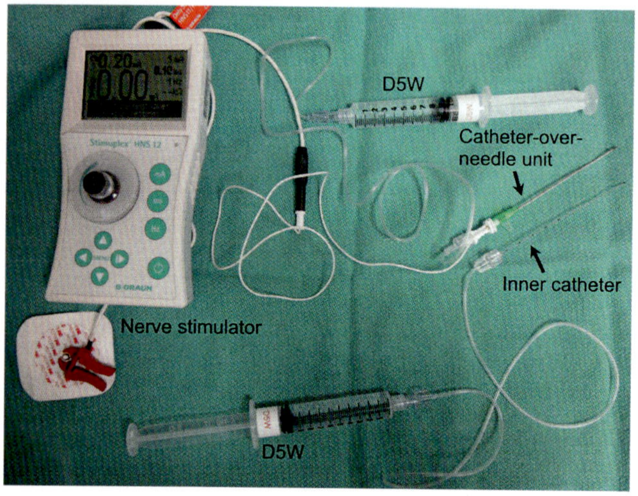

Fig. 5.5 Pajunk® catheter-over-needle assembly

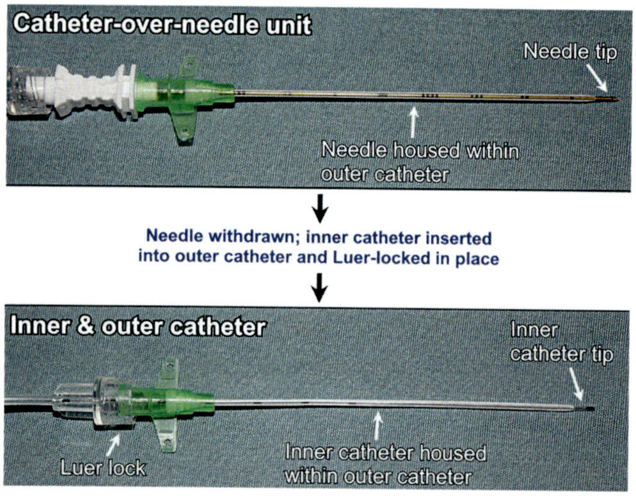

Fig. 5.6 Detail of Pajunk® catheter-over-needle components

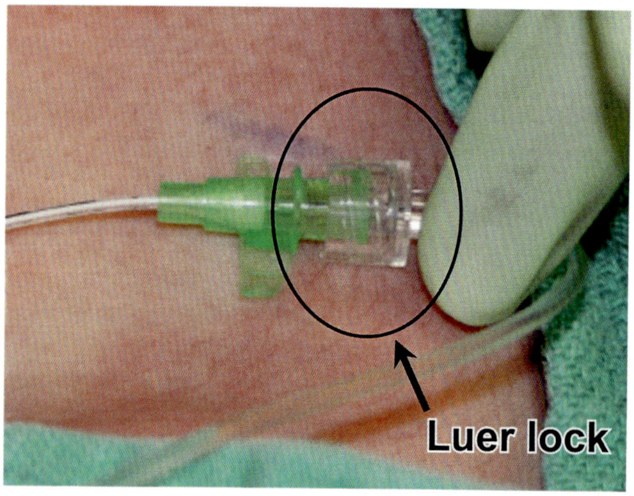

Fig. 5.7 Luer-lock holding together the inner and outer catheter

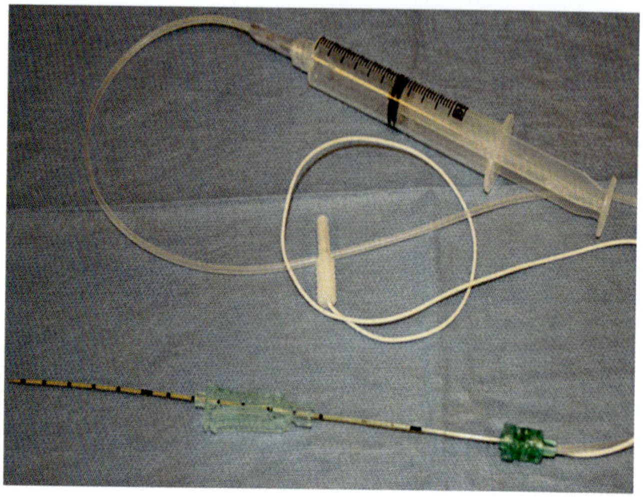

Fig. 5.8 B.Braun® catheter-over-needle assembly

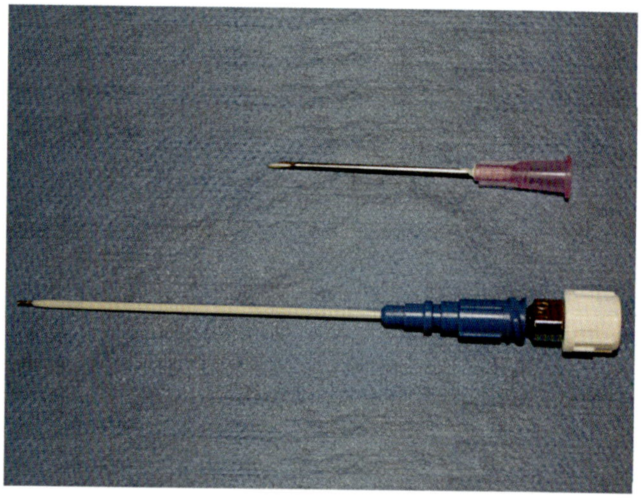

Fig. 5.9 Blunt and sharp needles from Arrow® catheter-over-needle assembly

5.2.2 Sterile Transducer Preparation

For peripheral nerve catheter insertion, it is important to have an appropriate sterile cover for the ultrasound transducer as well as for the cord so it does not contaminate the sterile field while scanning (see Chap. 4, Sect. 4.3). The following describes how to prepare a sterile transducer probe:

- Open the sterile sheath by placing two thumbs inside the sheath, and roll the length of the sheath up so that the sheath bunches up in the hand.
- Ensure plenty of sterile gel is applied on the inside of the sheath where the surface of the transducer is to be placed.
- Cover the transducer inside the sheath, and push the length of the sheath to cover the cord of the transducer (take care to avoid desterilizing the gloves).
- Pull an elastic band over the cord to hold the sheath on the cord.
- Stretch the surface of the sheath covering the transducer to avoid any air bubbles or creases before pulling an elastic band over the transducer to hold it in place. This will also minimize any sliding between the sheath and the transducer while scanning.

5.2.3 Choice of Injectates

5.2.3.1 During Catheter Insertion

To facilitate advancement of the catheter, a solution is injected through the Tuohy needle to expand the perineural space; however, the use of local anesthetics or conducting solution, such as normal saline, will abolish the capacity to stimulate. This is particularly important when stimulating catheters are used.

Hydrodissection using D5W, a nonconducting fluid, is useful for "dissecting" or "opening" of the perineural space. This facilitates catheter advancement while maintaining the ability to stimulate and may enhance the contrast at the tissue interface, potentially allowing for better visibility of both the needle and the catheter under ultrasound. Overaggressive hydrodissection is not advised since it may hinder electrical stimulation of the nerve by creating a potential mechanical barrier.

Local Anesthetics

Unlike in adults, the dose of local anesthetics is weight dependent in infants and children. In pediatric patients, after an initial bolus, the dosage recommended for continuous infusion is 0.1–0.2 mL/kg/h of either bupivacaine or levobupivacaine (0.125–0.25 %) or ropivacaine (0.15–0.2 %). The lower rates are generally used for upper extremity catheters and the higher rates for lower extremity catheters. If necessary, the infusion rate may be adjusted up to a maximum of 0.2 mg/kg/h for infants of less than 6 months and 0.4 mg/kg/h in children of more than 6 months.

5.3 Technique

When inserting peripheral nerve catheters, aseptic technique should always be observed in order to reduce the risk of infection. All the equipment should be ready as described in Chap. 1.

The key practical techniques for insertion of peripheral nerve catheters are as follows:

- An assistant who is trained in regional anesthesia with experience in monitoring pediatric patients under sedation or general anesthesia should be present. This is important not only for monitoring the child during catheter insertion but to assist with the nerve stimulator and the injectate.
- Routine monitoring such as electrocardiography, noninvasive blood pressure, pulse oximetry, capnography, and end-tidal gas monitoring (especially for those in whom anesthesia is maintained on volatile agents) is applied.
- Emergency drugs such as atropine, ephedrine, and succinylcholine are drawn up, and resuscitation drugs such as epinephrine and Intralipid are available if needed.
- There should be oxygen supply and an Ambu® bag (or Bagger) available.
- Intravenous access should be established.
- The child should either be sedated with titrated doses of midazolam and/or fentanyl or induced under general anesthetic. If nerve stimulation is used for identifying the target nerve or for the stimulating catheter, use of muscle relaxants should be avoided.
- Patient is placed in a suitable position for peripheral nerve catheter placement.
- The height of the bed and the position of the ultrasound machine should be placed in an ergonomically friendly fashion.
- Pre-procedure scanning is helpful to determine the optimal ultrasound machine settings such as gain, depth, scanning mode, and focus range. Scanning can also identify any abnormal anatomy in advance.
- Ensure all the equipment is gathered and prepared as outlined earlier in this chapter.
- The skin should be cleaned with a sterile solution and the area draped.
- The probe is covered with sterile gel which is then covered with the long sterile probe sleeve. An elastic band can be applied to minimize slipping of the sheath against the transducer and to prevent air bubbles from accumulating.

Traditional non-stimulating nerve block catheter and stimulating nerve block catheter insertion techniques

- The catheter is prepared, kept in a sterile towel, and placed on the sterile field. It must be within easy reach of the operator during the procedure.
- The Tuohy needle is attached to the extension tubing and flushed with D5W.
- Sterile gel is applied to the skin.
- The ultrasound probe is used to identify the target nerve.
- If the patient is sedated, local anesthetics can be injected to raise a skin wheal at the site of planned needle entry.
- The Tuohy needle can be inserted in plane or out of plane with respect to the probe axis.
  - When an in-plane approach is used, there is a good view of the advancement of the needle. If the nerve runs perpendicular to the needle insertion, the tip of the catheter should be placed underneath or above the nerve rather than parallel to the nerve.
  - When an out-of-plane approach is used, tissue movement can be appreciated as the needle is advanced. On sliding the probe proximally and distally from the needle insertion site, the cross section of the tip of the needle can be appreciated when the hyperechoic dot disappears and reappears as the probe is slid proximally and distally. An out-of-plane technique allows the catheter to be placed parallel to the nerve if the nerve runs parallel to the direction of needle insertion.
- For both in-plane and out-of-plane techniques, D5W can be used to hydrodissect the tissue plane to confirm the position of the needle tip, provide a space for the advancement of the catheter, and create a better contrast medium for visualization of the needle.

Methods used to confirm the catheter tip location differ between the non-stimulating and the stimulating nerve block catheters. Ultrasound can be used to help ascertain the non-stimulating catheter tip, whereas both nerve stimulation and ultrasound can be used to determine the stimulating catheter tip in relation to the nerve.

5.3.1 Confirming Catheter Tip Location with Ultrasonography

When using ultrasound to determine the location of the catheter tip, the transducer may be placed along the length of the catheter as it is aspirated, allowing movement of the column of fluid within the catheter to be observed. Injecting D5W through the catheter to expand the hypoechoic area may also help to locate the catheter tip.

If the movement of the fluid column in the catheter can be observed on aspiration but no spread of the injectate is in view, the catheter may be too deep into the tissue and may need to be pulled back. One can also use the markings along the catheter to note the depth of the catheter in the tissue.

Doppler color flow is another useful method to determine tissue movement upon injection of agitated D5W through the catheter.

As previously mentioned, it is always good practice to observe the spread of the injectate delivered via the peripheral nerve catheter to visually confirm the position of the catheter tip. This practice should be employed whether a stimulating catheter is used or not.

5.3.2 Confirming Catheter Tip Location with Nerve Stimulation

- Since the stimulating catheter is to be inserted beyond the tip of the needle, the length of the needle and the extension tubing should be noted to ensure an accurate stimulation response elicited by the catheter independent from the needle.
- The nerve stimulator should be set at 0.5 mA since a higher current not only causes discomfort to the patient but can also cause muscle twitches which displace the probe and the needle.
- When the tip of the needle is at the desired position, negative aspiration for blood should be confirmed and a small amount of D5W should be injected. It is important to observe the spread of the solution since it provides information on the location of the needle tip. If hydrodissection is not observed, the needle tip may be in an intravascular position.
- The injection of D5W should amplify the motor response.
- The extension tubing is then removed and the nerve stimulator is disconnected from the Tuohy needle.
- The catheter, with the stimulation port attached to the nerve stimulator, is inserted through the Tuohy needle.
- The catheter should be advanced beyond the tip of the Tuohy needle and the subsequent motor response observed.
- In order to place the nerve block catheter tip in proximity to the nerve, the specific motor response pertaining to the sensory distribution of the nerve should be observed.
- It is possible for the catheter to be advanced too far, causing it to coil. This can be seen by an increase in the motor response on further advancement of the catheter. If this is noted, the catheter should be pulled back until ideal motor stimulation is achieved.

5.3.3 Catheter-Over-Needle Assembly Insertion

- An appropriate length catheter-over-needle assembly is the key to success. Therefore, it is useful to perform a prescan to estimate the distance between skin puncture and the nerve.
- Both the catheter-over-needle assembly and the inner catheter should each be primed with 10 mL of D5W.
- Sterile gel is applied to the skin.
- Ultrasound probe is used to identify the target nerve.
- Local anesthetic is used to raise a skin wheal at the site of planned needle entry.
- 21G catheter-over-needle (of the chosen length) can be inserted in plane or out of plane.
- Nerve stimulator at a current of 0.2 mA can be attached to monitor for the absence of motor response. This will help to prevent intraneural needle insertion.
- As the tip of the needle is in the desired position, injection of D5W can be used to ascertain the spread. Hydrodissection with D5W or local anesthetic can be used.
- The needle is removed while the outer catheter remains in situ.
- The inner catheter is introduced within the outer catheter and is Luer-locked in place (Fig. 5.7).
- The spread of the injectate via the inner catheter tip can be confirmed under ultrasound. This is relatively easy to do since the ultrasound probe can be held at all times during the catheter insertion (with a single operator) and the inner catheter is inserted the same place as the needle which has been removed.

Clinical Pearls

Catheter insertion can be performed using in-plane or out-of-plane approach (see Chap. 4) with the nerve imaged in a short axis (cross-sectional view) or long axis (longitudinal view). However, if the nerve is imaged in short axis and an in-plane approach is used, the catheter should not be threaded too far beyond the Tuohy needle tip when using the traditional catheter insertion technique. Note that this is *not* an issue if the catheter-over-needle approach is used.

It seems logical to scan the nerve in a long axis and use an in-plane approach such that the catheter travels parallel to the nerve. However, it is not always easy to scan the nerve in a long axis since the course of the nerve may not be straight or it may become more superficial or deep. Therefore, it is important to apply the knowledge of anatomy when selecting the most appropriate plane to scan the nerve.

5.3.4 Securing the Catheter

It is important to secure the peripheral nerve catheter in place both for inpatient and ambulatory care. This can be done in several ways:

- Applying cyanoacrylate (e.g., Dermabond®) at the entrance site of the catheter.
- Subcutaneous tunneling before fixation with occlusive dressing.
- Securing the dressing more effectively (e.g., with Tegaderm™) by removing all of the gel before applying skin glue, such as Mastisol or cyanoacrylate glue.
- The catheter-over-needle can be secured with a normal IV dressing and a caution label, such that the catheter is clearly marked as a peripheral nerve block catheter (Fig. 5.10).

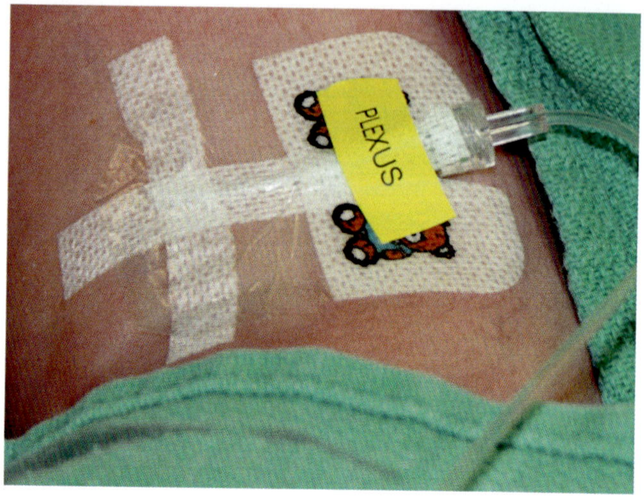

Fig. 5.10 Catheter-over-needle secured with IV dressing and clearly marked as a peripheral nerve block catheter

5.4 Examples of Common Peripheral Nerve Catheterization Procedures Used in Children

5.4.1 Infraclavicular Nerve Block Catheterization

5.4.1.1 Position

Supine with arm adducted, elbow flexed, and forearm placed on the abdomen

5.4.1.2 Transducer

SLA "hockey stick" (25 mm, 13–6 MHz) for smaller children or linear probe (38 mm, 13–6 MHz) for older/larger children

5.4.1.3 Surface Landmark

Coracoid process and clavicle

5.4.1.4 Sonoanatomy

The axillary artery is deep to the pectoralis major and minor muscles. The lateral cord of the brachial plexus lies superior to the artery, the posterior cord lies posterior to the artery, and the medial cord lies posterior and medial to the artery. The axillary vein lies just caudad to the artery.

5.4.1.5 In-Plane Approach

Place the transducer just medial to the coracoid process, caudad to the clavicle, in a longitudinal or parasagittal position. Insert a 5 cm, 18G–20G insulated Tuohy needle in a cephalad-to-caudad direction. Aim to position the catheter just next to the posterior cord and posterior to the artery. Beware of the pleura medially to the transducer.

5.4.1.6 Motor Response to Nerve Stimulation

Flexion or extension of wrist or fingers

> **Clinical Pearl**
> Sometimes the arm can be abducted 90° at the shoulder and elbow to increase visibility of the cords.

5.4.1.7 Clinical Evidence

Continuous infraclavicular brachial plexus block was described for pain control in two pediatric patients undergoing orthopedic procedures [1]. Another case report used ultrasound-guided continuous infraclavicular block to produce sympathectomy of extended duration, resulting in a long-term positive outcome in a 9-year-old with traumatic amputation of the hand [2].

5.4.2 Femoral Nerve Block Catheterization

5.4.2.1 Position

Supine

5.4.2.2 Transducer Selection

Linear probe (38 mm, 13–6 MHz) or SLA "hockey stick" (25 mm, 13–6 MHz), depending on the size of the child

5.4.2.3 Surface Landmark

Inguinal crease

5.4.2.4 Sonoanatomy

Identify the femoral artery. If the profunda femoris artery is in view, scan proximally until only one artery is present. The hyperechoic femoral nerve is lateral to the femoral artery, superficial to the iliopsoas muscle, and just deep to the hyperechoic line of the fascia iliaca.

5.4.2.5 In-Plane Approach

Place the transducer just below the inguinal crease. Insert an appropriately sized insulated Tuohy needle (e.g., 5 cm, 18G–20G) lateral to the femoral nerve. The needle shaft and tip should be in view. Aim to place the catheter just deep to the femoral nerve on its medial aspect.

5.4.2.6 Out-of-Plane Approach

As with the in-plane technique, place the transducer just below the inguinal crease. Insert an appropriately sized insulated Tuohy needle perpendicular to the transducer. Only the cross section of the needle shaft can be seen. Aim to place the needle tip just deep to the fascia iliaca. Hydrodissection will help to confirm that the injectate is introduced at the correct tissue layer and will also help to open up the space. Advance the catheter 1–3 cm beyond the needle tip, depending on the age and size of the child, so that it lies parallel to the nerve.

5.4.2.7 Motor Response to Nerve Stimulation

Sartorius and midline "dancing of the patella" (quadriceps) twitches are both accepted.

> **Clinical Pearl**
> If two branches of the femoral nerve are observed after hydrodissection, aim for the deeper branch.

5.4.2.8 Clinical Evidence

The evidence supporting the use of femoral nerve catheter in children is limited. There is a recent case report on its use in intractable pain from a chronic dislocated hip in a 12-year-old girl [3].

5.4.3 Sciatic Nerve Block Catheterization

5.4.3.1 Subgluteal Approach

Position
Lateral

Transducer
Linear probe (38 mm, 13–6 MHz)

Surface Landmark
Greater trochanter and ischial tuberosity

Sonoanatomy
Identify the acoustic shadows cast by the greater trochanter and the ischial tuberosity. The sciatic nerve is in cross section lateral to the long head of the biceps femoris muscle.

In-Plane Approach
Place the transducer with one end on the greater trochanter and the other end on the ischial tuberosity. Insert an appropriately sized insulated Tuohy needle (e.g., 5 cm, 18G–20G) perpendicular to the probe. Aim to place the needle tip just above the sciatic nerve, and advance the catheter 1–3 cm beyond the needle tip, depending on the age and size of the child.

Motor Response to Nerve Stimulation
Plantar flexion or dorsiflexion of the foot

> **Clinical Pearls**
> The current of the nerve stimulator needs to be increased as the catheter is advanced.
> Rotating the Tuohy needle 90° sometimes allows for better advancement of the catheter.

Clinical Evidence
Compared with other blocks, there are more clinical studies and case reports on continuous subgluteal sciatic nerve blocks in children for correction of congenital defects, orthopedic oncology surgery, osteotomy, and amputation [4, 5]. Each has demonstrated successful results with minimal side effects.

5.4.3.2 Popliteal Approach

Position
Lateral

Transducer
Linear probe (38 mm, 13–6 MHz)

Surface Landmark
Knee crease

Sonoanatomy
The sciatic nerve at the popliteal region is just medial to the biceps femoris muscle. Be aware of the popliteal vessels just medial and anterior to the sciatic nerve. Scan proximally and distally to identify where the sciatic nerve divides into the tibial nerve and the common peroneal nerve.

Out-of-Plane Approach
Place the transducer just above the knee crease; the sciatic nerve is usually divided at this point. Scan proximally until the sciatic nerve has just divided. Insert an appropriately sized insulated Tuohy needle (e.g., 5 cm, 18G–20G) perpendicular to the probe and aim to place the needle tip at a point when the sciatic nerve just split. The catheter can then be advanced 1–3 cm beyond the needle tip, depending on the age and size of the child.

Motor Response
Plantar flexion or dorsiflexion of the foot

> **Clinical Pearl**
> It is better to direct the catheter cephalad to enable its proximal placement along the sciatic nerve.

Clinical Evidence
There are prospective studies and case reports demonstrating the efficacy of continuous popliteal sciatic nerve blocks [6–9]. One study also demonstrated reduced adverse effects compared to epidural analgesia [10]. A recent study evaluating the adverse effects of continuous peripheral nerve block found a significant association of persistent insensate extremity with continuous popliteal nerve block [11]; however, this could be secondary to the volume and concentration of local anesthetic used in this confined perineural space. Ilfeld et al. [12] reported a lower incidence of insensate extremity in adults with a lower infusion rate of local anesthetic, such as 4 mL/h of 0.4 % ropivacaine.

5.5 Summary

Continuous peripheral nerve catheters have been shown to help aid in pain control, especially in managing challenging cases in the pediatric population. Ultrasonography enables visualization of the spread of injectate in real time, while stimulating catheters use the principles of physics to guide their placement. The catheter-over-needle technique increases the precision of catheter tip placement without the need for over-feeding the catheter. With these recent technological advancements, the risk of peripheral nerve catheter placement in anesthetized children is relatively low.

References

1. Dadure C, Raux O, Troncin R, Rochette A, Capdevila X. Continuous infraclavicular brachial plexus block for acute pain management in children. Anesth Analg. 2003;97:691–3.
2. Loland VJ, Ilfeld BM, Abrams RA, Mariano ER. Ultrasound-guided perineural catheter and local anesthetic infusion in the perioperative management of pediatric limb salvage: a case report. Pediatr Anesth. 2009;19:905–7.
3. Nayak S, Roberts S, Cunliffe M. Management of intractable pain from a chronic dislocated hip in an adolescent. Pediatr Anesth. 2008;18:357–8.
4. van Geffen GJ, Gielen M. Ultrasound-guided subgluteal sciatic nerve blocks with stimulating catheters in children: a descriptive study. Anesth Analg. 2006;103:328–33.
5. van Geffen GJ, Pirotte T, Gielen MJ, Scheffer G, Bruhn J. Ultrasound-guided proximal and distal sciatic nerve blocks in children. J Clin Anesth. 2010;22:241–5.
6. Dadure C, Pirat P, Raux O, Troncin R, Rochette A, Ricard C, Capdevila X. Perioperative continuous peripheral nerve blocks with disposable infusion pumps in children: a prospective descriptive study. Anesth Analg. 2003;97:687–90.
7. Dadure C, Acosta C, Capdevila X. Perioperative pain management of a complex orthopedic surgical procedure with double continuous nerve blocks in a burned child. Anesth Analg. 2004;98:1653–5.
8. Dadure C, Bringuier S, Raux O, Rochette A, Troncin R, Canaud N, Lubrano-Lavadera JF, Capdevila X. Continuous peripheral nerve blocks for postoperative analgesia in children: feasibility and side effects in a cohort study of 339 catheters. Can J Anesth. 2009;56: 843–50.
9. Ludot H, Berger J, Pichenot V, Belouadah M, Madi K, Malinovsky JM. Continuous peripheral nerve block for postoperative pain control at home: a prospective feasibility study in children. Reg Anesth Pain Med. 2008;33:52–6.
10. Dadure C, Bringuier S, Nicolas F, Bromilow L, Raux O, Rochette A, Capdevila X. Continuous epidural block versus continuous popliteal nerve block for postoperative pain relief after major podiatric surgery in children: a prospective, comparative randomized study. Anesth Analg. 2006;102:744–9.
11. Saporito A, Sturini E, Petri J, Borgeat A, Aguirre JA. Case report: unusual complication during outpatient continuous regional popliteal analgesia. Can J Anesth. 2012;59:958–62.
12. Ilfeld BM, Loland VJ, Gerancher JC, Wadhwa AN, Renehan EM, Sessler DI, Shuster JJ, Theriaque DW, Maldonado RC, Mariano ER. The effects of varying local anesthetic concentration and volume on continuous popliteal sciatic nerve blocks: a dual-center, randomized, controlled study. Anesth Analg. 2008;107:701–7.

Suggested Reading

Bosenberg AT. New developments in paediatric regional anaesthesia. South Afr J Anaesth Analg. 2008;14:81–3.

Dhir S, Ganapathy S. Use of ultrasound guidance and contrast enhancement: a study of continuous infraclavicular brachial plexus approach. Acta Anaesthesiol Scand. 2008;52:338–42.

Ecoffey C, Lacroix F. Pediatric regional anesthesia update: results in a French survey. In: Rawal N, Ivani G, editors. Highlights in regional anesthesia and pain therapy XVII. Geneva: Kenes International; 2008. p. 162–3.

Ganapathy S. Regional block catheter insertion using ultrasonography and stimulating catheters. In: Tsui BC, editor. Atlas of ultrasound and nerve stimulation-guided regional anesthesia. New York: Springer; 2007. p. 215–23.

Giaufre E, Dalens B, Gombert A. Epidemiology and morbidity of regional anesthesia in children: a one-year prospective survey of the French-language society of pediatric anesthesiologists. Anesth Analg. 1996;83:904–12.

Ivani G, Codipietro L, Gagliardi F, et al. A long term infusion via a sciatic catheter in a 3-years-old-boy. Pediatr Anesth. 2003;13: 718–21.

Ivani G, Mossetti V. Continuous central and perineural infusions for postoperative pain control in children. Curr Opin Anesthesiol. 2010;23:637–42.

Koscielniak-Nielsen ZJ, Rasmussen H, Hesselbjerg L. Long-axis ultrasound imaging of the nerves and advancement of perineural catheters under direct vision: a preliminary report of four cases. Reg Anesth Pain Med. 2008;33:477–82.

Lonnqvist PA, Morton NS. Postoperative analgesia in infants and children. Br J Anaesth. 2005;95:59–68.

Tsui BCH, Kropelin B, Ganapathy S, Finucane B. Dextrose 5% in water: fluid medium for maintaining electrical stimulation of peripheral nerves during stimulating catheter placement. Acta Anaesthesiol Scand. 2005;49:1562–5.

Tsui BC, Wagner A, Finucane B. Electrophysiologic effect of injectates on peripheral nerve stimulation. Reg Anesth Pain Med. 2004;29: 189–93.

Part II

Considerations in Pediatric Regional Anesthesia

Pain Assessment in Children Undergoing Regional Anesthesia

6

Bruce D. Dick, Kathy Reid, Michelle J. Verrier, and Alex Baloukov

Contents

B.D. Dick, PhD, R Psych (✉)
Division of Pain Medicine, Department of Anesthesiology and Pain Medicine, Stollery Children's Hospital, University of Alberta, 2-150 Clinical Sciences Building, Edmonton, AB T6G 2B7, Canada
e-mail: bruce.dick@ualberta.ca

K. Reid, RN, MN, NP
Pediatric Anesthesia, Stollery Children's Hospital, 8440 – 112 St, Room 1C3.09, Edmonton, AB T6G2B7, Canada
e-mail: kathy.reid@albertahealthservices.ca

M.J. Verrier, BA
Department of Anesthesiology and Pain Medicine, University of Alberta, 2-150 Clinical Sciences Building, Edmonton, AB T6G 2G3, Canada
e-mail: mrheault@ualberta.ca

A. Baloukov, MPH
Faculty of Health Sciences, Simon Fraser University, Burnaby, BC, Canada
e-mail: abalouko@sfu.ca

B.C.H. Tsui, S. Suresh (eds.), *Pediatric Atlas of Ultrasound- and Nerve Stimulation-Guided Regional Anesthesia*, DOI 10.1007/978-0-387-79964-3_6

6.1 Background

Effective pain management is a key objective of proper patient care. Adequate pain management has the potential to improve health, facilitate healing, and reduce long-term negative results of pain after hospitalization [1]; poor pain management is inhumane and unethical. Inherent to good pain management is skilled pain assessment, and practice standards have been developed mandating effective pain assessment and management across the life span [2]. For example, effective pain assessment and management and staff education on these topics are now required for institutional accreditation in the United States [3].

Children are a particularly vulnerable clinical population who are at risk for poor pain management for a variety of reasons. A child's developmental level and ability to communicate play important roles in pain assessment and management [4]. The medical history of the child can also play an important role in pain assessment. Previous experience with medical procedures, particularly painful medical procedures, can markedly affect a child's response to pain, pain behaviors, and potentially even the child's perception of pain [5].

Sadly, not only are children vulnerable to undertreatment of pain, they are also especially at risk for experiencing negative consequences resulting from poor pain control. For example, neonates who experience less analgesia following painful procedures are more likely to experience augmented pain and increased behavioral changes during and following subsequent painful stimuli [6–8]. It has been found that these changes result from alterations in the central nervous system through processes such as central sensitization, windup, receptive field alteration, and even altered gene expression [9, 10]. Pain-related stress responses also affect hormonal responses, homeostatic function, immune function, infection rates, disease progression, and mortality rates [11, 12]. In addition, children often have less control over their environments and can be strongly affected by their parents' behaviors, including parental responses to medical settings and medical procedures [13].

In considering how to effectively assess pain in a clinical setting, there are many factors to be aware of and a variety of dimensions of pain that could potentially be assessed. Current pain theory falls within the widely validated biopsychosocial model. This chapter will discuss a number of important aspects of pain assessment in children undergoing medical procedures. An outline of validated measures is included along with practical guidelines for their use, and the importance of these guidelines for assessing biological, psychological, and social factors will be reviewed. These factors have the potential to impact a child's pain and the resulting response to pain in the clinical setting as well as following post-hospital discharge. The best practice standards based on current guidelines will also be reviewed and will be discussed with a particular focus on pain assessment relevant to regional anesthesia practice.

6.2 Principles of Pain Assessment in Infants and Children

Assessing pain in pediatric patients is often challenging due to the subjective personal nature of pain and the difficulty that children can have in verbally reporting pain. Pain is a multidimensional phenomenon, and pain measurement tools need to capture the many important aspects of pain. It is important to note that measurements of pain intensity, often used in acute care settings, are only one part of a comprehensive pain assessment [14]. Pain assessment tools should be reliable, valid, developmentally appropriate, clinically useful, and practical to use [15]. Utilizing multiple measures, such as behavioral and physiological data, may result in a more accurate assessment [16]. Several reliable and valid measures exist to assist in assessing pain in pediatric patients undergoing procedures, including self-reporting, behavioral observations, and physiological measures. The pain assessment tools included in the following section have been validated for use in pediatric patients experiencing acute postoperative pain.

6.3 Assessing Pain in Neonates and Infants

Neonates and infants under the age of 1 month often undergo painful interventions, including surgical procedures, venipunctures, and heel lances [17]. Assessing pain in this vulnerable population requires multidimensional measures, as infants are preverbal and cannot communicate their pain with words [18]. Recent reviews have shown that while over 40 tools have been developed for assessing pain in these children, no one tool has been identified as ideal [19–21]. Many of the tools such as the Neonatal Facial Coding System (NFCS) [22] and the Neonatal Infant Pain Scale (NIPS) [23] are useful for the assessment of short-term acute pain involved in medical procedures, such as venipunctures, but their usefulness for painful experiences of longer duration such as postoperative pain is limited [18]. Tools with demonstrated validity in assessing postoperative pain in neonates and infants include the Premature Infant Pain Profile (PIPP), the Neonatal Pain Agitation and Sedation Scale (N-PASS), and CRIES (Table 6.1). These tools will be described below, including information about their development, content, validation, and reliability.

Table 6.1 Pain assessment tools for neonates

Tool	Reference	Age range	Clinical indications for use	Guidelines for use	Advantages and disadvantages
PIPP	Stevens et al. [24]; McNair et al. [25]	28–40 weeks gestational age	Procedural pain, postoperative pain	Score ranges from 0 to 3 in each indicator, scores can range from 0 to 21 in infants less than 36 weeks gestation, maximum score 21 in infants over 36 weeks gestation	Includes cutoff scores for mild, moderate, and severe pain Multidimensional; 7 indicators, including two physiological, three behavioral, and two contextual
N-PASS	Hummel et al. [26]	0–100 days old; 23 weeks gestation and above	Ventilated and/or postoperative infants	Scoring determines whether infant is sedated or in pain	Multidimensional; 5 indicators, including four behavioral and one physiological. Measures sedation and pain on a continuum. Includes scoring criteria for corrected age. Has been validated in ventilated infants
CRIES	Krechel and Bildner [27]	32–60 weeks gestational age	Postoperative infants	Scoring ranges from 0 to 2 in each of the 5 indicators for a total score of 0–10	Multidimensional; 5 indicators, including two physiological and three behavioral

6.3.1 The Premature Infant Pain Profile (PIPP)

This tool consists of a seven-item, 4-point scale that measures behavioral, physiological, and contextual indicators [24] (Fig. 6.1). These measures include gestational age, behavioral state, oxygen saturation, brow bulge, eye squeeze, and nasolabial furrows. Initial reliability and validity testing involved procedural pain such as heel lance, circumcision, and venipuncture. Research on the PIPP has demonstrated construct validity of the tool as a measure of prolonged post-operative pain in premature infants who underwent surgical procedures [25].

Infant Study Number: ______________________
Date/time: ______________________
Event: ______________________

Process	Indicator	0	1	2	3	Score
Chart	Gestational age	36 weeks and more	32–35 weeks, 6 days	28–31 weeks, 6 days	less than 28 weeks	
Observe infant 15 s	Behavioral state	active/awake eyes open facial movements	quiet/awake eyes open no facial movements	active/sleep eyes closed facial movements	quiet/sleep eyes closed no facial movements	
Observe baseline Heart rate __ Oxygen saturation __						
Observe infant 30 s	Heart rate Max ___	0–4 beats/min increase	5–14 beats/min increase	15–24 beats/min increase	25 beats/min or more increase	
	Oxygen saturation Min ___	0–2.4 % decrease	2.5–4.9 % decrease	5.0–7.4 % decrease	7.5 % or more decrease	
	Brow bulge	None 0–9 % of time	Minimum 10–39 % of time	Moderate 40–69 % of time	Maximum 70 % of time or More	
	Eye squeeze	None 0–9 % of time	Minimum 10–39 % of time	Moderate 40–69 % of time	Maximum 70 % of time or More	
	Nasolabial furrow	None 0–9 % of time	Minimum 10–39 % of time	Moderate 40–69 % of time	Maximum 70 % of time or More	
					Total score	________

Fig. 6.1 Scoring method for the premature infant pain profile (PIPP) (Adapted from Stevens et al. [24]. With permission from Wolters Kluwer Health)

6.3.2 Neonatal Pain Agitation and Sedation Scale (N-PASS)

The N-PASS [26] consists of five indicators that have demonstrated reliability and validity as pain measures in various neonatal pain assessment scales (Fig. 6.2). These indicators are cry/irritability, behavior state, facial expression, extremities/tone, and vital signs. The tool was tested on infants in the neonatal intensive care unit who had received surgical procedures [26]. The infants ranged in postnatal age from 0 to 100 days, and gestational age ranged from 23 to 40 weeks. Convergent validity, assessed by correlation with the PIPP, was 0.83 at high pain scores and 0.61 at low pain scores. Inter-rater reliability was high (0.85–0.95). The N-PASS is validated up to 3 years of age.

N-PASS:

Neonatal Pain, Agitation, & Sedation Scale

Assessment Criteria	Sedation		Sedation/Pain	Pain / Agitation	
	-2	-1	0/0	1	2
Crying Irritability	No cry with painful stimuli	Moans or cries minimally with painful stimuli	No sedation/ No pain signs	Irritable or crying at intervals Consolable	High-pitched or silent-continuous cry Inconsolable
Behavior State	No arousal to any stimuli No spontaneous movement	Arouses minimally to stimuli Little spontaneous movement	No sedation/ No pain signs	Restless, squirming Awakens frequently	Arching, kicking Constantly awake or Arouses minimally / no movement (not sedated)
Facial Expression	Mouth is lax No expression	Minimal expression with stimuli	No sedation/ No pain signs	Any pain expression intermittent	Any pain expression continual
Extremities Tone	No grasp reflex Flaccid tone	Weak grasp reflex ↓ muscle tone	No sedation/ No pain signs	Intermittent clenched toes, fists or finger splay Body is not tense	Continual clenched toes, fists, or finger splay Body is tense
Vital Signs HR, RR, BP, SaO_2	No variability with stimuli Hypoventilation or apnea	< 10% variability from baseline with stimuli	No sedation/ No pain signs	↑ 10-20% from baseline SaO_2 76-85% with stimulation - quick ↑	↑ > 20% from baseline SaO_2 ≤ 75% with stimulation - slow ↑ Out of sync/fighting vent

Premature Pain Assessment: + 1 if <30 weeks gestation / corrected age

Fig. 6.2 N-PASS assessment table. Used with permission

6.3.3 CRIES

CRIES [27] is a tool that measures five physiological and behavioral variables: C-crying, R-requires increased oxygen administration, I-increased vital signs, E-expression, and S-sleepiness (Fig. 6.3). The tool was tested on infants between 32 and 60 weeks gestational age who underwent surgical procedures, including insertion of ventriculoperitoneal shunts and thoracotomies. Construct validity was established by comparing scores pre- and post-analgesia administration. Inter-rater reliability was found to be acceptable ($r=0.72$).

Date/time						
Crying - Chracteristic cry of pain is high pitched. 0 – No cry or cry that is not high-pitched 1 – Cry high pitched but baby is easily consolable 2 – Cry high pitched but baby is inconsolable						
Requires O_2 for SaO_2 <95 % - Babies experiencing pain manifest decreased oxygenation. Consider other cause of hypoxemia, e.g., oversedation, atelectasis, pneumothorax) 0 – No oxygen required 1 – <30 % oxygen required 2 – >30 % oxygen required						
Increased vital signs (BP* and HR*) - Take BP last as this may awaken child making other assessments difficult 0 – Both HR and BP unchanged or less than baseline 1 – HR or BP increased but increase in <20 % of baseline 2 – HR or BP is increased >20 % over baseline.						
Expression - The facial expression most often associated with pain is a grimace. A grimace may be characterized by brow lowering, eyes squeezed shut, deepening naso-labial furrow, or open lips and mouth. 0 – No grimace present 1 – Grimace alone is present 2 – Grimace and non-cry vocalization grunt is present						
Sleepless - Scored based upon the infant's state during the hour preceding this recorded score. 0 – Child has been continuously asleep 1 – Child has awakened at frequent intervals 2 – Child has been awake constantly						
Total score						

Fig. 6.3 CRIES neonatal pain assessment tool. Used with permission

6.3.4 Assessing Postoperative Pain in Infants and Young Children

Although most children over the age of 18 months are verbal, their ability to communicate pain may still be limited to crying or to providing information only about the presence or absence of pain. Assessing pain in infants and preschool age children is best accomplished by measures that include behavioral manifestations of pain. Tools that have shown reliability and validity in assessing postoperative pain in infants and young children include the Faces, Limb, Activity, Cry, and Consolability (FLACC) scale for hospital use and the Parents' Postoperative Pain Measure (PPPM) for use at home [28].

6.3.4.1 FLACC (Faces, Limb, Activity, Cry, and Consolability)

The FLACC [29] has been shown to be a reliable tool for measuring postoperative pain in young children (Fig. 6.4). The acronym FLACC incorporates the different domains of the assessment – Facial expression, Leg movement, Activity level, Cry, and Consolability. Each domain receives a score between 0 and 2 for a total score of between 0 and 10. Initial testing of the tool involved assessment of children between 2 months and 7 years of age who had undergone surgical procedures in the postanesthesia care unit. Inter-rater reliability was found to be high using simultaneous independent evaluations ($r=0.94$). Validity testing has demonstrated that FLACC scores decrease with analgesia administration in children under the age of 3 years [30].

6.3.4.2 Parents' Postoperative Pain Measure (PPPM)

The Parents' Postoperative Pain Measure [31] has been validated as a measure for home use in children who are discharged to home following day surgery procedures. This 15-item tool includes cutoff scores which show excellent sensitivity and specificity (>80 %) in determining clinically meaningful pain scores. The initial validation of this tool was completed on children ages 7–12 years undergoing procedures which were ranked by experts into three classes – highly painful (e.g., tonsillectomies), moderately painful (e.g., sinus surgeries), or little or no pain (e.g., myringotomies). Further validation of the PPPM [32] demonstrated that the tool is a reliable valid measure for home use on children between the ages of 2 and 6 years.

Categories	Scoring		
	0	1	2
Face	No particular expression or smile	Occasional grimace or frown, withdrawn, disinterested	Frequent to constant quivering chin, clenched jaw
Legs	Normal position or relaxed	Uneasy, restless, tense	Kicking, or legs drawn up
Activity	Lying quietly, normal position, moves easily	Squirming, shifting back and forth, tense	Arched, rigid or jerking
Cry	No cry (awake or asleep)	Moans or whimpers; occasional complaint	Crying steadily, screams or sobs, frequent complaints
Consolability	Content, relaxed	Reassured by occasional touching, hugging or being talked to, distractable	Difficult to console or comfort
Each of the five categories (F) Face; (L) Legs; (A) Activity; (C) Cry; (C) Consolability is scored from 0-2, which results in a total score between zero and ten.			

Fig. 6.4 FLACC pain assessment tool (Based on data from Ref. [29])

6.4 Assessing Pain in Children and Adolescents

Children over the age of 3 years can often provide reliable information about the intensity or severity of their pain using validated self-report scales. Much of the research related to pain assessment tools for this population has focused on the use of the scales in clinical trials rather than in clinical practice. The Pediatric Initiative on Methods, Measurement, and Pain Assessment in Clinical Trials (Ped-IMMPACT) by Stinson et al. [33] reviewed 34 self-report tools and found that while no single tool was optimal for all types of pain, six were shown to be reliable and valid for acute pain (Table 6.3). The Faces Pain Scale [34] and Faces Pain Scale-Revised [35] have both been shown to be reliable, valid, simple, easy to use, and require minimal instruction. Other recommended pain scales include the Oucher, the Pieces of Hurt, the Wong-Baker FACES Pain Scale, and the Visual analogue scale. Numeric rating scales are frequently used in clinic practice. Each of these scales is discussed below.

6.4.1 Faces Pain Scale-Revised

The Faces Pain Scale-Revised [35] has been translated into more than 40 languages and can be obtained free of charge for use in clinical practice. Obviously, it is important when using pain assessment tools with young verbal children to communicate in a language that they understand whenever possible. These pictorial scales with accompanying instructions have a series of six faces that the child points to, indicating how much they hurt or how sore they feel. This scale has strong psychometric properties and is widely used in research and clinical practice internationally.

6.4.2 Numeric Rating Scales (NRS)

Older children are often asked to rate their pain using these scales (Fig. 6.5). The NRS is generally composed of an 11-point numeric rating scale, with anchors of 0 (No Pain) and 10 (Worst Pain Imaginable). A recent publication by von Baeyer et al. [36] reviewed the use of the numeric rating scale to define age limits for which it would be appropriate and concluded that the scale is supported for use in children over the age of 8 years.

6.4.3 Oucher

The Oucher [37] consists of a numeric rating scale combined with six photographs of children's faces. Caucasian, African-American, Hispanic, First Nations (boy/girl), and Asian (boy/girl) versions are available. Using this scale, the child chooses the face that best reflects the pain level. The picture selection is then converted to a number between 0 and 10. The scale must be printed in color in order for the child to accurately see the faces, making it a more expensive tool to use.

6.4.4 Pieces of Hurt/Poker Chip Scale

The Pieces of Hurt, or Poker Chip Scale [38], consists of four chips or pieces of hurt. The child chooses how many pieces of hurt they are experiencing. The tool is difficult to use in postoperative care in hospitals because of infection control concerns and availability of poker chips on the unit.

6.4.5 Wong-Baker FACES Pain Scale

The Wong-Baker FACES Pain Scale [39] is a reliable and valid tool for assessing pain in children over 3 years of age. It is similar to the Faces Pain Scale-Revised in that it consists of a series of six cartoon faces depicting "no hurt" to "hurts worst." The child then chooses the face that best describes his/her pain. Recent research [40, 41] has found that children's pain ratings are influenced by the pictorial anchors, as the "no pain" face has a smile and the "most pain" face has tears. These findings suggest that the faces in this scale may measure pain affect rather than pain intensity.

6.4.6 Visual Analogue Scale (VAS)

The visual analogue scale (VAS) [42], which has several forms, is composed of a line with the words "no pain" and "worst" or "most pain" as anchors (Fig. 6.6). The line can be vertical or horizontal. The child is asked to mark a point on the line to indicate pain intensity. The VAS has been used extensively in research studies. It is not as clinically useful as a tool as it may be difficult to interpret and difficult to include in a chart document and requires careful explanation to the child. Debate continues as to optimal line length and the choice of anchor words.

6.4.7 Children's Hospital of Eastern Ontario Pain Scale (CHEOPS)

The Children's Hospital of Eastern Ontario Pain Scale [43] is a time-sampling behavioral pain scale. It looks for behaviors related to six items: cry, facial, child verbal, torso, touch, and legs. Each behavior listed under each item is given a numerical score and definition. The numerical scores are assigned based on the following criteria: 0 is behavior that is the antithesis of pain; 1 is behavior not indicative of pain, and not the antithesis of pain; 2 is behavior indication of mild or moderate pain; and 3 is behavior indicative of severe pain. Therefore, the total score can be from 4 to 13 for each time period sampled. It showed good inter-rater reliability, with average percentage of agreement by patients ranging from 90 to 99.5 %.

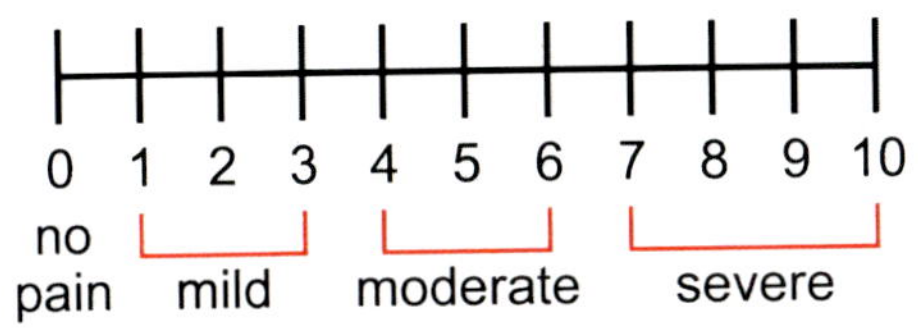

Fig. 6.5 Numeric rating scale (NRS)

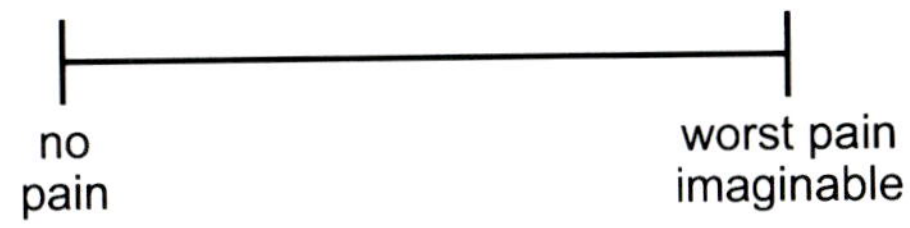

Fig. 6.6 Visual analogue scale (VAS). A 10-cm scale is recommended; the child marks a point along the scale that corresponds with his/her pain. A ruler is then used to determine the score by measuring the distance between the "no pain" anchor and the mark

6.5 Assessing Postoperative Pain in Critically Ill Children

Assessing postoperative pain in critically ill children in an intensive care unit requires multidimensional tools. If a critically ill child is not sedated, a self-report should be obtained where possible. However, for many of these children, sedation is a required part of their care, making valid assessment by self-reporting more difficult. The COMFORT scale [44, 45] (Fig. 6.7) was developed to assess distress in critically ill children. In many critically ill children, pain may be a contributor to the distress. The COMFORT scale consists of behavioral and physiological indicators. The tool requires extensive training of clinical staff but is one of the few tools validated for use in this population. The modified FLACC [46] is valid in measuring postoperative pain in intubated children. The Cry section is modified to reflect the facial expression associated with crying.

Patient Sticker

Date ______________ Time ______________

Observer ______________

Category	Description	Score
Alertness	• Deeply asleep (eyes closed, no response to changes in the environment)	❑ 1
	• Lightly asleep (eyes mostly closed, occasional responses)	❑ 2
	• Drowsy (child closes his or her eyes frequently, loss respansive to the environment)	❑ 3
	• Awake and alert (child responsive to the environment)	❑ 4
	• Awake and hyperalert (exaggerated responses to the environmental stimuli)	❑ 5
Calmness–Agitation	• Calm (child appears serene and franquil)	❑ 1
	• Slightly anxious (child shows slight anxiety)	❑ 2
	• Anxious (child appers agilated but remains in control)	❑ 3
	• Very anxious (child appears very agilated, just able to control)	❑ 4
	• Panicky (child appears severely distressed, with loss of control)	❑ 5
Respiratory response (score only in mechanically ventilated children)	• No spontaneous respiration	❑ 1
	• Spontaneous and ventilator respiration	❑ 2
	• Restlessness or resistance to ventilator	❑ 3
	• Active breathing against ventilator or regular coughing	❑ 4
	• Fighting against ventilator	❑ 5
Crying (score only in childran breathing spontaneously)	• Quiet breathing, no crying sounds	❑ 1
	• Occasional sobbing or moaning	❑ 2
	• Whining (monotone)	❑ 3
	• Crying	❑ 4
	• Screaming or shricking	❑ 5
Physical movement	• No movement	❑ 1
	• Occasional (3 or fewer) slight movements	❑ 2
	• Frequent (more than 3) slight movements	❑ 3
	• Vigorous movements limited to extremities	❑ 4
	• Vigorous movements including lorso and head	❑ 5
Muscle tone	• Muscles totally relaxed, no muscle tone	❑ 1
	• Reduced muscle tone, less resistance than normal	❑ 2
	• Normal muscle tone	❑ 3
	• Increased muscle tone and flexion of fingers and loes	❑ 4
	• Extreme muscle rigidity and flexion of fingers and loes	❑ 5
Facial tension	• Facial muscles totally relaxed	❑ 1
	• Normal facial tone	❑ 2
	• Tension evident in some facial muscles (not sustained)	❑ 3
	• Tension evident throughout facial muscles (sustained)	❑ 4
	• Facial muscle contorted and grimacing	❑ 5
	Total Score	

VAS (Visual Analogue Scale)
Put a mark on the line below to indicate how much pain you think the child has **at this very moment.**

no pain |————————————————| worst pain **VAS Score**

Treatment datails

Datails of child's condition

Assessments made
(before or after medication or standard assessment)

Fig. 6.7 COMFORT scale for pain assessment in critically ill children (Reprinted from van Dijk et al. [45]. With permission from Wolters Kluwer Health)

6.6 Assessing Postoperative Pain in Children with Cognitive Impairments

Assessing postoperative pain in children with cognitive impairments requires the use of multidimensional tools and parental input. It can be difficult to determine which behaviors are pain related in this population. The Non-Communicating Children's Pain Checklist-Postoperative Version (NCCPC-PV) by Breau et al. [47] (Fig. 6.8) demonstrated good inter-rater reliability and included cutoff scores to determine mild or moderate to severe pain. The tool requires a 10-min observation of behaviors in six domains – vocal, social, facial, activity, body and limbs, and physiological. The FLACC has also shown reliability and validity in assessing postoperative pain in children with cognitive impairments. Malviya et al. [48] utilized the FLACC as well as individualized behaviors identified by the parent for each child in assessing pain postoperatively in children aged 4–19 years with cognitive impairments.

Non-communicating Children's Pain Checklist – Postoperative Version (NCCPC-PV)

NAME: ______	UNIT/FILE #: ______	DATE: ______ (dd/mm/yy)
OBSERVER: ______	START TIME: ______ AM/PM	STOP TIME: ______ AM/PM

How ofetn has this child shown these behaviours in the last 10 minutes? Please circle a number for each behaviour. If an item does not apply to this child (for example, this child cannot reach with his/her hands), then indicate "not applicable" for that item.

0 = NOT AT ALL 1 = JUST A LITTLE 2 = FAIRLY OFTEN 3 = VERY OFTEN NA = NOT APPLICABLE

I. Vocal

1. Moaning, whining, whimpering (fairly soft)	0	1	2	3	NA
2. Crying (moderately loud)	0	1	2	3	NA
3. Screaming/yelling (very loud)	0	1	2	3	NA
4. A specific sound or word for pain (e.g., a word, cry or type of laugh)	0	1	2	3	NA

II. Social

5. Not cooperating, cranky, irritable, unhappy	0	1	2	3	NA
6. Less interaction with others, withdrawn	0	1	2	3	NA
7. Seeking comfort or physical closeness	0	1	2	3	NA
8. Being difficult to distract, not able to satisfy or pacify	0	1	2	3	NA

III. Facial

9. A furrowed brow	0	1	2	3	NA
10. A change in eyes, including: squinching of eyes, eyes opened wide, eyes frowing	0	1	2	3	NA
11. Turning down of mouth, not smiling	0	1	2	3	NA
12. Lips puckering up, tight, pouting, or quivering	0	1	2	3	NA
13. Clenching or grinding teeth, chewing or thrusting tongue out	0	1	2	3	NA

IV. Activity

14. Not moving, less active, quiet	0	1	2	3	NA
15. Jumping around, agitated, fidgety	0	1	2	3	NA

V. Body and Limbs

16. Floppy	0	1	2	3	NA
17. Stiff, spastic, tense, rigid	0	1	2	3	NA
18. Gesturing to or touching part of the body that hurts	0	1	2	3	NA
19. Protecting, favoring or guarding part of the body that hurts	0	1	2	3	NA
20. Flinching or moving the body part away, being sensitive to touch	0	1	2	3	NA
21. Moving the body in a specific way to show pain (e.g. head back, arms down, curls up, etc.)	0	1	2	3	NA

VI. Physiological

22. Shivering	0	1	2	3	NA
23. Change in color, pallor	0	1	2	3	NA
24. Sweating, perspiring	0	1	2	3	NA
25. Tears	0	1	2	3	NA
26. Sharp intake of breath, gasping	0	1	2	3	NA
27. Breath holding	0	1	2	3	NA

SCORE SUMMARY:

Category:	I	II	III	IV	V	VI	TOTAL
Score:							

Fig. 6.8 The Non-Communicating Children's Pain Checklist-Postoperative Version (NCCPC-PV). Used with permission

6.7 Summary

In summary, there are many tools available for assessing postoperative pain in children. Clinicians need to use tools that are reliable, valid, and easy to use. Many of the tools are designed to capture pain intensity, which is only one part of a comprehensive pain assessment. Figure 6.9 and the following tables summarize current tools for assessing pain in children of different age groups. Table 6.1 addresses tools for use in neonates, Table 6.2 addresses behavioral tools, and Table 6.3 addresses self-report tools. Whichever tool is chosen for use, it must be used regularly to effectively manage postoperative pain in children.

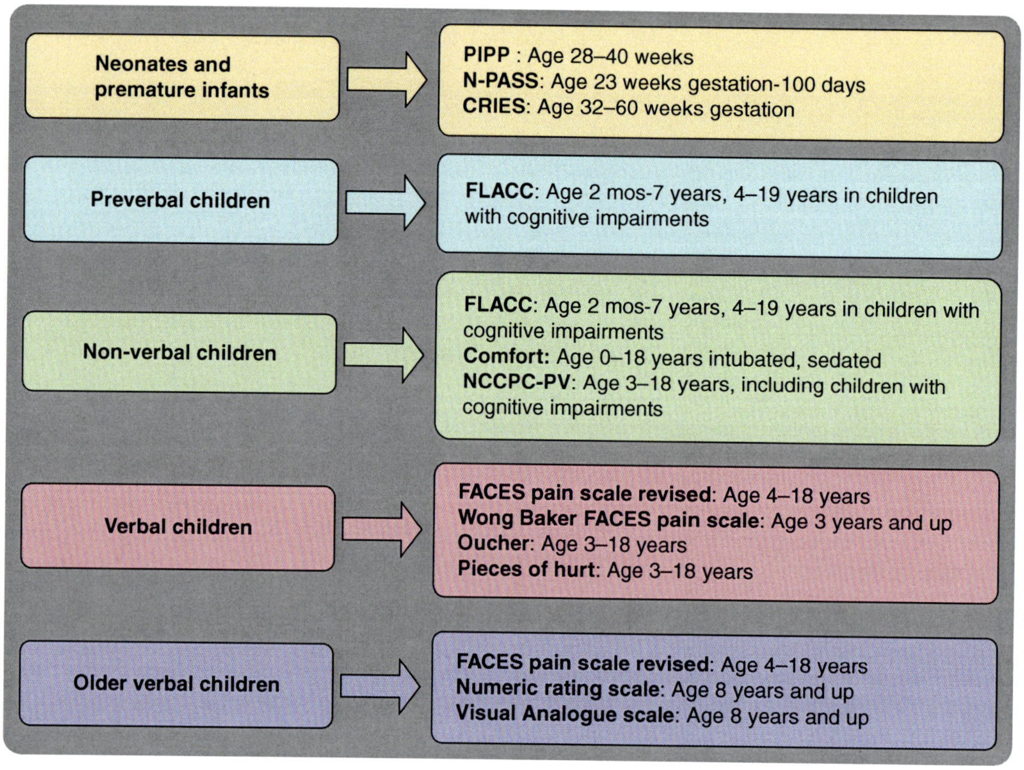

Fig. 6.9 Appropriate pain assessment scales for children of different age groups (See text for details)

Table 6.2 Behavioral pain assessment tools

Tool	Reference	Age range	Clinical indications for use	Guidelines for use	Advantages and disadvantages
FLACC	Merkel et al. [29]	2 months–7 years; ages 4–19 years for children with cognitive impairments	Postoperative pain	Scoring ranges from 0 to 2 in each of the 5 indicators for a total score of 0–10	Child needs to be observed for a minimum of 2 min while awake, 5 min while asleep. Five behavioral indicators
COMFORT	Ambuel et al. [44]	0–18 years	Postoperative pain	8 categories with scores for each of 1–5. Scoring between 8 and 40. Score determines optimal sedation in child	Multidimensional; 8 indicators, including six behavioral and two physiological. Requires extensive training. Only tool validated for use in intubated sedated children
NCCPC-PV	Breau et al. [47]	Children ages 3–18 years who are able to provide a verbal report including children with cognitive impairments	Postoperative pain	6 categories with indicators for a total of 27 indicators. Scores 0–3 or not applicable for each indicator scores are tabulated. A score of 11 or more is indicative of moderate to severe pain; a score of 6–10 is indicative of mild pain	Requires a 10-min observation time. More comprehensive than FLACC in that it includes five behavioral indicators and one physiological. Includes cutoff scores

Table 6.3 Self-reporting pain assessment tools

Tool	Reference	Age range	Clinical indications for use	Guidelines for use	Advantages and disadvantages
Faces Pain Scale-Revised	Hicks et al. [35]	4–18 years	Postoperative pain, acute procedural pain	Series of 6 faces depicting "no pain" to "most pain possible." Scoring 0–10	Simple, easy to use and explain. Translated into 32 languages and available on the Internet, although not all translations have been validated
Wong-Baker FACES Pain Scale	Wong and Baker [39]	3 years and older	Postoperative pain, procedural pain	Series of six faces ranging from smiling to crying. Scoring 0–5	Simple, easy to use, and readily available. Children have demonstrated a tendency to choose the anchors; may measure pain affect rather than pain intensity
Numeric rating scale	von Baeyer et al. [36]	8–18 years	Postoperative pain, procedural pain	11-point scale with 0 = no pain and 10 = most pain	Easy and quick to use. Does not require tools. Can be explained verbally
Visual analogue scale	Huskisson [42]	8 years and older	Procedural pain	Premeasured horizontal or vertical line, usually 100 mm in length. Child indicates pain intensity by marking a point along the line	Easy and quick to use. Limited clinical utility: difficult to interpret and document; requires careful explanation. Variability in length of line, use of marking, and choice of anchor words
Oucher	Beyer and Aradine [37]	3–18 years	Postoperative pain, procedural pain	Two scales; a series of 6 photographic faces and a 0–100-mm vertical numeric scale	Expensive (must be printed in color). Children should be screened to determine their ability to use the numeric rating scale
Pieces of Hurt	Hester [38]	3–18 years	Procedural pain	Four red plastic poker chips representing "little hurt" to "most hurt you could have." Child chooses the chip that represents his/her pain intensity. Scoring 0–4	Need to have poker chips. Infection control (cannot be used between patients); need to store chips at the bedside

6.8 Developmental, Familial, and Psychological Factors

6.8.1 Age

Historically, some have been tempted to erroneously conceptualize children as "mini-adults" when it came to formulating practice guidelines. It is now clear that many aspects of children's behavior are unique and dissimilar to corresponding behavior in adults. Age-related developmental changes interact with many factors that influence pain assessment. The effects of age in the context of pain assessment have been increasingly studied over the past 20 years. Some of these effects are clear and some are more subtle.

One of the most obvious and pertinent factors relevant to assessing a child's pain is the level of the child's ability to communicate the experience of pain. While self-report is the gold standard for pain assessment [49], this is often difficult or impossible for young children or for children with developmental delays. Further, as pain is by nature a subjective experience, reporting something as complex as one's pain experience is inherently challenging [50]. In addition to possible limitations in communicating information about pain being experienced, what a developing child understands when questioned about pain or the child's understanding of how to respond using pain assessment tools can be limited or qualitatively different from what the assessing adult understands. These differences can be a result of a number of factors including the child's level of communication sophistication, past pain experiences, and culture. Furthermore, a child who is ill and/or in pain may have more difficulty engaging effectively in tasks, particularly if those tasks are complex.

Neonates and Infants

There is considerable evidence from biological measures that newborns and infants experience pain at the same level of intensity as adults [51]. There is strong evidence from the use of physiological and behavioral measures that infants show enhanced acute pain responses [52]. It has long been known that as the number of painful procedures that a neonate or infant experiences increases, there can be a corresponding increase in anticipatory fear reactions related to cues for an upcoming medical procedure [53]. Obviously, given the very limited ability of an infant to communicate, physiological, biological, and observational measures must be relied upon to assess pain in very young children. In many cases, parents can provide valuable information based on behavioral observations of an infant that can be valid and reliable estimates of pain and distress.

Preschoolers

Preschool age children present with some remarkable abilities but also experience considerable challenges in many cases when trying to rate their pain. As children develop and as new skills are acquired in cognitive, motor, and social domains, new abilities emerge. Along with these abilities come unique response tendencies that correspond with a child's developmental stage. For example, it has been found that younger children tend to assign higher intensity scores to pain descriptors than older children [54]. It has also been noted that as cognitive skills such as seriation, classification, matching, and estimation develop, children are able to more reliably produce valid pain scores. The younger a child is, the greater the tendency that a child will be more egocentric and concrete and focus excessively on perceptually salient aspects of a scale [55]. Younger children such as those in the 3–4-year age range have been found to be more likely to choose endpoints of visual analogue or categorical scales [56]. It is also important to note that a child's ability to attend to and complete tasks such as pain ratings is affected by stressors [57]. This is particularly pertinent given the stressful nature of pain. As well, there also appears to be a strong developmental trend with regard to a child's ability to use words that label one's emotional state [58]. As a child's language skills become more sophisticated, his/her ability to provide valid and reliable pain reports also increases.

School-Age Children

As with the previously described age groups, as children in this age category develop, they become increasingly able to use language and conceptual thinking to more skillfully provide information related to pain assessment. It is during this developmental stage that children show increasing abilities to use many self-report scales. During this stage, children tend to use more complex conceptualizations and report more abstract and affective aspects of pain [4]. This ability can be noted between ages 7 and 10 years, becoming more established by the age of 11 years [59]. A wider range of self-report measures can be reliably used to obtain valid pain measures in this age range.

Adolescence

Adolescents show an increasing ability to describe and focus on the psychological and social impact of pain. Adolescents generally demonstrate increased cognitive flexibility, abstract thinking, and a broader vocabulary available to describe their experiences. They also tend to show increased concern about the personal and future relevance of a current pain experience as it pertains to disability and disfigurement [4].

6.8.2 Developmental Delays

Relevant to the discussion of a child's ability to report pain and an observer's ability to rate a child's pain is a discussion on unique challenges that exist when assessing pain in children with developmental delays or other forms of physical or mental impairment. Individuals with developmental disabilities are at risk of having their pain underestimated and undertreated due to their difficulties in verbal communication, cognitive impairment, and even motor skill deficits [60]. Malviya and colleagues found that few developmentally delayed children with postoperative pain were assessed for pain, and those who were assessed tended to receive fewer doses of analgesic medication [61]. This bias may be rooted in an incorrect belief that developmentally disabled children experience less pain or have higher pain tolerances [62]. Strong evidence exists that it is more likely that differences in apparent pain tolerance or pain behaviors are a result of differences in behavioral expression of pain [63]. This is especially pertinent as children in this population can be more likely to experience more frequent and particularly painful medical procedures due to other physical conditions [64, 65].

As is the case with very young children, parents and other caregivers who are familiar with a child with developmental disabilities have the potential to provide valuable and valid estimates of the child's pain experience. This information may simply not be measurable using existing pain assessment tools available in most hospital settings [64]. However, even caregiver reports have been found to be inconsistent and underestimate pain in this population [66, 67]. Fortunately, there is a growing body of research that has examined pain measurement in the developmentally disabled. There is evidence that observers, even those unfamiliar with a developmentally delayed child, can reliably assess pain in these children when provided with adequate information about the child in conjunction with the use of validated assessment measures [64].

6.8.3 Psychological Factors

Expectations

Assessing both a child's and parents' expectations with regard to the anticipated procedure can be a helpful aspect of pain assessment. An important part of understanding a child's expectations of pain is obtaining a history of the child's experience with previous painful procedures. Children who have experienced multiple previous painful procedures, particularly those who have received poor analgesia during those procedures, are at increased risk of developing higher levels of procedure- and pain-related anxiety [68]. This can lead to a vicious cycle where pain and anxiety amplify each other and thereby lead to heightened pain experience and pain behavior.

The impact of expectations on pain perception has been broadly established [69]. Cheng et al. reported that pain expectation, previous pain experience, and acceptance of pain accounted for 55 % of the variance in children's overall pain levels [70]. It has been found that children are prone to having difficulty in accurately estimating the amount of pain that they will experience [71]. Expectations related to a painful stimulus have been found to be associated with later pain ratings following a painful episode [72]. A subsequent study found that children who expected to have more pain postoperatively tended to report higher pain levels [73]. Of note, it has also been found that health-care providers can unintentionally affect an individual's perception of pain by doing such things as communicating personal expectations [74]. This highlights the importance of the care provider's approach to pain assessment and management while interacting with a child.

Anxiety, Fear of Pain, and Catastrophizing

Effective pain assessment includes an understanding of factors related to procedural and pain-related anxiety and fear. Pain-related fear and anxiety are natural and understandable consequences of pain and anticipating a painful procedure. It is important to understand that it can be difficult for children to separate their reactions to pain from their reactions to fear and anxiety [18]. However, this should not be used by clinicians as an excuse to deny appropriate analgesia due to a supposition that reported pain is psychosomatic or merely a manifestation of fear.

Anxiety has been established as a factor that can amplify one's pain experience [75]. Tsao and colleagues found that anxiety symptoms, anticipatory anxiety, and anxiety sensitivity accounted for 62 % of the variance when predicting a child's pain response to experimental pain [76]. Another study also found that pain catastrophizing predicts children's pain ratings for experimental pain [77]. An interesting study of postoperative pain in adolescents found that preoperative anxiety and anticipated pain levels predicted postoperative pain ratings and analgesic use [78]. These studies highlight some of the effects of pain-related anxiety and pain catastrophizing on pain. They emphasize the impact of anxiety and fear of pain on a child's perception of pain and should not be misinterpreted to suggest that appropriate analgesia should not be provided. Perception is reality for anyone experiencing pain, and assessing pain and pain-related anxiety effectively enables health-care providers to better understand and adequately manage pain.

Social and Family Factors

Understanding a child's family context is an obvious key factor in understanding a child's pain experience [79]. Children can be at risk for inaccurate assessment and poor pain management due to social and family factors. Accurate parental reports can play an important role in a child's care, putting a child at risk if those reports are not valid. Potential barriers include a parent's inability to accurately assess pain, parental fears regarding negative side effects of treatment, and inaccurate beliefs about the risk of addiction to analgesics [80, 81].

Palermo and Chambers have written an excellent review on important family variables relevant to pain assessment to take into account at the levels of the individual child, dyadic factors, and the family itself [13]. Working collaboratively with family members while using validated pain assessment tools has been found to result in effective pain assessment [47].

Schecter and colleagues found that parents' prediction of a child's pain response was the best predictor of distress during immunization, highlighting the potential value of parental input during pain assessment [82]. In addition, parents generally expect that their children's procedural pain be appropriately managed [83] and are therefore often highly motivated to assist health-care providers as needed during pain assessment.

Biases in Health-Care Providers

There is a rich collection of literature that clearly demonstrates humans' inherent tendency to individual bias. For example, a dated but relevant study found that physicians were biased to overestimate a child's cognitive level if the child is well dressed and does not have dysmorphic features [84]. There are a number of important issues that are worth noting for individuals involved in the medical care of children who experience pain due to disease and/or medical procedures.

A primary ongoing issue in pediatric pain assessment and management is the reluctance of some health-care providers to use analgesics (particularly opioids) to manage pain. Some of these biases result from misinformation based on outdated or biased perceptions [85]. Such biases can lead care providers to minimize pain when assessing it and attribute pain to other factors such as anxiety or other psychological factors. While it has been well established that stress and anxiety can exacerbate pain perception and pain behavior and impede pain coping [86, 87], a reluctance to use opioids or other analgesics according to established guidelines is unethical and inhumane.

In a survey of physicians across a variety of subspecialties, it was found that pediatricians tended to report a belief that pain was experienced at an earlier age than surgeons and family practitioners and were more likely to prescribe analgesics for pain than these other groups [88]. That same study also found that physicians tended to rate other subspecialty procedures as more painful than procedures from their own specialty. Another research found that physicians were far more likely to prescribe appropriate analgesics for the same medical problem in older patients compared to toddlers [89]. While these studies highlight physician bias in practice, these biases exist across specialties and disciplines. Awareness of one's own personal biases must be a priority for all care providers when assessing and managing a child's pain.

6.8.4 Gender

There have been a number of studies investigating the differences in pain response related to sex (physiological factors) and gender (psychosocial factors) in children. Several studies aimed at measuring relationships between sex and pain reactions have failed to observe any differences between boys and girls [90–92]. Other findings suggest that there are biological differences in ways males and females react to pain across the life span. For example, several researchers conclude that females have lower pain threshold and tolerances than males [93–95]. Sex differences in pain responses in adults have also been attributed to various biological differences in pain mechanisms, such as brain chemistry, metabolism, physical structures, and hormonal variations affecting pain transmission, pain sensitivity, and pain perception [94, 96]. Unfortunately, these findings are inconsistent in the pediatric population [97].

Further research on this subject has investigated gender-related differences, including pain behavior and characteristics influenced by sociocultural factors such as femininity and masculinity [98]. In these studies, females have commonly been found to report more severe levels of pain, more frequent pain, and pain of longer duration than males [96, 99, 100]. In addition, girls of various ages have been found to rate a greater difference between their ratings of unpleasantness of pain and pain intensity scores in comparison to boys, indicating that females may have a greater ability to discriminate different pain stimuli [101–103]. When analyzing these findings, it is essential to consider that differences in pain responses between genders could be attributed to differences in pain reporting styles. In multiple studies, girls consistently select more words to describe their pain than boys [54], which corresponds with findings suggesting greater verbal fluency and emotional expressiveness in girls.

While increased pain reactions and behaviors may be observed in females, this does not necessarily imply that they are experiencing more pain. It is possible that they could simply be more verbally expressive about their pain than males, which can be attributable to psychosocial factors [104]. Stereotypically, males in many cultures are expected to hold back on reporting pain. As a result there may be a greater social cost to openly express their experience of pain. This may teach boys to minimize pain responses, which in turn can lead society to expect less pain response from them. In some cultures, females are perceived to be weaker and to tolerate less pain, which invites them to express their pain more freely [105]. In a recent study on sex differences in parent and child pain ratings, researchers found that, although subjects of both genders correspondingly responded to pain in the presence of both parents, fathers were inclined to rate a higher pain score to their sons than daughters [106], which illustrates a societal expectation that may falsely contribute to differences observed in gender reactions to pain. Due to the inconsistency in the literature, it is important to consider the many factors that may influence pain responses and the various ways these can be interpreted when assessing a child's pain.

6.8.5 Cultural Factors

It is important to be aware of cultural factors and possible cultural stereotypes that can exist when assessing procedural pain in children. It is also important to note that subjective experience and coping strategies in response to pain in children can be unique across cultures. As well, some cultures conceptualize pain as positive, character building, or cleansing and welcome painful experiences for these and other reasons.

Studies that have examined pain in children from different cultures have shown some consistent findings. For example, differences have been found between children from cultural groups in their pain control and pain behaviors, but not in self-reported pain scores [107, 108]. Pfefferbaum and colleagues (1990) have noted that these differences may reflect biased descriptors included in observational instruments, which fail to capture pain behaviors unique to certain cultures [109]. Other findings suggest that self-report measures can accurately assess a child's level of pain regardless of his/her cultural background [110]. Gharaibeh and Abu-Saad (2002) argue that children have their own separate subculture mediated by common norms of growth and development, natural feelings and instinct, and common styles of nonverbal communication [110]. This line of thought supports the universal pain experience in children as mediated more by developmental maturation than by culture.

To maximize accurate assessment of children's pain that is also culturally sensitive, recent pediatric literature highlights the benefit of self-report measures [111, 112]. The researchers from these studies took Westernized self-report assessment tools, such as the Wong-Baker FACES Scale and Oucher Scale, and created new ethnic versions of these tools for a variety of cultures (African-American, Hispanic, and Lebanese). It is also worth noting that some original Western self-report assessment tools, including the Wong-Baker FACES Scale and Poker Chip Scale, were found to be reliable and appropriate for Jordanian-Muslim children between the ages of 3 and 14 [110]. In general, the new ethnic versions of each assessment tool achieved good correlations with existing reliable measures of pain, providing support for the use of these scales. As well, it was suggested that these culturally sensitive self-report measures foster a sense of respect between the medical team and patient's family, opening further communication that may help break down stereotypical barriers.

Conclusion

This chapter has reviewed current practice standards in assessing pain in children with a focus on practice relevant to regional anesthesia. Great progress has been made in the past 25 years in the field of pain assessment in children. However, it is also clear that a dearth of information exists on pain assessment specifically relevant to regional anesthesia.

References

1. Anand KJ, Hickey PR. Halothane-morphine compared with high-dose sufentanil for anesthesia and postoperative analgesia in neonatal cardiac surgery. N Engl J Med. 1992;326:1–9.
2. Canadian Pain Society. Accreditation pain standard: making it happen. Published by the Canadian Pain Society. 2005.
3. Joint Commission. Pain assessment and management; an organizational approach. Oakbrook Terrace: Joint Commission on Accreditation of Health care Organizations; 2000.
4. Gafney A, McGrath PJ, Dick BD. Measuring pain in children: developmental and instrument issues. In: Schecter N, Berde C, Yaster M, editors. Pain in infants, children, and adolescents. Philadelphia: Lippincott Williams & Wilkins; 2003. p. 128–41.
5. Taddio A, Katz J, Ilersich AL, Koren G. Effect of neonatal circumcision on pain response during subsequent routine vaccination. Lancet. 1997;349:599–603.
6. Fitzgerald M, Shaw A, MacIntosh M. Postnatal development of the cutaneous flexor reflex: comparative study of preterm infants and newborn rat pups. Dev Med Child Neurol. 1988;30:520–6.
7. Coggeshall RE, Jennings EA, Fitzgerald M. Evidence that large myelinated primary afferent fibers make synaptic contacts in lamina II of neonatal rats. Brain Res Dev Brain Res. 1996;92:81–90.
8. Porter FL, Grunau RE, Anand KJ. Long-term effects of pain in infants. J Dev Behav Pediatr. 1999;20:253–61.
9. Woolf CJ, Mannion RJ. Neuropathic pain: aetiology, symptoms, mechanisms, and management. Lancet. 1999;35:1959–64.
10. Mannion RJ, Woolf CJ. Pain mechanisms and management: a central perspective. Clin J Pain. 2000;16:S144–56.
11. Page GG, Ben Eliyahu S. The immune-suppressive nature of pain. Semin Oncol Nurs. 1997;13:10–5.
12. Mattila-Vuori A, Salo M, Iisalo E, Pajulo O, Viljanto J. Local and systemic immune response to surgery under balanced anaesthesia in children. Pediatr Anesth. 2000;10:381–8.
13. Palermo T, Chambers C. Parent and family factors in pediatric chronic pain and disability: an integrative approach. Pain. 2005;119: 1–4.
14. American Academy of Pediatrics and American Pain Society. The assessment and management of acute pain in infants, children and adolescents. Pediatrics. 2001;108:793–7.
15. McCaffery M, Pasero C. Pain: clinical manual. 2nd ed. St. Louis: Mosby; 1999.
16. Franck L. Nursing management of children's pain: current evidence and future directions for research. NT Res. 2003;8:330–53.
17. Goldschneider KR, Anand KS. Long term consequences of pain in neonates. In: Schechter NL, Berde CB, Yaster M, editors. Pain in infants, children and adolescents. 2nd ed. Philadelphia: Lippincott Williams and Wilkins; 2003.
18. Franck LS, Greenberg CS, Steven B. Pain assessment in infants and children. Pediatr Clin N Am. 2000;47:487–512.
19. Ranger M, Johnston C, Anand K. Current controversies regarding pain assessment in neonates. Semin Perinatol. 2007;31:283–8.
20. Duhn L, Medves J. A systematic integrative review of infant pain assessment tools. Adv Neonatal Care. 2004;4:126–40.
21. Gibbins S, Stevens B. State of the art: pain assessment and management in high risk infants. Newborn Infant Nurs Rev. 2001;1: 85–96.
22. Grunau R, Johnston C, Craig K. Neonatal facial and cry responses to invasive and non-invasive procedures. Pain. 1990;42:295–305.
23. Lawrence J, Alcock D, McGrath P, Kay J, MacMurray SB, Dulberg C. The development of a tool to assess neonatal pain. Neonatal Netw. 1993;12:59–66.
24. Stevens B, Johnston C, Petryshen P, Taddio A. Premature infant pain profile; development and initial validation. Clin J Pain. 1996;12:13–22.
25. McNair C, Ballantyne M, Dionne K, Stephens D, Stevens B. Postoperative pain assessment in the neonatal intensive care unit. Arch Dis Child Fetal Neonatal Ed. 2004;89:F537–41.
26. Hummel P, Puchalski M, Creech SD, Weiss MG. Clinical reliability and validity of the N-PASS: neonatal pain, agitation and sedation scale with prolonged pain. J Perinatol. 2008;28:55–60.
27. Krechel SW, Bildner J. CRIES; a new neonatal postoperative pain measurement score. Initial testing of validity and reliability. Pediatr Anesth. 1995;5:53–61.
28. von Baeyer CL, Spagrud LJ. Systematic review if observational (behavioral) measures of pain in children and adolescents aged 3 to 18 years. Pain. 2007;127:140–50.
29. Merkel S, Voepel-Lewis T. The FLACC; a behavioural scale for scoring postoperative pain in young children. Pediatr Nurs. 1997;23:293–7.
30. Manworren R, Hynan L. Clinical validation of FLACC; preverbal patient pain scale. Pediatr Nurs. 2003;29:140–6.
31. Chambers C, Reid G, McGrath PJ, Finley A. Development and preliminary validation of a postoperative pain measure for parents. Pain. 1996;68:307–13.
32. Chambers C, Finley GA, McGrath PJ, Walsh TM. The parents' postoperative pain measure: replication and extension to 2-6-year-old children. Pain. 2003;105:437–43.
33. Stinson J, Kavanagh T, Yamada J, Gill N, Stevens B. Systematic review of the psychometric properties, interpretability and feasibility of self-report pain intensity measures for use in clinical trials in children and adolescents. Pain. 2006;125:143–57.
34. Bieri D, Reeve R, Champion GD, Addicoat L, Ziegler J. The faces pain scale for the self-assessment of the severity of pain experienced by children: development, initial validation and preliminary investigation for ratio scale properties. Pain. 1990;41: 139–50.
35. Hicks CL, von Baeyer CL, Spafford P, van Korlaar I, Goodenough B. The faces pain scale – revised: toward a common metric in pediatric pain measurement. Pain. 2001;93:173–83.
36. von Baeyer C, Spagrud L, McCormick J, Neville K, Connelly M. Three new datasets supporting the use of the numeric rating scale (NRS-11) for children's self-reports of pain intensity. Pain. 2009;143:223–7.
37. Beyer J, Aradine C. Content validity of an instrument to measure young children's perceptions of the intensity of their pain. J Pediatr Nurs. 1986;1:386–95.
38. Hester N. The preoperational child's reaction to immunization. Nurs Res. 1979;28:250–5.
39. Wong D, Baker C. Pain in children; comparison of assessment scales. Pediatr Nurs. 1988;14:9–17.
40. Chambers C, Giesbrecht K, Craig K, Bennett S, Huntsman E. A comparison of faces scales for the measurement of pediatric pain: children's and parents' ratings. Pain. 1999;83:25–35.
41. Chambers C, Hardial J, Craig K, Court C, Montgomery C. Faces scales for the measurement of postoperative pain intensity in children following minor surgery. Clin J Pain. 2005;21:277–85.
42. Huskisson EC. Visual analogue scales. In: Melzack R, editor. Pain measurement and assessment. New York: Raven Press; 1983. p. 33–7.
43. McGrath PJ, Johnson G, Goodman JT, Schillinger J, Dunn J, Chapman J. CHEOPS: a behavioral scale for rating postoperative pain in children. In: Fields HL, Dubner R, Cervero F, editors. Proceedings of the fourth world congress on pain. New York: Raven Press; 1985. p. 395–402.
44. Ambuel B, Hamlett K, Marx C, Blumer J. Assessing distress in pediatric intensive care environments: the COMFORT scale. J Pediatr Psychol. 1992;17:95–109.
45. van Dijk M, Peters JW, van Deventer P, Tibboel D. The COMFORT behavior scale: a tool for assessing pain and sedation in infants. Am J Nurs. 2005;105:33–6.

46. Johansson M, Kokinsky E. The COMFORT behavioural scale and the modified FLACC scale in pediatric intensive care. Nurs Crit Care. 2009;14:122–30.
47. Breau LM, Finley GA, McGrath PJ, Camfield CS. Validation of the non-communicating children's pain checklist – postoperative version. Anesthesiology. 2002;96:528–35.
48. Malviya S, Voepel-Lewis T, Burke C, Merkel S, Tait A. The revised FLACC observational pain tool: improved reliability and validity for pain assessment in children with cognitive impairment. Pediatr Anesth. 2006;16:258–65.
49. Chambers C, Reid GJ, Craig KD, McGrath PJ, Finley GA. Agreement between child and parent reports of pain. Clin J Pain. 1998;14:336–42.
50. Merskey H, Bogduk N. Classification of chronic pain: descriptions of chronic pain syndromes and definitions of pain terms. 2nd ed. Seattle: IASP Press; 1994.
51. McCain GC, Morwessel NJ. Pediatric nurses' knowledge and practice related to infant pain. Issues Compr Pediatr Nurs. 1995;18:277–86.
52. Fitzgerald M. Pain in infancy: some unanswered questions. Pain Rev. 1995;2:77–91.
53. Levy DM. The infant's earliest memory of inoculation: a contribution to public health procedures. J Genet Psychol. 1960;96:3.
54. Abu-Saad HH, Kroonen E, Halfens R. On the development of a multidimensional Dutch pain assessment tool for children. Pain. 1990;43:249–56.
55. Flavell JH. The developmental psychology of Jean Piaget. New York: Von Nostrand Renhold; 1963.
56. Champion GD, Arts S, Abu-Saad HH, et al. Age-related responses to brief sharp physiological (needle) pain in children. Seventh World Congress on Pain. Seattle: IASP Publications; 1993. p. 512–3.
57. Lazarus RS, Folkman S. Stress, appraisal, and coping. New York: Springer; 1984.
58. Bloom L. Language acquisition in its developmental context. In: Damon W, editor. Handbook of child psychology. 5th ed. New York: Wiley; 1998.
59. Gafney A. Pain: perspectives in childhood. Dissertation. Cork: University College, 1987.
60. Oberlander TF, O'Donnell ME, Montgomery CJ. Pain in children with significant neurological impairment. Dev Behav Pediatr. 1999;20:235–43.
61. Malviya S, Voepel-Lewis T, Tait AR, Merkel S, Lauer A, Munro H, et al. Pain management in children with and without cognitive impairment following spine fusion surgery. Pediatr Anesth. 2001;453–8.
62. Biersdorff KK. Incidence of significantly altered pain experience among individuals with developmental disabilities. Am J Ment Retard. 1994;98:619–31.
63. Gilbert-MacLeod CA, Craig KD, Rocha EM, Mathias MD. Everyday pain responses in children with and without developmental delays. J Pediatr Psychol. 2000;25:301–8.
64. Breau LM, Camfield CS, McGrath PJ, Rosmus C, Finley GA. Measuring pain accurately in children with cognitive impairments: refinement of a caregiver scale. J Pediatr. 2001;138:721–7.
65. Carter B, McArthur E, Cunliff M. Dealing with uncertainty: parental assessment of pain in children with profound special needs. J Adv Nurs. 2002;38:449–57.
66. Doherty E, Yanni G, Conroy RM, Bresnihan B. A comparison of child and parent ratings of disability and pain in juvenile chronic arthritis. J Rheumatol. 1993;20:1563–6.
67. Breau LM, Camfield CS, McGrath PJ, Finley GA. The incidence of pain in children with severe cognitive impairments. Arch Pediatr Adolesc Med. 2003;157:1219–26.
68. Schecter NL, Berde CB, Yaster M. Pain in infants, children, and adolescents: an overview. In: Schecter N, Berde C, Yaster M, editors. Pain in infants, children, and adolescents. Philadelphia: Lippincott Williams & Wilkins; 2003. p. 3–18.
69. Cipher DJ, Fernandez E. Expectancy variables predicting tolerance and avoidance of pain in chronic pain patients. Behav Res Ther. 1997;35:437–44.
70. Cheng S, Foster RL, Hester NO. A review of factors predicting children's pain experiences. Issues Comp Pediatr Nurs. 2003;26:203–16.
71. von Baeyer CL, Carlson G, Webb L. Under prediction of pain in children undergoing ear piercing. Behav Res Ther. 1997;35:399–404.
72. Foster RL, Yucha CB, Zuk J, Vojir CP. Physiologic correlates of comfort in healthy children. Pain Manag Nurs. 2003;4:23–30.
73. Foster RL, Varni JW. Measuring the quality of children's postoperative pain management: initial validation of the child/parent total quality pain management (TQPM) instruments. J Pain Symptom Manage. 2002;23:201–10.
74. Melzack R, Wall PD. The challenge of pain. New York: Basic Books; 1982.
75. Asmundson GJ, Norton GR, Allerdings MD. Fear and avoidance in dysfunctional chronic back pain patients. Pain. 1997;69:231–6.
76. Tsao JC, Lu Q, Kim SC, Zeltzer LK. Relationships among anxious symptomatology, anxiety sensitivity, and laboratory pain responsivity in children. Cogn Behav Ther. 2006;35:207–15.
77. Lu Q, Tsao JC, Myers CD, Kim SC, Zeltzer LK. Coping predictors of children's laboratory-induced pain tolerance, intensity and unpleasantness. J Pain. 2007;8:708–17.
78. Logan DE, Rose JB. Is postoperative pain a self-fulfilling prophesy? Expectancy effects on preoperative pain and patient-controlled analgesia use among adolescent surgical patients. J Pediatr Psychol. 2005;30:187–96.
79. McGrath PJ. The family is the crucible. Pain. 2008;137:471–2.
80. Finley GA, McGrath PJ, Forward SP, McNeill G, Fitzgerald P. Parents' management of children's pain following 'minor' surgery. Pain. 1996;64:83–7.
81. Forward SP, Brown TL, McGrath PJ. Mothers' attitudes and behavior toward medication children's pain. Pain. 1996;67:469–74.
82. Schecter NL, Bernstein BA, Beck A, Hart L, Scherzer L. Individual differences in children's responses to pain: role of temperament and parental characteristics. Pediatrics. 1991;87:171–7.
83. Romsing J, Walther-Larsen S. Postoperative pain in children: a survey of parents' expectations and perceptions of their children's experiences. Pediatr Anesth. 1996;6:215–8.
84. Korsch B, Cobb K, Ashe B. Pediatrician's appraisals of patients' intelligence. Pediatrics. 1961;27:990–1003.
85. McGrath PJ, Unruh A. Pain in children and adolescents. Amsterdam: Elsevier; 1987.
86. Burckhardt CS, Clark SR, O'Reilly CA, Bennett. Pain-coping strategies of women with fibromyalgia: relationship to pain, fatigue, and quality of life. J Muscle Pain. 1997;5:5–21.
87. Fisher K, Johnston M. Emotional distress and control cognitions as mediators of the impact of chronic pain on disability. Br J Health Psychol. 1998;3:225–36.
88. Schecter NL, Allen DA. Physicians' attitudes towards pain in children. J Dev Behav Pediatr. 1986;7:350–4.
89. Hauswald M, Anison C. Prescribing analgesics: the effect of patient age and physician specialty. Pediatr Emerg Care. 1997;13:262–3.
90. Triplett JL, Ameson SW. The use of verbal and tactile comfort to alleviate distress in young hospitalized children. Res Nurs Health. 1979;2:17–23.
91. Owens ME, Todt EH. Pain in infancy: neonatal response to heel lance. Pain. 1984;20:77–86.
92. Harbeck C, Perterson L. Elephants dancing in my head: a developmental approach to children's concepts of specific pains. Child Dev. 1992;63:138–49.

93. Fillingim RB. Sex-related influences on pain: a review of mechanisms and clinical implications. Rehab Psychol. 2003;48:165–74.
94. Berkley KJ. Sex differences in pain. Behav Brain Sci. 1997;20: 371–80.
95. Vallerand AH. Gender differences in pain. Image J Nurs Sch. 1995;27:235–7.
96. Unruh AM. Gender variations in clinical pain experience. Pain. 1996;65:123–67.
97. Unruh AM, Campbell MA. Gender variation in children's pain experiences. In: McGrath PJ, Finley A, editors. Chronic and recurrent pain in children and adolescents. Seattle: IASP Press; 1999. p. 199–241.
98. Myers CD, Riley JL, Robinson ME. Psychosocial contributions to sex-correlated differences in pain. Clin J Pain. 2003;19:225–32.
99. Fillingim RB, Maixner W. Gender differences in the responses to noxious stimuli. Pain Forum. 1995;4:209–21.
100. Riley JL, Robinson ME, Wise E, Myers CD, Fillingim RB. Sex differences in the perception of noxious experimental stimuli: a meta analysis. Pain. 1998;74:181–7.
101. Zeltzer LK, Fanurik D, LeBaron S. The cold pressor pain paradigm in children: feasibility of an intervention model (Part II). Pain. 1989;37:305–13.
102. Goodenough B, Kampel L, Champion GD, Laubreaux L, Nicholas MK, Ziegler JB, McInerney M. An investigation of the placebo effect and age-related factors in the report of needle pain from venipuncture in children. Pain. 1997;72:383–91.
103. Goodenough B, Thomas W, Champion GD, Perrott D, Taplin JE, von Baeyer CL, Ziegler JB. Unraveling age effects and sex differences in needle pain: ratings of sensory intensity and unpleasantness of venipuncture pain by children and their parents. Pain. 1999;80:179–90.
104. Crook J. Women and chronic pain. In: Roy R, Tunks E, editors. Chronic pain: psychosocial factors in rehabilitation. Baltimore: Williams and Williams; 1982. p. 68–78.
105. Robinson ME, Riley JL, Myers CD, Papas RK, Wise EA, Waxenberg LB, Fillingim RB. Gender role expectations of pain: relationship to sex differences in pain. J Pain. 2001;2:251–7.
106. Moon EC, Chambers CT, Larochette A-C, Hayton K, Craig KD, McGrath PJ. Sex differences in parent and child pain ratings during an experimental child pain task. Pain Res Manag. 2008;13: 225–30.
107. Adams J. A methodological study of pain assessment in Anglo and Hispanic children with cancer. In: Tayler DC, Krane EJ, editors. Advances in research and therapy, vol. 15. New York: Raven Press; 1990. p. 43–51.
108. Bohannon A. Physiological, self-report and behavioral ratings of pain in 3-to 7-year-old African American and Anglo-American children. Unpublished doctoral dissertation: University of Miami. 1995.
109. Pfefferbaum B, Adams J, Aceves J. The influence of culture on pain in Anglo and Hispanic children with cancer. J Am Acad Child Adolesc Psychiatry. 1990;29:642–7.
110. Gharaibeh M, Abu-Saad H. Cultural validation of pediatric pain assessment tools: Jordanian perspective. J Transcult Nurs. 2002;13:12–8.
111. Beyer J, Knott C. Construct validity estimation for the African-American and Hispanic versions of the Oucher Scale. J Pediatr Nurs. 1998;13:20–31.
112. Zahr L, Puzantian H, Abboud M, Abdallah A, Shahine R. Assessing procedural pain in children with cancer in Beirut, Lebanon. J Pediatr Oncol Nurs. 2006;23:311–20.

Suggested Reading

Booker PD. The assessment of pain in children. In: Dalens BJ, editor. Pediatric regional anesthesia. Boca Raton: CRC Press; 1990. p. 71–86.

Malviya S, Polaner DM, Berde C. Acute pain. In: Cote CJ, Lerman J, Todres ID, editors. A practice of anesthesia for infants and children. 4th ed. Philadelphia: WB Saunders; 2009. p. 939–49.

Pediatric Pharmacological Considerations

7

Derek Dillane

Contents

D. Dillane, MB BCh BAO, MMedSci, FCARCSI
Department of Anesthesiology and Pain Medicine,
University of Alberta, 2-150 Clinical Sciences Building,
Edmonton, AB, Canada
e-mail: dillane@ualberta.ca

B.C.H. Tsui, S. Suresh (eds.), *Pediatric Atlas of Ultrasound- and Nerve Stimulation-Guided Regional Anesthesia*,
DOI 10.1007/978-0-387-79964-3_7

7.1 Introduction

The first amino-amide local anesthetic was developed by Swedish chemists Löfgren and Lundquist in 1943, and this xylidine derivative, which they called lidocaine, was first marketed in 1948 [1]. Lidocaine has been in clinical use for almost 60 years, is the most widely used local anesthetic worldwide, and remains one of the safest and most efficacious local anesthetic agents ever manufactured. One of its main drawbacks, however, is a short duration of action. The longer acting amino-amide, bupivacaine, was synthesized by Bo af Ekenstam in 1957 and introduced into clinical practice 10 years later [2]. It would take a further 10 years of clinical use before serious cardiac toxicity was reported, and this important safety issue led to the continuing search for a long-acting and safe agent. In the 1980s, the development of new, long-acting amides took advantage of the fact that most of these molecules have a chiral center. These three-dimensional stereoisomers have an identical chemical composition but differ in spatial orientation [3]. This led to the development of the single stereoisomers levobupivacaine and ropivacaine, first approved for clinical use in 1996.

7.2 Structure and Physiochemical Properties

All local anesthetics are weak bases. They have a molecular weight ranging from 220 to 288 Da [4]. Their formula consists of a lipophilic aromatic ring connected to a hydrophilic residue by a hydrocarbon chain. They are clinically classified as amino-esters or amino-amides depending on the link between the lipophilic ring and the hydrophilic tertiary amine (Fig. 7.1). Amino-ester local anesthetics are hydrolyzed in the plasma by cholinesterases, whereas the amides are metabolized in the liver by the cytochrome P450 enzyme system. The amino-amide group is most commonly used for pediatric regional anesthesia and, as such, will be the focus of this chapter.

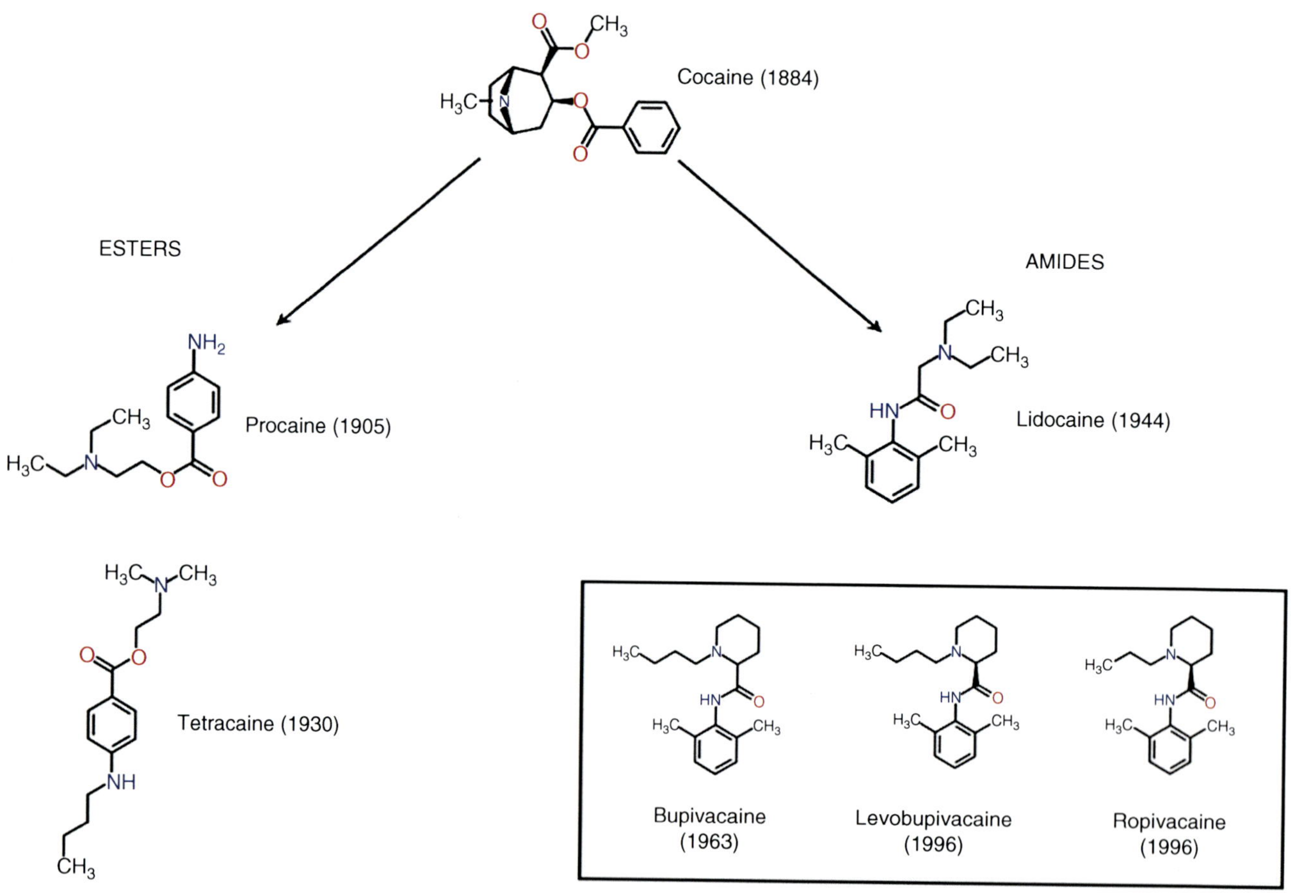

Fig. 7.1 Derivation of ester- and amide-class local anesthetics from cocaine. Shown are chemical structures and years in which each drug was first used

7.2.1 Onset of Action, Potency, and Duration

Being weak bases, local anesthetics exist in solution as both ionized (water soluble) and non-ionized (lipid soluble) molecules. Local anesthetics traverse phospholipid membranes in their non-ionized form. The degree of drug ionization is determined by the dissociation constant (pKa) and the pH of the surrounding fluid. The pKa of a molecule represents the pH at which 50 % of the molecules exist in a lipid-soluble form and 50 % in a water-soluble form. Local anesthetic molecules with a pKa that approaches physiologic pH have a higher concentration of the non-ionized lipid-soluble form. As the pKa of a drug increases, a greater proportion exists in the ionized hydrophilic form at physiological pH. Commonly used local anesthetics have a pKa between 7.8 (lidocaine) and 8.1 (ropivacaine and bupivacaine) (Table 7.1). Drugs with a lower pKa (e.g., lidocaine) exist to a greater degree in a non-ionized form and diffuse more easily across cell membranes. This explains why lidocaine has a faster *onset of action* than ropivacaine or bupivacaine. Moderately lipophilic drugs are most effective clinically due to the drug having to cross several membranes to reach its target site. At physiological pH, a significant fraction of the drug is in a non-ionized form and readily crosses the membrane to the cytosolic side of the nerve cell. Excessively lipophilic drugs remain in the first membrane encountered [6]. For the drug to effectively block the sodium channel, it must become re-ionized on the cytosolic side of the membrane.

Potency is directly related to lipid solubility which is expressed as lipid/water partition coefficient. Drugs with low lipid solubility need higher concentrations to produce a block of similar intensity to that produced by local anesthetics with higher lipid solubility (e.g., 2 % lidocaine (partition coefficient 43) vs. 0.5 % bupivacaine (partition coefficient 346)). *Duration of action* is largely determined by the degree of plasma protein binding.

Table 7.1 Comparative physicochemical properties of local anesthetics

Agent	Potency	pKa	Molecular weight (Da)	Toxic plasma concentration (μg/mL)	% protein binding
Lidocaine	1	7.8	234	>5	70
Prilocaine	1	7.8	220	>5	55
Mepivacaine	1	7.6	246	>5	77
Bupivacaine	4	8.1	288	>3	95
Levobupivacaine	4	8.1	288		>97
Ropivacaine	4	8.1	274	>4	94

Agent	% ionized at pH 7.4	Partition coefficient with h-octanol/buffer	Volume of distribution (L)	Clearance (L/min)
Lidocaine	25	43	91	0.95
Prilocaine	24	25	191	
Mepivacaine	39	21	84	9.78
Bupivacaine	17	346	73	0.47
Levobupivacaine	17	346	55	
Ropivacaine	17	115	59	0.44

7.2.2 Sodium Channel

Voltage-dependent Na^+ channels in nerves contribute to the control of membrane excitability and are responsible for action potential generation. When the cell membrane is depolarized by a few millivolts, sodium channels activate and inactivate within milliseconds (Fig. 7.2). Influx of sodium ions through the channel depolarizes the membrane further and initiates the action potential. Local anesthetics prevent neural excitation and subsequent propagation of action potential by inhibiting passage of Na^+ ions through these channels. The drug may access the Na^+ channel through the hydrophilic inner pore or traverse the hydrophobic cell membrane when the channel is closed [7]. The local anesthetic must be re-ionized to prevent passage of Na^+ ions. An equilibrium exists between the ionized and unionized forms in the Na^+ channel.

The voltage-gated sodium channel is a large, multimeric complex comprised of an α subunit and one or more smaller β subunits. The α subunit contains all the features necessary for a functional ion channel including voltage sensor, activation/inactivation gates, and ion pore. The β subunits play a role in membrane localization of the channel as well as modulation of channel gating [8]. Na^+ channels exist in a closed, open, and inactivated state [7]. Local anesthetics bind more tightly to the Na^+ channel during the open and inactivated state than the closed state. In effect, this means that they show high affinity for their site of action during high-frequency action potentials, such as those that occur during sensory transmission or motor activity [9]. This is a phenomenon known as frequency-dependent or use-dependent blockade.

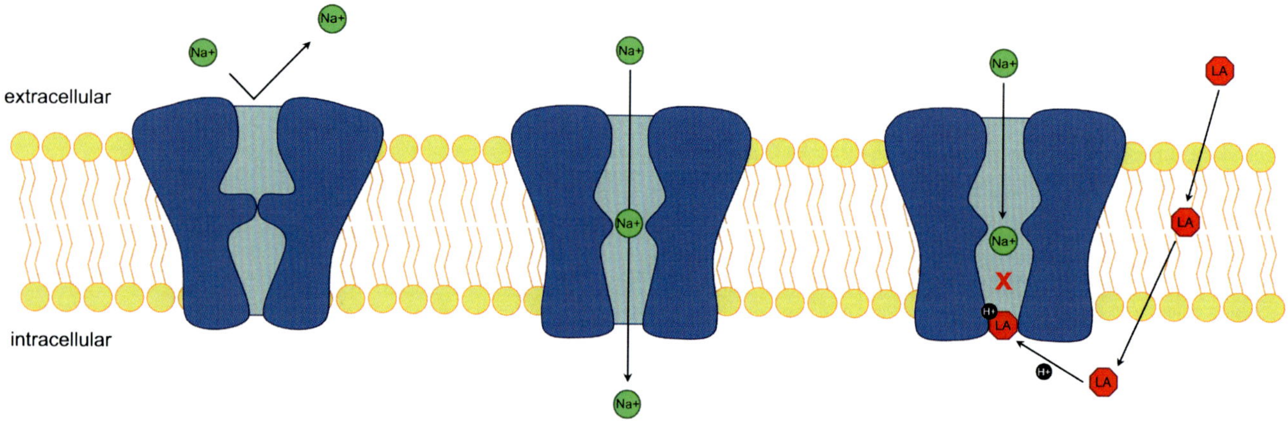

Fig. 7.2 Schematic diagram of a sodium channel in a neuron cell membrane. *Left*, the deactivated form is impermeable to sodium ions; *middle*, the activated form allows sodium ions to flow into the cell; *right*, the channel is blocked by local anesthetic. Local anesthetics traverse the phospholipid membrane in their non-ionized form. Drugs with a low pKa (e.g., lidocaine) exist to a greater degree in a non-ionized form and more readily cross the cell membrane. The drug must become re-ionized in the intracellular environment to effectively block the sodium channel

7.2.3 Physiological Considerations

The diameter and degree of myelination of a nerve fiber determines the nature of impulse conduction and the effectiveness of local anesthetic drugs. There are three major anatomical categories: myelinated somatic nerves (A fibers), myelinated preganglionic autonomic nerves (B fibers), and unmyelinated axons (C fibers). The A fibers are subdivided into four groups according to decreasing speed of impulse conduction and diameter (Table 7.2). The thinnest A fibers, the Aδ group, are responsible for pain and cold temperature transmission. Aγ fibers are responsible for muscle tone. C fibers are thinner than myelinated axons, have a much lower conduction velocity, and are also responsible for the transmission of pain signals. Aδ fibers are responsible for fast pain transmission, whereas C fibers are responsible for second or slow pain transmission [6]. Differential nerve blockade has been demonstrated in animal studies after administration of local anesthetic (i.e., fibers of smaller diameter are blocked before those of larger size with recovery from blockade occurring in the reverse order) [10]. Clinically, it is more likely that the action of local anesthetic on nerve fibers is multifactorial (e.g., peripheral versus core nerve fiber, state of activation of the nerve, length of nerve exposed to local anesthetic, and degree of myelination in addition to nerve diameter).

Myelination is not complete before the age of 12 years. The relative absence of a myelin sheath coupled with the smaller nerve fiber diameter may explain why infants and children are subject to prolonged motor blocks with local anesthetic solutions of lower concentration [4]. In addition, the endoneurium of developing nerves is loose and easily penetrated by local anesthetic molecules in both directions. This may account for both the shorter onset and shorter duration of effect of local anesthetic action in younger age groups. Beyond infancy, the endoneurium contains more connective tissue, making it more difficult for the local anesthetic to traverse [9].

Table 7.2 Classification and properties of peripheral nerve fibers

Nerve class	Aα	Aβ	Aγ	Aδ	B	C
Function	Motor	Pressure/touch	Proprioception/motor tone	Pain/temperature	Preganglionic autonomic	Pain/temperature
Diameter (μm)	12–20	5–12	1–4	1–4	1–3	0.5–1
Conduction speed (m/s)	70–120	30–70	10–30	12–30	10–15	0.5–1.2
Local anesthetic sensitivity (+++ most susceptible)	++	++	+++	+++	+++	+

7.3 Pharmacokinetics

Pharmacologists and anesthesiologists share a common interest in pharmacokinetics, but rather than being concerned with volumes of distribution and total body clearance, the pediatric anesthesiologist wants to know how much local anesthetic can be safely administered to produce an effective nerve block in a timely fashion. However, these empirical and abstract concepts are not mutually exclusive.

Unlike other therapeutic agents administered to infants and children, local anesthetics can be delivered directly to their site of action. Traditionally, a large volume and high concentration of local anesthetic has been injected to ensure adequate anesthesia and analgesia. This was, in part, due to the relatively small number of local anesthetic molecules thought to reach the target nerves. The nerve sheath or perineurium is a very effective diffusion barrier. A large fraction of the delivered agent is absorbed by the surrounding tissue or is removed by the systemic circulation. Direct measurement in an animal model demonstrates that <2–3 % of an injected dose enters the target nerve. In addition, more than 90 % of an injected dose is taken up by the systemic circulation within 30 min of injection [11]. Ultrasound guidance may allow for more accurate deposition, necessitating a smaller volume and dose of local anesthetic.

Neonates and infants present significant pharmacokinetic peculiarities possibly leading to an increased risk of toxicity. Immature hepatic metabolism and marked differences in serum protein binding serve to increase serum concentrations of unbound amide local anesthetic.

7.3.1 Absorption

Regional anesthesia in the pediatric population involves the injection of a relatively large volume of a concentrated local anesthetic solution into a compact anatomical space. The rate of absorption into the bloodstream is a major determinant of systemic toxicity. This has been studied predominantly for epidural/caudal anesthesia. Explicit detail on the kinetics of other routes of administration is lacking for this population. What is evident, though, for both central and peripheral blocks, is the more rapid rate of absorption from the cephalic parts of the body [4]; for example, a cervical epidural leads to higher plasma levels of local anesthetic than a caudal epidural. Similarly, absorption decreases from head to foot for peripheral conduction and infiltration blocks due to the relative difference in vascularity between these areas.

7.3.2 Absorption from Epidural Space

The main component of the epidural space is fat, which is an important determinant of local anesthetic systemic uptake. More lipophilic local anesthetic molecules will be retained to a greater degree by epidural fat leading to subsequent delayed absorption. It has been demonstrated in adults that after a single-shot epidural injection, 30 % of a dose of lidocaine and 50 % of a dose of bupivacaine remained in the epidural space for 3 h after injection [12]. The time to maximum peak plasma concentration (T_{max}) in infants for lidocaine and bupivacaine is 30 min after caudal or lumbar epidural injection [13]. Ropivacaine T_{max} is longer in infants than in children and longer in children compared to adults. In children aged 1–2 years, ropivacaine T_{max} is 115 min, whereas in children aged 5–8 years, ropivacaine T_{max} is closer to the adult value of 30 [14]. The vasoconstrictive properties of ropivacaine may contribute to its prolonged absorption from the epidural space. After T_{max} has been achieved, the rate of absorption slows down significantly so that it becomes longer than that of elimination, leading to a flip-flop effect in plasma drug concentration [4]. This continuous, protracted systemic absorption during the elimination phase, in combination with the buffering effect of plasma protein binding, limits the plasma concentration of unbound drug and is protective against toxicity.

7.3.3 Absorption from Other Routes of Administration

Absorption rates at different block sites are directly related to local blood flow and inversely related to local tissue binding [15]. As a consequence, plasma uptake is faster from the more vascular intercostal space or the axilla than from the caudal space. Vascular uptake of local anesthetic after intercostal nerve block occurs more rapidly than with any other regional technique [16]. Despite recently published epidemiologic data indicating up to a fivefold increase in the utilization of peripheral nerve blockade in the pediatric population, specific pharmacokinetic data are lacking [17]. Ilioinguinal-iliohypogastric nerve blockade is the only peripheral block whose kinetics have been reported with any degree of regularity. Significantly higher plasma concentrations of both bupivacaine and ropivacaine have been reported in one study following ilioinguinal-iliohypogastric nerve block as compared to caudal blockade [18]. Times to peak plasma concentration were much faster for both drugs following ilioinguinal-iliohypogastric nerve block. The narrow inter-fascial space at this block location may facilitate absorption. This, coupled with greater uptake of local anesthetic into epidural fat, may account for the lower plasma levels seen after caudal injection.

7.3.4 Distribution

Local anesthetics are distributed to the tissues and body fluid compartments after systemic absorption to the plasma. Volume of distribution (Vd) is a mathematical expression which depicts the distribution characteristics of a drug in the body. It is a measure of the degree to which a drug is delivered by the plasma to the organs and tissues of the body. Drugs with a small calculated Vd have a high concentration of drug in the plasma, have a concomitant low tissue concentration, and are more likely to accumulate to toxic levels. Drugs with a larger Vd are subject to slower elimination. Vd is influenced by degree of ionization/lipophilicity, plasma protein binding, and molecular size [19]. Since local anesthetics are weak bases that have dissociation constants (pKa values) above physiological pH, more than 75 % of the commonly used amide local anesthetic drugs exist in a hydrophilic ionized form at physiological pH (Table 7.1). Hence, they are highly water-soluble molecules but are less likely to cross lipid cell membranes. As a result of the delayed systemic absorption of local anesthetic drugs, it is impossible to calculate a volume of distribution with any accuracy. One study found bupivacaine to have a higher Vd in neonates and infants [20], which may be related to the higher fraction of unbound drug to plasma protein (see next section). Following adult epidural anesthesia, ropivacaine appears to have a smaller Vd than bupivacaine [21, 22], and indirect evidence points to a similarly reduced Vd in infants. Following single-shot caudal anesthesia, peak concentration of ropivacaine is higher than bupivacaine [23]. Two further studies have demonstrated that Vd of ropivacaine appears slightly smaller before the age of four [14, 24].

Local anesthetic is distributed to organs according to their vascular density. The local anesthetic is taken up within each organ according to the tissue-plasma partition coefficient (Table 7.3). The lungs play an important buffering role by taking the full impact of drug-laden venous blood. A variety of investigational techniques, including autoradiography, scintillation counts, and tissue assays, confirm the lung's ability to quickly extract local anesthetic [25], although this buffering action of the lung is saturable.

Table 7.3 Tissue-blood partition coefficients (lidocaine)

Organ	Tissue-plasma λ	Tissue-blood λ
Spleen	3.5	–
Lung	3.1	5.4
Kidney	2.8	–
Stomach	2.4	–
Fat	2.0	2.9
Brain	1.2	1.7
Heart	1.0	–
Muscle	0.7	0.9
Liver	0.6	2.9
Skin	0.6	–
Bone	0.4–0.9	–

Based on data from de Jong [59]

7.3.5 Plasma Protein Binding

Local anesthetics bind tightly to serum proteins, greatly limiting the free fraction of available drug. This is clinically relevant as it is only the free or unbound fraction that is bioactive (i.e., readily available to cross cell membranes to become active at the sodium channel). Volume of distribution (see above) is inversely related to protein binding. Drugs which are highly protein-bound have limited passage into tissues resulting in a high drug plasma concentration and a low Vd. In adults, lidocaine is up to 70 % protein bound while bupivacaine, levobupivacaine, and ropivacaine are over 90 % protein bound [19].

Three principal blood components are involved in local anesthetic binding: the plasma proteins alpha-1-acid glycoprotein (AAG), human serum albumin (HSA), and erythrocytes. Like most weak bases, local anesthetics bind mainly to AAG. AAG has a greater affinity for binding local anesthetic by an order of magnitude of 5,000–10,000 compared to albumin [26]. Capacity for binding is relatively low, however, and saturation occurs at clinically relevant concentrations. Even though albumin is the most abundant plasma protein (50–80 times more abundant than AAG), it has a low affinity for amide local anesthetic drugs [4]. By virtue of its enormous binding capacity (it is almost unsaturable), together with its abundance, the role of HSA becomes significant when AAG is saturated.

AAG concentration is very low at birth (less than 30 % of the adult concentration) and progressively increases to adult levels during the first year of life [5]. The unbound fraction of local anesthetic is higher during infancy which increases susceptibility to toxicity. Conversely, a consequence of this high free drug concentration is a greater hepatic clearance than would be expected with immature hepatic microsomal metabolism.

AAG is a major acute-phase protein, and its concentration rapidly increases in the first 24–48 h after surgery. The resulting AAG level *in infants* remains lower than that which is present in children and adults, but the subsequent decrease in free drug concentration may provide some protection against toxicity in the early postoperative period. This elevation in AAG levels may diminish on the third postoperative day, leading to a sudden rise in the unbound fraction, which can precipitate toxicity. A total cessation or reduction in the infusion dose of local anesthetic has been recommended in the neonatal age group beyond 48 h [9].

Affinity for red blood cells is low and not saturable. This may be considered as a buffer system when toxic concentrations occur. It is especially relevant in infants with a low AAG concentration. It is important to remember that infants have a physiologic anemia which reduces storage capacity and favors increased fraction of unbound drug [26].

7.3.6 Hepatic Metabolism

Local anesthetics undergo extensive hepatic biotransformation prior to renal excretion. Clearance is low at birth and does not reach adult levels until 6–9 months [27, 28]. The terminal half-life of amide local anesthetics is three to eight times longer in neonates when compared to adults [4]. Amide local anesthetics are metabolized in the liver by oxidative pathways involving the cytochrome P450 enzyme superfamily (Fig. 7.3). Lidocaine and bupivacaine are metabolized mainly by CYP3A4, an enzyme system which is not fully mature at birth. However, most biotransformation activities are achieved by CYP3A7, an enzyme which is present only in the fetus and during the first months of life [29].

Ropivacaine is metabolized by CYP1A2, which is not fully functional before the age of 3 years. Consequently, it is reasonable to assume that bupivacaine clearance should be at or near normal adult levels from birth and that ropivacaine clearance should be markedly deficient; however, this is not the case. Clearance of bupivacaine is markedly deficient at birth and increases slightly in the first year of life. Conversely, ropivacaine clearance is not very low at birth; however, it does not fully reach adult values before the age of 5 years [14]. This enzymatic immaturity is clinically relevant to a limited extent but does not preclude the use of local anesthetics in neonates and infants.

Only a small fraction of unmetabolized amide local anesthetic is excreted in the urine. Thus, renal dysfunction affects local anesthetic clearance less than hepatic failure, notwithstanding the accumulation of potentially harmful metabolites [25]. The clearance of one of the main metabolites of ropivacaine, 2,6-pipecoloxylidide (PPX), is decreased in uremic patients. Its cardiotoxicity in rat studies is reported as half that of bupivacaine.

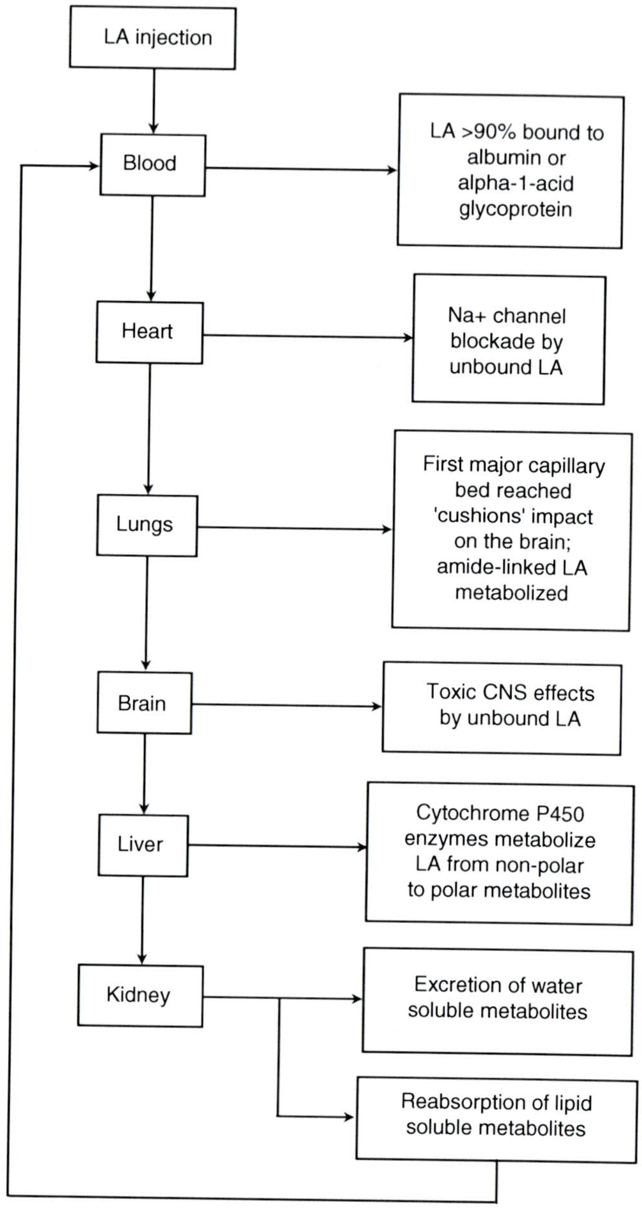

Fig. 7.3 Sites of local anesthetic action and metabolism following plasma absorption. Local anesthetic molecules are bound to plasma proteins, and this limits the free fraction of available drug. The unbound fraction is metabolized in the liver by the cytochrome p450 enzyme superfamily

7.4 Toxicity

Local anesthetics have the same toxic effects in infants and children as those seen in adults. The major toxic effects are on the cardiovascular and central nervous systems. In the adult patient, neurologic toxicity occurs at lower concentrations followed by cardiac toxicity at higher concentrations. This is not always true for bupivacaine, an assumption which may be broadened to include the entire spectrum of local anesthetic toxicity in the pediatric population. Early signs of cerebral toxicity are subjective (dizziness, drowsiness, tinnitus). These will not be related by the young or anesthetized child (and most pediatric blocks are performed under anesthesia or heavy sedation). Moreover, general anesthesia itself raises the cerebral toxicity threshold, and neuromuscular blockade will preclude the onset of generalized tonic-clonic seizures. Consequently, the first manifestation of an accidental intravascular injection or rapid absorption may be cardiovascular collapse (Table 7.4) [9].

Table 7.4 Dosage recommendations for regional blocks in pediatric patients

Route of administration	Recommended agent	Maximum dose single shot	Maximum dose reinjection	Maximum dose continuous
Caudal epidural	Bupivacaine[a] Bupivacaine with epinephrine	2 mg/kg 2.5 mg/kg	Not recommended	
Lumbar epidural	Bupivacaine with epinephrine Bupivacaine	1.25–1.75 mg/kg	0.75–1 mg/kg	Infants 1 month–1 year: 0.2–0.25 mg/kg/h 1–4 years old: 0.25–0.35 mg/kg/h 4 years: 0.25–0.4 mg/kg/h
Peripheral blocks	Lidocaine Lidocaine with epinephrine	6 mg/kg 7 mg/kg		As for lumbar epidural

[a]Use bupivacaine-equivalent doses (i.e., 1:1) for ropivacaine and levobupivacaine

7.4.1 Central Nervous System Toxicity

Local anesthetics readily cross the blood-brain barrier to disrupt cerebral function. The central toxic response is specifically related to plasma levels of local anesthetic in the central nervous system (CNS) and their effect on the complex interplay between excitatory and inhibitory pathways that facilitate neurotransmission. Initially, there is a generalized excitatory phase, as manifested by seizure activity. This initial phase appears to be the result of blocking inhibitory pathways in the amygdala which allow excitatory neurons to function unopposed. When levels of local anesthetic in the CNS increase further, both inhibitory and excitatory pathways (being more resistant to the effects of local anesthetic toxicity) are inhibited, leading to CNS depression, a reduced level of consciousness, and eventually coma.

The reported incidence of cerebral toxicity is low. Two large surveys (each greater than 20,000 regional anesthesia procedures in the pediatric population) indicate that the incidence of seizures is <0.01–0.05 % [30, 31]. There have been several case reports of children experiencing seizures after a regional anesthesia procedure, most of which involved continuous lumbar or caudal epidural anesthesia with bupivacaine [32–35]. Bupivacaine is associated with seizures at blood levels as low as 4.5–5.5 μg/mL. Rather alarmingly on occasion, these toxic blood levels were reached even after adhering to the recommended therapeutic range [32, 34]. Cerebral toxicity is associated with lidocaine, prilocaine, and mepivacaine at blood levels of 5–10 μg/mL.

7.4.2 Cardiac Toxicity

The potentially devastating sequelae of cardiovascular toxicity may be the first manifestation of local anesthetic toxicity in infants and children, although the overall incidence in this population is remarkably low. Several large series of regional anesthesia procedures in infants and children report no cases of cardiovascular toxicity [32, 35–37]. A prospective study of more than 24,000 regional anesthesia procedures reported four patients who developed a cardiac arrhythmia, and none of these progressed to cardiac arrest or collapse [31].

For obvious ethical reasons, most available information on this subject comes from animal studies and case reports. The principal mechanism relates to the blockade of myocardial voltage-dependent sodium channels leading to an increase in the PR interval and QRS duration, provoking a dose-dependent prolongation of conduction time and eventual depression of spontaneous pacemaker activity. Persistent sodium channel blockade predisposes to reentrant arrhythmias. Subtle T-wave changes on the electrocardiogram may progress to ventricular arrhythmias, the most malignant being torsades de pointes. These arrhythmias may subsequently be followed by ventricular fibrillation. Alternatively, profound bradycardia may ensue, followed by asystole [4]. Because of their higher heart rate, neonates and infants may be more susceptible to the use-dependent blockade of sodium channels produced by bupivacaine. These electrophysiological effects are compounded by a direct negative inotropic effect of local anesthetic drugs. A number of the reported fatalities due to cardiovascular toxicity resulting from the use of bupivacaine in caudal anesthesia were associated with doses in excess of the recommended therapeutic range [38, 39]. Nevertheless, there have been reports of cardiovascular collapse requiring resuscitation in infants who received caudally administered bupivacaine within the recommended dose range [40, 41].

The levorotatory isomer (S-) of bupivacaine has less potential for cardiac toxicity than the dextrorotatory one (R+) or racemic mixture of both [25]. This led to the development of the single stereoisomers levobupivacaine and ropivacaine. It has been purported that lidocaine blocks sodium channels in a "fast-in/fast-out" fashion, whereas bupivacaine blocks these channels in either a "slow-in/slow-out" manner in low concentrations or a "fast-in/slow-out" manner at higher concentrations [42]. Ropivacaine, on the other hand, has been shown to block sodium channels in a "fast-in/medium-out" fashion [43]. The dissociation constant (between ligand and receptor) for bupivacaine is almost ten times longer than that of lidocaine, resulting in a prolonged and near irreversible cardiac depressant effect [42]. There is a positive correlation between local anesthetic lipid solubility and inhibition of cardiac contractility – further evidence for the clinically relevant finding that ropivacaine is less toxic than racemic bupivacaine [44]. In vitro studies appear to concur with animal studies which have demonstrated that bupivacaine has the most potent myocardial depressant effect, followed by ropivacaine and lidocaine [45].

The true equipotency ratio between the enantiomeric agents has been the subject of much conjecture. Results from a number of animal and clinical studies would suggest a rank order of potency of ropivacaine < levobupivacaine < bupivacaine [3]. This suggests that any theoretical cardioprotective benefit derived from ropivacaine would be negated by the clinical need for higher doses due to its lower potency. The difference in potency does not appear to be clinically relevant for surgical blocks (both peripheral and epidural) when the newer agents are used at concentrations of 0.5–0.75 %, with the clinical profile of the nerve block being similar to that obtained with racemic bupivacaine. However, the lower potency of ropivacaine becomes relevant when used for postoperative analgesia with both epidural and continuous peripheral nerve blockade. For this application, 0.2 % ropivacaine appears to be as effective as 0.125–0.15 % levobupivacaine, which in turn is identical to racemic bupivacaine [3].

7.4.3 Treatment of Toxicity

Immediate intervention at the earliest sign of toxicity is of prime importance and improves the chances of successful treatment. General supportive measures are warranted, including Advanced Life Support Guidelines (ACLS) and more specific measures directed at local anesthetic toxicity. All patients subject to a regional anesthesia procedure must have electrocardiography, pulse oximetry, and blood pressure monitoring. Acute morbidity from seizure activity is due in large part to airway complications. Hypoxia, hypercarbia, and acidosis all worsen prognosis. Consequently, airway control must be achieved prior to management of seizure activity. Seizure control can be achieved with midazolam (0.05–0.2 mg/kg) or small doses of propofol if there are no signs of cardiovascular instability. The approach to cardiovascular collapse must be similarly methodical and must prioritize oxygenation and ventilation. Increasing the heart rate may be imperative in infants especially in the presence of profound intraventricular block. Though contentious as to its effect on long-term survival, epinephrine has been recommended for the treatment of cardiac toxicity [4, 46]; however, careful titration is required with individual boluses of less than 1 μg/kg in order to avoid ventricular fibrillation or tachycardia. Vasopressin is contraindicated for the treatment of local anesthetic-induced cardiovascular collapse.

Experimental animal studies and clinical case reports suggest that lipid emulsion is effective in the reversal of local anesthetic toxicity [47–49]. Intralipid® 20 % is a Food and Drug Administration-approved hyperalimentation source comprised of soybean oil, glycerol, and egg phospholipids. The mechanism of action of lipid emulsion in the reversal of local anesthetic toxicity has not been fully elucidated but may act as a circulating lipid sink extracting lipophilic local anesthetic from plasma or tissues [50]. Alternatively, it may facilitate the reversal of local anesthetic inhibition of myocardial fatty acid oxidation, thereby restoring the myocardial adenosine triphosphate (ATP) supply [51]. Lipid emulsion may act as a direct inotrope by increasing intracellular myocardial calcium [52]. Weinberg et al. conducted the original research involving the successful resuscitation of rats in whom cardiovascular collapse was induced with intravenous bupivacaine [47], and these findings were successfully repeated in a canine model of bupivacaine toxicity [50]. It would take a further 8 years after publication of the original animal studies before the appearance of the first clinical case report of the successful use of lipid emulsion in the treatment of bupivacaine-induced cardiac toxicity [48]. Its successful use has subsequently been reported for the treatment of toxicity induced by ropivacaine [53], levobupivacaine [54], and mepivacaine [55, 56]. It has had a favorable outcome in the treatment of a 13-year-old child when administered for ropivacaine- and lidocaine-induced ventricular arrhythmia following posterior lumbar plexus blockade [57].

Intralipid 20 % should be administered as a bolus of 1.5 mL/kg over 1 min followed immediately by an infusion at a rate of 0.25 mL/kg/min. It is important that chest compressions continue to allow the lipid to circulate. Two further boluses of 1.5 mL/kg with 5 min between boluses may be considered if the initial response is inadequate. The infusion may be continued until hemodynamic stability is restored. The rate may be increased to 0.5 mL/kg if blood pressure remains low (Fig. 7.4).

In light of the current evidence, it would appear prudent to ensure immediate availability of Intralipid 20 % in areas where regional anesthesia is performed. For patients in cardiac arrest due to local anesthetic toxicity and who are being resuscitated following current ACLS guidelines, it is appropriate to administer lipid emulsion. It is equally justifiable to administer lipid emulsion to patients displaying overt neurologic toxicity in an attempt to preempt cardiac toxicity.

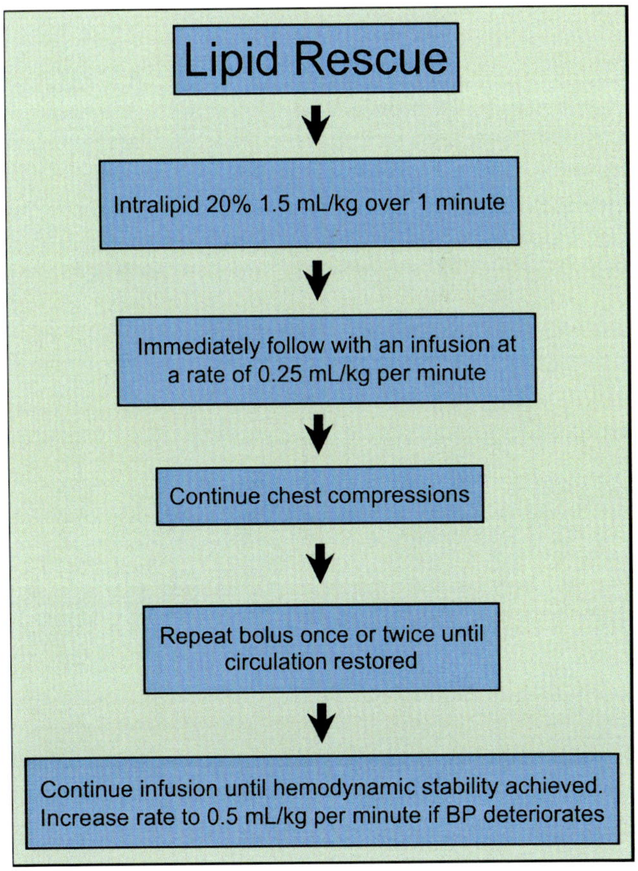

Fig. 7.4 Pathway for use of Intralipid® in treating local anesthetic toxicity

7.4.4 Prevention of Toxicity

Unintentionally high blood levels of local anesthetic lead to a spectrum of neurological and cardiac complications with potentially devastating effect. This usually results from unintentional intravascular injection and may be prevented by careful observation of a number of safety steps. Slow, incremental injection of an appropriate dose of a safe agent should be standard practice. The dose should be determined according to age and lean body mass and modified according to physical status. Higher plasma concentrations may occur after injection into a vascular area. There are no corresponding pediatric data, but in adults, the highest plasma levels are achieved after intercostal nerve blocks, followed by caudal, epidural, brachial plexus, femoral, and sciatic blockade. The use of a vasoconstrictor will serve to reduce the rate of uptake in addition to prolonging the block. An epinephrine concentration of 1:200,000 or less is appropriate. The authors prefer to add epinephrine (1:200,000) to a dextrose solution, the primary purpose of which is ultrasonographic observation of the spread of injectate. This is used in 0.5–1 mL increments as a test dose prior to injection of local anesthetic. A rise in heart rate of ten beats per minute or more is indicative of intravascular injection.

The use of ultrasound-guided regional anesthesia may be as important for local anesthetic systemic toxicity as the pharmacological advances of previous decades. For the first time in the century-old practice of regional anesthesia, it is now possible to visualize the target neural structure, potential vascular hazards, and the spread of local anesthetic solution. This allows for more accurate deposition of smaller volumes of local anesthetic. The largest registry in the ultrasound era (over 25,000 peripheral nerve blocks) reports a reduction in local anesthetic systemic toxicity of 65 % when ultrasound guidance is used [58]. The use of ultrasound does not negate the need for the more conventional safety mechanisms but when used in combination with them makes for an entirely more scientific proposition.

7.5 Dosing

- Clearance is reduced in infants less than 6 months of age, and dosing must be modified accordingly.
- Infants less than 6 months have a larger Vd. Despite this, care is needed with reinjection and infusion. When the compartments are saturated, the reduced drug clearance in this age group can rapidly lead to toxic drug levels.
- After 1–2 years of age, the higher ratio of liver volume to total body volume leads to a higher clearance ratio. It is safe to administer higher doses than in adults.
- In children over 30 kg, regardless of age, dose should be reduced to adult dose.
- Local anesthetic doses need to be modified in the presence of pathology which affects drug clearance (e.g., liver or cardiac disease).

References

1. Löfgren N, Lundqvist B. Studies on local anaesthetics II. Svensk Kemisk Tidskrift. 1946;58:206–17.
2. Ekenstam BEB, Petterson G. Local anaesthetics: I. N-alkyl pyrrolidine and N-alkyl piperidine carboxylic acid amides. Acta Chem Scand. 1957;11:1183–90.
3. Casati A, Putzu M. Bupivacaine, levobupivacaine and ropivacaine: are they clinically different? Best Pract Res Clin Anaesthesiol. 2005;19:247–68.
4. Mazoit JX. Pharmacology of local anesthetics. In: Bissonnette BJD, editor. Pediatric anesthesia: principles and practice. 1st ed. New York: McGraw-Hill; 2002. p. 302–37.
5. Mazoit J-X, Lonnqvist P-A. Local anesthetics and their adjuncts. In: Hatch S, editor. Textbook of pediatric anesthesia. 3rd ed. Boca Raton: CRC Press; 2007. p. 211–25.
6. Schulman JM, Strichartz GR. Local anesthetic pharmacology. In: Golan DE, Tashjian Jr AH, Armstrong EJ, Armstrong AW, editors. Principles of pharmacology. 3rd ed. Philadelphia: Lippincott Williams & Wilkins; 2012. p. 147–60.
7. Bruhova I, Tikhonov DB, Zhorov BS. Access and binding of local anesthetics in the closed sodium channel. Mol Pharmacol. 2008;74:1033–45.
8. Amir R, Argoff CE, Bennett GJ, Cummins TR, Durieux ME, Gerner P, et al. The role of sodium channels in chronic inflammatory and neuropathic pain. J Pain. 2006;7:S1–29.
9. Ramamurthi RJ, Krane EJ. Local anesthetic pharmacology in pediatric anesthesia. Tech Reg Anesth Pain Manag. 2007;11:229–34.
10. Strichartz GR, Pastijn E, Sugimoto K. Neural physiology and local anesthetic action. In: Cousins MJ, Carr DB, Horlocker TT, Bridenbaugh PO, editors. Neural blockade in clinical anesthesia and pain medicine. 4th ed. Philadelphia: Lippincott Williams & Wilkins; 2009. p. 26–47.
11. Berde C. Local anesthetics in infants and children: an update. Pediatr Anesth. 2004;14:387–93.
12. Burm AG, Vermeulen NP, van Kleef JW, de Boer AG, Spierdijk J, Breimer DD. Pharmacokinetics of lignocaine and bupivacaine in surgical patients following epidural administration. Simultaneous investigation of absorption and disposition kinetics using stable isotopes. Clin Pharmacokinet. 1987;13:191–203.
13. Mazoit JX, Dalens BJ. Pharmacokinetics of local anaesthetics in infants and children. Clin Pharmacokinet. 2004;43:17–32.
14. Lonnqvist PA, Westrin P, Larsson BA, Olsson GL, Lybeck A, Huledal G, et al. Ropivacaine pharmacokinetics after caudal block in 1-8 year old children. Br J Anaesth. 2000;85:506–11.
15. Tucker GT. Pharmacokinetics of local anaesthetics. Br J Anaesth. 1986;58:717–31.
16. Rothstein P, Arthur GR, Feldman HS, Kopf GS, Covino BG. Bupivacaine for intercostal nerve blocks in children: blood concentrations and pharmacokinetics. Anesth Analg. 1986;65:625–32.
17. Rochette A, Dadure C, Raux O, Capdevila X. Changing trends in paediatric regional anaesthetic practice in recent years. Curr Opin Anaesthesiol. 2009;22:374–7.
18. Ala-Kokko TI, Karinen J, Raiha E, Kiviluoma K, Alahuhta S. Pharmacokinetics of 0.75% ropivacaine and 0.5% bupivacaine

after ilioinguinal-iliohypogastric nerve block in children. Br J Anaesth. 2002;89:438–41.
19. Stoelting RK, Hillier SC. Pharmacokinetics and pharmacodynamics of injected and inhaled drugs. In: Stoelting RK, Hillier SC, editors. Pharmacology and physiology in anesthetic practice. 4th ed. Philadelphia: Lippincott Williams & Wilkins; 2006. p. 3–41.
20. Mazoit JX, Denson DD, Samii K. Pharmacokinetics of bupivacaine following caudal anesthesia in infants. Anesthesiology. 1988;68: 387–91.
21. Emanuelsson BM, Zaric D, Nydahl PA, Axelsson KH. Pharmacokinetics of ropivacaine and bupivacaine during 21 hours of continuous epidural infusion in healthy male volunteers. Anesth Analg. 1995;81:1163–8.
22. Morrison LM, Emanuelsson BM, McClure JH, Pollok AJ, McKeown DW, Brockway M, et al. Efficacy and kinetics of extradural ropivacaine: comparison with bupivacaine. Br J Anaesth. 1994;72:164–9.
23. Luz G, Innerhofer P, Haussler B, Oswald E, Salner E, Sparr H. Comparison of ropivacaine 0.1% and 0.2% with bupivacaine 0.2% for single-shot caudal anaesthesia in children. Pediatr Anesth. 2000;10:499–504.
24. Hansen TG, Ilett KF, Reid C, Lim SI, Hackett LP, Bergesio R. Caudal ropivacaine in infants: population pharmacokinetics and plasma concentrations. Anesthesiology. 2001;94:579–84.
25. Aberg G. Toxicological and local anaesthetic effects of optically active isomers of two local anaesthetic compounds. Acta Pharmacol Toxicol (Copenh). 1972;31:273–86.
26. Dalens BJ, Truchon R. Neural blockade for pediatric surgery. In: Cousins MJ, Carr DB, Horlocker TT, Bridenbaugh PO, editors. Neural blockade in clinical anesthesia and pain medicine. 4th ed. Philadelphia: Lippincott Williams & Wilkins; 2009. p. 595–629.
27. Dalens BJ, Mazoit JX. Adverse effects of regional anaesthesia in children. Drug Saf. 1998;19:251–68.
28. Luz G, Innerhofer P, Bachmann B, Frischhut B, Menardi G, Benzer A. Bupivacaine plasma concentrations during continuous epidural anesthesia in infants and children. Anesth Analg. 1996; 82:231–4.
29. Mazoit JX, Baujard C. Paediatric caudal and epidural analgesia. Curr Opin Anaesthesiol. 2002;15:533–6.
30. Berde CB. Convulsions associated with pediatric regional anesthesia. Anesth Analg. 1992;75:164–6.
31. Giaufre E, Dalens B, Gombert A. Epidemiology and morbidity of regional anesthesia in children: a one-year prospective survey of the French-Language Society of Pediatric Anesthesiologists. Anesth Analg. 1996;83:904–12.
32. Bosenberg AT. Epidural analgesia for major neonatal surgery. Pediatr Anesth. 1998;8:479–83.
33. Agarwal R, Gutlove DP, Lockhart CH. Seizures occurring in pediatric patients receiving continuous infusion of bupivacaine. Anesth Analg. 1992;75:284–6.
34. Peutrell JM, Hughes DG. A grand mal convulsion in a child in association with a continuous epidural infusion of bupivacaine. Anaesthesia. 1995;50:563–4.
35. Wood CE, Goresky GV, Klassen KA, Kuwahara B, Neil SG. Complications of continuous epidural infusions for postoperative analgesia in children. Can J Anesth. 1994;41:613–20.
36. Dalens B, Hasnaoui A. Caudal anesthesia in pediatric surgery: success rate and adverse effects in 750 consecutive patients. Anesth Analg. 1989;68:83–9.
37. Veyckemans F, Van Obbergh LJ, Gouverneur JM. Lessons from 1100 pediatric caudal blocks in a teaching hospital. Reg Anesth. 1992;17:119–25.
38. McGown RG. Caudal analgesia in children. Five hundred cases for procedures below the diaphragm. Anaesthesia. 1982;37: 806–18.
39. Matsumiya N, Dohi S, Takahashi H, Kondo Y, Naito H. Cardiovascular collapse in an infant after caudal anesthesia with a lidocaine-epinephrine solution. Anesth Analg. 1986;65:1074–6.
40. Ved SA, Pinosky M, Nicodemus H. Ventricular tachycardia and brief cardiovascular collapse in two infants after caudal anesthesia using a bupivacaine-epinephrine solution. Anesthesiology. 1993;79: 1121–3.
41. Freid EB, Bailey AG, Valley RD. Electrocardiographic and hemodynamic changes associated with unintentional intravascular injection of bupivacaine with epinephrine in infants. Anesthesiology. 1993;79:394–8.
42. Clarkson CW, Hondeghem LM. Mechanism for bupivacaine depression of cardiac conduction: fast block of sodium channels during the action potential with slow recovery from block during diastole. Anesthesiology. 1985;62:396–405.
43. Veering BT. Complications and local anaesthetic toxicity in regional anaesthesia. Curr Opin Anaesthesiol. 2003;16:455–9.
44. Heavner JE. Cardiac toxicity of local anesthetics in the intact isolated heart model: a review. Reg Anesth Pain Med. 2002;27: 545–55.
45. Reiz S, Haggmark S, Johansson G, Nath S. Cardiotoxicity of ropivacaine–a new amide local anaesthetic agent. Acta Anaesthesiol Scand. 1989;33:93–8.
46. Carpenter TC, Stenmark KR. High-dose epinephrine is not superior to standard-dose epinephrine in pediatric in-hospital cardiopulmonary arrest. Pediatrics. 1997;99:403–8.
47. Weinberg GL, VadeBoncouer T, Ramaraju GA, Garcia-Amaro MF, Cwik MJ. Pretreatment or resuscitation with a lipid infusion shifts the dose-response to bupivacaine-induced asystole in rats. Anesthesiology. 1998;88:1071–5.
48. Rosenblatt MA, Abel M, Fischer GW, Itzkovich CJ, Eisenkraft JB. Successful use of a 20% lipid emulsion to resuscitate a patient after a presumed bupivacaine-related cardiac arrest. Anesthesiology. 2006;105:217–8.
49. Weinberg G. LipidRescue. 2012. Available from: www.lipidrescue.org.
50. Weinberg G, Ripper R, Feinstein DL, Hoffman W. Lipid emulsion infusion rescues dogs from bupivacaine-induced cardiac toxicity. Reg Anesth Pain Med. 2003;28:198–202.
51. Picard J, Meek T. Lipid emulsion to treat overdose of local anaesthetic: the gift of the glob. Anaesthesia. 2006;61:107–9.
52. Ozcan MS, Weinberg G. Intravenous lipid emulsion for the treatment of drug toxicity. J Intensive Care Med. 2014;29:59–70.
53. Litz RJ, Popp M, Stehr SN, Koch T. Successful resuscitation of a patient with ropivacaine-induced asystole after axillary plexus block using lipid infusion. Anaesthesia. 2006;61:800–1.
54. Foxall G, McCahon R, Lamb J, Hardman JG, Bedforth NM. Levobupivacaine-induced seizures and cardiovascular collapse treated with intralipid. Anaesthesia. 2007;62:516–8.
55. Litz RJ, Roessel T, Heller AR, Stehr SN. Reversal of central nervous system and cardiac toxicity after local anesthetic intoxication by lipid emulsion injection. Anesth Analg. 2008;106:1575–7.
56. Warren JA, Thoma RB, Georgescu A, Shah SJ. Intravenous lipid infusion in the successful resuscitation of local anesthetic-induced cardiovascular collapse after supraclavicular brachial plexus block. Anesth Analg. 2008;106:1578–80.
57. Ludot H, Tharin JY, Belouadah M, Mazoit JX, Malinovsky JM. Successful resuscitation after ropivacaine and lidocaine-induced ventricular arrhythmia following posterior lumbar plexus block in a child. Anesth Analg. 2008;106:1572–4.
58. Barrington MJ, Kluger R. Ultrasound guidance reduces the risk of local anesthetic systemic toxicity following peripheral nerve blockade. Reg Anesth Pain Med. 2013;38:289–97.
59. de Jong RH, editor. Local anesthetics. St. Louis: Mosby-Year Book; 1994. p. 165.

Suggested Reading

Ecoffey C. Narcotics and non-narcotic analgesics. In: Dalens BJ, editor. Pediatric regional anesthesia. Boca Raton: CRC Press Inc.; 1990. p. 127–41.

Haberer JP, Dalens BJ. Local anesthetics and additives. In: Dalens BJ, editor. Pediatric regional anesthesia. Boca Raton: CRC Press Inc.; 1990. p. 91–126.

Mather SJ. Biology and pharmacology: some differences. In: Peutrell JM, Mather SJ, editors. Regional anaesthesia for babies and children. Oxford: Oxford University Press; 1997. p. 33–48.

Murat I. Pharmacology. In: Dalens B, editor. Regional anesthesia in infants, children, and adolescents. Philadelphia: Lippincott Williams & Wilkins; 1995. p. 67–125.

Suresh S, Polaner DM, Cote CJ. Regional Anesthesia. In: Cote CJ, Lerman J, Anderson BJ, Eds. 5th ed. Philadelphia: WB Saunders; 2013. p. 835–879.

Complications of Regional Anesthesia in the Pediatric Population

8

Adam M. Dryden and Ban C.H. Tsui

Contents

A.M. Dryden, MD, FRCPC
Department of Anesthesiology and Pain Medicine,
University of Alberta Hospital, Edmonton, AB, Canada
e-mail: dryden@ualberta.ca

B.C.H. Tsui, Dip Eng, BSc (Math), B Pharm, MSc, MD, FRCPC (✉)
Department of Anesthesiology and Pain Medicine,
Stollery Children's Hospital/University of Alberta Hospital,
2-150 Clinical Sciences Building, Edmonton, AB T6G 2G3, Canada
e-mail: btsui@ualberta.ca

B.C.H. Tsui, S. Suresh (eds.), *Pediatric Atlas of Ultrasound- and Nerve Stimulation-Guided Regional Anesthesia*,
DOI 10.1007/978-0-387-79964-3_8

8.1 General Principles

An adverse event rarely occurs as a result of a single factor (Fig. 8.1). Rather, complications occur as a result of an accumulation of factors spanning multiple domains. Thus, it is critical that all steps be taken to mitigate risk as best as possible to decrease the likelihood of an adverse event. The most important factors for prevention are the patient, the practitioner, the place, the procedure, and, finally, proper consent (Table 8.1).

Not all patients are ideal candidates for regional anesthesia, and one needs to select their patient carefully (Table 8.2). A complete anesthetic history must be sought prior to deciding which anesthetic options to offer the patient and their family. Patient-specific contraindications to regional anesthesia have been covered in other chapters. In short, extra consideration must be given to patients with respiratory difficulties, hemodynamic disturbances, cardiac abnormalities, clotting disorders, or preexisting neurological conditions prior to offering a regional technique. One must be prepared to detail the extraordinary risks of performing a block in a patient who may have relative contraindications to a particular technique and to communicate these risks to the family in a relevant manner. Preexisting deficits must be documented prior to undertaking a procedure. Careful consideration must be given to the behavioral tendencies of a child when regional anesthesia is offered as the sole modality of anesthesia, and the practitioner must be prepared to induce general anesthesia at any point should the child become uncooperative during the procedure. When an awake block is placed in a pediatric patient, the patient and parents should be given the option of having the parents present for reassurance and guidance during the procedure. Additionally, patients who are unable to tolerate a likely adverse event should not be offered a particular procedure (e.g., an interscalene block in a patient with poor respiratory reserve).

Prior to performing a block, the anesthetist should be highly skilled in regional technique or be under the direct guidance of a well-trained regional anesthetist. Familiarity with the equipment and the drugs alone are not enough to facilitate a safe block. When performing a block, there are always many possible outcomes, and the practitioner should have the requisite skill to anticipate and manage each and every one of the outcomes. Anesthetists performing regional anesthesia in a pediatric patient should know how to use the technology and tools at hand to decrease the chances of an adverse outcome.

Blocks must be placed in the safest environment possible. The majority of pediatric blocks are placed under general anesthesia, and as such the standard monitors must be placed prior to the initiation of any block. For those regional techniques performed in the awake pediatric patient, we advocate for the procedure being done in the operating room or in a dedicated block area. Again, the patient must have complete cardiopulmonary monitoring throughout all stages of the block. Resuscitation equipment and drugs must be readily available wherever regional anesthesia is being performed. Monitoring by well-trained staff must also be available in the postanesthetic recovery unit. The nursing staff must be familiar with the blocks being performed and know when and who to call for assistance. They must be able to reassure the child who wakes up with inability to move or with numbness from a block placed for postoperative analgesia. Finally, staff should be able to recognize an adverse event as early as possible since early recognition and diagnosis will facilitate the best outcomes for the child.

The safest and least invasive procedure should be chosen to accomplish a given task. As a general rule, distal blocks tend to produce fewer and less severe adverse outcomes than proximal or central blocks. Regional anesthesia should be induced with as few needle passes as possible. To facilitate this, we always recommend the use of nerve stimulators and appropriate ultrasound probes (as detailed in each of the block chapters) when possible. There has been much discussion in the literature attempting to characterize the additional level of safety offered by these technological advances, although there is still insufficient evidence to support this conclusion [1]. Despite this, block placement based solely on landmarks, paresthesia, and loss of resistance is difficult to endorse when these technological modalities have revolutionized the practice of regional anesthesia [2].

Finally, consent should be discussed with the patient and the parents, and this discussion should be documented. Serious complications such as convulsions, cardiac toxicity, spinal cord/nerve injury leading to paralysis or neurologic deficit, pneumothorax, hematoma, infection, cardiac arrest, and death must be disclosed, although less than half of anesthetists routinely disclose these risks prior to a neuraxial or peripheral nerve block [3]. Less serious, but common, adverse effects (e.g., nausea, pruritus, urinary retention) should also be disclosed. Pediatric patients should be as involved in the discussion and decision as appropriately possible. The steps involved in performing a block must be explained in age-appropriate language; this is especially true should the block be performed in an awake child. The decision to accept the risks of a regional anesthesia procedure ultimately lie with the parents and the child, and their views must be respected. Although time is often extremely limited, establishing good patient rapport is critical. This is especially true should an adverse event occur. Litigation often occurs with an adverse event in the setting of poor communication. Should an adverse event occur, disclosure should be as immediate, thorough, and truthful as possible. The management plan for the complication should be outlined with assurance that the best interests of the child are paramount.

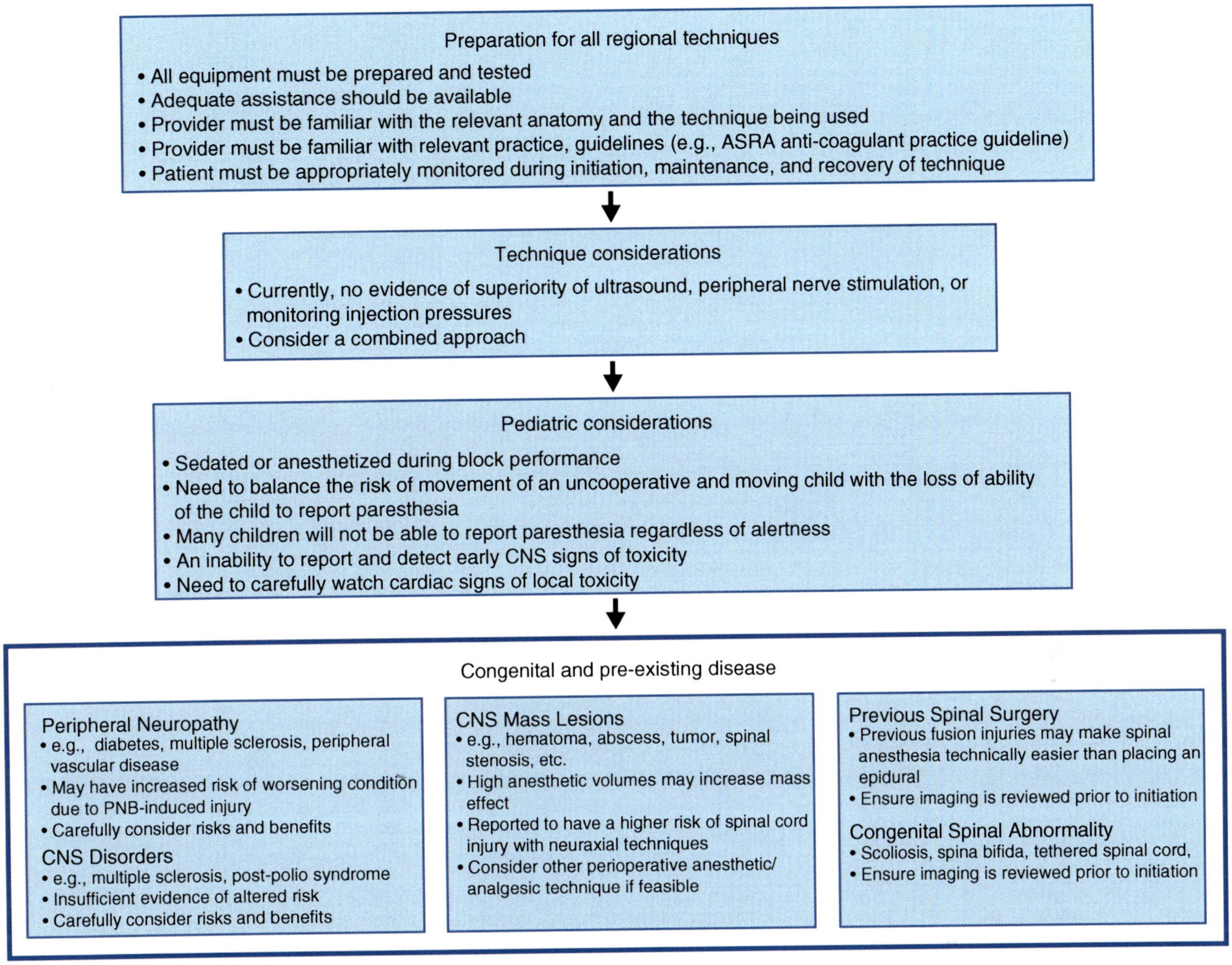

Fig. 8.1 General principles for performing regional anesthesia in pediatric patients

Table 8.1 Maintaining a standard of care during regional anesthesia practice

Maintaining standard of care
• Preoperative patient selection
• Appropriate parental and parent consent
• Using appropriate equipment and technique
• Monitoring regional anesthesia practice
• Accurate and meticulous anesthesia documentation
• Postoperative communication and follow-up visit

Table 8.2 Patient selection factors

Factors involved in patient selection	Relative contraindications	Absolute contraindications
Patient cooperation	Consider safety of maintaining catheter postoperatively when using a continuous catheter technique	Parental and patient refusal
Anatomic and physiologic considerations	Anatomical anomalies; technical challenges: small structures	
Anesthetic considerations		Lack of experience and skills; lack of appropriate equipment for performing the block (e.g., nerve stimulator, ultrasound, proper size of needle); lack of appropriate equipment for resuscitation and monitoring (e.g., oxygen, mask, drugs, etc.)
Coexisting diseases	Preexisting progressive neurological disease; comatose states; sepsis; coagulopathy	Infection at the site of injection; allergy to local anesthetics; coagulopathy [although an International Normalized Ratio (INR) of <2 is acceptable for ophthalmic procedures]
Surgical procedures	Lengthy procedures that outlast the duration of action of the local anesthetic (single injection techniques – should consider performing block at the end of the procedure)	

8.2 Adverse Events Related to Local Anesthetics

8.2.1 Allergic Reactions

8.2.1.1 Introduction

True allergic reactions to local anesthetics are, thankfully, rare. The full spectrum of allergic signs and symptoms ranging from skin irritation to anaphylaxis are indeed possible, though reports are scarce [4, 5]. The likelihood of an allergic reaction is higher with local anesthetics belonging to the amino-ester class. Reactions to preservatives (e.g., methylparaben, metabisulfite) are also possible [6].

8.2.1.2 Prevention

Preventing a de novo allergic reaction is not possible. One must, however, ensure that a detailed history is taken from the patient and parents detailing previous exposures to local anesthetics (e.g., dentist's appointments, emergency room visits) and that the chart is reviewed for documented allergies. When a family history of an allergic reaction to a local anesthetic is provided, the anesthetist should fully characterize the incident, including the offending agent and the consequence thereof. A positive family history does not preclude the use of a particular agent but should increase the level of vigilance in monitoring for a possible adverse event.

One can, however, prevent a mild local reaction from transforming into an anaphylactic reaction with careful monitoring and early intervention. As the majority of blocks are performed in the deeply sedated or anesthetized child, careful monitoring of the site of injection is required for early recognition of local reactions. Continuous cardiopulmonary monitoring is required during the initial stages of a block, and particular attention should be made to ventilator pressures (in the ventilated child), as bronchospasm can occur prior to hemodynamic alterations.

8.2.1.3 Management

The management of an allergic reaction should be tailored to the presentation. For mild local reactions (e.g., pruritus, erythema), an antihistamine is often sufficient in children who cannot tolerate the symptoms. When the symptoms remain mild but become systemic (e.g., nausea, vomiting), then one should consider the addition of a corticosteroid to systemic and complete (i.e., H1 and H2 receptors) antihistamine blockade. Finally, true anaphylaxis (e.g., hypotension, bronchospasm) should be managed as per Pediatric Advanced Life Support guidelines with maintenance of a patent airway, supplemental oxygenation, and cardiovascular support, bearing in mind that anaphylaxis requires epinephrine (0.01 mg/kg s.c. or i.m.) for successful treatment.

8.2.2 Systemic Toxic Reactions

8.2.2.1 Introduction

As with allergic reactions, severe systemic toxic reactions to local anesthetics are so exceedingly rare that quantification of the risks of such a reaction is virtually impossible. In three studies that attempted quantification, each with an excess of 20,000 patients, the occurrence of such events was estimated at less than 0.05 % [7–9]. The specific presentations included in this category include cardiovascular disturbances (both electrical and hemodynamic) as well as neural insults (seizures and neurotoxicity).

8.2.2.2 Prevention

The pattern of systemic toxic reactions is no different in children than it is in adults, but the presentation can be vastly different. One of the major reasons for this is that when a child is heavily sedated or anesthetized, initial irritability and seizures will not be evident when performing initial blocks. The first signs may in fact be dysrhythmias, hypotension, or even cardiac arrest. The ability to detect inadvertent intravascular injection of local anesthetics is also altered in the pediatric population. Resting heart rates in neonates and infants are so high that a bolus dose of a local anesthetic with epinephrine does not increase the heart rate to a reliably detectable level [10, 11]. Some advocate for vagolysis with atropine prior to injection of epinephrine containing local anesthetic to increase the sensitivity of intravascular injection, while others advocate for the use of isoproterenol [12, 13]. Monitoring T wave height may also provide an early warning system for a systemic toxic reaction (Fig. 8.2). Indeed, detecting an increase in impedance with a nerve stimulator following an injection of D5W prior to the administration of a local anesthetic can be used to rule out intravascular injection [14, 15]. At the very least, one must carefully aspirate prior to the injection of a local anesthetic and repeat the aspiration after any change in needle position.

In any event, it is important for the clinician to recognize the early CNS indicators of inadvertent intravascular injection, as they may occur during continuous anesthetic infusion via peripheral or epidural catheters (Table 8.3).

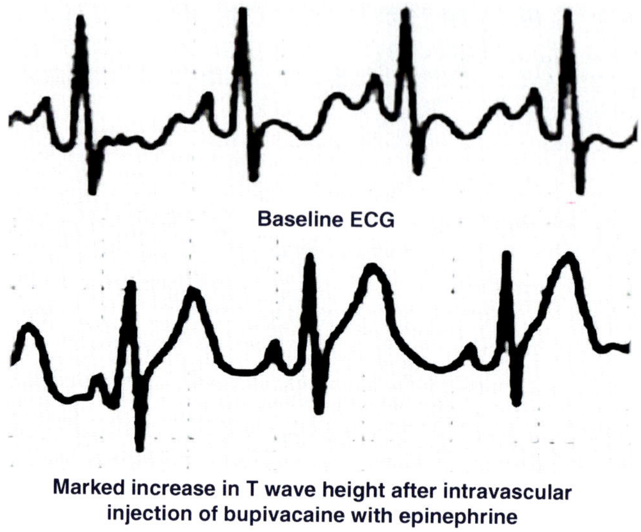

Fig. 8.2 Representative ECG readings showing normal baseline ECG (*top*) and ECG after intravascular injection of local anesthetic (*bottom*). Monitoring T wave height can help warn of systemic local anesthetic toxicity

Table 8.3 Signs of early accidental intravascular injection during continuous local anesthetic infusion

Early signs[a]	Late signs
• Light-headedness	• Muscle twitching
• Tinnitus	• Drowsiness
• Blurred vision	• Generalized tonic-clonic convulsions
• Perioral numbness	

[a]Detection of these signs can be challenging due to communication barriers with pediatric patients

8.2.2.3 Nervous System Toxicity and Management

The toxicity to the nervous system from local anesthetics comes in two forms: CNS toxicity (seizures) and local neural toxicity. Fortunately, the incidence of each remains rare. In two large studies, the incidence of seizures or convulsions following any regional anesthesia in infants and children was estimated at 0.01–0.05 % [9]. Case reports, however, are present in the literature. In one of the first accounts of the use of a caudal block in children with lidocaine, convulsions were reported in two children [16]. Seizures caused by bupivacaine have been also reported in association with continuous infusions [17, 18] and after a top up [19].

The management of seizures induced by local anesthetics remains unclear. There has been a case report of the successful halting of a bupivacaine-induced seizure with a dose of phenytoin [20]. Since the incidence is so low, it is difficult to devise standardized management recommendations. One must always be guided by basic resuscitation principles (i.e., circulation, airway, breathing). The particular agent used to halt seizure activity will be guided by local practice patterns and personal comfort – there is no conclusive evidence for the use of phenytoin compared to benzodiazepines. There are early reports that the use of lipid emulsions may halt seizure activity in an adult patient [21], although this has not yet been reported in the pediatric population. This treatment modality has the advantage of possibly aborting the syndrome of local anesthetic systemic toxicity and preventing the development of life-threatening cardiovascular consequences. Nevertheless, insufficient evidence exists for this method to be uniformly recommended.

Local anesthetics are also directly toxic to neural structures and can result in an irreversible blockade if used at high enough concentrations [22]. Reports suggestive of direct local anesthetic toxicity are difficult to tease out of the literature, and neurological injuries reported are more likely due to direct injury by needles or ischemia from embolized air as a result of a loss of resistance technique. Some have suggested that the young pediatric patient may, theoretically, be at a higher risk for neural toxicity as myelination is not complete until at least two years of age. In children, there is always the possibility that our ability to detect neural injury is lower since we must rely solely on clinical exams and parental history for detection. Furthermore, the plasticity of the nervous system is so great in these patients that the insult may be fully recovered before it was ever detected. Regardless, long-term morbidity is not evident from direct toxicity from local anesthetics.

8.2.2.4 Cardiovascular Toxicity and Management

Cardiovascular toxicity of local anesthetics is the final step in the presentation of local anesthetic toxicity and, as such, is one of the rarest manifestations. In a prospective study performed by Giaufre et al. [9] of over 24,000 infants and children, only four dysrhythmias (0.017 %) were reported, which is within the same order of magnitude reported by a previous retrospective study [23].

Local anesthetics exert their effect by blocking sodium channels. A portion of this block is a use-dependent block – the faster the sodium channels cycle through open, closed, and inactivated conformations, the higher the probability that they will be blocked by the anesthetic. It is this same mechanism that contributes to the dysrhythmias induced by local anesthetics. In case reports, the predominant pattern of presentation of cardiac toxicity in infants and children is ST-segment elevation followed by elevation of T waves and subsequent bradycardia and ventricular dysrhythmias [11, 24, 25]. Complete cardiovascular collapse follows [26].

The initial steps to managing a patient in which local anesthetic systemic toxicity is suspected are no different than any other resuscitation. Airway, respiratory, and cardiovascular support as outlined by Pediatric Advanced Life Support should be followed. A helpful mnemonic, SAVED (*S*top injection, *A*irway, *V*entilation, *E*valuate circulation, *D*rugs; Fig. 8.3), was published in the adult literature and is also relevant in the pediatric population [27]. Once the patient's airway is appropriately controlled and the respiratory status has been optimized, the next step is management of the cardiovascular toxicity. As the child presenting with cardiovascular toxicity is often bradycardic and hypotensive, appropriate support in the form of fluid boluses (10–20 mL/kg of an isotonic crystalloid), epinephrine (0.01 mg/kg), and chest compressions should be provided.

One of the more novel methods of treating cardiovascular toxicity is the use of a lipid emulsion such as Intralipid® (see Chap. 7). Recent studies demonstrate improved hemodynamics and survival in animal models of bupivacaine toxicity with the administration of intravenous lipid emulsion [28, 29]. There are two proposed mechanisms of action. One is that the lipid emulsions function to remove local anesthetic molecules from binding sites responsible for cardiovascular depression [30], effectively acting as a "sink" for the anesthetic drug. Evidence also exists that lipid emulsions act by reversing the local anesthetic inhibition on myocardial fatty acid oxidation [31]. By doing this, they restore myocardial adenosine triphosphate supplies, allowing the cardiomyocytes to regain normal electrical and mechanical function. In the adult population, the use of lipid emulsions has been reported to treat local anesthetic-induced cardiac arrest due to bupivacaine, levobupivacaine, ropivacaine, and mepivacaine [32–34]. The use of lipid emulsions in pediatrics has only recently been reported. The first report of the use of lipid emulsions in a pediatric patient was in a 13-year-old girl by Ludot et al. [35]. Fifteen minutes after placing a posterior lumbar plexus block with lidocaine and ropivacaine under general anesthesia, a wide, complex tachycardia was noted and attributed to the use of local anesthetics. A 20 % lipid emulsion was administered at a dose of 3 mL/kg resulting in the restoration of normal hemodynamic parameters and a normalization of the electrocardiogram. Since then, Shah et al. [36] have reported the successful use of a 20 % lipid emulsion at a dose of 2 mL/kg to reverse hypotension and tachycardia attributed to the use of bupivacaine, which was not responsive to two doses of epinephrine (0.02 mg/kg) in a 40-day-old male infant. Currently, the upper limit of safe dosing is unclear, and whether ideal dosing varies among neonates, infants, and children is still unclear. Moreover, whether doses need to be adjusted in those with comorbidities has also not been elucidated. At this time, the recommended dosing for Intralipid® 20 % is a bolus of 1.5 mL/kg i.v. over 1 min, followed by infusion of 0.25 mL/kg/min. Compressions should be maintained to circulate the lipid. Bolus doses can be administered every 3–5 min to a total of 3 mL/kg. Lipid emulsions should be administered (during resuscitation) to patients in cardiac arrest due to local anesthetic toxicity and perhaps even preemptively to those exhibiting neurologic toxicity.

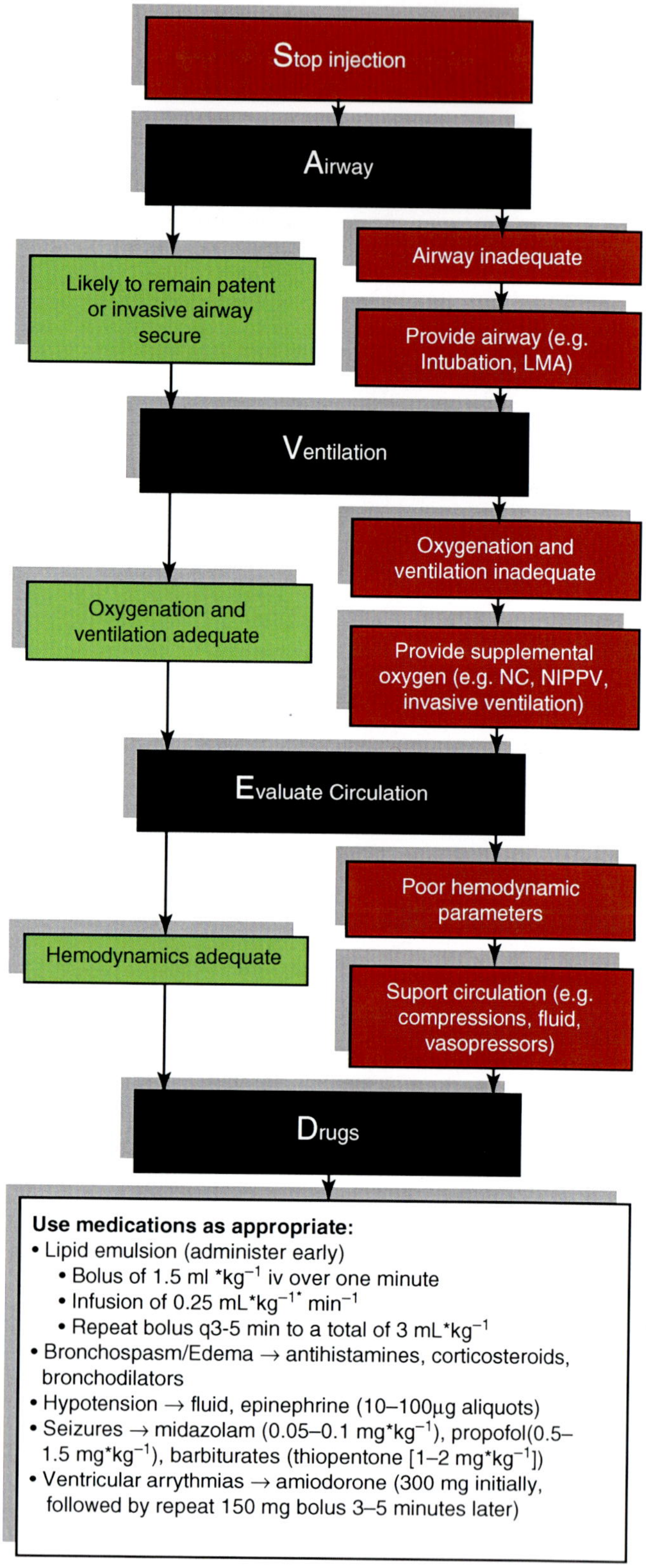

Fig. 8.3 The SAVED pathway for management of local anesthetic systemic toxicity

8.2.2.5 Summary

Serious adverse events resulting from the use of local anesthetics remain quite rare. Management guidelines are as scarce as the case reports which support them. That being said, when faced with a case of local anesthetic systemic toxicity or an allergic reaction, the consequences are dire and are true anesthetic emergencies. Basic principles in the management of adverse events from local anesthetics include [37]:

- Bronchodilators, antihistamines, and corticosteroids are often required in the treatment of allergic reactions.
- Endotracheal intubation and ventilation are required to correct acidosis and prevent hypoxia and hypercarbia, which can further worsen the child's condition.
- Profound hypotension can occur in both allergic reactions and systemic toxicity and can respond to fluid boluses and vasopressors (e.g., epinephrine).
- Decreased cardiac contractility is a core feature and can be improved with epinephrine.
- Chest compressions and defibrillation are often required to restore organ perfusion and should be instituted as necessary.
- Effective resuscitation in this setting is difficult, and atrioventricular pacing and cardiopulmonary bypass are additional options in refractory cases.
- Lipid emulsion therapy can be lifesaving and can be considered early. Lipid emulsions should be available in locations where local anesthetics are used in potentially toxic doses, regardless of the age of the patient [38].
- Seizures can be managed with benzodiazepines, propofol, barbiturates, or phenytoin. Lipid emulsions are an emerging therapy for seizure treatment in this context.

8.3 Complications Related to Regional Anesthesia Equipment

8.3.1 Introduction

Ideally, any piece of equipment introduced into our repertoire will function to decrease the overall morbidity and mortality of performing any procedure. While many of the tools used in regional anesthesia are designed to do just that, there are always new and sometimes unexpected complications introduced with every new piece of technology. We also cannot ignore the fact that the basic instrument of regional anesthesia, the hollow needle, is a fundamentally risky device. The reports of harm to children from the equipment routinely used to perform blocks are exceedingly rare, and the large safety studies done to date in this patient population reveal an excellent safety record.

8.3.2 Adverse Events Caused by Needles

8.3.2.1 Needle Trauma to the Peripheral Nerve

In a prospective study of over 24,000 patients, not one permanent peripheral neural injury was reported as a result of needle penetration [9]. In an adult population, Auroy et al. [39] reported an incidence of permanent nerve injury caused by peripheral nerve blocks to be about 0.02 %, and this finding has been validated in a smaller, more recent study [40]. Assuming that the incidence is similar in the pediatric population, one would have expected that perhaps five to ten pediatric patients in large safety studies would have experienced permanent neural injury, but this has not been the case. There are several possible reasons for this. Perhaps our ability to detect neural injury is diminished in the young child, as history may prove less reliable and is not available in the infant or neonate. In the adult patient, neural injury is almost always accompanied with paresthesia or pain upon injection of local anesthetic, which raises suspicion of intraneural injection and neural trauma. This reporting is not possible in the sedated or anesthetized child and is perhaps unreliable in the immature child; as a result, we do not go looking for transient or permanent neural injuries. In the adult patient, however, there is insubstantial evidence that performing nerve blocks in awake patients results in less neural injury than performing them in anesthetized patients [41]. It is also possible that the child's immature nervous system is able to adapt to a neural insult and recover function before it is detectable.

Our ability to prevent peripheral neural trauma may account for the low incidence. Needle selection is one particular method of prevention (Table 8.4). Common sense dictates that damage caused by a small-gauge needle is less than that caused by a larger-gauge one. The recommendation for the use of blunt needles in regional anesthesia was made by Selander et al. [42] in 1977. It was thought that blunt needles were less likely to penetrate neural structures and that resultant intraneural injections would be less likely. Although there are no clinical trials supporting recommendations as to what type of needle is best for regional anesthesia procedures in any age range, small-gauge, short, blunt needles are recommended if possible. The likelihood of neural damage can also be decreased with low injection pressures. Even if the needle is placed within the nerve sheath, the majority of trauma may be related to the pressure of injection. Rapid, high-pressure injections should be avoided. A practical way to do this is to aspirate air above the injectate in a syringe and to monitor the volume of the air during injection using a compressed air injection technique (CAIT) (Chap. 1, Fig. 1.9). Injection pressure should be decreased if the volume of air decreases to less than half of its original volume [43]. Finally, one would assume that one of the primary modalities of preventing neural injury would be to use either nerve stimulation or ultrasound to rule out intraneural injection. While we recommend the use of both of these technologies (as described elsewhere in this book), it remains difficult to prove that they in fact decrease intraneural injection and neural trauma from needles [37, 44]. Neural damage as a result of peripheral nerve blocks is rare, and as such, demonstrating the safest approach will prove difficult.

As discussed in Chap. 2, recent literature has suggested that by measuring differences in electrical impedance of tissues, it may be possible to distinguish between extraneural and intraneural injection during administration of peripheral nerve blocks. This difference in impedance is thought to relate to the different tissue compositions and water contents of extraneural and intraneural tissue. However, further research is needed to determine whether this technique can be utilized in peripheral nerve blocks in humans as a method to avoid intraneural injection.

Regardless of the safety record of needles with respect to the peripheral nerve, when neurological sequelae are present in a child who has undergone a regional anesthesia procedure, it is the duty of the anesthesiologist to rule out iatrogenic neural injury. Neural symptoms can include motor, sensory, and autonomic dysfunction in a specific neural territory. When these symptoms are found, other causes must be considered. Patient positioning, surgical trauma, and tourniquet application are all possible causes and must be considered. Neural injury caused by the needle may not necessarily be due to laceration, but rather to high-pressure injections which may cause mechanical destruction of the neural fascicular architecture, damage, and subsequent scarring [45]. As indicated previously in this chapter, the substance being injected is also a potential source of injury.

Thus, when a neurologic injury is suspected, a thorough history must be taken, a complete physical examination must be performed and documented, and all stages of the operative period scrutinized. Consultation should be sought with neurological specialists to determine the best and quickest way to achieve a diagnosis. During this time, disclosure to the patient and parents must be timely and thorough. Oftentimes, imaging in the form of an MRI is the primary modality of diagnosis. The anesthesiologist, neurologist, neurosurgeon, and radiologist must work as a team to arrive at a diagnosis before permanent injury occurs. Electrodiagnostic techniques (such as nerve conduction studies, electromyography and evoked potentials) can also be useful under the guidance of a neurologist. Experience from the adult population suggests that should a neurological deficit persist at the time of discharge, most will resolve in 4–6 weeks, and the majority (>99 %) are resolved within one year. The paucity of reports from the pediatric literature suggests that permanent peripheral nerve injury is almost unheard of.

Table 8.4 Suggested methods/equipment for reducing nerve injuries when performing regional anesthesia

Methods/equipment for reducing the risk of nerve injuries
• Needle type: small gauge, short beveled
• Patient: awake with appropriate level of sedation
• Nerve stimulation: use accurate nerve stimulators and insulated nerve needles (current ≥0.2 mA)
• Ultrasound: direct visualization of nerves and surrounding structures by using high-resolution ultrasound equipment if available
• Paresthesia: injection should be stopped and needle repositioned if persistent
• High injection pressure: avoid rapid and high-pressure injections (pressure <20 psi)
• Local anesthetic: avoid high concentrations (i.e., lidocaine 2 % or bupivacaine 0.75 %)

8.3.2.2 Needle Trauma to the Spinal Cord

Spinal cord injury following a peripheral or neuraxial block is a feared complication. In the adult literature, there are multiple examples of permanent spinal cord injuries following peripheral nerve blocks [46–48]. There are, however, no such case reports in the pediatric literature. In the 2010 ADARPEF study, complications from over 30,000 regional anesthesia procedures were reported over a 1-year period, and not one permanent spinal cord injury was reported [8]. This is in contrast to the reporting of one permanent neurological deficit in a 3-month-old child in a study following over 10,000 epidurals over a 5-year period [49].

Prevention of needle trauma to the spinal cord is critical. In adults, most cases of permanent neuraxial injury involve deviations from recommended practice. As such, when deviating from the standard practice, the anesthetist should consider it carefully and document the justification for doing so. One of the key ways of preventing neuraxial injury is to increase the distance of the needle from the spinal cord by performing a peripheral block. There are already reports [8] of a large shift away from neuraxial techniques in favor of peripheral blocks in pediatric regional anesthesia. One particular institution reported a decrease in the use of neuraxial anesthesia in pediatric patients from 97 to 24.9 % of cases over the past 17 years [50]. Although placement of epidurals in anesthetized adults remains controversial [41, 51–53], it seems quite clear that this practice is the accepted – and safe – standard in the pediatric population. The reason for this disparity remains unclear.

Knowing the position of the needle tip at all times is key to the prevention of spinal cord injury. This begins with a well-studied technique and a detailed understanding of the anatomy involved for performance of a particular block. Even with technological aids, placing needles without the prerequisite knowledge is tempting fate. Although difficult to prove from the literature, techniques involving nerve stimulation and ultrasound for monitoring needle tip placement are useful tools. As described in other chapters, both techniques can be used for a variety of peripheral and neuraxial procedures and have the potential to decrease the likelihood of a devastating spinal cord injury.

Should it occur, there is no specific treatment for primary needle damage to the spinal cord. When suspected, the initial step in the management of spinal cord injury is the recognition and identification of neural dysfunction. It is important to rule out acute and reversible causes of spinal cord injury (Fig. 8.4). This includes nerve compression from hematomas, as they must be identified and dealt with early (within 6–8 h) to avoid the development of permanent paraplegia or quadriplegia. All causes of neural injury must be investigated, including surgical causes (ligation of spinal cord vessels during abdominal or thoracic surgery, injury to the femoral nerve during pelvic surgery, injury to the lateral cutaneous nerve of the thigh during retraction near the inguinal ligament, and fibular head pressure causing neurapraxia of the lateral popliteal nerve), patient positioning, preexisting conditions, and the regional anesthesia procedure. As with peripheral nerve injuries, neurology and radiology specialists must be consulted immediately and a team approach used to arrive at the correct diagnosis. Each of these specialties has a very useful body of knowledge when dealing with these situations. An emergent MRI is often used to arrive at the correct diagnosis, and management is often guided by the consultant neurologist and neurosurgeon.

Fig. 8.4 Decision tree for management of neural dysfunction and possible spinal cord injury

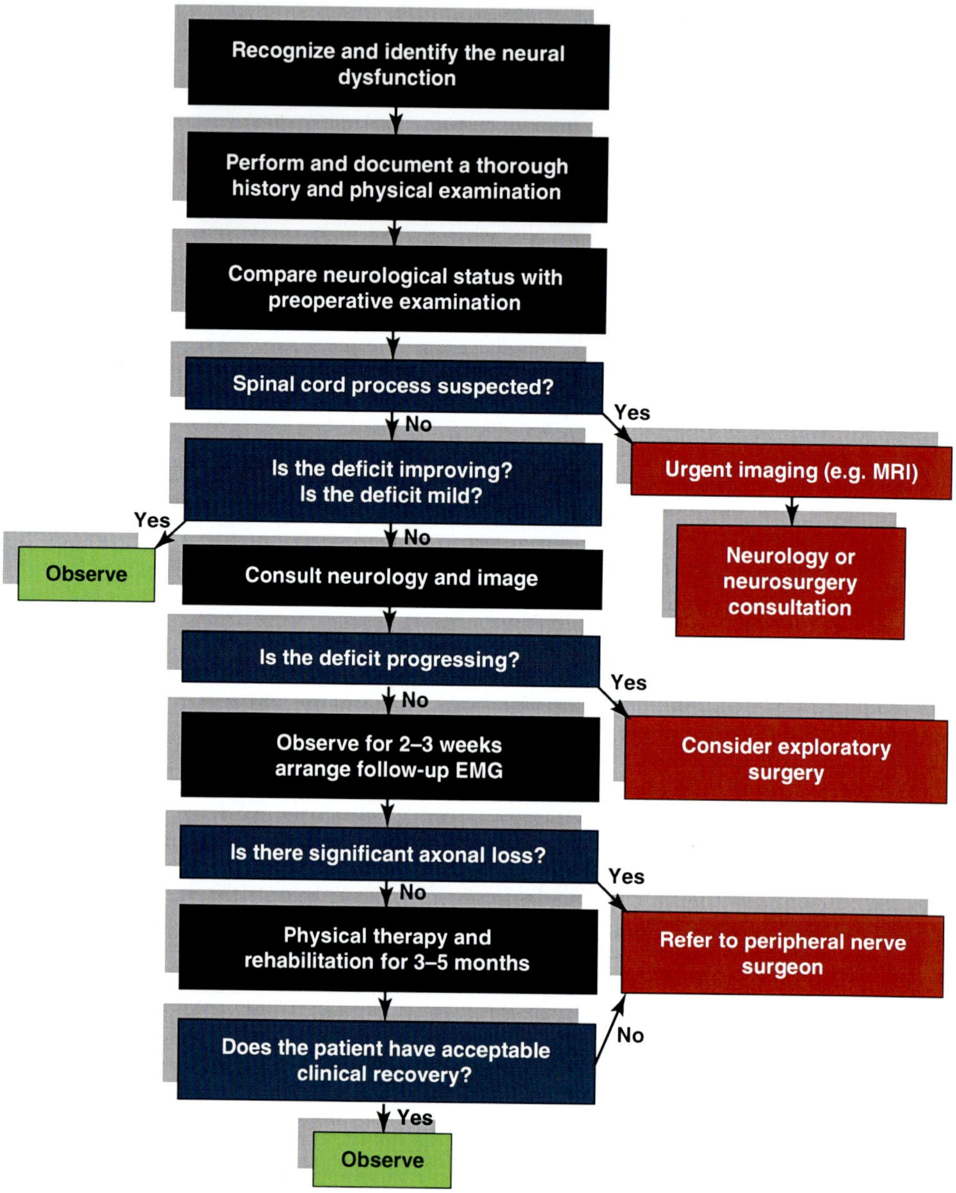

8.3.2.3 Needle Trauma to Pleura

Regional techniques involving needles moving towards the lung, particularly the supraclavicular approach, involve the risk of pneumothorax. The risk of pneumothorax in the pediatric population is difficult to quantify, and it is even difficult to glean from the adult literature, with some studies reporting incidences in the range of 5 % and others quoting positive radiologic evidence in up to 25 % of patients [54, 55]. Other approaches to the brachial plexus are often sought for this very reason. With the advent of ultrasound, there is renewed interest in the supraclavicular block. In a series [56] of 40 children (>5 years old), 40 ultrasound-guided supraclavicular blocks were placed without a clinically significant pneumothorax, and Pande et al. [57] reported the successful use of ultrasound in performing nearly 200 supraclavicular blocks without incidence of pneumothorax. These studies are too small to detect the true incidence but provide evidence that the practice of supraclavicular blocks is being revisited with some success.

As always, a detailed understanding of the anatomy can help prevent a pneumothorax. Simultaneously visualizing the pleura and the needle moving towards the target can decrease the likelihood of a pneumothorax. These blocks should never be placed bilaterally. When performing high risk blocks on patients scheduled for same-day surgery, the signs and symptoms of pneumothorax (sudden onset chest pain, shortness of breath) should be clearly conveyed to the patient and parents, and they should be instructed to present to their nearest emergency department should these symptoms occur. Using ultrasound to detect pneumothorax has been well described in the adult population, but there is no data for such use in the pediatric literature (Fig. 8.5).

In the event of a pneumothorax, the patient should be placed on 100 % oxygen until stabilized, and positive pressure ventilation should be halted as soon as feasible. Continuous monitoring is required in the initial stages to rule out the presence of a tension pneumothorax leading to cardiovascular collapse. N_2O should also be avoided as it can result in an increase in pneumothorax size. A chest tube or pleural catheter is often required if the lung has lost approximately one-fourth of its volume. Needle decompression may be required in the event of a tension pneumothorax while thoracostomy supplies are being prepared.

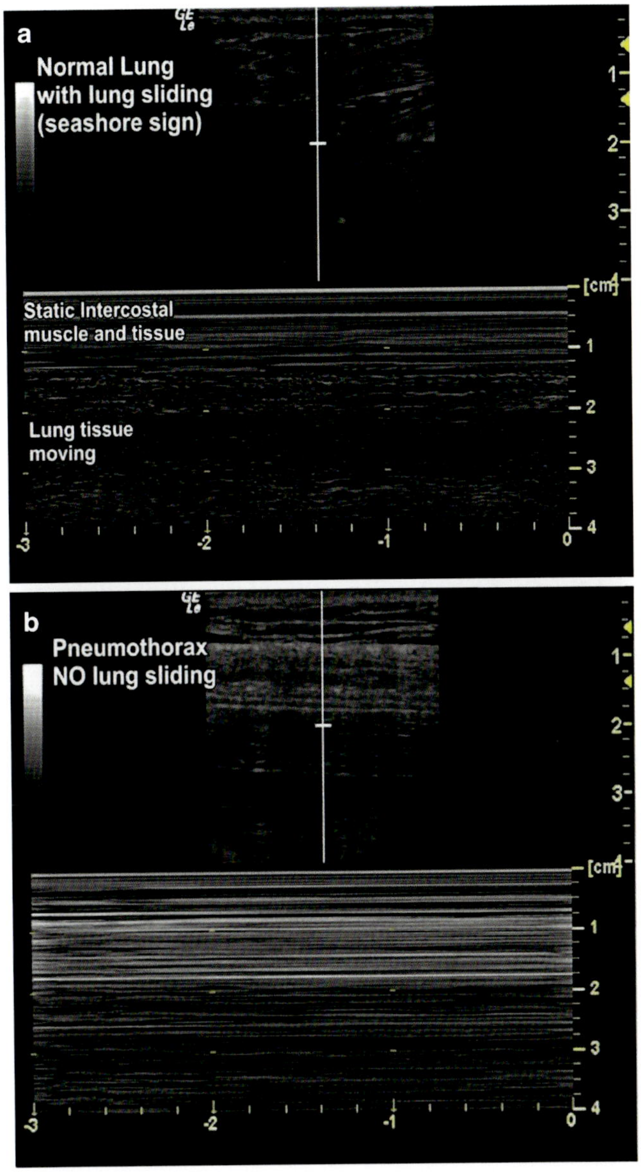

Fig. 8.5 Ultrasound images of lung sliding to assess for pneumothorax. Normal lung sliding (**a**) can be visualized on ultrasound; in the case of needle trauma to the pleura, lung sliding can no longer be visualized (**b**), suggesting possible pneumothorax

8.3.3 Adverse Events Caused by Nerve Stimulators

Patients undergoing a regional anesthesia procedure can describe the sensation from nerve stimulators in a variety of ways. Words such as "funny," "tingly," "tapping," and sometimes even "pain" are used. Both patients and parents will often ask if the electricity from the nerve stimulator is harmful in any way. There are no published reports of any harm caused by nerve stimulators in any population. Nerve stimulators have the ability to malfunction, but there are no instances of electricity-induced burns or neurapraxia reported. Nerve stimulators can therefore be considered a piece of equipment that only adds to the safety of the regional anesthetic procedure being performed.

8.3.4 Adverse Events Caused by Ultrasound Probes

Whenever an imaging modality is suggested, the potential harm from ionizing radiation that has been publicized springs to mind. This is especially true in the minds of parents looking to prevent long-term sequelae from medical procedures. As detailed in Chap. 3, ultrasound probes do not produce ionizing radiation; rather, they use high-frequency sound waves to generate echoes and subsequent images. Ultrasound waves have the potential to transfer energy by increasing the rate of vibration of the substrate being examined. In fact, this is a common therapeutic tool in physiotherapy. At the wavelengths and powers typically used in regional anesthetic practice, this effect is negligible and there are no reports of an ultrasound-induced burn.

Ultrasound probes may incite a false sense of security when placing an unfamiliar block, leading to unnecessary risk. We advocate for the use of ultrasound whenever possible, but only in the hands of a practitioner who also has the requisite anatomic and procedural knowledge coupled with the experience (or under the guidance of an anesthetist with the experience) to place the block in the safest way possible and to manage potential complications. Ultrasound probes can also act as a fomite. We recommend following manufacturers' guidelines to sterilize ultrasound probes between patients and to always cover the ultrasound probe in a sterile fashion when placing blocks (see Chap. 4).

8.3.5 Summary

Much of the potential harm in regional anesthesia arises from the fundamental instrument, the needle. Until such time that we are able to deliver local anesthetics to target tissues without tissue penetration, we must accept this risk and make every effort to mitigate it.

8.4 Block Complications

8.4.1 Introduction

The use of regional anesthesia in pediatrics has been increasing dramatically over the past 20 years; as a result, we are likely to see a higher number of complications. This is an emerging area of study. As it currently stands, there are a limited number of high-quality studies of significant enough power to detect infrequent minor and major complications, and developing management guidelines is difficult. We must draw on the experiences of our adult regional anesthesia colleagues and translate it to our patient group while continuing to build a body of literature to guide future actions.

8.4.2 Complications of Peripheral Nerve Blocks

8.4.2.1 Phrenic Nerve Paralysis and Paresis

These complications have gone unreported in the pediatric literature despite the overwhelming incidence in the adult literature. Estimates of temporary hemidiaphragmatic paresis following supraclavicular and interscalene blocks range in the order of 50–100 % [58]. A permanent phrenic nerve palsy has even been reported as a result of an interscalene block [59]. The difference in patient and block selection likely explains the absence of reports in pediatric patients. There were an insufficient number of blocks above the clavicle in a group of over 2,000 pediatric patients to even report [8]. Should these blocks be performed, some evidence exists that using low volumes of local anesthetics, coupled with ultrasound guidance, can decrease the risk of hemidiaphragmatic paralysis [60]. Bilateral blocks above the clavicle are contraindicated. Recently, it was demonstrated that a bolus injection of normal saline through an interscalene catheter originally used for a brachial plexus block was sufficient to resolve inadvertent phrenic nerve palsy and restore diaphragmatic function [61].

8.4.2.2 Hematoma and Subsequent Sequelae

Inadvertent puncture of blood vessels while performing peripheral nerve blocks is relatively common. Transarterial techniques are described elsewhere in this book as an accepted method of delivering local anesthetics. Preventing vessel penetration is done with anatomical understanding and visualization techniques (ultrasound). Prior to block placement, a history ruling out clotting disorders must also be elicited, as regional anesthesia is relatively contraindicated in this patient group. In the event of a vascular puncture, the needle should be removed (oftentimes, the block can still be placed safely and effectively). Pressure should be applied to the site until bleeding ceases and the hematoma stops expanding. The site should be continuously monitored throughout the case and in the postanesthetic care unit. Pulses and compartment pressures should also be monitored clinically distal to the site of hematoma to rule out compartment syndrome (Table 8.5). Should compartment syndrome be suspected, orthopedic surgery and plastic surgery should be consulted for diagnosis and management. In the case of admitted patients, an order should also be left for the nursing unit to continue intermittent monitoring of limb pulses, pain, pressure, and paresthesia as the block fades. For same-day surgery patients, these same instructions should be given to the caregivers of the child.

Serious complications arising from peripheral hematomas are rare. The only significant reporting of hematomas in the pediatric population following peripheral nerve blocks are those following dorsal penile nerve blocks. The most recent Cochrane Review of dorsal penile nerve blocks revealed that there were no serious sequelae as a result of hematomas [62]. There has also been a report of a bowel wall hematoma following an ilioinguinal-iliohypogastric nerve block in a 6-year-old girl without serious consequences [63].

Table 8.5 Causes of compartment syndrome

Causes of compartment syndrome
• Excessive tourniquet pressures
• Allergic reactions
• Undiagnosed Raynaud's disease
• Sickle cell disease
• Intra-arterial injection
• Drug administration error

8.4.2.3 Bacterial Infection

Any time the skin is penetrated with a foreign object, there is the potential for the introduction of an infection. Preventing bacterial infection is done by ensuring the block is placed in a clean environment (either an operating room or a dedicated block room). Sterile technique must be used at all times with the patient and tools draped and covered appropriately. Patients and their parents should be warned of the potential for infection and should report to a medical caregiver should the child develop localized erythema, pain around the puncture site, fevers, chills, or purulent discharge. Infections can be treated as per local antibiotic guidelines with drainage of abscesses as required. The actual risk of infection in the setting of sterile technique and peripheral nerve blocks in pediatric patients has yet to be quantified.

8.4.3 Complications of Neuraxial Blocks

8.4.3.1 Hematoma

Epidural hematoma following neuraxial anesthesia is rare. The incidence is estimated to be less than 1 in 150,000 cases of neuraxial anesthesia in adult patients [64]. Although specifically tailored for the adult population, guidance from the American Society of Regional Anesthesia is available [64]. In the pediatric literature, reports are scarce and none of the large pediatric studies have demonstrated this risk, although they are likely insufficiently powered if the incidence is in the range of 0.0007 %, as in the adult population. Should the child experience bilateral lower limb weakness with back pain, consideration should be given to a centrally compression lesion. MRI is the primary modality of diagnosis and early neurology and neurosurgical consultation is advised, lest the deficit become permanent.

8.4.3.2 Infection

Epidural abscesses are a rare but potentially devastating complication. In the adult literature, the incidence has been estimated at between 0 and 0.005 % [65, 66]. Large studies in the pediatric population have failed to show any cases of epidural abscesses [8]. There were, however, two reports of epidural abscesses in the UK audit of over 10,000 epidurals [49]. Presentation is variable, but one should be suspicious if a child complains of back pain with localized tenderness and fever developing days after the puncture. Leukocytosis can also be present. The consequences of an unrecognized abscess are dire; progressive weakness and paraplegia can develop if untreated. Meningitis may also develop, a case of which was also reported in the UK study [49]. Antibiotic regimes should be tailored to local guidelines. When the tips of caudal catheters were cultured, Gram-negative bacteria were present, with *Staphylococcus epidermidis* being the most common microorganism colonized on the skin and catheters of lumbar and caudal epidurals [67]. Prompt surgical consultation is recommended for consideration of abscess drainage. While the overall infection rate associated with caudal epidural catheters is quite low, fixing the catheter with an occlusive dressing in a cephalad direction is recommended to reduce the risk of contamination by stool and urine [68, 69].

8.4.3.3 Total Spinal Anesthesia

An excessive dose of local anesthetic injected into the subarachnoid space results in total spinal anesthesia. Typically, this is the result of an unintentional injection of a dose of local anesthetic intended for the epidural space. It may also be seen when a small epidural dose or a large spinal dose of local anesthetic enters the subarachnoid space. Minimizing this adverse event is possible with the use of ultrasound as well as nerve stimulation (Chap. 2, Table 2.2) [70]. In adult patients, total spinal anesthesia is seen in 0.2 % of patients undergoing epidural anesthesia [71]. Out of 1,100 pediatric epidurals, one child experienced a total spinal anesthetic [8]. This was recognized in the recovery room as the child did not initiate spontaneous breathing and was treated successfully with 4 h of monitored ventilation. Inability to breathe, combined with possible hemodynamic instability, is the typical presentation pattern. Resuscitation with endotracheal intubation, mechanical ventilation, and vasopressor therapy may be required. Recovery may take between 30 min and 6 h, depending on the agent used and the dose administered. Cerebrospinal fluid lavage via an epidural catheter has been used to successfully treat a total spinal in a 14-year-old child [72]. In this case, the patient recovered within 30 min.

8.4.3.4 Subdural Injections

The subdural space is a potential space between the dura and the arachnoid that extends from the level of the second sacral vertebra up to the floor of the third ventricle. The subdural space differs from the epidural space in that it is both extra- and intracranial. This space envelops the cranial and spinal nerves for a short distance and is widest in the cervical area. The incidence of subdural injections of local anesthetic drugs is reported to range from 0.1 to 0.8 % [73], although it is infrequently reported in the pediatric population. The epidural stimulation test can provide information about the location of the needle or catheter in the subdural space [74, 75]. When suspected a radiopaque dye can be used to diagnose subdural catheter placement. The progression of the block in a subdural injection is variable and can present as a "patchy" block with a slow onset of motor and sensory blockade. Respiratory insufficiency is possible and supportive ventilation and sedation can be required until the block subsides.

8.4.3.5 Post-Dural-Puncture Headache

Post-dural-puncture headache (PDPH) is a relatively common phenomenon in the adult population. It was previously thought that PDPH did not occur in the pediatric population [76]. Possible explanations previously offered included lower CSF pressure, lower hydrostatic pressure when upright, and differences in the elasticity of the dural matter in these different age groups. This, however, has proven untrue. In fact, the incidence of PDPH in children is quoted between 2 and 15 % [77].

The symptoms of PDPH remain the same in the pediatric population. The International Headache Society defines a PDPH as a headache occurring within 7 days of a lumbar puncture and resolving within 14 days and is worse in the upright position [78]. Other symptoms may include nausea, vomiting, and various optical and auditory phenomena. The primary difference between the two populations is the ability to verbalize these symptoms. Children may exhibit a wide range of behaviors instead of vocalizing and describing their symptoms. Thus, children should be questioned routinely following dural puncture, and caregivers should be provided information on possible manifestations of PDPH.

Prevention of PDPH is possible with knowledge of the factors that influence the incidence of PDPH. In pediatrics, links have been demonstrated between headaches and needle gauge, bevel design, and orientation. The importance of bevel orientation was demonstrated following dural penetration with an epidural needle and confirmed in a study showing no difference in the incidence of PDPH when comparing 22G and 25G needles, as long as the bevel was oriented vertically [79, 80]. Needle design is also a factor in the development of PDPH; blunt-pointed needles (e.g., Sprotte, Whitacre) are linked to a reduced incidence of PDPH as opposed to sharp, cutting-point needles (e.g., Quincke). This has been demonstrated in the pediatric population [77].

Initial treatment is to utilize conservative measures such as bed rest and oral hydration, despite little evidence to support them. Analgesics (acetaminophen, nonsteroidal anti-inflammatories) can also be used for symptomatic treatment. Caffeine can also be used and has been shown to be effective in the adult population, although there is some controversy [81, 82]. Autologous epidural blood patching (EBP), introduced by Gormley in 1960, remains one of the most effective treatments for PDPH [83]. Success rates for EBPs are approximately 85 % and rise to 98 % after a second patch. It has suggested that the blood acts as a sealant, plugging the hole created by the needle, thus preventing further CSF leakage. Another possibility is the counterpressure theory whereby the injected blood increases the epidural pressure increasing CSF pressure.

EBPs are not commonly reported in the pediatric population. Case reports have suggested the use of between 3 and 8.5 mL, and a small series in adolescents suggested using a volume of 0.2–0.3 mL/kg [84–87]. A caudal blood patch has been reported by Kowbel in a 4-year-old child who developed a subarachnoid cutaneous fistula following repeated lumbar punctures for chemotherapy [88]. A lumbar EBP has been performed in a 7-year-old child [85]. Furthermore, there has been one case reported of cervical dural puncture treated successfully with a lumbar EBP [89]. A CSF leak of 5 weeks' duration in a 3-year-old child was quickly and successfully treated with an EBP after repair was attempted with invasive techniques [90]. When performed successfully, pain dissipates within 10–15 min. This procedure is not without risk, and side effects such as transient bradycardia, lumbovertebral syndrome, and facial palsy have been reported [91–94].

8.4.3.6 Hypotension

Hypotension following neuraxial blockade in young pediatric patients is almost unheard of [95]. This is likely due to the immaturity of the autonomic nervous system and decreased reliance on sympathetic tone to maintain blood pressure. As such, hypotension following neuraxial blockade should prompt the practitioner to consider other such causes, including those related to surgery and other unrecognized bleeding, local anesthetic toxicity, anaphylaxis, and total spinal anesthesia. In the older adolescent, a decrease in blood pressure can be seen following a neuraxial block and should be treated as it is in adults, with fluids, positioning (Trendelenburg), and sympathomimetics.

8.4.4 Summary

Complications from neuraxial blocks in pediatric patients are surprisingly rare, and there are almost no reports of mortality as sequelae. However, the recent ADARPEF study indicates that the complication rate of central blocks is six times higher than that of peripheral blocks [8]. Given this fact, peripheral blocks must always be considered for anesthesia. Management of the majority of these complications remains supportive, and in the event of a space-occupying lesion (abscess or hematoma), consultation with neurology and neurosurgical specialists should be considered early.

Conclusion

A review of the potential complications of pediatric regional anesthesia is provided. In this relatively understudied group, new complications will emerge as sample sizes increase and more patients are offered regional anesthesia. In the interim, we must take some of our guidance from our adult regional anesthesia colleagues. Fortunately, the practice of regional anesthesia in pediatrics is quite safe. Reports of adverse events are few and far between, and those that do exist are rarely associated with long-term consequences. Every effort must be made to maintain this excellent safety record. We can prevent complications by carefully selecting our patients, ensuring that practitioners are well trained, that areas in which blocks are performed are the safest possible, that the safest procedure is chosen, and that proper consent is given by both the patient and caregivers. Management and assessment must be carried out promptly whenever any complication is suspected (Table 8.6).

Table 8.6 Suggested steps for evaluating neurological injury

Suggested steps involved in evaluating neurological injury
• Recognize and identify the neural dysfunction
• The history of any new or intensifying neural dysfunction in the absence of further anesthetic injection must be considered as a warning sign of possible neural injury
• When neural damage is suspected, a careful history assessment and a physical examination must be carried out promptly
• The sequence and onset of the symptoms must be determined
• The nature of pain, motor weakness, sensory deficit, and sphincter control should be compared to information obtained preoperatively about the patient's baseline neurologic status; such information may provide clues to the cause of injury and appropriate management
• Symptoms/signs of spinal cord compression must be dealt with urgently (within 6–12 h); otherwise, permanent paraplegia or quadriplegia may occur
• A thorough postoperative follow-up should be completed, even if a neurologic injury is not suspected
• Consider surgical causes:
○ Surgical trauma to neural structures from retractors, a scalpel blade, or tension within the surgical site may not have been mentioned to the anesthesiologist
○ Long-acting local anesthetics may have been injected by the surgeon
○ Compartment syndrome resulting from edema or bleeding around the wound caused by dressings or casts can compromise neural function
○ Vascular injury during the surgery could result in nerve injury (e.g., spinal cord injury after thoracic aneurysm repair). Because of this, it is probably desirable to let the block subside after aortic surgery
○ Patient positioning must be reviewed to rule out direct pressure (e.g., peroneal nerve at the fibular head) or tension on nerves (e.g., traction on the brachial plexus from hyperextension of the shoulder during thoracotomy); improper patient positioning may produce nerve injury that might otherwise be attributed to a regional anesthetic mishap
• Consider anesthetic causes:
○ The details of anesthesia management should be thoroughly reviewed, especially if portions of the anesthetic care were delivered by other anesthesiologists
○ Drug choice, dose, and last time of administration should be recorded
○ Duration of nerve blockade should be noted; a long duration of blockade can result in neural injury
○ High concentrations of agents probably increase the risk of neural complications
○ Multiple nerve-blocking attempts can increase the risk of injury
○ In awake patients, the presence of paresthesia during needle insertion and the subsequent injection of local anesthetic can be a warning sign indicating neural injury
○ For cooperative teenagers, the level of sedation must be appropriate without compromising the ability to observe a paresthesia. In younger patients, regional anesthesia often needs to be performed under general anesthetic

References

1. Rubin K, Sullivan D, Sadhasivam S. Are peripheral and neuraxial blocks with ultrasound guidance more effective and safe in children? Paediatr Anaesth. 2009;19:92–6.
2. Lonnqvist PA. Is ultrasound guidance mandatory when performing paediatric regional anaesthesia? Curr Opin Anaesthesiol. 2010;23:337–41.
3. Brull R, Wijayatilake DS, Perlas A, et al. Practice patterns related to block selection, nerve localization and risk disclosure: a survey of the American Society of Regional Anesthesia and Pain Medicine. Reg Anesth Pain Med. 2008;33:395–403.
4. Gunter JB. Benefit and risks of local anesthetics in infants and children. Paediatr Drugs. 2002;4:649–72.
5. Dalens BJ, Mazoit JX. Adverse effects of regional anaesthesia in children. Drug Saf. 1998;19:251–68.
6. Curley RK, Macfarlane AW, King CM. Contact sensitivity to the amide anesthetics lidocaine, prilocaine, and mepivacaine. Case report and review of the literature. Arch Dermatol. 1986;122:924–6.
7. Berde CB. Convulsions associated with pediatric regional anesthesia. Anesth Analg. 1992;75:164–6.
8. Ecoffey C, Lacroix F, Giaufre E, Orliaguet G, Courreges P. Epidemiology and morbidity of regional anesthesia in children: a follow-up one-year prospective survey of the French-Language Society of Paediatric Anaesthesiologists (ADARPEF). Paediatr Anaesth. 2010;20:1061–9.
9. Giaufre E, Dalens B, Gombert A. Epidemiology and morbidity of regional anesthesia in children: a one-year prospective survey of the French-Language Society of Pediatric Anesthesiologists. Anesth Analg. 1996;83:904–12.
10. Fisher QA, Shaffner DH, Yaster M. Detection of intravascular injection of regional anaesthetics in children. Can J Anesth. 1997;44:592–8.
11. Freid EB, Bailey AG, Valley RD. Electrocardiographic and hemodynamic changes associated with unintentional intravascular injection of bupivacaine with epinephrine in infants. Anesthesiology. 1993;79:394–8.
12. Sethna NF, Sullivan L, Retik A, et al. Efficacy of simulated epinephrine-containing epidural test dose after intravenous atropine during isoflurane anesthesia in children. Reg Anesth Pain Med. 2000;25:566–72.
13. Perillo M, Sethna NF, Berde CB. Intravenous isoproterenol as a marker for epidural test-dosing in children. Anesth Analg. 1993;76:178–81.
14. Tsui BCH, Kropelin B. The electrophysiological effect of dextrose 5 % in water on single-shot peripheral nerve stimulation. Anesth Analg. 2005;100:1837–9.
15. Chin J, Tsui BC. No change in impedance upon intravascular injection of D5W. Can J Anesth. 2010;57:559–64.
16. Fortuna A. Caudal analgesia: a simple and safe technique in paediatric surgery. Br J Anaesth. 1967;39:165–70.
17. Agarwal R, Gutlove DP, Lockhart CH. Seizures occurring in pediatric patients receiving continuous infusion of bupivacaine. Anesth Analg. 1992;75:284–6.
18. Peutrell JM, Hughes DG. A grand mal convulsion in a child in association with a continuous epidural infusion of bupivacaine. Anaesthesia. 1995;50:563–4.
19. Bosenberg AT. Epidural analgesia for major neonatal surgery. Paediatr Anaesth. 1998;8:479–83.
20. Maxwell LG, Martin LD, Yaster M. Bupivacaine-induced cardiac toxicity in neonates: successful treatment with intravenous phenytoin. Anesthesiology. 1994;80:682–6.
21. Foxall G, McCahon R, Lamb J, Hardman JG, Bedforth NM. Levobupivacaine-induced seizures and cardiovascular collapse treated with Intralipid. Anaesthesia. 2007;62:516–8.
22. Lambert LA, Lambert DH, Strichartz GR. Irreversible conduction block in isolated nerve by high concentrations of local anesthetics. Anesthesiology. 1994;80:1082–93.
23. Flandin-Blety C, Barrier G. Accidents following extradural analgesia in children. The results of a retrospective study. Paediatr Anaesth. 1995;5:41–6.
24. McCloskey JJ, Haun SE, Deshpande JK. Bupivacaine toxicity secondary to continuous caudal epidural infusion in children. Anesth Analg. 1992;75:287–90.
25. McGown RG. Caudal analgesia in children. Five hundred cases for procedures below the diaphragm. Anaesthesia. 1982;37:806–18.
26. Matsumiya N, Dohi S, Takahashi H, Kondo Y, Naito H. Cardiovascular collapse in an infant after caudal anesthesia with a lidocaine-epinephrine solution. Anesth Analg. 1986;65:1074–6.
27. Faccenda KA, Finucane BT. Complications of regional anaesthesia: incidence and prevention. Drug Saf. 2001;24:413–42.
28. Weinberg G, Ripper R, Feinstein DL, Hoffman W. Lipid emulsion infusion rescues dogs from bupivacaine-induced cardiac toxicity. Reg Anesth Pain Med. 2003;28:198–202.
29. Weinberg GL, VadeBoncouer T, Ramaraju GA, Garcia-Amaro MF, Cwik MJ. Pretreatment or resuscitation with a lipid infusion shifts the dose-response to bupivacaine-induced asystole in rats. Anesthesiology. 1998;88:1071–5.
30. Weinberg G. Lipid rescue resuscitation from local anaesthetic cardiac toxicity. Toxicol Rev. 2006;25:139–45.
31. Picard J, Meek T. Lipid emulsion to treat overdose of local anaesthetic: the gift of the glob. Anaesthesia. 2006;61:107–9.
32. Rosenblatt MA, Abel M, Fischer GW, Itzkovich CJ, Eisenkraft JB. Successful use of a 20 % lipid emulsion to resuscitate a patient after a presumed bupivacaine-related cardiac arrest. Anesthesiology. 2006;105:217–8.
33. Litz RJ, Popp M, Stehr SN, Koch T. Successful resuscitation of a patient with ropivacaine-induced asystole after axillary plexus block using lipid infusion. Anaesthesia. 2006;61:800–1.
34. Leskiw U, Weinberg GL. Lipid resuscitation for local anesthetic toxicity: is it really lifesaving? Curr Opin Anaesthesiol. 2009;22:667–71.
35. Ludot H, Tharin JY, Belouadah M, Mazoit JX, Malinovsky JM. Successful resuscitation after ropivacaine and lidocaine-induced ventricular arrhythmia following posterior lumbar plexus block in a child. Anesth Analg. 2008;106:1572–4, table of contents.
36. Shah S, Gopalakrishnan S, Apuya J, Martin T. Use of Intralipid in an infant with impending cardiovascular collapse due to local anesthetic toxicity. J Anesth. 2009;23:439–41.
37. Dillane D, Finucane BT. Local anesthetic systemic toxicity. Can J Anesth. 2010;57:368–80.
38. Neal JM, Bernards CM, Butterworth JF, et al. ASRA practice advisory on local anesthetic systemic toxicity. Reg Anesth Pain Med. 2010;35:152–61.
39. Auroy Y, Narchi P, Messiah A, et al. Serious complications related to regional anesthesia: results of a prospective survey in France. Anesthesiology. 1997;87:479–86.
40. Barrington MJ, Watts SA, Gledhill SR, et al. Preliminary results of the Australasian Regional Anaesthesia Collaboration: a prospective audit of more than 7000 peripheral nerve and plexus blocks for neurologic and other complications. Reg Anesth Pain Med. 2009;34:534–41.
41. Bernards CM, Hadzic A, Suresh S, Neal JM. Regional anesthesia in anesthetized or heavily sedated patients. Reg Anesth Pain Med. 2008;33:449–60.
42. Selander D, Dhuner KG, Lundborg G. Peripheral nerve injury due to injection needles used for regional anesthesia. An experimental study of the acute effects of needle point trauma. Acta Anaesthesiol Scand. 1977;21:182–8.
43. Tsui BC, Li LX, Pillay JJ. Compressed air injection technique to standardize block injection pressures. Can J Anesth. 2006;53:1098–102.

44. Neal JM. Ultrasound-guided regional anesthesia and patient safety: an evidence-based analysis. Reg Anesth Pain Med. 2010;35:S59–67.
45. Deschner S, Borgeat A, Hadzic A. Neurologic complications of peripheral nerve blocks: mechanisms and management. In: Hadzic A, editor. Textbook of regional anesthesia and acute pain management. New York: McGraw-Hill; 2007. p. 969–78.
46. Barutell C, Vidal F, Raich M, Montero A. A neurological complication following interscalene brachial plexus block. Anaesthesia. 1980;35:365–7.
47. Passannante AN. Spinal anesthesia and permanent neurologic deficit after interscalene block. Anesth Analg. 1996;82:873–4.
48. Winnie AP, Håkansson L, Buckój P. Plexus anesthesia Volume I: perivascular techniques of Brachial Plexus Block. Philadelphia: WB Saunders; 1983.
49. Llewellyn N, Moriarty A. The national pediatric epidural audit. Paediatr Anaesth. 2007;17:520–33.
50. Rochette A, Dadure C, Raux O, et al. A review of pediatric regional anesthesia practice during a 17-year period in a single institution. Paediatr Anaesth. 2007;17:874–80.
51. Kao M-C, Tsai S-K, Tsou M-Y, et al. Paraplegia after delayed detection of inadvertent spinal cord injury during thoracic epidural catheterization in an anesthetized elderly patient. Anesth Analg. 2004;99:580–3.
52. Rose JB. Spinal cord injury in a child after single-shot epidural anesthesia. Anesth Analg. 2003;96:3–6.
53. Bromage PR, Benumof JL. Paraplegia following intracord injection during attempted epidural anesthesia under general anesthesia. Reg Anesth Pain Med. 1998;23:104–7.
54. Brand L, Papper EM. A comparison of supraclavicular and axillary techniques for brachial plexus blocks. Anesthesiology. 1961;22:226–9.
55. De Jong RH. Local anesthetics. St. Louis: Mosby-Year Book; 1994.
56. De Jose MB, Banus E, Navarro Egea M, et al. Ultrasound-guided supraclavicular vs infraclavicular brachial plexus blocks in children. Paediatr Anaesth. 2008;18:838–44.
57. Pande R, Pande M, Bhadani U, Pandey CK, Bhattacharya A. Supraclavicular brachial plexus block as a sole anaesthetic technique in children: an analysis of 200 cases. Anaesthesia. 2000;55:798–802.
58. Neal JM, Moore JM, Kopacz DJ, et al. Quantitative analysis of respiratory, motor, and sensory function after supraclavicular block. Anesth Analg. 1998;86:1239–44.
59. Robaux S, Bouaziz H, Boisseau N, Raucoules-Aime M, Laxenaire MC. Persistent phrenic nerve paralysis following interscalene brachial plexus block. Anesthesiology. 2001;95:1519–21.
60. Riazi S, Carmichael N, Awad I, Holtby RM, McCartney CJ. Effect of local anaesthetic volume (20 vs 5 ml) on the efficacy and respiratory consequences of ultrasound-guided interscalene brachial plexus block. Br J Anaesth. 2008;101:549–56.
61. Tsui BC, Dillane D. Reducing and washing off local anesthetic for continuous interscalene block. Reg Anesth Pain Med 2014;39: 175–6.
62. Brady-Fryer B, Wiebe N, Lander JA. Pain relief for neonatal circumcision. Cochrane Database Syst Rev. 2004;3:CD004217.
63. Frigon C, Mai R, Valois-Gomez T, Desparmet J. Bowel hematoma following an iliohypogastric-ilioinguinal nerve block. Paediatr Anaesth. 2006;16:993–6.
64. Horlocker TT, Wedel DJ, Benzon H, et al. Regional anesthesia in the anticoagulated patient: defining the risks (the second ASRA Consensus Conference on Neuraxial Anesthesia and Anticoagulation). Reg Anesth Pain Med. 2003;28:172–97.
65. Kane RE. Neurologic deficits following epidural or spinal anesthesia. Anesth Analg. 1981;60:150–61.
66. Moen V, Dahlgren N, Irestedt L. Severe neurological complications after central neuraxial blockades in Sweden 1990–1999. Anesthesiology. 2004;101:950–9.
67. Kost-Byerly S, Tobin JR, Greenberg RS, et al. Bacterial colonization and infection rate of continuous epidural catheters in children. Anesth Analg. 1998;86:712–6.
68. Bubeck J, Boos K, Krause H, Thies K-C. Subcutaneous tunneling of caudal catheters reduces the rate of bacterial colonization to that of lumbar epidural catheters. Anesth Analg. 2004;99:689–93.
69. Tsui BCH, Wagner A, Cave D, Kearney R. Thoracic and lumbar epidural analgesia via the caudal approach using electrical stimulation guidance in pediatric patients: a review of 289 patients. Anesthesiology. 2004;100:683–9.
70. Tsui BC, Suresh S. Ultrasound imaging for regional anesthesia in infants, children, and adolescents: a review of current literature and its application in the practice of neuraxial blocks. Anesthesiology. 2010;112:719–28.
71. Dawkins CJ. An analysis of the complications of extradural and caudal block. Anaesthesia. 1969;24:554–63.
72. Tsui BCH, Malherbe S, Koller J, Aronyk K. Reversal of an unintentional spinal anesthetic by cerebrospinal lavage. Anesth Analg. 2004;98:434–6.
73. Lubenow T, Keh-Wong E, Kristof K, Ivankovich O, Ivankovich AD. Inadvertent subdural injection: a complication of an epidural block. Anesth Analg. 1988;67:175–9.
74. Tsui BC, Gupta S, Emery D, Finucane B. Detection of subdural placement of epidural catheter using nerve stimulation. Can J Anesth. 2000;47:471–3.
75. Lena P, Martin R. Subdural placement of an epidural catheter detected by nerve stimulation. Can J Anesth. 2005;52:618–21.
76. Janssens E, Aerssens P, Alliet P, Gillis P, Raes M. Post-dural puncture headaches in children. A literature review. Eur J Pediatr. 2003;162:117–21.
77. Apiliogullari S, Duman A, Gok F, Akillioglu I. Spinal needle design and size affect the incidence of postdural puncture headache in children. Paediatr Anaesth. 2010;20:177–82.
78. Evans RW, Armon C, Frohman EM, Goodin DS. Assessment: prevention of post-lumbar puncture headaches: report of the therapeutics and technology assessment subcommittee of the american academy of neurology. Neurology. 2000;55:909–14.
79. Norris MC, Leighton BL, DeSimone CA. Needle bevel direction and headache after inadvertent dural puncture. Anesthesiology. 1989;70:729–31.
80. Lybecker H, Moller JT, May O, Nielsen HK. Incidence and prediction of postdural puncture headache. A prospective study of 1021 spinal anesthesias. Anesth Analg. 1990;70:389–94.
81. Camann WR, Murray RS, Mushlin PS, Lambert DH. Effects of oral caffeine on postdural puncture headache. A double-blind, placebo-controlled trial. Anesth Analg. 1990;70:181–4.
82. Halker RB, Demaerschalk BM, Wellik KE, et al. Caffeine for the prevention and treatment of postdural puncture headache: debunking the myth. Neurologist. 2007;13:323–7.
83. Gormley JB. Treatment of post spinal headache. Anesthesiology. 1960;21:565.
84. Liley A, Manoharan M, Upadhyay V. The management of a post-dural puncture headache in a child. Paediatr Anaesth. 2003;13: 534–7.
85. Roy L, Vischoff D, Lavoie J. Epidural blood patch in a seven-year-old child. Can J Anesth. 1995;42:621–4.
86. Ylonen P, Kokki H. Management of postdural puncture headache with epidural blood patch in children. Paediatr Anaesth. 2002;12:526–9.
87. Ylonen P, Kokki H. Epidural blood patch for management of post-dural puncture headache in adolescents. Acta Anaesthesiol Scand. 2002;46:794–8.
88. Kowbel MA, Comfort VK. Caudal epidural blood patch for the treatment of a paediatric subarachnoid-cutaneous fistula. Can J Anesth. 1995;42:625–7.

89. Colonna-Romano P, Linton P. Cervical dural puncture and lumbar extradural blood patch. Can J Anesth. 1995;42:1143–4.
90. Sanders JC, Gandhoke R, Moro M. Lumbar epidural blood patch to treat a large, symptomatic postsurgical cerebrospinal fluid leak of 5 weeks duration in a 3-year-old. Anesth Analg. 2004;98:629–31.
91. Andrews PJ, Ackerman WE, Juneja M, Cases-Cristobal V, Rigor BM. Transient bradycardia associated with extradural blood patch after inadvertent dural puncture in parturients. Br J Anaesth. 1992;69:401–3.
92. Palmer JH, Wilson DW, Brown CM. Lumbovertebral syndrome after repeat extradural blood patch. Br J Anaesth. 1997;78:334–6.
93. Perez M, Olmos M, Garrido FJ. Facial nerve paralysis after epidural blood patch. Reg Anesth. 1993;18:196–8.
94. Seeberger MD, Urwyler A. Lumbovertebral syndrome after extradural blood patch. Br J Anaesth. 1992;69:414–6.
95. Murat I, Delleur MM, Esteve C, et al. Continuous extradural anaesthesia in children. Clinical and haemodynamic implications. Br J Anaesth. 1987;59:1441–50.

Suggested Reading

Ecoffey C. Pediatric regional anesthesia. In: Gregory GA, Andropoulos DB, editors. Gregory's pediatric anesthesia. 5th ed. Chichester: Wiley-Blackwell; 2012. p. 439–41.

Fincuane BT, editor. Complications of regional anesthesia. 2nd ed. New York: Springer; 2007.

Horlocker TT. Neurologic complications of regional anesthesia. In: Dureja GP, Madan R, Kaul HL, editors. Regional anaesthesia and pain management: current perspectives. New Delhi: Elsevier; 2000. p. 104–14.

Neal J, Rathmell JP, editors. Complications in regional anesthesia and pain medicine. 2nd ed. Philadelphia: Lippincott Williams & Wilkins; 2013.

Pawar DK. Complications of paediatric regional anesthesia. In: Dureja GP, Madan R, Kaul HL, editors. Regional anaesthesia and pain management: current perspectives. New Delhi: Elsevier; 2000. p. 124–6.

Part III

Clinical Anatomy

Clinical Anatomy of the Head and Neck

9

Glenn Merritt, Anil H. Walji, and Ban C.H. Tsui

Contents

G. Merritt, MD
Department of Anesthesiology, University of Colorado Hospital and Children's Hospital Colorado, Aurora, CO, USA
e-mail: Merrittmd@aol.com

A.H. Walji, MD, PhD
Division of Anatomy, Department of Surgery, Faculty of Medicine and Dentistry, University of Alberta, Edmonton, AB, USA

B.C.H. Tsui, Dip Eng, BSc (Math), B Pharm, MSc, MD, FRCPC (✉)
Department of Anesthesiology and Pain Medicine, Stollery Children's Hospital/University of Alberta Hospital, 2-150 Clinical Sciences Building, Edmonton, AB T6G 2G3, Canada
e-mail: btsui@ualberta.ca

B.C.H. Tsui, S. Suresh (eds.), *Pediatric Atlas of Ultrasound- and Nerve Stimulation-Guided Regional Anesthesia*,
DOI 10.1007/978-0-387-79964-3_9

9.1 Clinical Anatomy of Trigeminal Nerve

- The trigeminal nerve (cranial nerve V), the largest of the cranial nerves, is fundamentally *the* sensory nerve of the head and supplies sensory innervation to the entire face all the way from the lambdoidal suture on the vertex of the skull to the bottom of the chin. Of its three major divisions, the *ophthalmic* and *maxillary* nerves are purely sensory, while the *mandibular* nerve is a mixed sensory and motor nerve, the motor fibers being distributed primarily to the muscles of mastication. In addition, the trigeminal nerve acts as a conduit for postganglionic parasympathetic fibers from the ciliary, pterygopalatine, mandibular, and otic ganglia in the head. The preganglionic fibers destined for these ganglia arise from the oculomotor nerve (for the ciliary ganglion), facial nerve (for the pterygopalatine and submandibular ganglia), and glossopharyngeal nerve (for the otic ganglion).
- The sensory and motor roots of the trigeminal nerve arise from the ventral aspect of the base of the pons. Sensory branches are sent to the large semilunar (trigeminal, semilunar, or Gasserian) ganglion, which lies in a shallow depression, recess, or cleft in the meningeal layer of dura (trigeminal or Meckel's cave; trigeminal fossa) in the middle cranial fossa on the dorsal surface of the petrous temporal bone near its tip or apex. The ganglion's anterior aspect gives rise to three main divisions: the ophthalmic (V1), maxillary (V2), and mandibular (V3) nerves (Fig. 9.1).
- A smaller motor root lies underneath the main trigeminal ganglion and supplies motor fibers to the mandibular nerve. These motor fibers supply mostly the muscles of mastication, namely, the masseter, temporalis, medial and lateral pterygoids, as well as the anterior belly of the digastric, mylohyoid, tensor tympani, and tensor veli palatini muscles.
- The three major divisions of the trigeminal nerve exit the cranium through three distinct foramina – the *ophthalmic* nerve enters the orbit through the superior orbital fissure, where it divides into its three main branches, the frontal, lacrimal and nasociliary nerves. The *maxillary* nerve passes through the foramen rotundum to cross over the top of the pterygopalatine fossa and then enters the floor of the orbit through the inferior orbital fissure. After exiting the skull through the foramen rotundum, the maxillary nerve courses anteriorly over the pterygopalatine fossa and enters the floor of the orbit through the infraorbital fissure as the infraorbital nerve; the infraorbital nerve courses in the infraorbital canal, and descending branches include the greater palatine, lesser palatine, and nasopalatine and superior alveolar nerves. The *mandibular* nerve courses into the infratemporal fossa through the foramen ovale and divides into its two major branches, the lingual nerve and inferior alveolar nerve. The terminal branches of these three divisions, destined for the face, namely, the supraorbital, infraorbital, and mental nerves, exit the skull through the supraorbital, infraorbital, and mental foramina, respectively, and usually lie vertically in-line with each other in the plane of the pupil (neonate, Fig. 9.2a; adolescent, Fig. 9.2b). The greater palatine, lesser palatine, and nasopalatine nerves exit the palate through corresponding foramina of the posterior aspect of the secondary palate and anterior aspect of the primary palate. Although the terminal branches are the nerves that we focus on for many common regional anesthesia blocks, it is important to remember that each of the trigeminal divisions send branches internally to supply the oral and nasal mucosa as well as the mucosa of the paranasal sinuses external branches to supply the lateral aspect of the face.

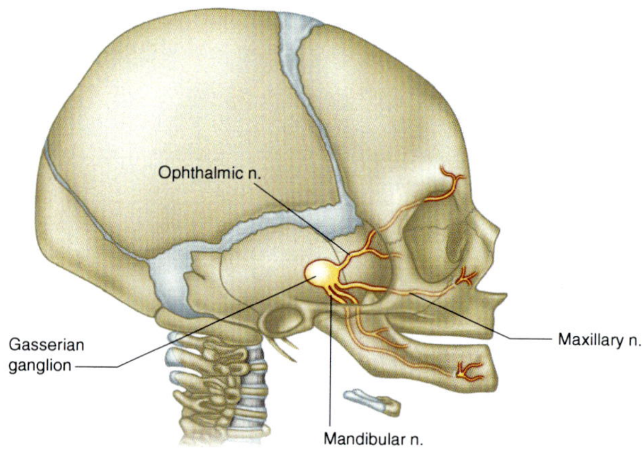

Fig. 9.1 Major branches of the trigeminal nerve: ophthalmic, maxillary, and mandibular nerves. The roots of the trigeminal nerve arise from the base of the pons and form the Gasserian ganglion

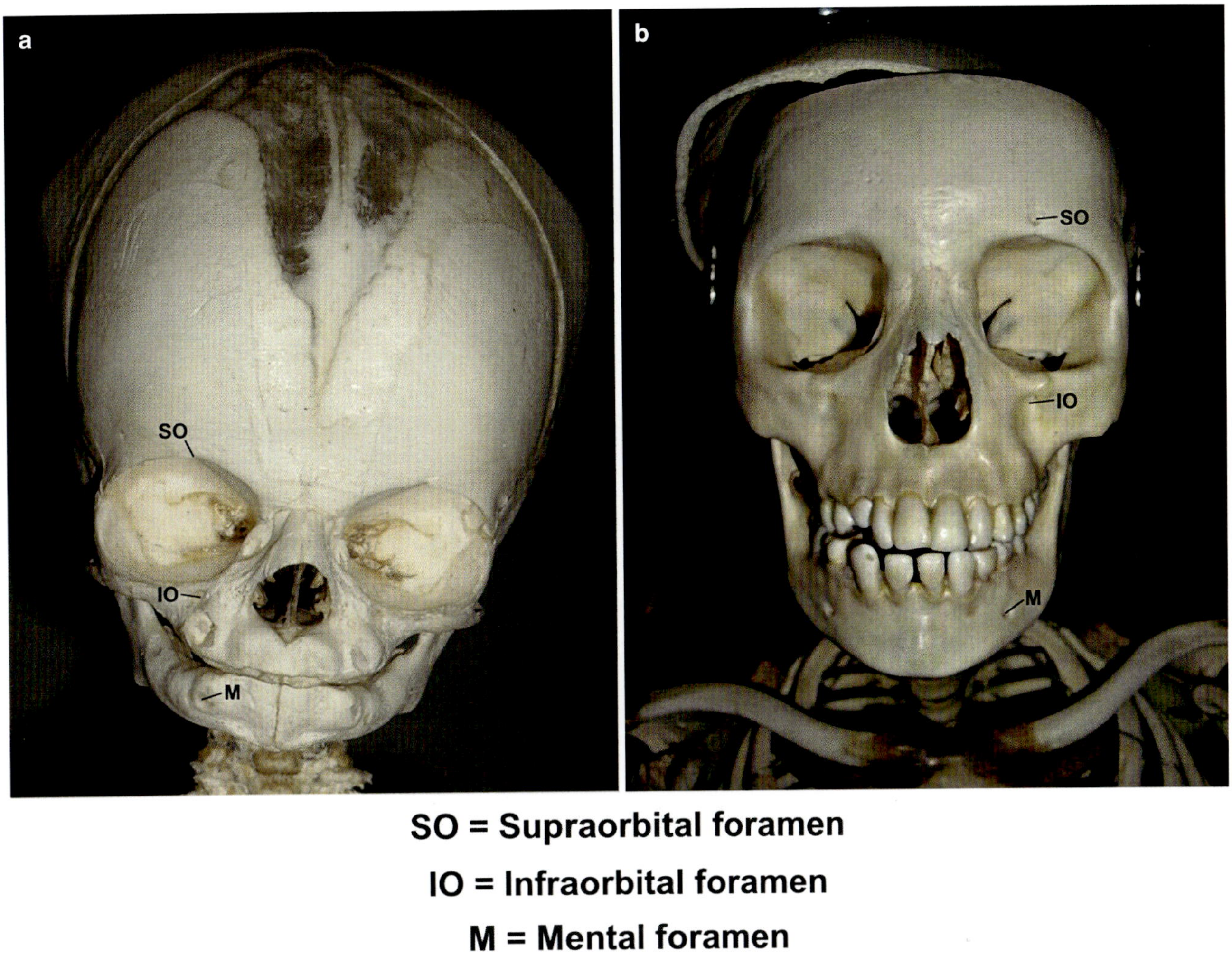

Fig. 9.2 Neonate (**a**) and adolescent (**b**) skull models depicting three distinct foramina, through which branches of the trigeminal nerve exit the cranium. The ophthalmic, maxillary, and mandibular nerves exit through the supraorbital foramen (*SO*), infraorbital foramen (*IO*), and mental foramen (*M*), respectively

9.1.1 Ophthalmic Nerve (V1 Division of the Trigeminal Nerve, Pure Sensory)

- The uppermost ophthalmic branch of the trigeminal nerve is a pure sensory nerve and passes through the superior orbital fissure (sphenoidal fissure) into the orbit.
- The nerve divides into three main branches – lacrimal, frontal, and nasociliary – just prior to entering the orbit through the superior orbital fissure.
- The *lacrimal* nerve is the smallest of the three divisions. It enters the orbit through the superior orbital fissure and communicates with the zygomaticotemporal branch of the maxillary nerve. It courses through the lateral aspect of the orbit over the lateral rectus muscle. The lacrimal nerve then enters the lacrimal gland and innervates it with parasympathetic secretomotor fibers (from the zygomaticotemporal nerve) and the adjoining conjunctiva with sensory fibers. The nerve eventually pierces the orbital septum to innervate the skin of the lateral aspect of the upper eyelid, joining with filaments from the facial nerve.
- The division's largest branch, the *frontal* nerve, courses anteriorly through the orbit along the upper surface of the levator palpebrae superioris muscle and bifurcates into its terminal sensory branches, the larger supraorbital nerve laterally and the smaller supratrochlear nerve medially.
- The *supraorbital* nerve courses anteriorly between the levator palpebrae superioris and the periosteum of the orbital roof, continues anteromedially towards the trochlea, exits the orbit through the supraorbital foramen (or notch in some cases), and finally curves superiorly into the forehead before branching into its medial and lateral branches. Anesthesia of the supraorbital nerve blocks the conjunctiva and skin of the upper eyelid as well as the ipsilateral upper forehead as far back as the lambdoidal suture (Figs. 9.3 and 9.4). It also supplies sensory fibers to the mucous membrane of the frontal air sinuses.
- The *supratrochlear* nerve traverses the orbit along the same plane as the supraorbital nerve but just medial to it, passes over the trochlea, and enters the front of the face via the frontal notch (or just medial to the supraorbital foramen or notch). It then courses superiorly into the forehead. As it passes through the orbit, the nerve sends a branch to join the infratrochlear branch of the nasociliary nerve. This nerve supplies sensation to the medial part of the upper eyelid, the conjunctiva, and the lower-middle forehead (Fig. 9.4).
- The *nasociliary* nerve is the intermediate branch (in terms of size) of the frontal nerve and passes obliquely through the orbit to reach its medial aspect. Its anterior and posterior ethmoidal branches pass through the ethmoidal foramina to enter the cranium. The nerve then travels on the upper surface of the cribriform plate of the ethmoid bone underneath the dura mater and descends through a slitlike opening in the crista galli to enter the nasal cavity. The nasociliary nerve supplies two internal nasal branches that innervate the lateral wall of the nasal cavity and the mucous membrane of the front part of the nasal septum.
- The *ethmoidal branches* also supply the mucosa lining the ethmoid air cells. The posterior branch leaves the orbit through the posterior ethmoidal foramen and innervates the sphenoidal sinus. The nasociliary nerve terminates in the infratrochlear and anterior ethmoidal branches; the former supplies the conjunctiva and skin of the medial aspect of the upper eyelid, while the latter supplies the anterior and middle ethmoid cells and then sends two internal branches that innervate the mucous membranes of the front part of the nasal septum and lateral nasal wall. The anterior ethmoidal branch eventually exits the face as the external nasal nerve, which innervates the skin of the nasal ala and apex of the nose.

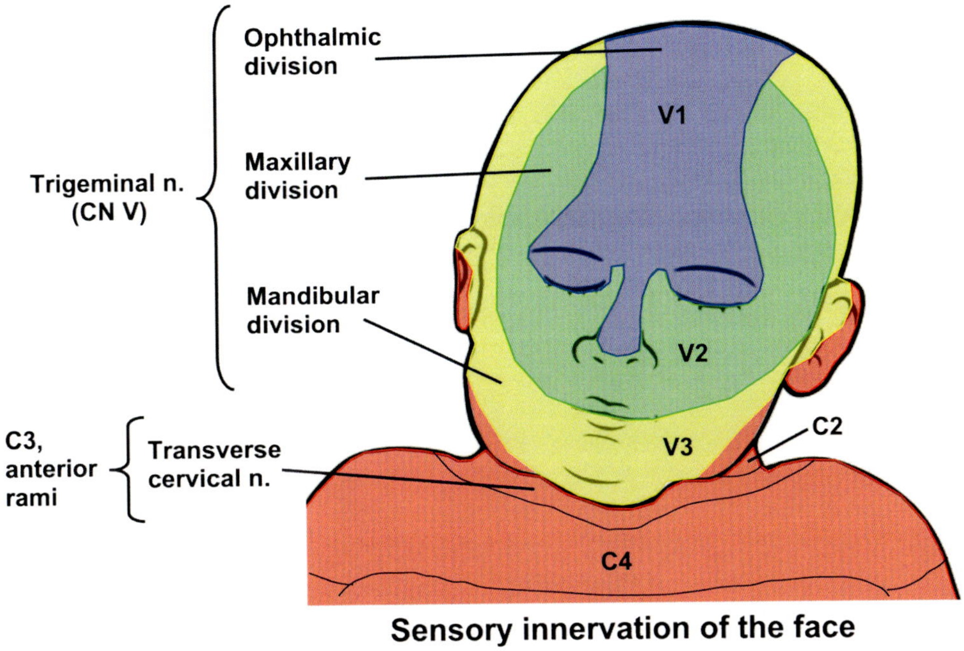

Fig. 9.3 Cutaneous innervation by the trigeminal nerve and cervical plexus

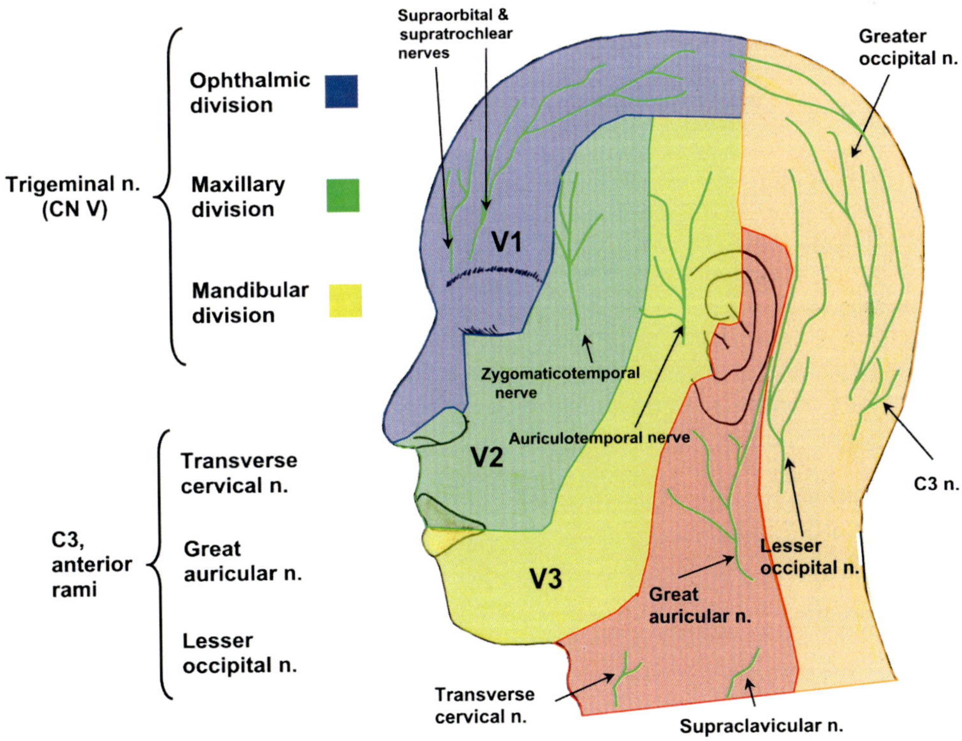

Fig. 9.4 Cutaneous innervation by the trigeminal nerve, cervical plexus, and dorsal nerve roots

9.1.2 Maxillary Nerve (V2 Division of the Trigeminal Nerve, Pure Sensory)

- The maxillary nerve, like the ophthalmic, also contains purely sensory fibers. It exits the skull through the foramen rotundum, courses beneath the skull base anteriorly, and crosses over the upper part of the pterygopalatine (sphenopalatine) fossa (medial to the lateral pterygoid plate on each side) before entering the orbit through the inferior orbital fissure as the infraorbital nerve (Fig. 9.5).
- Suspended from the nerve as it courses over the pterygopalatine fossa is the *parasympathetic pterygopalatine*, or more commonly called *sphenopalatine ganglion*, which lies within the fossa. Several branches of the maxillary nerve appear to arise from the pterygopalatine ganglion; however, the nerve fibers within them simply pass through the sphenopalatine ganglion without synapsing. Although they seem to be branches of the ganglion, they are in reality branches of the maxillary nerve just coursing through the ganglion and very intimately associated with it.
- During its course through the infraorbital groove and/or canal in the floor of the orbit, the maxillary nerve gives off two superior alveolar (dental) branches (the middle and anterior superior alveolar nerves) that supply the maxillary teeth and gingivae before terminating as the infraorbital nerve, which surfaces onto the face through the infraorbital foramen (Fig. 9.5).
- The *middle* and *anterior superior alveolar* (dental) nerves arise from the main trunk of the nerve as it passes through the infraorbital groove and/or canal, while the *posterior superior alveolar* nerve is given off just before it enters the floor of the orbit. The nerve pierces the infratemporal surface of the maxilla to run under the mucous membrane of the maxillary sinus, which it supplies. It then breaks up into small branches to form the posterior part of the superior dental plexus to supply the maxillary molars. Branches given off from within the pterygopalatine fossa include the zygomatic nerve to the orbit (with its zygomaticotemporal and zygomaticofacial branches), the short sphenopalatine (pterygopalatine) nerves, and the posterior superior alveolar (dental) nerve (Fig. 9.5).
- The *zygomaticofacial* nerve passes along the inferolateral aspect of the orbit and exits through a foramen in the zygoma to supply the skin on the cheek. The zygomaticofacial nerve merges with nerve fibers from the palpebral branches of the maxillary nerve and zygomatic branches from the facial nerve to form a plexus. The *zygomaticotemporal* nerve sends a branch to join the lacrimal nerve, providing parasympathetic, secretomotor innervation to the lacrimal gland. The *posterior superior alveolar* nerve also arises high in the pterygopalatine fossa before the maxillary nerve enters the infraorbital groove. The nerve then pierces the infratemporal surface of the maxilla to course under the mucous membrane of the maxillary sinus which it supplies. The posterior, anterior, and middle superior alveolar (dental) nerves form the superior dental plexus, which innervates the maxillary teeth and gingivae. Together with the infraorbital nerve, these superior alveolar nerves also supply sensory innervation to the mucosa lining the maxillary sinus.
- The *palatine* nerves (Fig. 9.6), the greater (anterior) and lesser (middle and posterior), are the terminal sensory endings of the maxillary nerve and emerge as branches from the pterygopalatine ganglion. The sensory fibers within them pass through the ganglion without synapsing. They are distributed to the roof of the mouth, the soft palate, the palatine tonsil, and the mucous membrane lining the nasal cavity. The branches descend through the pterygopalatine (greater palatine) canal and emerge on the hard palate; the anterior branch emerges through the greater palatine foramen (Fig. 9.6), while the middle/posterior branches emerge via a minor/lesser palatine foramen (an opening behind the greater palatine foramen). The sensory supply of the greater branch includes the gums and the mucosa and glands of the hard palate; the sensory supply of the lesser branches includes the uvula, the tonsils, and the soft palate.
- *Nasal branches* (also arising from the ganglion) enter the nasal cavity through the sphenopalatine foramen to be distributed in lateral and medial groups to the posterior aspects of the superior and middle nasal conchae laterally and the posterior part of the roof of the nasal septum medially. The largest of these nerves is the *nasopalatine* (long sphenopalatine) nerve which courses anteroinferiorly on the nasal septum and then descends through the incisive foramen in the anterior aspect of the hard palate to be distributed to the roof of the mouth (Fig. 9.6).
- The *pharyngeal* nerve arises from the posterior aspect of the pterygopalatine ganglion and courses through the palatovaginal canal to supply the mucosa of the nasopharynx just posterior to the opening of the Eustachian (auditory, pharyngotympanic) tube.
- The terminal *infraorbital* nerve passes through the inferior orbital fissure into the floor of the orbit, where it courses through the infraorbital groove and/or canal (just below the eye and lateral to the nose), and reaches the facial surface of the maxilla. It then divides into the inferior palpebral nerves (lower eyelid), external and internal nasal nerves (wings or ala of the nose), and medial and lateral branches of the superior labial nerve (upper lip).
- The infraorbital nerve innervates the lower eyelid and upper lip, including the philtrum, the lateral portion of the nasal cavity and the skin of the cheek. Blockade of the infraorbital nerve produces anesthesia of the middle third of the ipsilateral face (Fig. 9.5).

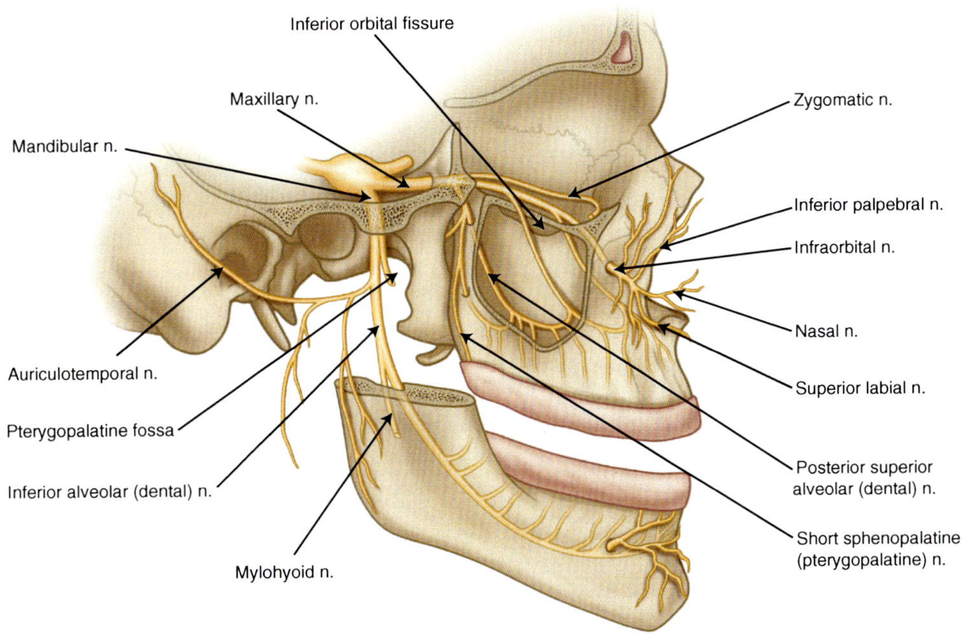

Fig. 9.5 Anatomy of the maxillary and mandibular nerves

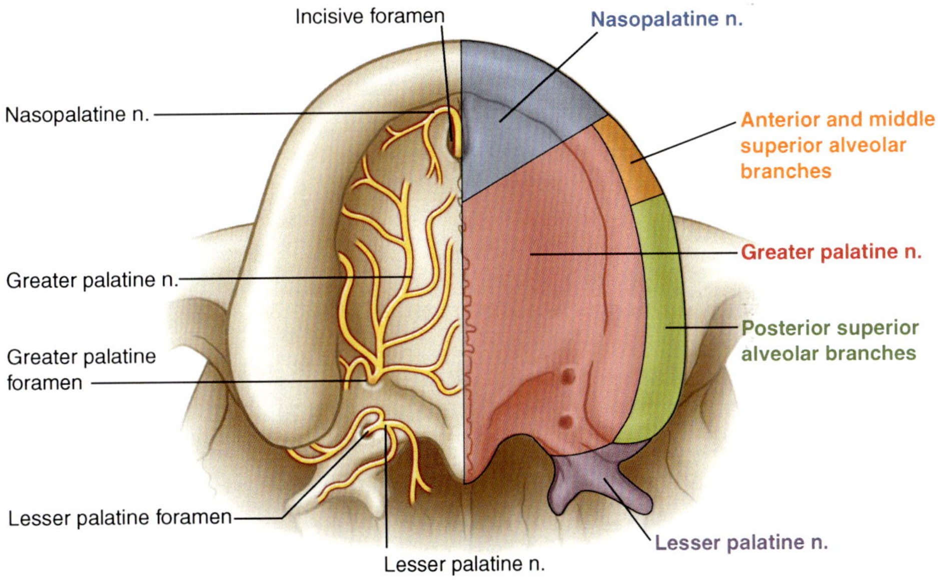

Fig. 9.6 *Left side*: the greater and lesser palatine nerves emerge on the hard palate from the greater and lesser palatine foramen, respectively. The nasopalatine nerve emerges from the incisive foramen. *Right side*: sensory innervation of the hard palate

9.1.3 Mandibular Nerve (V3 Division of the Trigeminal Nerve, Sensory and Motor to Muscles of Mastication)

- The mandibular nerve is the third and largest branch of the trigeminal and the only mixed nerve (i.e., with both a sensory and a motor component). It exits the skull posterior to the maxillary nerve (Fig. 9.5) through the foramen ovale, enters the infratemporal fossa, and forms a short, thick trunk, which divides quickly into a small, mainly motor, anterior trunk and a large, mainly sensory, posterior trunk.
- The main sensory posterior (mandibular) trunk receives a few filaments from the motor root, and its branches are the *auriculotemporal*, *lingual*, and *inferior alveolar* (dental) nerves.
- The anterior trunk of the mandibular nerve gives rise to the *buccal* nerve (sensory) and the *masseteric*, *deep temporal*, and *lateral pterygoid* nerves (motor).
- The main branch (posterior trunk) continues as the *inferior alveolar* (dental) nerve medial to the ramus of the mandible. After giving off the nerve to the mylohyoid, the inferior alveolar nerve enters the mandibular canal through the mandibular foramen, which is guarded by a tongue-shaped process of bone called the lingula (used as a landmark for locating the nerve during an inferior alveolar nerve block) (Fig. 9.5). Within the mandibular canal the nerve courses inferiorly and anteriorly to innervate the mandibular teeth and gingivae. The nerve then curves anteriorly to follow the body and anterior aspect of the mandible and exits through the mental foramen, located on the mental process of the mandible, giving off the incisive nerve and its terminal branch – the *mental* nerve.
- Other terminal nerves of the posterior trunk include the *lingual* nerve (lying under the lingual mucosa and supplying the mucosa of the floor of the mouth, mandibular gingivae, and general sensation to the anterior two-thirds of tongue) and the *auriculotemporal* nerve (dividing into superficial temporal branches behind the temporomandibular joint to supply the joint, the external acoustic meatus and auricle of the ear, and the scalp over the temple). The auriculotemporal nerve usually has two roots encircling the middle meningeal artery within the infratemporal fossa.
- The *mental* nerve, with its three branches (one ascending to reach the chin and two descending to innervate the skin and mucous membrane of the lower lip), is the primary target of anesthesia.
- The mandibular nerve also supplies the skin of the temporal region, lower jaw, and chin (Figs. 9.4 and 9.5); the mandibular gingival and labial mucosae; and the meninges of the middle cranial fossa.

9.2 Clinical Anatomy of the Cervical Plexus

- The cervical plexus is a mixed spinal nerve plexus in the neck formed from the anterior (ventral) rami of the first four cervical nerves.
- Sensory and motor fibers supplying the neck and posterior scalp arise from these four cervical (C1–C4) spinal nerves (Fig. 9.7). The cervical plexus is unique in that it divides early into cutaneous branches (penetrating the cervical fascia to supply the skin and subcutaneous tissues of the neck) and muscular branches (deeper branches which innervate the neck muscles, the diaphragm and joints of the cervical spine), which can be blocked separately. The branches of the plexus provide sensory innervation to the skin and subcutaneous tissues of the anterior and lateral aspects of the neck; part of the posterior scalp; the skin inside, above, and posterior to the external ear; and the posterior aspect and lower third of the auricle or pinna of the ear (Fig. 9.4). The cervical plexus lies deep to the sternocleidomastoid muscle (Fig. 9.8) and internal jugular vein, but is anterior to the scalenus medius and levator scapulae muscles.
- Each ramus (except the first) divides into ascending and descending parts that unite in communicating loops; the first or C2 and C3 loop supplies superficial sensory branches to the head and neck; the second or C3 and C4 loop gives rise to cutaneous nerves supplying the shoulder region and upper thorax as well as muscular (motor) branches which go deep to supply the muscles. C3, C4, and C5 anterior rami form the phrenic nerve which supplies the diaphragm (its sole motor supply), as well as the fibrous pericardium, mediastinal pleura and diaphragmatic pleura and peritoneum with sensory fibers.
- Motor branches innervating the strap muscles of the neck (sternohyoid, sternothyroid, and omohyoid) emerge from the ansa cervicalis, a neural loop formed from the joining of the *descendens hypoglossi* (C1) and *descendens cervicalis* (C2 and C3) which form the *ansa cervicalis* usually embedded within the anterior aspect of the carotid sheath deep to the sternocleidomastoid.
- Classic cervical plexus anesthesia can be achieved by injecting along the tubercles of the transverse processes of the cervical vertebrae, producing both motor and sensory blockade. The transverse processes of the cervical vertebrae form peculiar elongated troughs for the emergence of the cervical spinal nerve roots (Fig. 9.9). These troughs lie immediately lateral to an aperture for the cephalad passage of the vertebral artery, the foramen transversarium. At the lateral end of the transverse process, the trough is guarded by an anterior and a posterior tubercle, the anterior of which can often easily be palpated.

- These tubercles also serve as the attachment sites for the anterior and middle scalene muscles, which form a compartment for the cervical plexus as well as the brachial plexus immediately below. The compartment at this level is less developed than the one formed around the brachial plexus.
- The deep muscular branches curl anteriorly around the lateral border of the scalenus anterior and proceed caudally and medially. Many branches serve the deep anterior neck muscles; other branches include the superior root of the ansa cervicalis, the trapezius branch of the plexus, and the phrenic nerve. These deep muscular branches also supply the sternocleidomastoid muscle as they pass behind it.
- The sensory fibers emerge from behind the scalenus anterior muscle but are separate from the motor branches and continue laterally to emerge superficially under the posterior border (clavicular head) of the sternocleidomastoid muscle at about its midpoint (Erb's point). The branches, including the lesser occipital nerve, great auricular nerve, transverse cervical nerve, and supraclavicular nerves (medial, intermediate and lateral [posterior] branches), innervate the skin on the anterior and posterior aspects of the neck and shoulder (Fig. 9.8).
- After arising from the second and third cervical nerve roots, the great auricular nerve ascends up to the angle of the mandible and gives off anterior and posterior branches to supply the skin over the parotid gland and the mastoid process (Fig. 9.8).

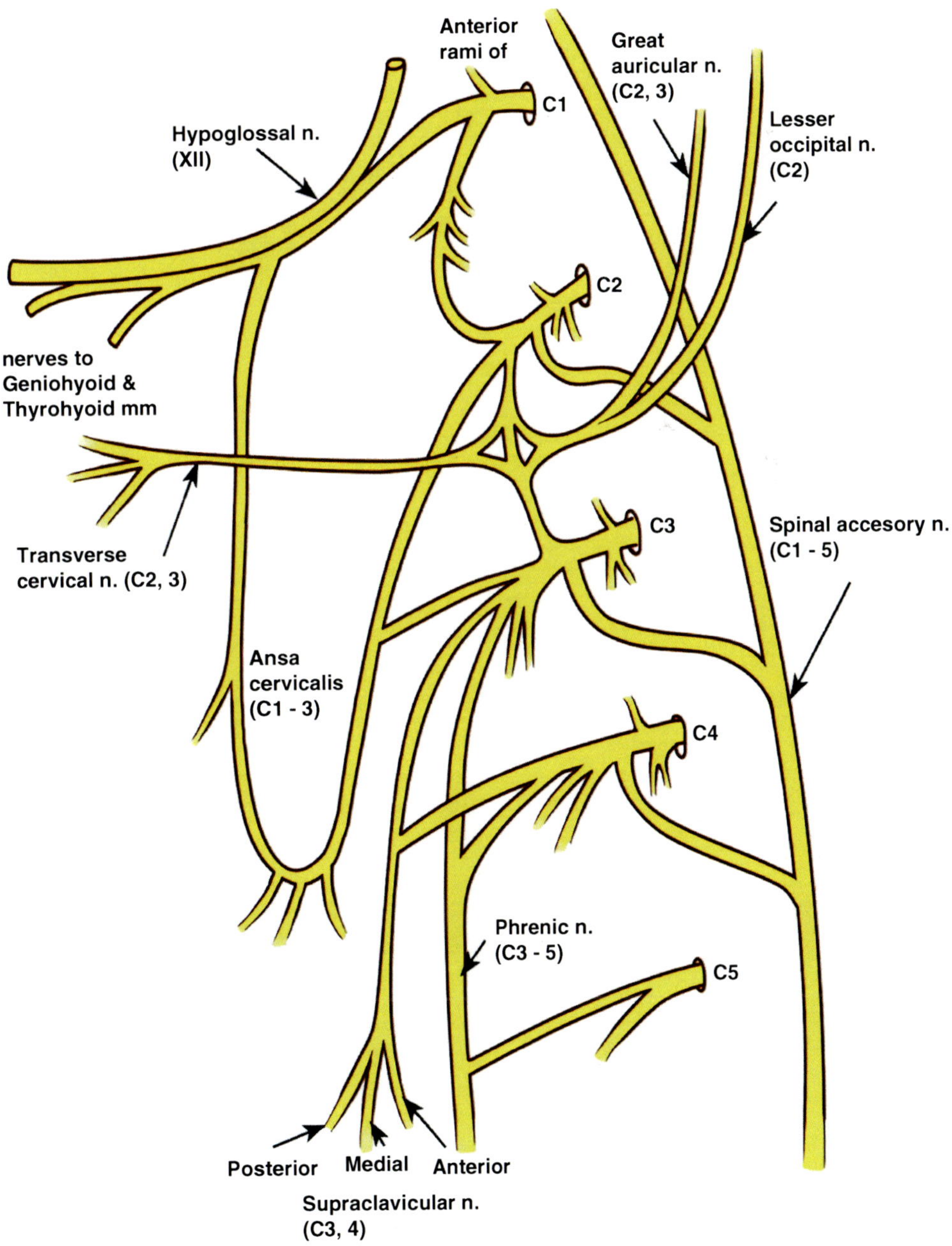

Fig. 9.7 Schematic of the cervical plexus, which arises from the anterior primary rami of C1–C4

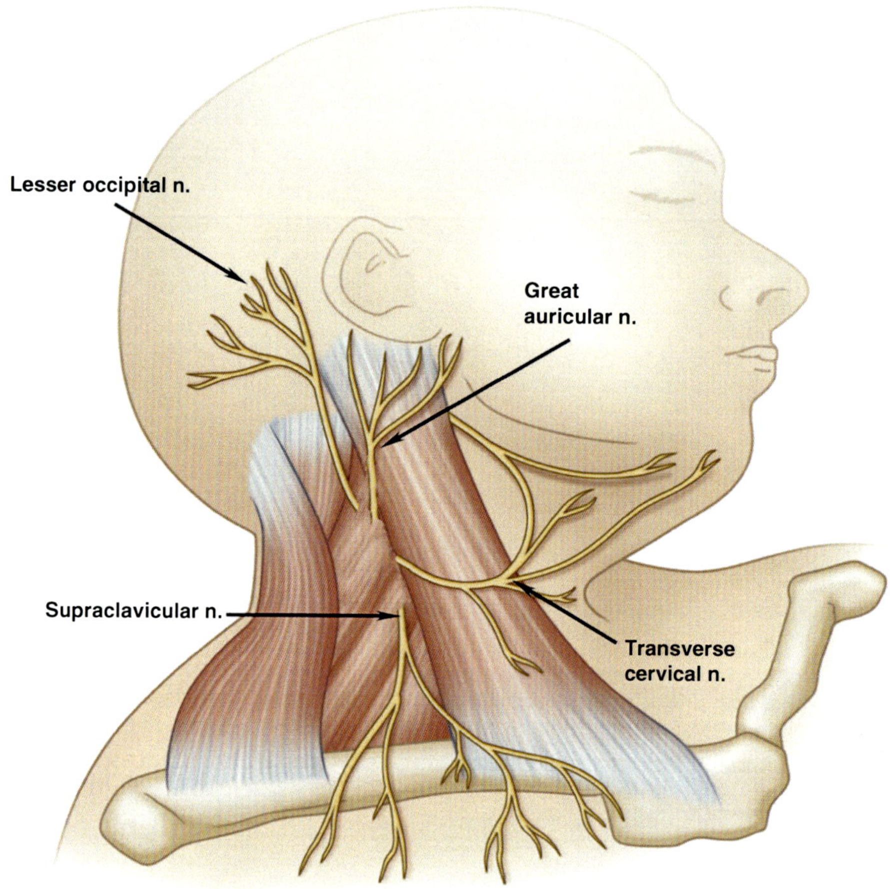

Fig. 9.8 Cutaneous innervation by the superficial cervical plexus

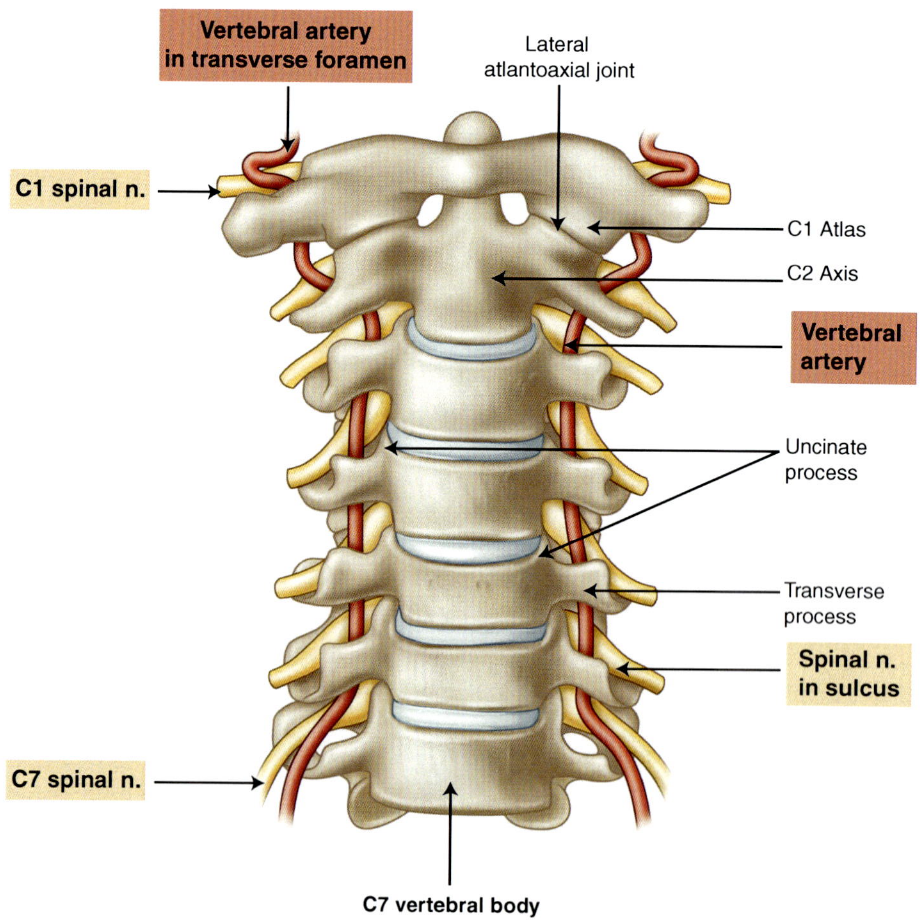

Fig. 9.9 Nerve roots of the cervical plexus emerging from the troughs formed by the transverse processes, posterior and lateral to the vertebral artery

9.3 Clinical Anatomy of Occipital Nerves

The posterior scalp over the occipital region is innervated by sensory fibers of the greater and lesser occipital nerves.

9.3.1 Lesser Occipital Nerve (C2)

- This nerve arises from the second (sometimes also the third) anterior cervical ramus and is a superficial (cutaneous) nerve. It traverses cephalad from the posterior edge of the sternocleidomastoid muscle towards the top of the head, where it pierces the deep fascia and ascends the scalp behind the auricle, dividing into several branches (Fig. 9.10).

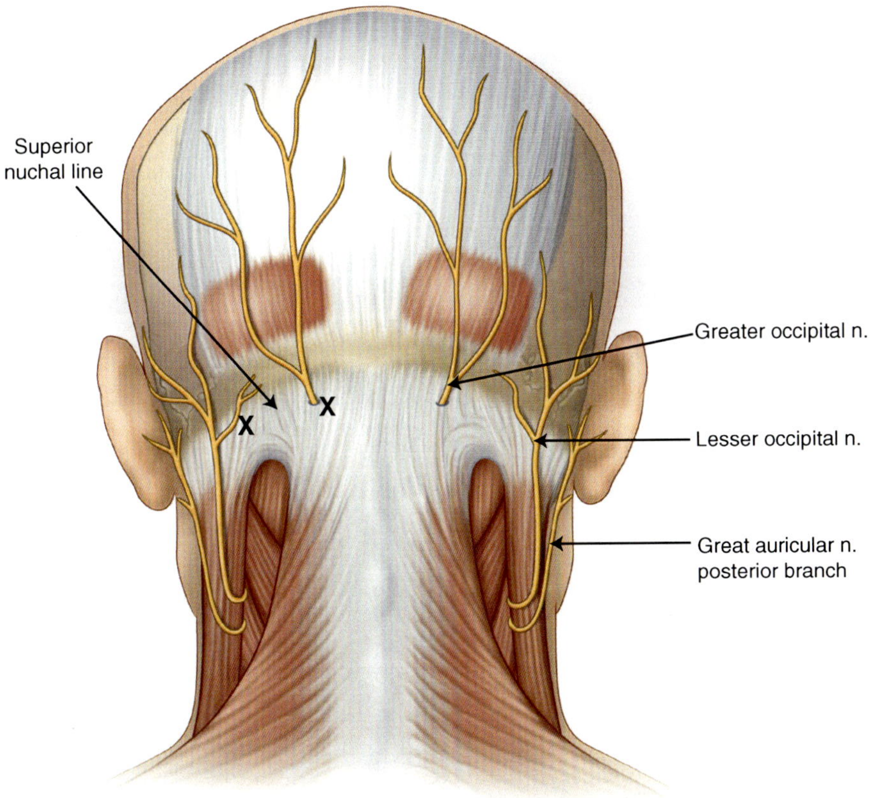

Fig. 9.10 Greater and lesser occipital nerve distributions. Sites of needle insertion are marked with X

9.3.2 Greater Occipital Nerve (C2)

- The greater occipital nerve arises from the *posterior ramus* of the second cervical spinal nerve as its medial branch (the cervical plexus arises from the anterior rami) and travels in a cranial direction, medial to the occipital artery (Fig. 9.10), to reach the skin at a location within the aponeurosis of the trapezius muscle just inferior to the superior nuchal line. At this point, it provides branches medially to supply the head and laterally to supply the skin of the scalp in the area behind the auricle (post-auricular area). It supplies motor fibers to the semispinalis capitis muscle. The lateral branch supplies the splenius, longissimus, and semispinalis capitis muscles.

9.4 Clinical Anatomy of the Nerve of Arnold

- The Nerve of Arnold is the sensory auricular branch of the vagus nerve. It arises from the jugular (superior) ganglion of the vagus nerve. Soon after its origin, it is joined by a filament from the petrous (inferior) ganglion of the glossopharyngeal nerve, after which it passes behind the internal jugular vein and enters the mastoid canaliculus on the lateral wall of the jugular fossa. Passing through the substance of the temporal bone, it crosses the facial canal about 4 mm (in adult) above the stylomastoid foramen, where it gives off an ascending branch which joins the facial nerve. The nerve then passes through the tympano-mastoid fissure between the mastoid process and the temporal bone, becomes superficial, and divides into two branches. One branch joins the posterior auricular nerve, while the other travels to the skin of the posterior auricular area and to the posterior wall and floor of the external acoustic meatus which it supplies with sensory innervation (Fig. 9.11). The nerve also provides sensory innervation to the inferior portion of the outer aspect of the tympanic membrane.

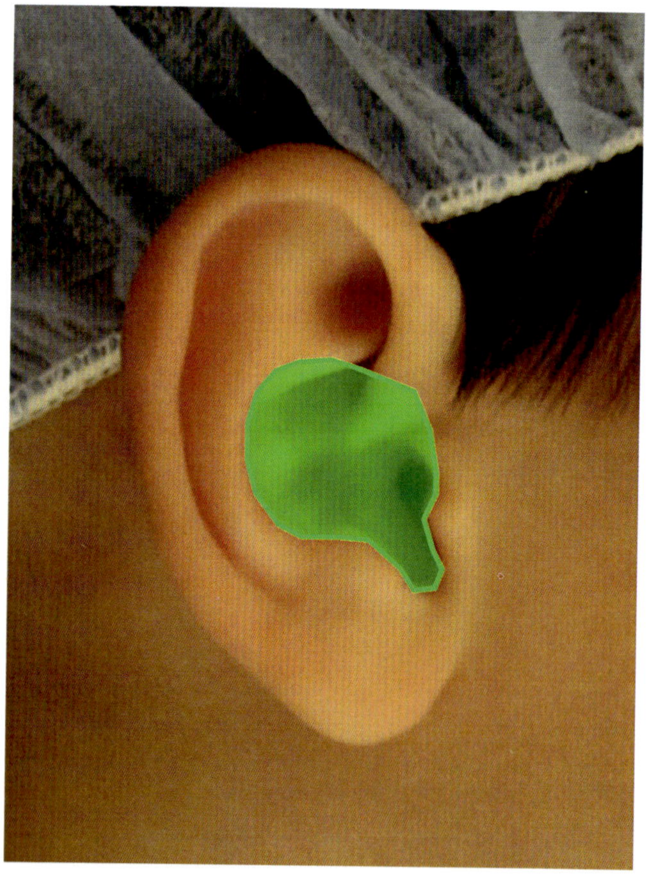

Fig. 9.11 Sensory distribution of the Nerve of Arnold, indicated by *green*-shaded area

Suggested Reading

Chapter 28: Neck. In: Standring S, editor. Gray's anatomy. 40th ed. London: Churchill Livingstone; 2008. p. 455–62.

Chapter 29: Face and scalp. In: Standring S, editor. Gray's anatomy. 40th ed. London: Churchill Livingstone; 2008. p. 492–5.

Clinical Anatomy of the Brachial Plexus

10

Anil H. Walji and Ban C.H. Tsui

Contents

A.H. Walji, MD, PhD
Division of Anatomy, Department of Surgery,
Faculty of Medicine and Dentistry,
University of Alberta, Edmonton, AB, Canada

B.C.H. Tsui, Dip Eng, BSc (Math), B Pharm, MSc, MD, FRCPC (✉)
Department of Anesthesiology and Pain Medicine,
Stollery Children's Hospital/University of Alberta Hospital,
2-150 Clinical Sciences Building, Edmonton,
AB T6G 2G3, Canada
e-mail: btsui@ualberta.ca

B.C.H. Tsui, S. Suresh (eds.), *Pediatric Atlas of Ultrasound- and Nerve Stimulation-Guided Regional Anesthesia*,
DOI 10.1007/978-0-387-79964-3_10

10.1 Brachial Plexus: Overview

The brachial plexus is a spinal nerve plexus in the neck, shoulder, and axilla that provides innervation to the skin, subcutaneous tissues, and muscles of the entire upper limb from the shoulder to the fingers, as well as articular innervation to the shoulder, elbow, and wrist joints. It is one of the largest somatic plexuses in the body, and its components, namely, the roots, trunks, divisions, cords, and terminal nerves, are arranged proximo-distally in a regional fashion; the roots are *paravertebral* in location, the trunks by and large *interscalene*, the divisions *subclavian*, the cords *axillary,* and the nerves *brachial*. Surgical anesthesia and postoperative analgesia can be achieved from local anesthetic blockade of the brachial plexus at any point along its course.

The interscalene and periclavicular block approaches (e.g., supraclavicular, intersternocleidomastoid, and subclavian perivascular) target the brachial plexus at the root and trunk levels, while the infraclavicular, axillary, and peripheral approaches target the cords and terminal nerves of the brachial plexus.

This chapter highlights the clinical anatomy of the brachial plexus itself, while the anatomy and distribution of the peripheral nerves are discussed at length in a subsequent chapter (Chap. 14). Chapter 14 also provides an overview and detailed description of the clinically relevant anatomy of the brachial plexus as well as that of the dermatomes, myotomes, osteotomes, and innervation of major joints of the upper extremity.

The five roots of the brachial plexus arise in a paravertebral location from the anterior (primary) rami of C5–T1 spinal nerves and exit from the intervertebral foramina, above the transverse processes of the corresponding cervical vertebrae (Fig. 10.1). The plexus may receive variable contributions from C4 and T2. When C4 makes a large contribution, T1 is reduced, forming a *prefixed* brachial plexus (*C4 to C8*); however, in some cases, the contribution from C5 may be reduced and that from T2 increased, leading to a *postfixed* plexus (*C6 to T2*).

After exiting the intervertebral foramina, the roots traverse through the interscalene groove or triangle (scalene hiatus) before forming the trunks and entering the floor of the posterior triangle of the neck (supraclavicular fossa). In the posterior triangle, the plexus is covered only by platysma, deep fascia, and skin and is palpable, especially in thin individuals. The anterior and middle scalene muscles lie immediately anterior and posterior respectively to the plexus in the interscalene region, forming the so-called interscalene groove or triangle. The plexus at this level consists of upper (superior), middle, and lower (inferior) *trunks* and is enclosed within the interscalene fascial sheath. Most commonly, the upper trunk is formed by the convergence of C5 and C6, while C7 becomes the middle trunk, and C8 and T1 converge to make the lower trunk. The trunks are crossed by the external jugular vein, the superficial (transverse) cervical and suprascapular arteries (branches of the thyrocervical trunk that can function as external collaterals of the subclavian artery), the inferior belly of the omohyoid, and the supraclavicular nerves as they course inferolaterally.

At and above the level of the interscalene groove (C6), the plexus lies posterolateral to the internal jugular vein and common carotid artery. As the plexus emerges between the scalene muscles, its proximal part is cephalad to the third part of the subclavian artery and its lower trunk posterior to it. The plexus then courses behind the medial two thirds of the clavicle where it is also posterior to the subclavius muscle and suprascapular vessels. Near the midpoint of the clavicle, the plexus and the subclavian artery are separated from the subclavian vein by the tendinous insertion of the anterior scalene muscle (Fig. 10.2).

Coursing distally, each of the three trunks then branches into anterior and posterior divisions deep to the clavicle (subclavian location), following which the divisions reunite to form three cords in the axilla (axillary location) and five major terminal nerves in the upper arm (brachial location) (Fig. 10.3). The three cords of the plexus, namely, lateral, medial, and posterior, are named for their relationship to the second part of the axillary artery. Within the axilla, the brachial plexus is enclosed together with the first part of the axillary artery and axillary vein within the fibrous *axillary sheath*, a continuation of the prevertebral layer of deep cervical fascia. The major terminal nerves and their branches can been seen in Fig. 10.4.

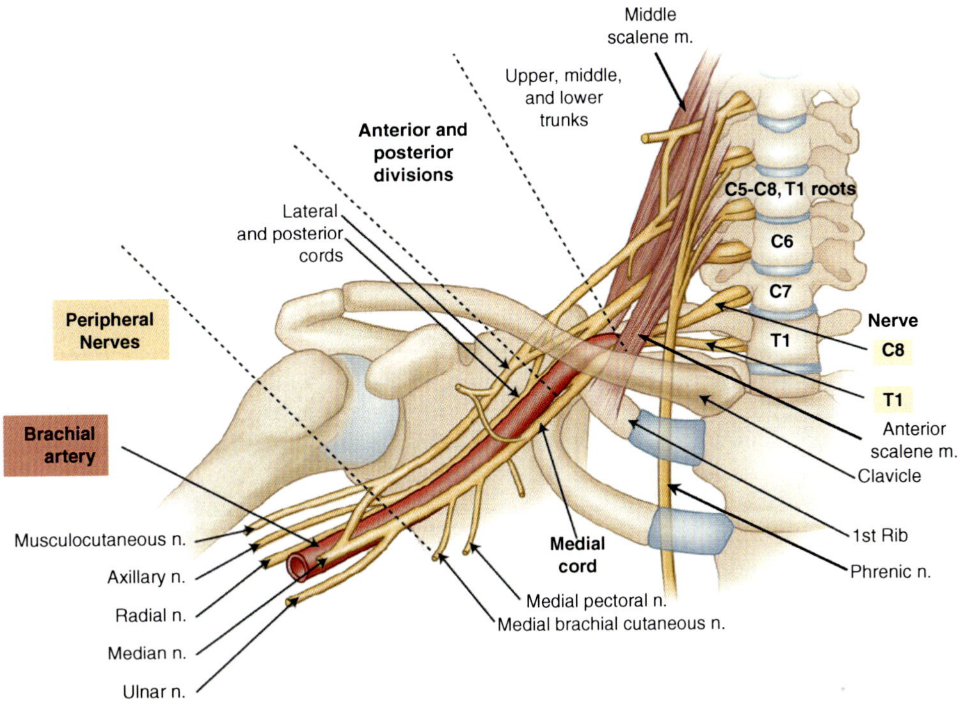

Fig. 10.1 Anatomy of the brachial plexus

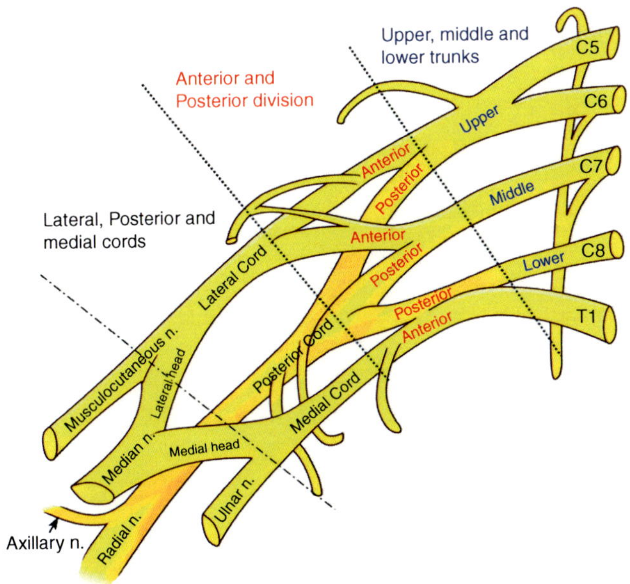

Fig. 10.2 Course of the brachial plexus at the interscalene groove and under the clavicle

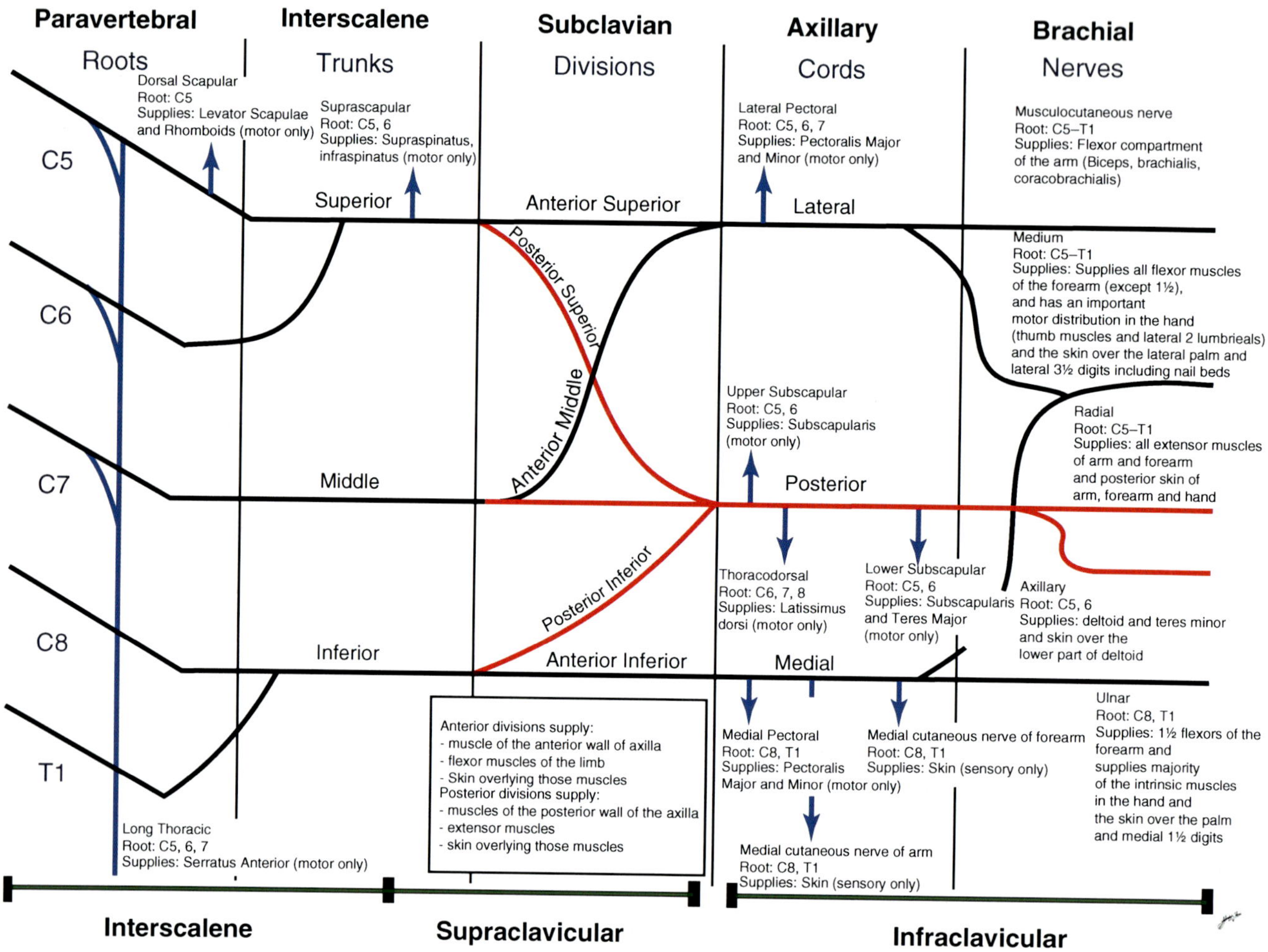

Fig. 10.3 Schematic diagram of the brachial plexus

Fig. 10.4 A "map" of the brachial plexus showing sensory and motor supply, terminal nerves, and targets of interscalene, supraclavicular, and infraclavicular blocks

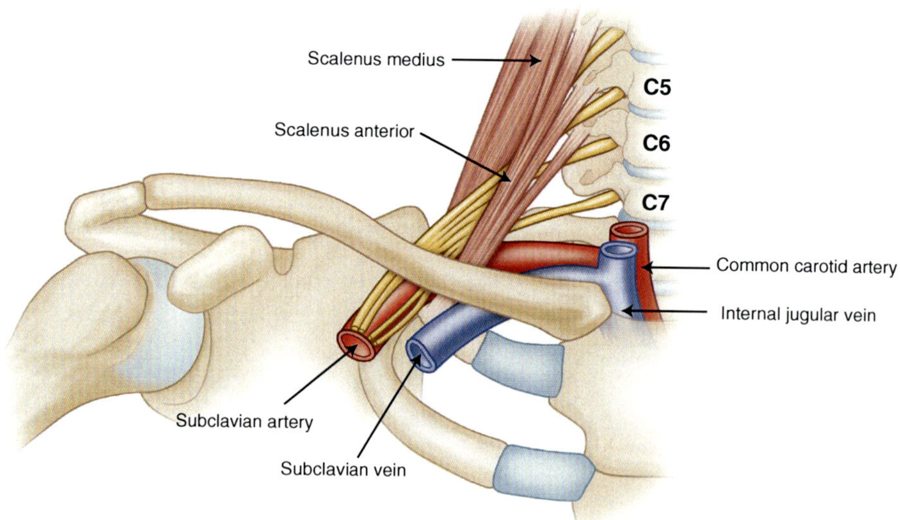

10.2 Branches of the Brachial Plexus

From proximal to distal, the plexus is distributed regionally and consists of five *roots* (paravertebral), three *trunks* (interscalene), two *divisions* per trunk (subclavian), three *cords* (axillary), and five major *terminal nerves* (brachial) (Figs. 10.3 and 10.4).

Branches arising from the roots and trunks of the brachial plexus are generally classified as "supraclavicular" branches, while those arising from the cords are referred to as "infraclavicular" branches.

- *Root branches (supraclavicular):*
  - Nerve to longus cervicis muscle (C5–C8)
  - Nerve to longus colli and scalene muscles (C5–C8)
  - Contribution to phrenic nerve (C5)
  - Dorsal scapular nerve [nerve to rhomboids] (C5)
- *Trunk branches (supraclavicular)*:
  - Nerve to subclavius (superior trunk, C5, C6)
  - Suprascapular nerve (superior trunk, C5, C6)
  - Long thoracic nerve [posterior thoracic nerve] (C5–C7)
- *Cord branches (infraclavicular)*:
  - Lateral cord
    - Lateral pectoral nerve (C5–C7); *musculocutaneous* nerve (C5–C7); lateral root (head) of *median* nerve (C5–C6, C7)
  - Medial cord
    - Medial pectoral nerve (C8, T1); medial cutaneous nerve of arm (medial brachial cutaneous nerve, C8, T1); medial cutaneous nerve of forearm (medial antebrachial cutaneous nerve, C8, T1); medial root (head) of *median* nerve (C8, T1); *ulnar* nerve (C7–C8, T1)
  - Posterior cord
    - Upper subscapular nerve (C5, C6); thoracodorsal nerve (C6–C8); lower subscapular nerve (C5, C6); axillary nerve (C5, C6); *radial* nerve (C5–C8, T1)

Selective clinically relevant nerves will be described in more detail below with respect to their origins, course, and function as related to clinical practice.

10.2.1 Branches from the Roots (Ventral Rami)

10.2.1.1 Phrenic Nerve

Strictly speaking, the phrenic nerve is not part of the brachial plexus; however, due to its close relationship to the plexus, the nerve has to be considered from a clinical perspective since it plays an important role and has significant clinical implications when performing brachial plexus block. The phrenic nerve arises from the anterior rami of spinal nerves C3, C4, and C5 (*C3, C4 and C5 keep the diaphragm alive*!) and normally descends in a superolateral to inferomedial direction on the anterior surface of the scalenus anterior muscle (subject to anatomic variation) deep to the prevertebral fascia, before passing under the clavicle and through the superior thoracic aperture into the superior mediastinum, passing just medial to and in front of the internal thoracic (mammary) artery. Once within the thoracic cavity, both right and left phrenic nerves descend anterior to the pulmonary hila together with the pericardiophrenic vessels (branches of the internal thoracic or mammary vessels) in the plane between the fibrous pericardium medially and the mediastinal pleura laterally on their way to the diaphragm which they pierce to supply. The right phrenic pierces the diaphragm's central tendon near the caval orifice, while the left phrenic traverses the muscular portion of the left hemidiaphragm and lies somewhat more anterior than the right.

Innervation	*Motor*: diaphragm (*the phrenic is the sole motor supply to the diaphragm*)
	Sensory: fibrous pericardium, parietal layer of serous pericardium, mediastinal parietal pleura, diaphragmatic parietal pleura, and diaphragmatic parietal peritoneum

10.2.1.2 Dorsal Scapular Nerve

Originating from the ventral ramus of C5, this nerve passes through the scalenus medius and courses behind the levator scapulae before running with the deep branch of the dorsal scapular artery to terminate in the rhomboids, which it supplies.

Innervation	*Motor*: rhomboid major, rhomboid minor, levator scapulae (occasionally)
	Sensory: none

10.2.2 Branches from the Trunks

10.2.2.1 Long Thoracic Nerve

This nerve has contributions from the roots of C5–C7. Contributions from C5 and C6 pierce the scalenus medius and join within or lateral to the muscle; the nerve then descends dorsal (posterior) to the brachial plexus and first part of the axillary artery. The C7 contribution, when present, emerges between the scalenus medius and scalenus anterior muscles before joining with the C5 and C6 contributions near the superior border of the serratus anterior muscle. The nerve then crosses the superior border of the serratus anterior to reach its lateral surface before descending on the muscle to supply each of its digitations and to terminate at its lower border.

Innervation	*Motor*: serratus anterior
	Sensory: none

10.2.2.2 Nerve to the Subclavius

Small but deserving of mention is the nerve to the subclavius. Arising from where the ventral rami of C5 and C6 join, this small filament travels anterior to the main plexus, passing anterior to the third part of the subclavian artery, and is usually connected in some capacity to the phrenic nerve before passing above the subclavian vein to supply the subclavius muscle.

Innervation	*Motor* – subclavius
	Sensory – none

10.2.2.3 Suprascapular Nerve

A large branch of the superior trunk, this nerve arises from the anterior rami of C5 and C6; travels laterally, deep to the trapezius and omohyoid muscles; and enters the supraspinous fossa through the suprascapular notch beneath the superior transverse scapular ligament. Coursing deep to the supraspinatus and supplying it, the nerve then curves around the lateral border of the spine of the scapula (spinoglenoid notch) and, with the supraclavicular artery, reaches the infraspinous fossa, where it supplies the infraspinatus and provides articular branches to the capsule of the glenohumeral (shoulder) and acromioclavicular joints. A cutaneous branch, though rare, may pierce the deltoid close to the tip of the acromion and become superficial to supply the skin of the shoulder and upper arm within the region supplied by the axillary nerve.

Innervation	*Motor*: supraspinatus, infraspinatus
	Sensory: when present, supplies skin on lateral aspect of shoulder, proximal third of arm; *articular* innervation to shoulder and acromioclavicular joints

10.2.3 Branches from the Cords

10.2.3.1 Lateral Pectoral Nerve

With contributions from the C5 to C7 anterior rami, the lateral pectoral nerve can either arise from the anterior divisions of the upper and middle trunks or have a single origin from the lateral cord. It passes anterior to the axillary artery and vein before piercing the clavipectoral fascia and terminating on the deep surface of the pectoralis major muscle, which it supplies. A filament from the nerve loops in front of the axillary artery (ansa pectoralis) and joins with the medial pectoral nerve to send fibers to the pectoralis minor muscle.

Innervation	*Motor*: pectoralis major, some to pectoralis minor
	Sensory: none

10.2.3.2 Medial Pectoral Nerve

Arising from the medial cord, with contributions from C8 and T1, this nerve travels from its origin posterior to the axillary artery and then swings anteriorly between the axillary artery and vein to join with the filament from the lateral pectoral nerve anterior to the axillary artery. It enters the deep surface of the pectoralis minor and supplies it; usually some branches will travel around the inferior border of the pectoralis minor to terminate in the pectoralis major.

Innervation	*Motor*: pectoralis minor, some to pectoralis major
	Sensory: none

10.2.3.3 Upper and Lower Subscapular Nerves

The upper (superior) subscapular nerve (C5 and C6) arises from the posterior cord and usually enters the subscapularis quite high to supply it; frequently it may be double.

The lower (inferior) subscapular nerve (C5 and C6) arises further down, also from the posterior cord, and is the larger of the two nerves. It supplies the inferior portion of the subscapularis and terminates in the teres major which it also supplies.

Innervation	*Motor*: subscapularis, usually also the teres major
	Sensory: none

10.2.3.4 Thoracodorsal Nerve

Arising from the posterior cord between the subscapular nerves, the thoracodorsal nerve has contributions from C6 to C8. It travels initially with the subscapular artery then with the thoracodorsal artery along the posterior wall of the axilla to the deep surface of the latissimus dorsi, which it supplies before terminating at the muscle's lower border.

Innervation	*Motor*: latissimus dorsi
	Sensory: none

10.2.4 Terminal Nerves

10.2.4.1 Axillary Nerve

The axillary nerve (C5, C6), also known as the circumflex humeral nerve, arises from the posterior cord of the brachial plexus and initially lies posterior to the axillary artery, lateral to the radial nerve, and anterior to the subscapularis (Figs. 10.5, 10.6, and 10.7). The nerve then courses inferiorly to the lower border of the subscapularis where it winds posteriorly through the quadrangular space, underneath the capsule of the shoulder joint, together with the posterior circumflex humeral vessels to reach the back of the shoulder and deltoid region. The quadrangular intermuscular space is bounded laterally by the neck of the humerus, medially by the long head of the triceps, and superiorly and inferiorly by the teres minor and major muscles, respectively. Here, the nerve divides into anterior, posterior, and collateral branches.

The anterior branch travels around the surgical neck of the humerus with the posterior circumflex humeral vessels, deep to the deltoid, and as far as the anterior border of this muscle. It supplies the deltoid and also gives off several small cutaneous branches which travel through the deltoid to the skin overlying its lower part on the lateral aspect of the shoulder.

The posterior branch supplies the posterior aspect of the deltoid and teres minor. It usually lies medial to the anterior branch in the quadrangular space. It travels posteromedially along the attachment of the lateral head of the triceps, generally inferior to the rim of the glenoid cavity. It then gives a branch to the teres minor, which enters the muscle through its inferior surface. The posterior branch also gives rise to the upper (superior) lateral cutaneous nerve of the arm, which pierces the deep fascia on the lower aspect of the posterior border of the deltoid and sends cutaneous branches to the overlying skin. Although this nerve usually supplies the posterior aspect of the deltoid, the deltoid can also be supplied by the anterior branch. The main trunk of the axillary nerve supplies an articular branch to the capsule of the shoulder joint just below the subscapularis. The collateral branch to the long head of the triceps arises just prior to the termination of the posterior cord.

Innervation	*Motor*: deltoid, teres minor, and long head of the triceps
	Sensory: *articular* innervation to the shoulder joint, cutaneous innervation to the skin of the shoulder over the lower portion of deltoid and upper portion of the long head of the triceps

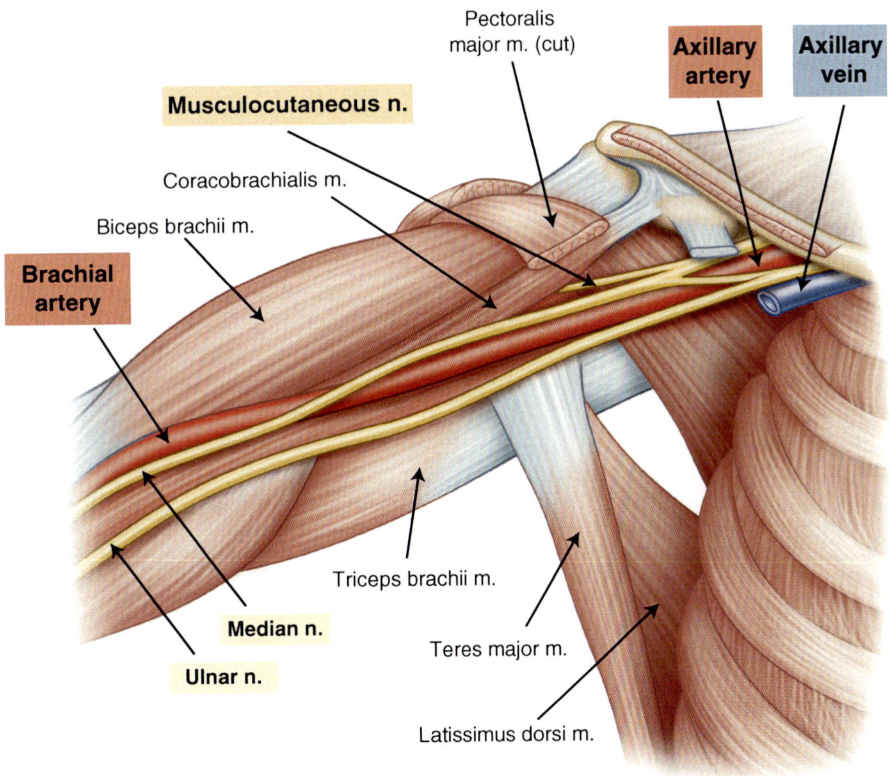

Fig. 10.5 Peripheral nerves and vessels of the upper extremity

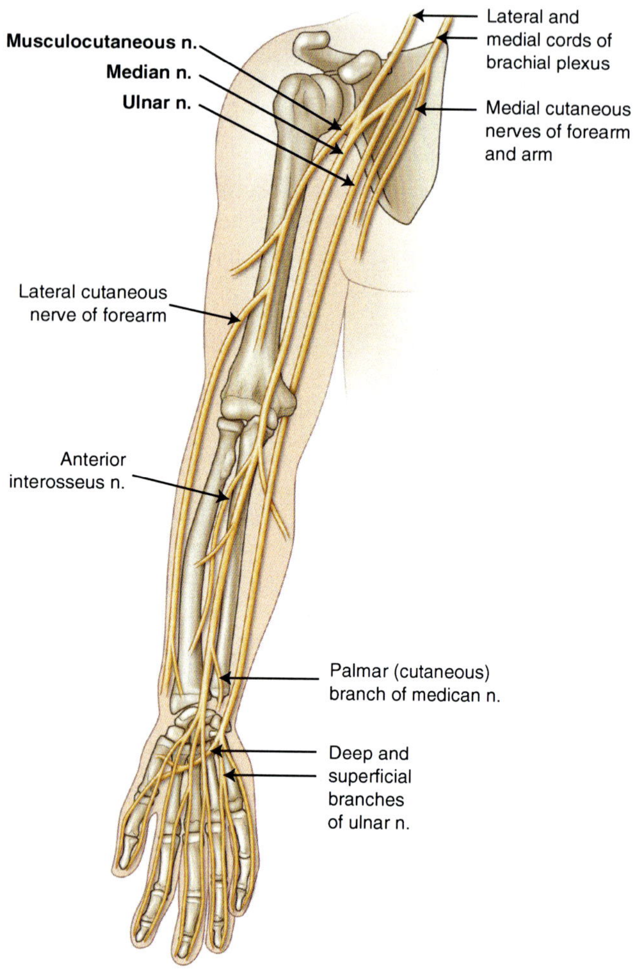

Fig. 10.6 Peripheral nerves of the upper extremity: medial and lateral cords

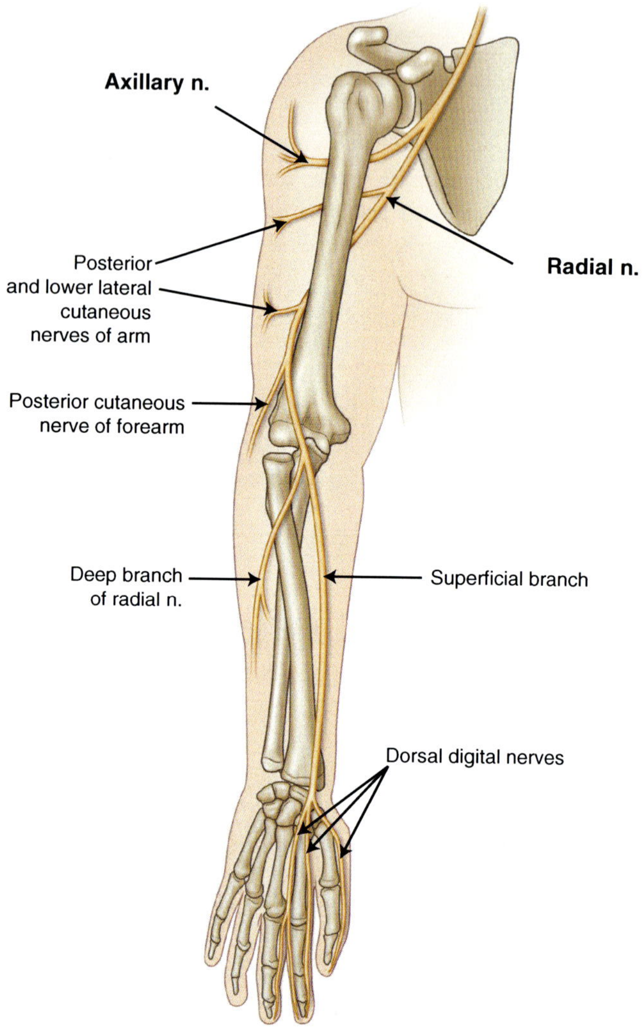

Fig. 10.7 Peripheral nerves of the upper extremity: posterior cords

10.2.4.2 Musculocutaneous Nerve

Arising from the lateral cord of the brachial plexus opposite the lower border of the pectoralis minor and derived from the anterior rami of C5 to C7, this nerve usually pierces the coracobrachialis and passes obliquely between the biceps brachii and the brachialis to the lateral aspect of the arm (Figs. 10.6 and 10.7). It supplies the coracobrachialis, biceps brachii, and most of brachialis (a small lateral portion of the muscle is supplied by the radial nerve [C7]). At about the level of the elbow, it pierces the deep fascia lateral to the tendon of the biceps brachii and continues as the lateral cutaneous nerve of the forearm. The branch to the coracobrachialis usually comes off before the nerve enters the muscle; these fibers may also arise directly from the lateral cord. The branch to the brachialis gives off an articular branch to the capsule of the elbow joint. It also supplies a small branch to the periosteum of the humerus which courses with the nutrient artery.

Innervation	*Motor*: coracobrachialis, biceps brachii, most of brachialis, occasionally pronator teres
	Sensory: skin of lateral forearm, articular innervation to the elbow, small branch to humerus

10.2.4.3 Lateral Cutaneous Nerve of the Forearm

A continuation of the musculocutaneous nerve after it has supplied the muscles in the anterior arm, this nerve pierces the deep fascia lateral to the biceps brachii tendon and descends along the radial (lateral) border of the forearm deep to the median cubital and cephalic veins to reach the wrist (Fig. 10.6). It supplies sensory innervation to the skin and subcutaneous tissues of the anterolateral forearm up to the lateral aspect of the wrist, with communicating branches around the radial border of the forearm to the posterior cutaneous nerve of the forearm (from the radial nerve) and the superficial terminal branch of the radial nerve. At the wrist, the lateral cutaneous nerve of the forearm lies anterior to the radial artery, courses to the base of the thenar eminence, and ends in cutaneous branches with communications to the palmar cutaneous branch of the median nerve and terminal branches of the radial nerve.

Innervation	*Motor*: none
	Sensory: skin of anterolateral forearm up to lateral aspect of wrist

10.2.4.4 Medial Cutaneous Nerve of the Arm

Arising from the medial cord of the brachial plexus (C8 and T1), this nerve passes through the axilla close to the axillary vein and communicates with the intercostobrachial nerve (Fig. 10.6). It then descends medial to the brachial artery and basilic vein, piercing the deep fascia at the mid-upper arm to supply the skin on the lower third of the medial aspect of the arm and terminate in cutaneous branches around the elbow, some reaching as far as the olecranon.

Innervation	*Motor*: none
	Sensory: skin on the lower third of the medial aspect of the arm, skin over the medial epicondyle and olecranon

10.2.4.5 Medial Cutaneous Nerve of the Forearm

Similar to the medial cutaneous nerve of the arm, this nerve also arises from the medial cord (C8 and T1). It courses between the axillary artery and vein, and as it leaves the axilla, it sends a branch that pierces the deep fascia to supply the skin over the biceps brachii nearly as far as the elbow. From its origin, the nerve courses downwards medial to the brachial artery before piercing the deep fascia together with the basilic vein midway down the arm and dividing into anterior and posterior branches. The anterior branch generally passes in front of the median cubital vein, traveling anteromedially in the forearm and connecting with the palmar cutaneous branch of the ulnar nerve. The posterior branch travels across the forearm medial to the basilic vein, anterior to the medial epicondyle, and curves to the back of the forearm to descend along its medial (ulnar) border to the wrist. It terminates by communicating with the medial cutaneous nerve of the arm, the posterior cutaneous nerve of the forearm, and the dorsal branch of the ulnar nerve.

Innervation	*Motor*: none
	Sensory: skin on medial aspect of lower third of arm and forearm

10.2.4.6 Median Nerve

The median nerve is formed from the lateral and medial cords of the brachial plexus via the lateral (C5–C7) and medial (C8 and T1) roots of the median nerve respectively (Figs. 10.5, 10.6, 10.8, and 10.9). These roots surround the third part of the axillary artery, generally uniting in front of it. The median nerve then enters the upper arm lateral to the brachial artery, crossing over the artery anteriorly at the level of the insertion of the coracobrachialis. From there, it courses down the arm medial to the artery into the cubital fossa, at which point it lies deep to the bicipital aponeurosis and superficial to the brachialis, which separates it from the elbow joint capsule.

During its course in the arm, the median nerve gives off vascular vasomotor (sympathetic) branches to the brachial artery, articular branches to the elbow, and proximal radio-ulnar joints and muscular branches (usually given off proximally near the elbow) to the superficial flexor muscles in the anterior compartment of the forearm (except flexor carpi ulnaris). It usually sends a branch to the pronator teres a variable distance proximal to the elbow. The median nerve then leaves the cubital fossa and courses between the two heads of the pronator teres to enter the forearm, which it does by passing underneath a tendinous arch between the radial and humero-ulnar heads of the flexor digitorum superficialis (FDS) muscle. Here it may get compressed between the two heads of pronator teres (*pronator syndrome*) leading to weakness of wrist and digit flexors and pronation. From there, it travels distally adherent to the deep surface of the FDS but superficial to the flexor digitorum profundus muscle. Near the wrist it emerges approximately 5 cm proximal to the flexor retinaculum just lateral to the tendons of the flexor digitorum superficialis and between them and the tendon of flexor carpi radialis. When present, the tendon of palmaris longus lies just medial to the nerve at the wrist, the median nerve peeking out laterally from behind it.

In the forearm, the median nerve gives off two branches; the anterior interosseous nerve and the palmar cutaneous branch. The *anterior interosseous* branch forms posteriorly as the nerve traverses between the two heads of the pronator teres (where it may also be compressed in pronator syndrome) and travels deep along the anterior aspect of the interosseous membrane (hence the name) together with the anterior interosseous artery. It terminates at the level of the pronator quadratus, which it supplies, and also innervates the remaining two muscles of the deep anterior compartment of the forearm, namely, the flexor pollicis longus and the lateral half of flexor digitorum profundus (which provides tendons to the index (second) and middle (third) fingers). The *palmar cutaneous* branch arises just proximal to the flexor retinaculum (thus, it is usually spared in carpal tunnel syndrome) and either pierces it or the deep fascia before branching into lateral and medial divisions. The lateral divisions connect with the lateral cutaneous nerve of the forearm and innervate the thenar skin, while the medial branches innervate the palmar skin in the center of the palm and connect with palmar cutaneous branches of the ulnar nerve. It is important to note that many possible communicating branches can exist simultaneously, even from the anterior interosseous nerve, which helps to explain anomalous innervation commonly found within the hand.

The median nerve then passes deep to the flexor retinaculum, within the *carpal tunnel*, into the palm, where it divides into five or six branches which are variable in number and position. The nerve may get compressed in *carpal tunnel syndrome* (an entrapment neuropathy) leading to pain, tingling and numbness along its distribution in the hand, with atrophy of the thenar muscles if long-standing. The *recurrent (motor)* branch comes off the lateral side of the nerve and may be the first palmar branch or a terminal branch unto itself. The recurrent motor branch is extremely important as it supplies the muscles of the thenar eminence, responsible for moving the thumb. Its terminal portion may give a branch to the first dorsal interosseous muscle, which may be its only supply or shared with that from the ulnar nerve. The nerve continues as the common and proper palmar digital branches, providing cutaneous innervation to the first three and a half digits anteriorly and the second through fourth digits dorsally from their tips to the distal interphalangeal joints. In addition, the median nerve also sends motor branches to first, second, and occasionally third lumbricals.

Innervation	*Motor (median nerve)*: pronator teres, flexor carpi radialis, palmaris longus (when present), flexor digitorum superficialis
	Anterior interosseous nerve: lateral half of flexor digitorum profundus, flexor pollicis longus, pronator quadratus
	Median nerve in the hand: opponens pollicis, abductor pollicis brevis, flexor pollicis brevis, and lumbricals (1, 2, and occasionally 3)
	Sensory: *articular* innervation to capsule of elbow joint, skin on radial side of the wrist anteriorly and palm, palmar surface of the thumb and index and middle fingers and radial side of ring finger, skin distal to DIP joints of thumb, index, middle, and radial side of ring fingers dorsally. *Vascular* to brachial artery

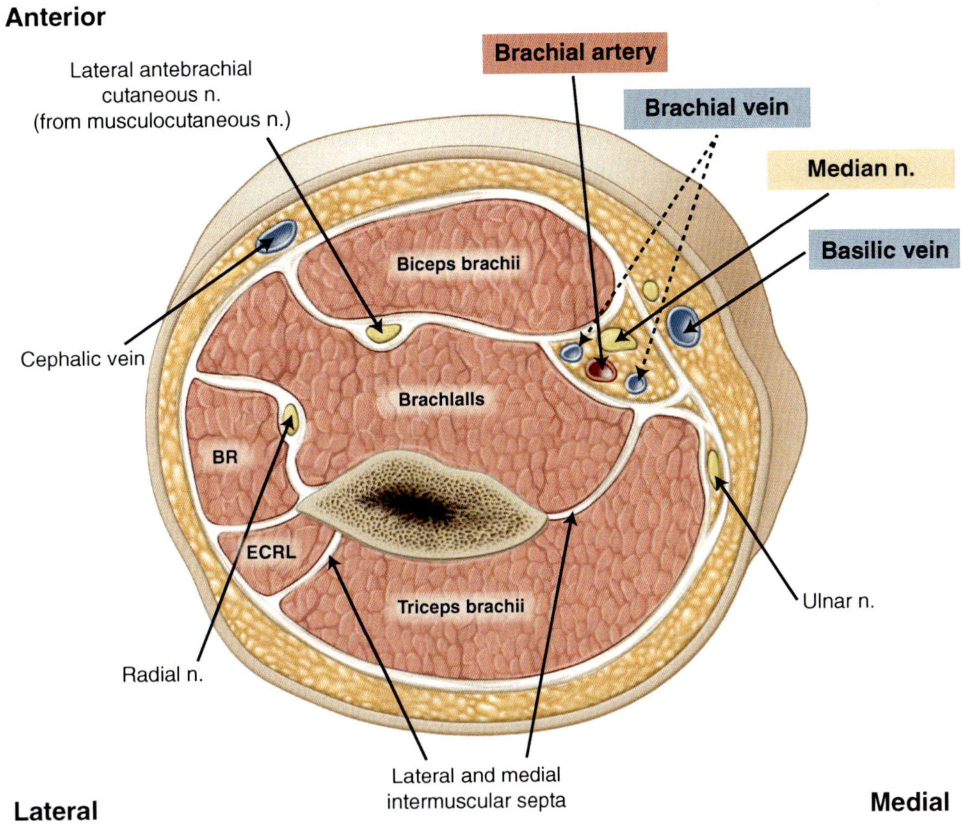

Fig. 10.8 Cross section of the arm showing positions of major muscles, blood vessels, and nerves. *BR* brachioradialis, *ECRL* extensor carpi radialis longus muscle

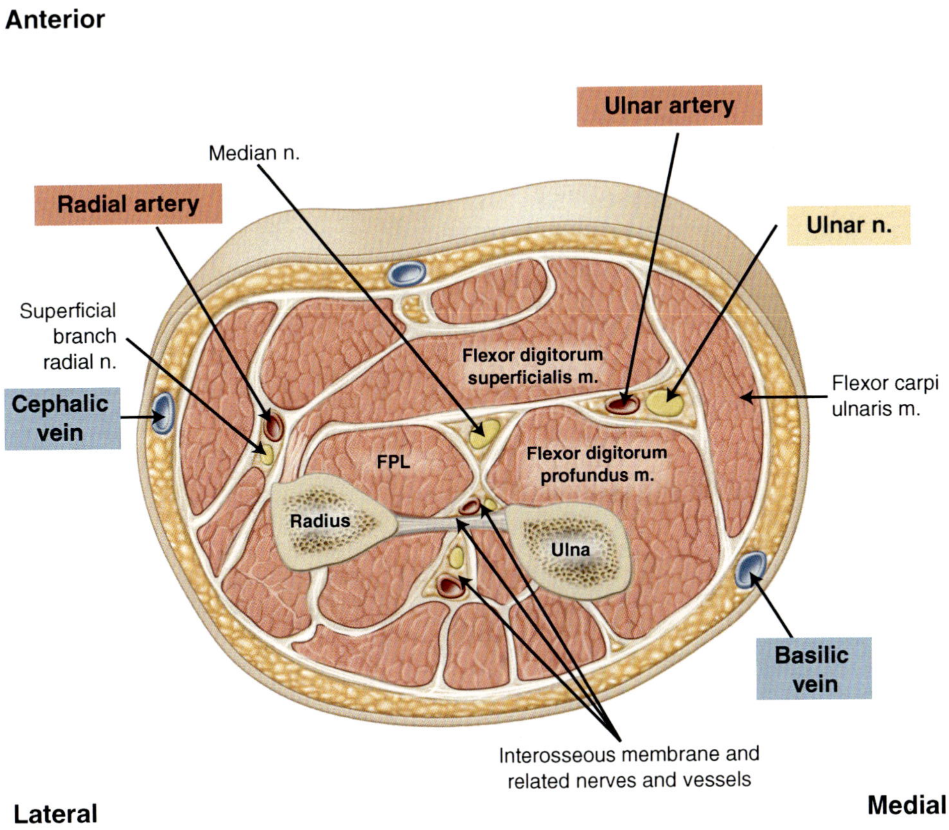

Fig. 10.9 Cross section of the distal forearm showing location of ulnar nerve with respect to ulnar artery. *FPL* flexor pollicis longus muscle

10.2.4.7 Ulnar Nerve

The ulnar nerve arises from the medial cord of the brachial plexus from C8 and T1 and an occasional contribution from C7 (Figs. 10.6, 10.9, and 10.10). Initially, the nerve courses between the axillary artery and vein and then lies along the medial aspect of the brachial artery up to the midpoint of the humerus, where it pierces the medial intermuscular septum, passes posteriorly, and then descends along the anterior surface of the medial head of the triceps brachii muscle. It then passes behind the medial epicondyle of the humerus (in the condylar groove) where it is very superficial and can be rolled against the bone. If jarred against the epicondyle, characteristic tingling sensations result ("funny bone"). It has no branches in the arm. Just beyond the medial epicondyle, the nerve enters the forearm between the two heads of the flexor carpi ulnaris which it supplies. Here, the nerve lies medial to the elbow joint, superficial to the fibrous joint capsule and the ulnar collateral ligament. The nerve may also get compressed in the osseofibrous tunnel formed by the tendinous arch connecting the ulnar and humeral heads of the flexor carpi ulnaris (*cubital tunnel syndrome*) leading to numbness and tingling along its distribution in the hand.

The nerve then descends through the medial aspect of forearm, coursing somewhat anteriorly and coming to lie deep to and between the flexor carpi ulnaris and flexor digitorum superficialis muscles. As it courses through the middle of the forearm between these muscles, it approaches the ulnar artery on its lateral aspect; the artery, distant from it in the upper third of the forearm, comes to lie close to the nerve and just lateral to it in the lower half to two thirds of the forearm (Fig. 10.9). The nerve and artery lie directly anterior to the ulna at the junction of the lower third and upper two thirds of the forearm (Fig. 10.10). In the forearm, the ulnar nerve supplies the flexor carpi ulnaris and the medial half of flexor digitorum profundus which provides tendons to the ring (fourth) and little (fifth) fingers. Approximately 5 cm proximal to the wrist the ulnar nerve gives off its *dorsal cutaneous* branch which continues distally into the hand after passing anterior to the flexor retinaculum, just lateral to the pisiform bone and posteromedial to the ulnar artery. The ulnar nerve then passes under the superficial part of the flexor retinaculum (within Guyon's canal) with the ulnar artery and divides into its *superficial* and *deep terminal* branches. The ulnar artery lies anterolateral to the nerve at the wrist.

The dorsal branch continues distally and posteriorly beneath the flexor carpi ulnaris before piercing the deep fascia and dividing into two, often three dorsal digital branches along the medial aspect of the back of the wrist and hand.

The superficial terminal branch supplies the palmaris brevis and skin on the medial aspect of the palm and divides into two palmar digital nerves; one supplying the medial side of the fifth (little) finger and the other supplying the adjoining sides of the fifth (little) and fourth (ring) fingers through a common digital nerve.

The deep terminal branch courses with the deep branch of the ulnar artery as it passes between the abductor digiti minimi and flexor digiti minimi, perforating the opponens digiti minimi to follow the deep palmar arch deep to the long flexor tendons. It supplies the muscles of the hypothenar eminence controlling the fifth finger, and as it crosses the hand from medial to lateral, it sends branches to the interossei and to the third and fourth lumbricals. The nerve terminates by supplying the adductor pollicis, the first palmar interosseous and flexor pollicis brevis (usually). It sends articular twigs to the wrist joint capsule and to intercarpal, carpometacarpal, and metacarpophalangeal joints. It also sends vasomotor (sympathetic) branches to the ulnar and palmar arteries.

Innervation	*Motor*: flexor carpi ulnaris, medial half of flexor digitorum profundus, lumbricals 3 and 4, opponens digiti minimi, flexor digiti minimi, abductor digiti minimi, all the interossei, adductor pollicis, flexor pollicis brevis (usually)
	Sensory: cutaneous innervation to fifth digit and medial half of fourth, extending to just proximal to the wrist, both dorsal and ventral. Articular branches to wrist joint, intercarpal, carpometacarpal, and interphalangeal joints
	Vasomotor: to ulnar and palmar arteries

Fig. 10.10 Median and ulnar nerve pathways in the anterior forearm

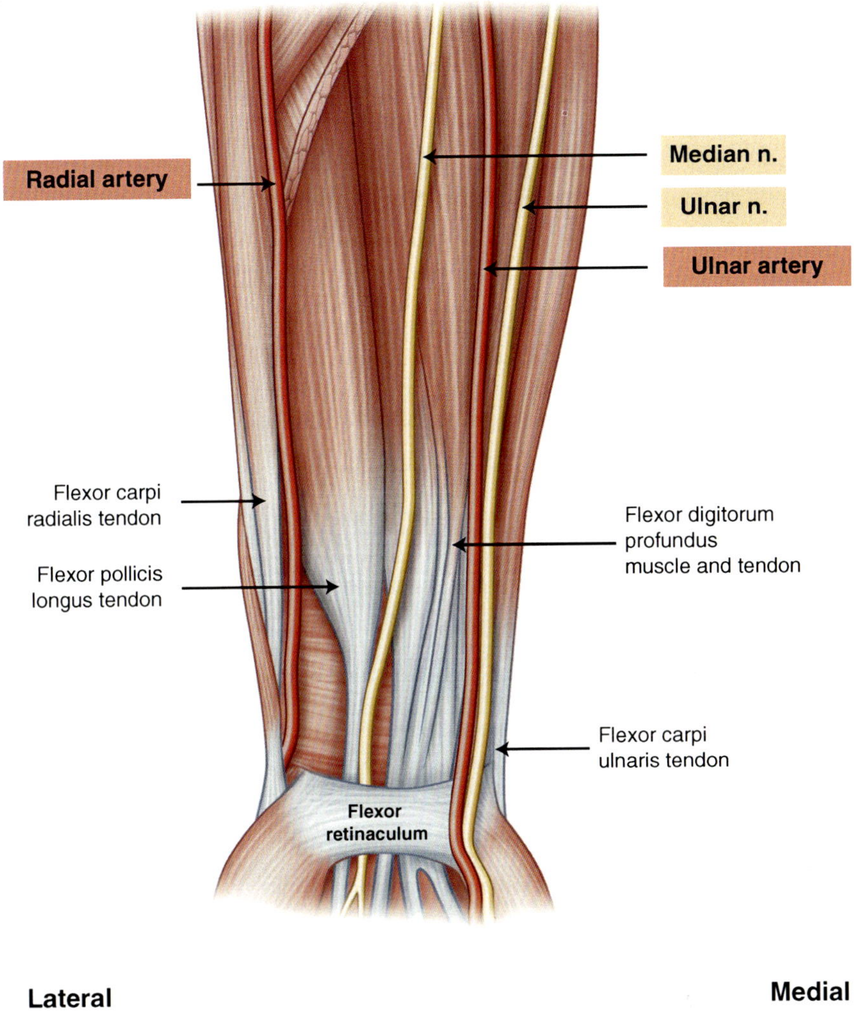

10.2.4.8 Radial Nerve

The radial nerve is the largest branch of the brachial plexus and arises from the posterior cord (C5–C8) (Figs. 10.7 and 10.11). It emerges from the posterior aspect of the plexus and lies posterior to the third part of the axillary artery and the proximal portion of the brachial artery. The nerve descends within the axilla (where it gives rise to the posterior cutaneous nerve of the arm), coursing across the subscapularis and the tendons of teres major and latissimus dorsi (it lies on the insertion of this latter muscle). It then passes between the medial and lateral heads of the triceps brachii muscle through the triangular interval together with the profunda brachii artery (deep brachial artery), giving rise to the posterior cutaneous nerve of the forearm and the lower (inferior) lateral cutaneous nerve of the arm. Here, lying posteromedial to the profunda brachii artery, it descends obliquely across the posterior aspect of the humerus along the radial (spiral) groove at the level of the insertion of the deltoid muscle. Here it may be compressed by badly fitted crutches and plaster casts, prolonged resting of the arm on the back rest of a chair or over the edge of the operating table if the arm is not positioned correctly. It may also get injured in mid-shaft fractures of the humerus. Compression of the radial nerve in the radial groove results in wrist drop due to weakness or paralysis of wrist and digit extensors ("*Saturday night palsy*"). The nerve then reaches the lateral margin of the humerus above the elbow, pierces through the lateral intermuscular septum, and crosses over the lateral epicondyle of the humerus to enter the anterior compartment of the arm in a deep groove between the brachialis and brachioradialis muscles proximally and the extensor carpi radialis longus muscle distally (Fig. 10.11). Muscular branches of the radial nerve supply the triceps brachii, anconeus, brachioradialis, and extensor carpi radialis longus muscles. Articular branches supply the capsule of the elbow joint.

In front of the lateral epicondyle of humerus, the nerve divides into its two terminal branches, the superficial terminal or radial (sensory) and the deep terminal or posterior interosseous (motor) nerves. The *superficial terminal* branch travels inferiorly beneath the brachioradialis and lateral to the radial artery and curves around the lateral side of the radius before eventually piercing the deep fascia dorsally at approximately the level of the wrist. From here, it divides into four or five dorsal digital nerves, often communicating with posterior and lateral cutaneous nerves of the forearm. The *posterior interosseous nerve* travels to the posterior aspect of the forearm around the lateral aspect of the radius, passing through the supinator muscle between its two heads and supplying it. Emerging from the supinator, the deep branch courses between the deep and superficial forearm extensors inferiorly, which it supplies (except extensor carpi radialis longus which is supplied by the main radial nerve). At the distal border of the extensor pollicis brevis, the nerve travels deep to descend along the interosseous membrane and terminate at the dorsal aspect of the carpus, supplying articular innervation to the wrist and hand.

Innervation	*Motor (main radial nerve)*: triceps brachii, anconeus, brachioradialis, extensor carpi radialis longus
	Posterior interosseous nerve: extensor carpi radialis brevis, supinator, extensor carpi ulnaris, extensor digiti minimi, extensor digitorum, extensor indicis, extensor pollicis brevis, abductor pollicis longus, extensor pollicis longus
	Sensory: skin of posterior arm and forearm, posterior hand laterally near the base of the thumb, and the dorsal aspect of the index finger and the lateral half of the ring finger up to the distal interphalangeal crease
	Articular: elbow, wrist, distal radio-ulnar, some intercarpal and carpometacarpal joints

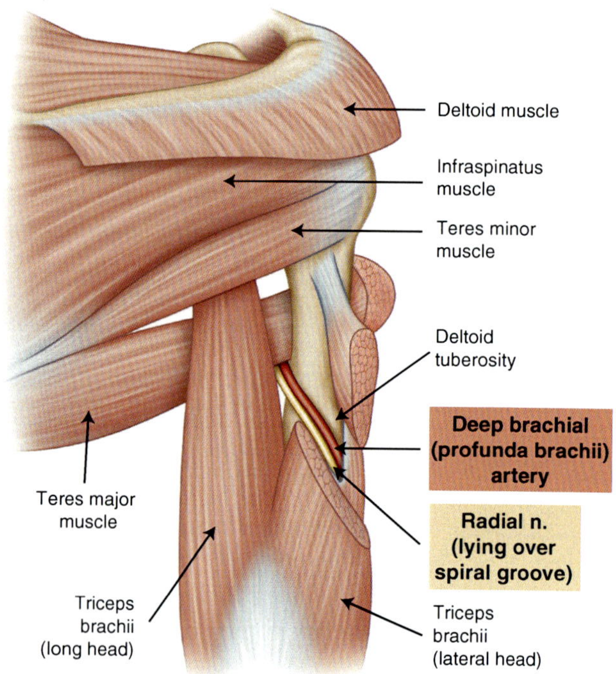

Fig. 10.11 Route of the radial nerve between the medial and lateral heads of the triceps brachii muscle. The nerve travels deep to the brachial artery and then follows the path of the spiral groove beyond the deltoid tuberosity

Suggested Reading

Chapter 45. Pectoral girdle and upper limb: overview and surface anatomy. In: Standring S, Johnson D, editors. Gray's anatomy, 40th ed. London: Churchill Livingstone; 2008. p. 780–90.

Chapter 45. Pectoral girdle, shoulder region and axilla. In: Standring S, Johnson D, editors. Gray's anatomy, 40th ed. London: Churchill Livingstone; 2008. p. 818–22.

Schuenke M, Schulte E, Schumacher U. The brachial plexus. In: Ross LM, Lamperti ED, editors. Thieme atlas of anatomy: general anatomy and musculoskeletal system. Stuttgart: Georg Thieme Verlag; 2006. p. 314–27.

Clinical Anatomy of the Lumbar Plexus

11

Anil H. Walji and Ban C.H. Tsui

Contents

A.H. Walji, MD, PhD
Division of Anatomy, Department of Surgery,
Faculty of Medicine and Dentistry, University of Alberta,
Edmonton, AB, Canada

B.C.H. Tsui, Dip Eng, BSc (Math), B Pharm, MSc, MD, FRCPC (✉)
Department of Anesthesiology and Pain Medicine,
Stollery Children's Hospital/University of Alberta Hospital,
2-150 Clinical Sciences Building, Edmonton,
AB T6G 2G3, Canada
e-mail: btsui@ualberta.ca

B.C.H. Tsui, S. Suresh (eds.), *Pediatric Atlas of Ultrasound- and Nerve Stimulation-Guided Regional Anesthesia*,
DOI 10.1007/978-0-387-79964-3_11

11.1 Lumbar Plexus

The lumbar plexus (Fig. 11.1) lies on the posterior abdominal wall in the retroperitoneum and is formed within the substance of the psoas major muscle from the union of the anterior primary rami of L1–L3 and most of L4 spinal nerves (Fig. 11.2). In some cases the plexus also receives a small branch from T12 (termed "pre-fixed" plexus) or a contribution from L5 (termed "post-fixed" plexus). The first lumbar nerve emerges between the first and second lumbar vertebrae; the last (L5) emerges between the fifth lumbar vertebra and the base of the sacrum (body of the first sacral vertebra) (Fig. 11.3). The lumbar spinal nerves (anterior rami) usually lie within the substance of the psoas major muscle immediately after exiting the intervertebral foramina (Fig. 11.4). In some cases, the plexus may lie posterior to the muscle. In the lumbar region, the psoas major has posterior attachments to the transverse processes and anterior attachments to the lips of the vertebral bodies, intervertebral discs, and intervening tendinous arches. The lumbar plexus lies between these two masses and is thus contained within the "psoas compartment" and lies in the same coronal (frontal) plane as the intervertebral foramina.

The nerves of the lumbar plexus are responsible for supplying motor innervation to the transversus abdominis and internal oblique muscles, the cremaster muscle in the male, muscles making up the posterior abdominal wall, and muscles in the anterior and medial compartments of the thigh. In addition, they provide sensory innervation to the skin of the posterolateral gluteal and suprapubic regions, anterior and medial thigh, and the external genitalia.

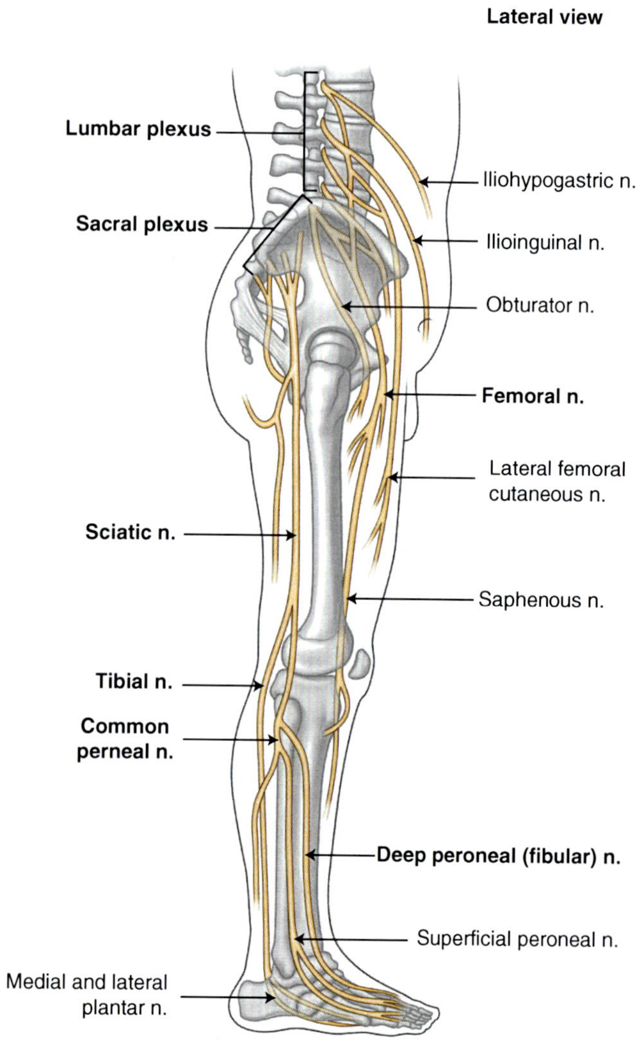

Fig. 11.1 Nerves of the lower extremity

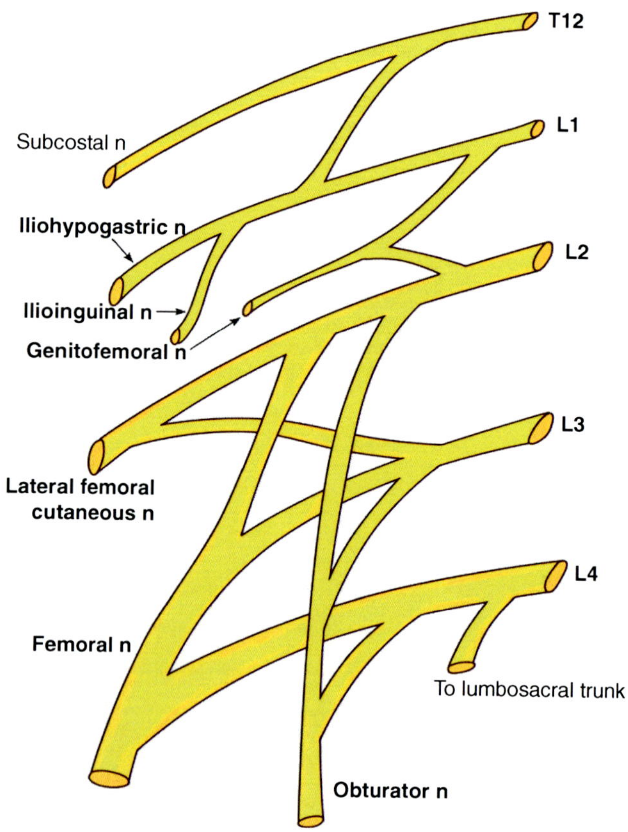

Fig. 11.2 Schematic diagram of the lumbar plexus

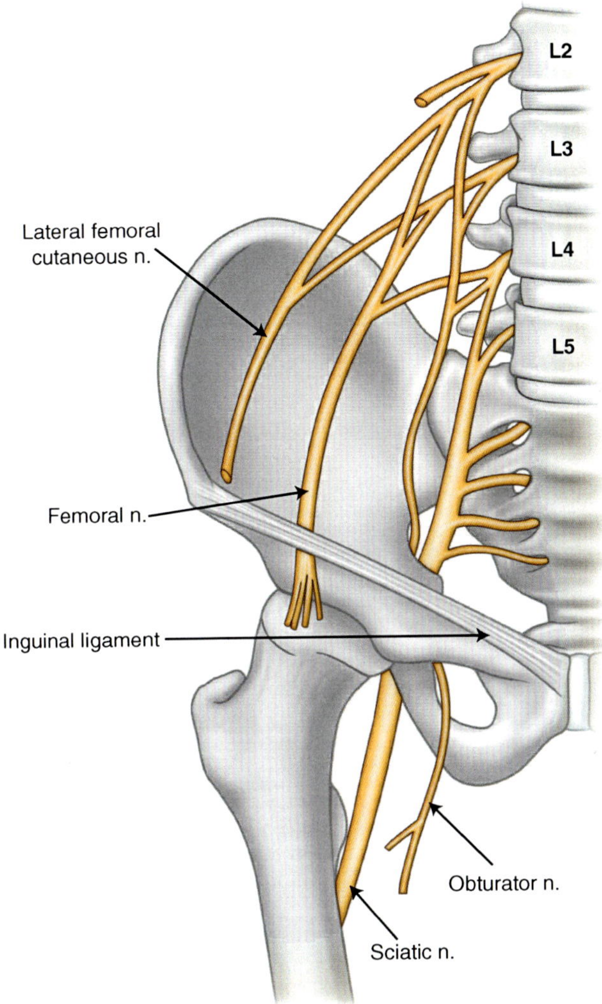

Fig. 11.3 Lumbar and sacral plexuses within the skeleton

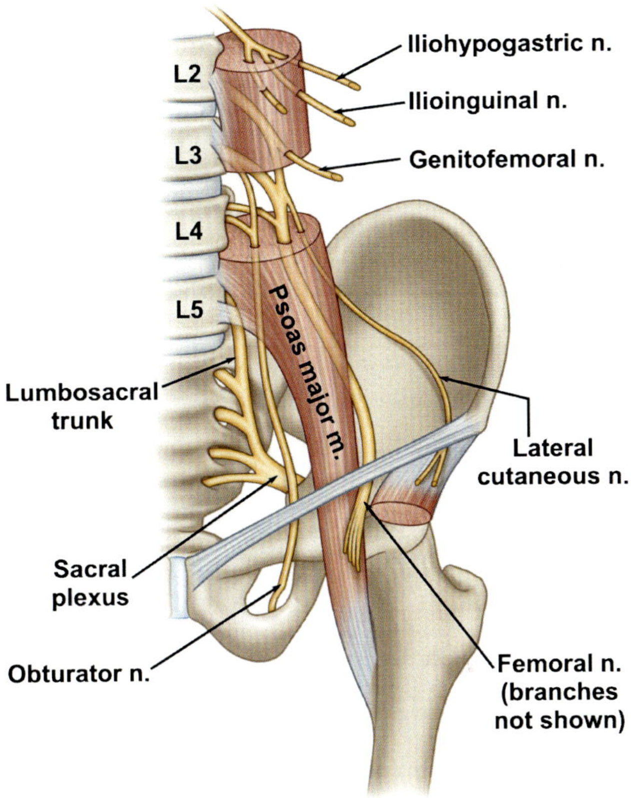

Fig. 11.4 Major branches of the lumbar plexus

11.1.1 Branches of the Lumbar Plexus

The plexus gives rise to direct muscular branches which supply the quadratus lumborum (T12; L1 to L4), psoas major (L2 to L4), psoas minor (L1), and iliacus (L2, L3) muscles as well as six major terminal nerves, as described below (Figs. 11.4 and 11.5).

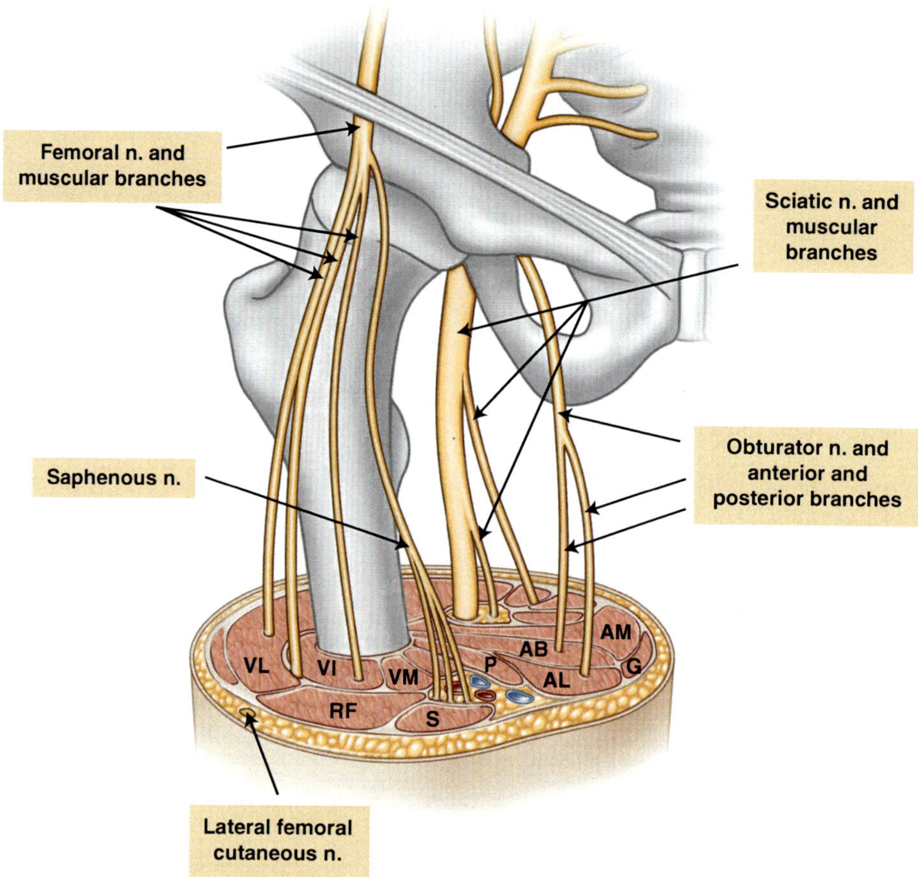

Fig. 11.5 Branches of the lumbar plexus in the upper thigh (anterior view). *VL* vastus lateralis, *VI* vastus intermedius, *RF* rectus femoris, *VM* vastus medialis, *S* sartorius, *P* pectineus, *AB* adductor brevis, *AL* adductor longus, *AM* adductor magnus, *G* gracilis

11.1.2 Iliohypogastric Nerve

A branch of the L1 nerve root (anterior ramus), the iliohypogastric nerve (Fig. 11.6), emerges from behind the upper part of the psoas major and courses laterally along the posterior abdominal wall underneath the subcostal nerve (T12). It crosses posterior to the inferior pole of the kidney obliquely, sandwiched between it and the anterior surface of the quadratus lumborum muscle. The nerve then pierces the posterior aspect of the transversus abdominis to run anteriorly along the iliac crest in the plane between the transversus abdominis and the internal oblique, dividing into its lateral and anterior cutaneous branches. The lateral branch pierces the internal and external oblique muscles above the iliac crest to be distributed to the posterolateral skin of the gluteal region. The anterior branch continues between the transversus abdominis and the internal oblique muscles and supplies them, coursing above and parallel to the inguinal ligament. It then pierces the internal oblique just medial to the anterior superior iliac spine and exits through the aponeurosis of the external oblique above the superficial inguinal ring to become cutaneous and supply the skin of the suprapubic region. The iliohypogastric nerve often has communicating branches with the subcostal (T12) and ilioinguinal (L1) nerves.

Innervation	*Motor*: transversus abdominis and internal oblique, including the conjoint tendon
	Sensory: posterolateral gluteal skin, suprapubic skin

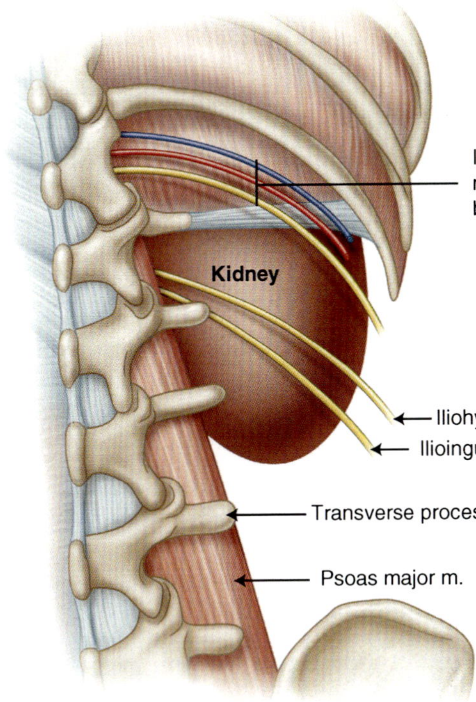

Fig. 11.6 Psoas major muscle compartment, highlighting the ilioinguinal and iliohypogastric nerves

11.1.3 Ilioinguinal Nerve

Another branch of the L1 nerve root, the ilioinguinal nerve (Fig. 11.6), is smaller than the iliohypogastric nerve. The nerve emerges from beneath the lateral border of the upper part of the psoas major with or just below the iliohypogastric nerve (the two may arise as a common trunk and split more distally at a variable distance) and crosses the inferior pole of the kidney obliquely just below the iliohypogastric nerve anterior to the quadratus lumborum. It then pierces the transversus abdominis near the anterior aspect of the iliac crest and enters the internal oblique, supplying it, after which it travels through the inguinal canal below the spermatic cord. The nerve emerges from the canal, lying inferior to the cord, through the superficial inguinal ring to be distributed to the skin on the proximal medial aspect of the thigh and the external genitalia. The nerve occasionally joins the iliohypogastric nerve as it enters the transversus abdominis, or it may be absent altogether, in which case the iliohypogastric nerve takes over supply to the associated areas.

Innervation	*Motor*: internal oblique, transversus abdominis
	Sensory: skin over the pubic symphysis, skin on proximal medial thigh, and upper part of scrotum/skin over the base of the penis (in males) or the mons pubis and lateral aspects of the labia majora (in females)

11.1.4 Genitofemoral Nerve

The genitofemoral nerve, with contributions from the L1 and L2 nerve roots, originates within the substance of the psoas major muscle. The nerve pierces through the muscle approximately at the level of L3/L4 and travels retroperitoneally along the muscle's anterior surface before dividing into its genital and femoral branches at the level of L5 or S1. It can also divide within the psoas major, emerging as two distinct nerves.

The *genital branch* crosses the external iliac artery and enters the inguinal canal through its deep ring and, in males, travels within the spermatic cord where it supplies the cremaster muscle; it then courses towards the scrotum to supply the scrotal skin. In females, the nerve travels within the inguinal canal and follows the round ligament of the uterus to the labia majora. The nerve ends in cutaneous branches to the skin over the mons pubis and labia majora. The *femoral branch* travels along the anterior surface of the lower part of the psoas major, courses lateral to the external iliac artery, and passes behind the inguinal ligament before entering the femoral sheath lateral to the femoral artery. It supplies vasomotor filaments to the femoral artery and then pierces the anterior lamina of the femoral sheath and fascia lata (deep fascia of the thigh) to supply the skin over the proximal part of the femoral triangle, where it terminates.

Innervation	*Motor*: cremaster muscle in males
	Sensory: scrotum in males, skin over mons pubis and labia majora in females, skin of anteromedial thigh/proximal, skin over proximal, lateral aspect of femoral triangle
	Vascular: vasomotor branches to femoral artery

11.1.5 Lateral Femoral Cutaneous Nerve (Lateral Cutaneous Nerve of Thigh)

This nerve is formed from the posterior branches of L2 and L3 anterior rami. The nerve emerges from behind or through the lateral border of the psoas major muscle and courses subperitoneally towards the anterior superior iliac spine, crossing the iliacus muscle obliquely on its anterior surface under the fascia iliaca. As it does so, it supplies the parietal peritoneum overlying the iliacus muscle. The nerve then enters the thigh through or below the inguinal ligament, approximately 1 cm medial to the anterior superior iliac spine (depending on the size and age of the subject). Here, it may be compressed by waistbands of tight clothing, tight belts, or abdominal obesity, leading to pain and/or paresthesias along the lateral aspect of the thigh (*meralgia paresthetica*). On the right side of the body, the nerve passes posterolateral to the cecum, and on the left, it traverses behind the lower part of the descending colon. The nerve then either pierces or lies on top of the sartorius muscle before dividing into its anterior and posterior branches.

The *anterior branch* becomes subcutaneous about 8–10 cm distal to the anterior superior iliac spine (in the average adult) and supplies the skin of the anterolateral thigh as far down as the knee. The *posterior branch* pierces the fascia lata more proximally than the anterior and courses posterolaterally to supply the skin over the posterolateral aspect of the thigh extending from the greater trochanter to mid-thigh, sometimes also including the skin over the gluteal region.

Innervation	*Motor* :none
	Sensory: skin on anterior and lateral thigh as far as the knee, skin on posterolateral thigh, sometimes skin over gluteal region

11.1.6 Femoral Nerve

The femoral nerve, with contributions from the posterior divisions of L2, L3, and L4 anterior rami, is the largest branch of the lumbar plexus. It descends through the substance of the psoas major muscle and emerges from its lower lateral border, coursing inferiorly between the psoas major medially and the iliacus laterally, deep to the iliac fascia. It then courses downwards behind the inguinal ligament somewhat deep and lateral to the femoral artery (Figs. 11.5, 11.7, and 11.8) to enter the femoral triangle in the proximal portion of the thigh. At the level of the femoral triangle and just below the inguinal ligament, one can use the mnemonic N-A-V-E-L from lateral to medial (*n*erve-*a*rtery-*v*ein-*e*mpty space [femoral canal]-*l*ymphatics) to determine the location of the various structures therein. Posterior to the inguinal ligament, the nerve is outside the femoral sheath and separated from the artery by a portion of the psoas major. While still within the abdomen, the nerve supplies muscular branches to the iliacus and pectineus muscles, as well as a small vascular (vasomotor) branch to the proximal part of the femoral artery. The nerve to the pectineus usually arises from the medial aspect of the femoral nerve near the inguinal ligament and runs behind the femoral sheath to enter the muscle through its anterior surface.

The femoral nerve divides right after passing beneath the inguinal ligament, remaining as a single nerve trunk only for a short distance. In the proximal thigh, the femoral nerve bifurcates into anterior and posterior divisions around the lateral circumflex femoral artery. The *anterior division* gives rise to the medial and intermediate cutaneous nerves of the thigh, supplying the skin on the anteromedial thigh, and provides motor branches to the sartorius muscle. The *posterior division* supplies motor innervation to the rectus femoris and vastus lateralis, intermedius (including the articularis genu, a small muscle attaching to the top of the suprapatellar bursa and sometimes fused with the vastus intermedius), and medialis muscles, as well articular innervation to the hip and knee joints. It also gives rise to the *saphenous nerve* (Fig. 11.9), the largest terminal cutaneous branch of the femoral nerve. The saphenous nerve arises within the femoral triangle and travels inferiorly deep to the sartorius muscle within the subsartorial (adductor, Hunter's) canal to the medial aspect of the knee, where it pierces the fascia lata between the tendons of sartorius and gracilis to become subcutaneous. Here it supplies the skin of the pre- and peripatellar regions of the knee. The nerve then continues inferiorly along the medial aspect of the leg together with the long (great) saphenous vein, supplies the skin along the medial aspect of the leg up to the ankle, and terminates in two branches; one along the medial aspect of the ankle, and the other passing anterior to the ankle and along the medial side of the foot ending just proximal to the big (great) toe; these branches supply the skin on the medial aspects of the ankle and foot up to the first metatarsophalangeal (MP) joint. The saphenous nerve has communicating branches with the lateral, intermediate, and medial cutaneous nerves of the thigh and the prepatellar plexus.

Vascular (vasomotor) branches of the femoral nerve supply the femoral artery and its branches.

Innervation	*Motor*: iliacus, pectineus, sartorius, quadriceps femoris, articularis genu
	Sensory: skin of anterior and medial thigh, pre- and peripatellar skin, skin on medial aspect of lower leg, medial aspect of ankle and foot up to 1st MP joint. Articular innervation to the hip and knee joints
	Vascular: vasomotor filaments to proximal femoral artery and its branches

Fig. 11.7 Relationship between the femoral nerve, artery, and vein deep to the inguinal ligament

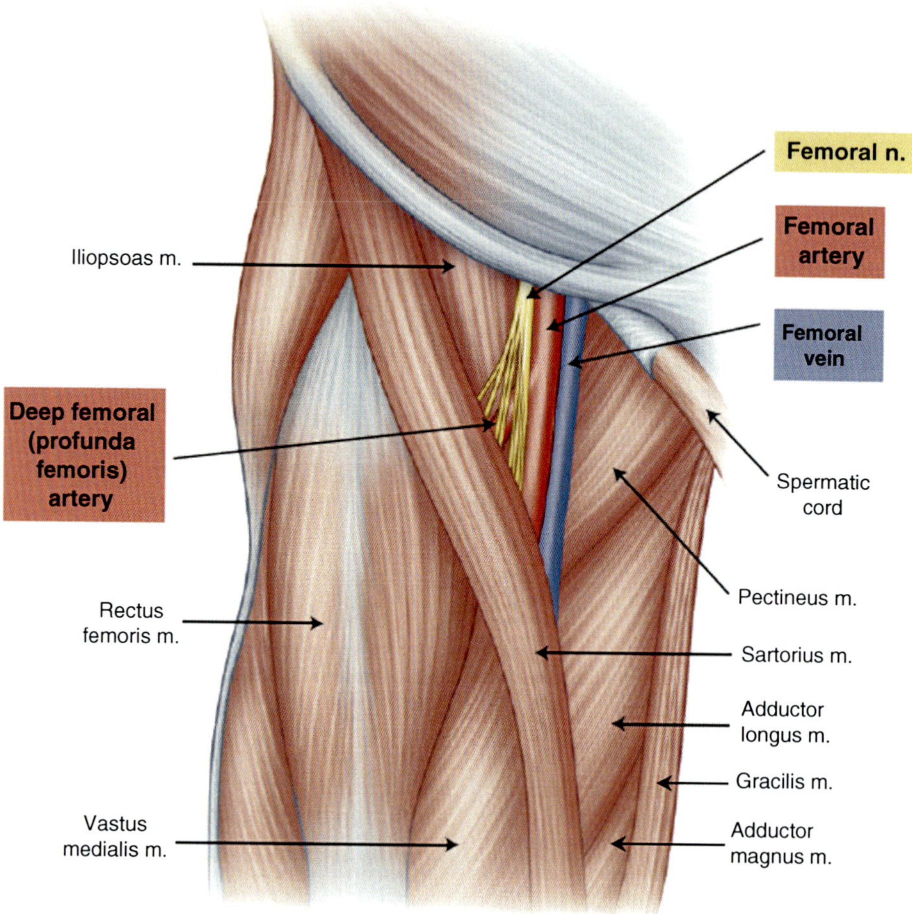

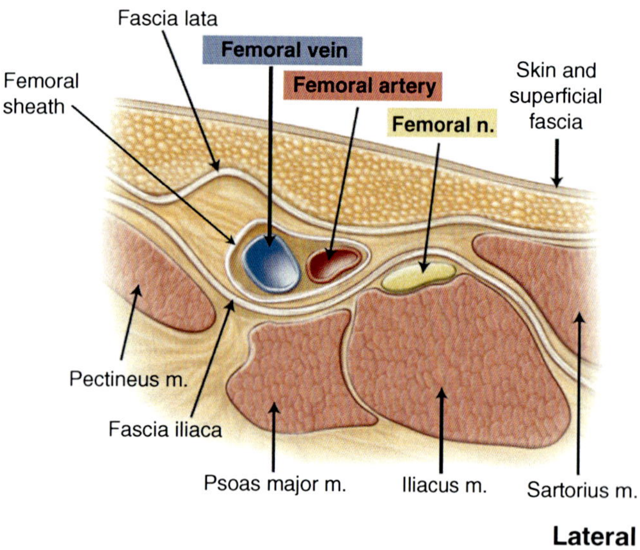

Fig. 11.8 Cross section at the block location below the inguinal crease. The femoral nerve lies deep to the fascia lata and fascia iliaca (iliopectineal fascia) and is separated from the artery and vein(s) by the latter

11.1.7 Obturator Nerve

The obturator nerve arises from the anterior divisions of L2, L3, and L4 anterior rami (Figs. 11.4 and 11.5). The nerve emerges from the medial border of the psoas major muscle at the pelvic brim and courses behind the common iliac vessels and lateral to the internal iliac vessels. It then descends anteriorly along the pelvic side wall on the obturator internus muscle, anterosuperior to the obturator vessels, towards the obturator canal, through which it enters the upper part of the medial aspect of the thigh. It divides into its anterior and posterior branches near the obturator foramen, just lateral to the pubic tubercle. Proximally, these branches are separated by the obturator externus, more distally by the adductor brevis.

The *anterior branch* passes into the thigh anterior to the obturator externus and descends in front of the adductor brevis but behind the pectineus and adductor longus muscles, alongside the femoral artery, which it may supply with vasomotor branches (Figs. 11.5 and 11.9). Near the obturator foramen, it sends an articular branch to the hip joint. As it courses behind the pectineus, it supplies it (often), the adductor longus, brevis (usually), and gracilis muscles. Its terminal cutaneous branches emerge at the lower border of adductor longus to supply the skin on the medial aspect of the thigh. The *posterior branch* pierces the obturator externus muscle through its anterior surface, supplies it, and then courses behind the adductor brevis muscle to descend on the anterior aspect of the adductor magnus muscle (medial to the anterior branch). It supplies the adductor magnus and the adductor brevis, when the brevis is not innervated by the anterior division. It usually sends an articular branch to the knee joint which either perforates through the distal portion of the adductor magnus or traverses the adductor hiatus with the femoral artery. It then traverses the adductor canal with the femoral artery (and vein) to enter the popliteal fossa. Here the nerve courses with the popliteal artery (with vascular filaments to it) along the back of the knee and terminates as an articular branch that pierces the oblique popliteal ligament to supply the posterior capsule of the knee joint. The posterior branch is not thought to provide any cutaneous innervation.

The obturator nerve and its branches can be quite variable in their course and distribution; occasionally, a small *accessory obturator nerve*, arising from the anterior rami of L3 and L4, may be present, supplying the pectineus and articular branches to the hip joint.

Innervation	*Motor*: obturator externus, adductors longus, brevis, and magnus, pectineus (usually), and gracilis
	Sensory: skin on medial distal thigh, articular innervation to the hip and knee joints
	Vascular: vasomotor to popliteal artery

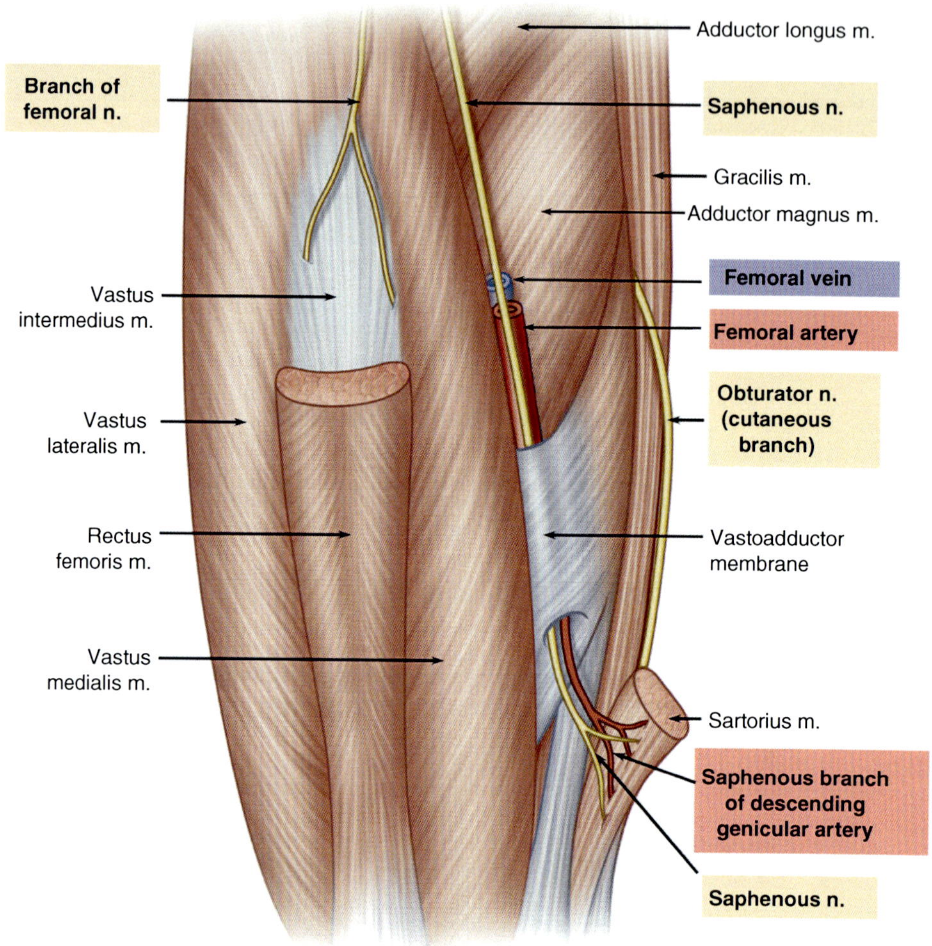

Fig. 11.9 Location of major vessels and nerves within the thigh

Suggested Reading

Borley NR. Posterior abdominal wall and retroperitoneum. In: Standring S, editor. Gray's anatomy. 40th ed. London: Churchill Livingstone; 2008. p. 1078–81.

Mahadevan V. Pelvic girdle and lower limb: overview and surface anatomy. In: Standring S, editor. Gray's anatomy. 40th ed. London: Churchill Livingstone; 2008. p. 1336–40.

Mahadevan V. Pelvic girdle, gluteal region and thigh. In: Standring S, editor. Gray's anatomy. 40th ed. London: Churchill Livingstone; 2008. p. 1382–3.

Schuenke M, Schulte E, Schumacher U. The nerves of the lumbar plexus. In: Ross LM, Lamperti ED, editors. Thieme atlas of anatomy: general anatomy and musculoskeletal system. Stuttgart: Georg Thieme Verlag; 2006. p. 472–5.

Clinical Anatomy of the Sacral Plexus

12

Anil H. Walji and Ban C.H. Tsui

Contents

A.H. Walji, MD, PhD
Division of Anatomy, Department of Surgery,
Faculty of Medicine and Dentistry, University of Alberta,
Edmonton, AB, Canada

B.C.H. Tsui, Dip Eng, BSc (Math), B Pharm, MSc, MD, FRCPC (✉)
Department of Anesthesiology and Pain Medicine,
Stollery Children's Hospital/University of Alberta Hospital,
2-150 Clinical Sciences Building, Edmonton,
AB T6G 2G3, Canada
e-mail: btsui@ualberta.ca

B.C.H. Tsui, S. Suresh (eds.), *Pediatric Atlas of Ultrasound- and Nerve Stimulation-Guided Regional Anesthesia*,
DOI 10.1007/978-0-387-79964-3_12

12.1 Sacral Plexus

The sacral plexus (Fig. 12.1) provides innervation to the skin, subcutaneous tissues, and muscles of the gluteal region, posterior thigh, leg, and foot, as well as articular innervation to the hip, knee, and ankle joints. The plexus is located within the pelvis and is formed from the fusion of the lumbosacral trunk (L4 and L5) with the anterior (primary) rami of sacral spinal nerves S1 to S3 and part of S4 (Fig. 12.1). The lumbosacral trunk is formed from the union of a branch of L4 with the anterior ramus of L5 and courses along the medial border of the psoas major muscle. The trunk passes over the pelvic brim, crosses anterior to the sacroiliac joint, and joins with the anterior ramus of S1. The anterior primary rami of S1–S3, after exiting through the anterior sacral foramina, join the lumbosacral trunk to form the *sciatic nerve*, the largest nerve of the sacral plexus and the widest nerve in the body. The anterior rami of sacral nerves S2 (partial), S3, and S4 join to form the *pudendal nerve*, the other terminal nerve of the plexus. Other branches of the plexus include the superior and inferior gluteal nerves, posterior femoral cutaneous nerve, and direct muscular branches. These rami lie on the anterior aspect of the piriformis muscle and converge toward the greater sciatic foramen, through which they exit as nerves to enter the gluteal region, perineum, and posterior thigh.

The sacral plexus itself lies anterior to the piriformis and between it and the endopelvic fascia (thus, it is extraperitoneal). Anterior to the plexus are the internal iliac vessels, the ureters, and the sigmoid colon on the left and distal ileal loops on the right. The superior gluteal vessels pass between the lumbosacral trunk (L4, L5) and S1 or between the S1 and S2 roots. The inferior gluteal vessels pass either between the roots of S1 and S2 or between S2 and S3 (the gluteal vessels generally follow the course of the sacral nerves in the frontal plane).

The *sciatic nerve* exits through the greater sciatic foramen to enter the gluteal region on its way to the posterior compartment of the thigh. The *pudendal nerve* and internal pudendal vessels course from the greater to the lesser sciatic foramina, crossing the sacrospinous ligament posteriorly near its attachment to the ischial spine. As they transit through the gluteal region on their way into the perineum, they lie superficial to the sacrospinous ligament but deep to the sacrotuberous ligament. Finally, the plexus gives off several direct muscular branches, including nerves to the piriformis, obturator internus, superior and inferior gamelli, and quadratus femoris muscles.

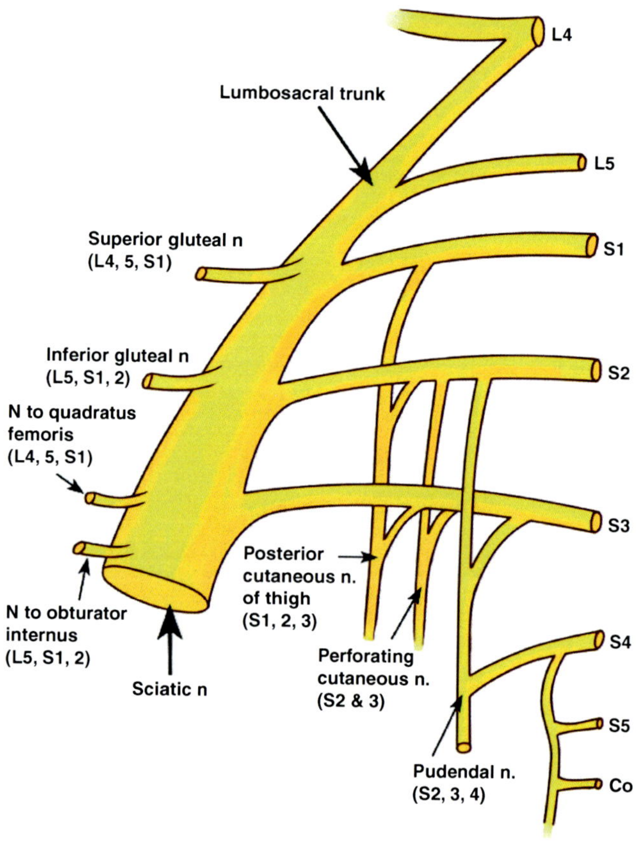

Fig. 12.1 Schematic diagram of the lumbosacral trunk and the sacral plexus

12.2 Direct Muscular Branches of the Sacral Plexus

12.2.1 Nerve to the Piriformis

The *nerve to the piriformis* usually arises from the posterior branches of S1 and S2 anterior rami (occasionally only S2) and enters the muscle through its anterior surface to supply it.

12.2.2 Nerve to Obturator Internus and Gemellus Superior

Arising from the anterior branches of L5, S1, and S2 anterior rami, this nerve leaves the pelvis through the greater sciatic foramen below the piriformis, supplies a branch to the gemellus superior, crosses the ischial spine, re-enters the pelvis (perineum) through the lesser sciatic foramen, and supplies the obturator internus by piercing it through its pelvic surface.

12.2.3 Nerve to Quadratus Femoris and Gemellus Inferior

This nerve arises from the anterior branches of L4, L5, and S1 anterior rami, exits the pelvis via the greater sciatic foramen below the piriformis, crosses the ischial tuberosity deep to the sciatic nerve, and supplies branches to the gemellus inferior and quadratus femoris as well as an articular branch to the capsule of the hip joint.

12.3 Major Terminal Nerves of the Sacral Plexus

12.3.1 Superior Gluteal Nerve

The *superior gluteal nerve* is formed from the posterior (dorsal) branches of L4, L5, and S1 anterior rami. The nerve leaves the pelvis via the greater sciatic foramen above the piriformis along with the superior gluteal artery and vein to enter the gluteal region, where it splits into superior and inferior branches. The superior branch travels with the upper ramus of the deep branch of the superior gluteal artery to supply the gluteus medius and sometimes the gluteus minimus. The inferior branch travels with the lower ramus of the deep branch of the superior gluteal artery across the gluteus minimus, supplying it and the gluteus medius and terminating in the tensor fasciae latae, which it also supplies.

Innervation	*Motor* – gluteus medius and minimus, tensor fasciae latae
	Sensory – none

12.3.2 Inferior Gluteal Nerve

The *inferior gluteal nerve* arises from the posterior branches of L5, S1, and S2 anterior rami. The nerve leaves the pelvis through the greater sciatic foramen below the piriformis muscle and enters the gluteal region, where it divides into several branches that enter the gluteus maximus through its deep surface to supply it.

Innervation	*Motor* – gluteus maximus
	Sensory – none

12.3.3 Posterior Femoral Cutaneous Nerve

Arising from the posterior branches of S1 and S2 and anterior branches of S2 and S3 anterior rami, the *posterior femoral cutaneous nerve* leaves the pelvis via the greater sciatic foramen below the piriformis and courses inferiorly deep to the gluteus maximus with the inferior gluteal artery, lying either medial or posterior to the sciatic nerve. The nerve continues down the posterior aspect of the thigh deep to the fascia lata but superficial to the long head of the biceps femoris. When the nerve reaches the posterior aspect of the knee, it pierces the deep fascia and travels with the small (short) saphenous vein to the mid-calf where its terminal branches communicate with the sural nerve. This is a purely cutaneous (sensory) nerve supplying the skin over the gluteal region, perineum, posterior thigh, and upper leg.

As the nerve crosses the lower border of the gluteus maximus, three or four *gluteal branches* (also known as the inferior clunial nerves) wind around the muscle's inferior border to supply the skin over its lower lateral aspect. The *perineal branch* supplies the skin on the upper medial aspect of the thigh, crosses the ischial tuberosity, pierces the fascia lata, and terminates in cutaneous branches to the skin of the scrotum and labia majora.

Innervation	*Motor* – none
	Sensory – cutaneous innervation to the gluteal region, perineum, back of thigh, and back of proximal leg

12.3.4 Sciatic Nerve

The *sciatic nerve* is formed within the pelvis from the fusion of the lumbosacral trunk (L4–L5) with the anterior rami of S1–S3. A flattened oval shape in cross section, the sciatic nerve is the widest, thickest, and largest peripheral nerve in the human body and at least 2 cm wide at its origin in the average adult. The sciatic nerve, although appearing as one nerve, is really two nerves, the tibial and common peroneal (fibular) nerves, enclosed within a common epineural sheath.

The nerve leaves the pelvis through the greater sciatic foramen below the piriformis (generally) and descends just medial to the midpoint of an imaginary line drawn between the greater trochanter of the femur and the ischial tuberosity along the back of the thigh (Fig. 12.2). It is accompanied medially by the posterior femoral cutaneous nerve and the inferior gluteal vessels. Proximally, the nerve lies deep to the gluteus maximus, resting first on the posterior surface of the ischium and then coursing inferiorly posterior to the obturator internus, gamelli, and quadratus femoris muscles to enter the back of the thigh, where it divides. Inferior to the lower border of the gluteus maximus, the nerve is relatively superficial, after which it lies on the posterior aspect of the adductor magnus under the cover of the long head of the biceps femoris muscle (Fig. 12.3).

The nerve generally divides into the tibial nerve medially and the common peroneal (fibular) nerve laterally near the apex of the popliteal fossa (approximately two thirds of the way down the thigh) (Fig. 12.4). The point where it divides, however, is variable and can be at a more proximal location or anywhere between the piriformis muscle and the popliteal fossa or, occasionally, even more distally. In about 2 % of the population, the nerve pierces the piriformis. Its surface projection on the back of the thigh is along an imaginary line drawn from just medial to the midpoint between the greater trochanter and ischial tuberosity to the superior apex of the popliteal fossa.

Muscular branches are distributed to the hamstrings (biceps femoris, semimembranosus, and semitendinosus muscles) and the hamstring (ischial) part of the adductor magnus muscle, mostly through its tibial division (see below). *Articular branches* arise from the proximal portion of the nerve (sometimes directly from the sacral plexus) and are distributed to the posterior aspect of the hip joint capsule. *Cutaneous branches* arise mostly from the tibial and common peroneal (fibular) divisions and supply the skin on the posterior and lateral aspects of the leg and lateral and plantar aspects of the foot (see below).

Innervation	*Motor* – biceps femoris, semimembranosus, semitendinosus, ischial (hamstring) portion of adductor magnus, muscles of the entire leg and foot through its tibial and common peroneal (fibular) divisions
	Sensory – articular innervation to the hip, cutaneous innervation to the skin of the entire lower leg and foot (with exception of the medial aspect supplied by the saphenous branch of the femoral nerve)

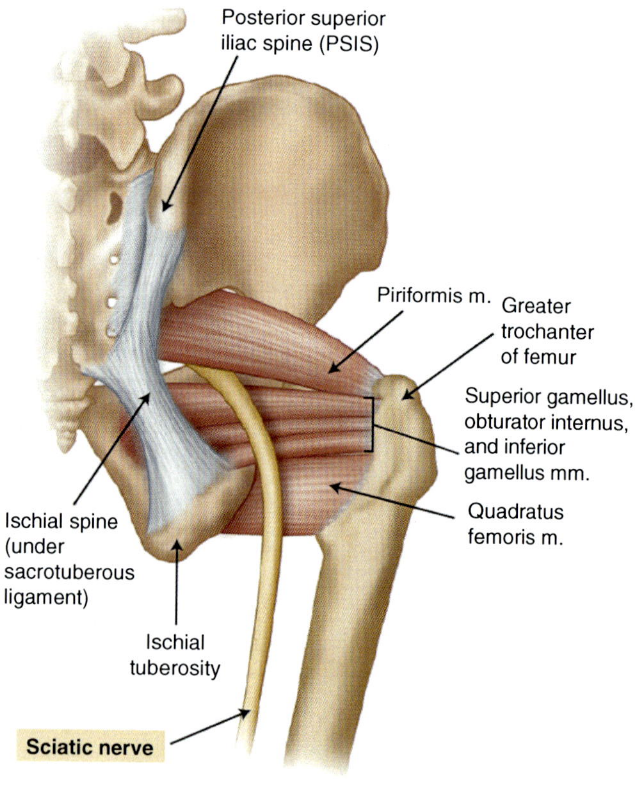

Fig. 12.2 Initial course of the sciatic nerve

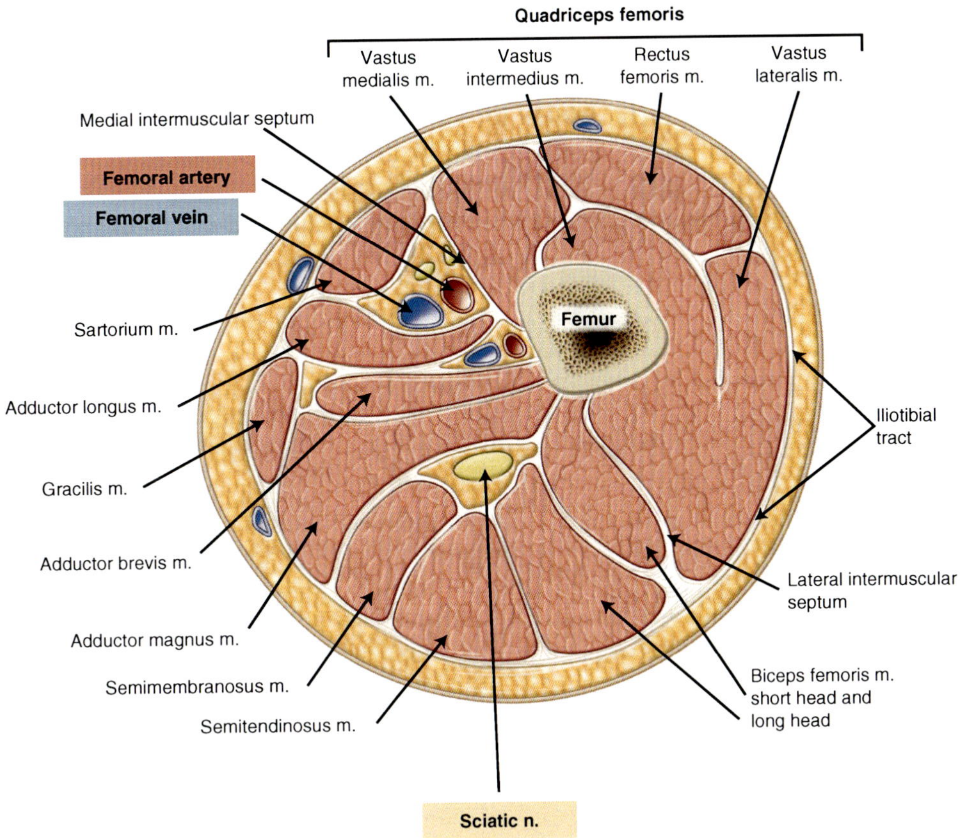

Fig. 12.3 Cross section of the thigh showing position of the sciatic nerve with respect to major muscles, vessels, and femur

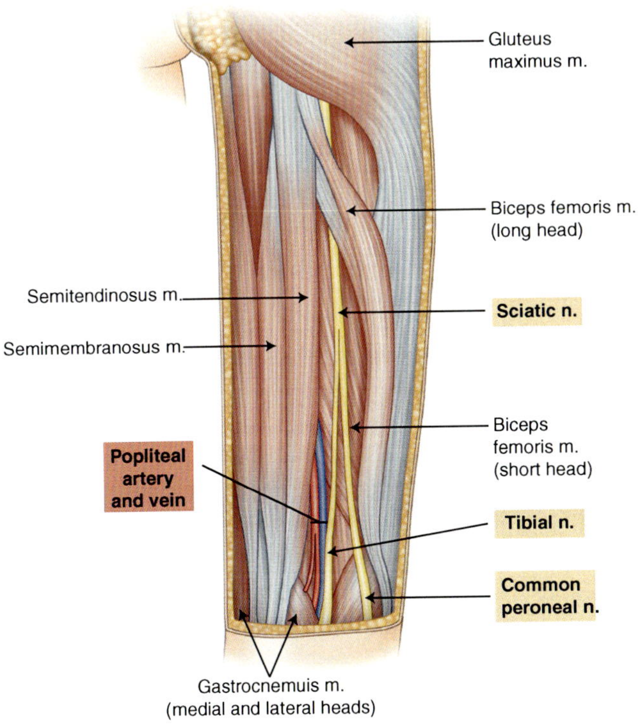

Fig. 12.4 Course and division of the sciatic nerve in the posterior thigh

12.3.5 Tibial Nerve

The *tibial* (*medial popliteal*) *nerve* is the larger of the two divisions of the sciatic nerve and arises from the anterior branches of the anterior rami of the fourth and fifth lumbar and first to third sacral nerves (L4, L5, S1, S2, and S3). It splits off from the sciatic generally near the apex (proximal aspect) of the popliteal fossa, about two thirds of the way down the thigh, although the split may occur anywhere between the piriformis and the popliteal fossa. The nerve courses inferiorly through the posterior compartment of the thigh and popliteal fossa to the lower border of the popliteus muscle, after which it passes deep (anterior) to the tendinous arch of the soleus with the popliteal artery to enter the posterior compartment of the leg. In the back of the thigh, the nerve is overlapped proximally by the semimembranosus and semitendinosus muscles medially and the biceps femoris muscle laterally. Within the popliteal fossa, the nerve becomes more superficial, while lower down, near the base (distal aspect) of the fossa, it is covered by both heads of the gastrocnemius muscle. Within the popliteal fossa, the nerve courses lateral to the popliteal vessels, becoming superficial to them at the level of the knee joint, and crosses to the medial side of the popliteal artery near the base of the fossa. Branches given off within the fossa include muscular branches, articular branches, and the cutaneous sural nerve.

Muscular branches in the popliteal fossa supply the gastrocnemius, plantaris, soleus and popliteus muscles; in the leg they supply the soleus, tibialis posterior, flexor digitorum longus and flexor hallucis longus muscls. Articular branches accompany the superior and inferior medial and middle genicular vessels to supply the posteromedial capsule of the knee joint including the oblique popliteal ligament.

The *sural nerve* travels inferiorly between the heads of the gastrocnemius, piercing the deep fascia in the leg proximally where it is usually joined (the point of union is variable) by a sural communicating branch from the common peroneal (fibular) nerve. Some sources term this the lateral sural cutaneous nerve and the main trunk from the tibial the medial sural cutaneous nerve. From here, the sural nerve descends subcutaneously close to the small (short) saphenous vein, lateral to the calcaneal tendon, toward the space between the lateral malleolus and the calcaneus. It then travels around the lateral malleolus inferiorly and along the lateral aspect of the foot, ending as the lateral dorsal cutaneous nerve. The sural nerve supplies cutaneous innervation to the skin on the posterior and lateral aspects of the distal third of the leg and the skin on the lateral aspect of the foot up to the little toe. It communicates with the posterior femoral cutaneous nerve in the leg and with the superficial peroneal (fibular) nerve on the dorsum of the foot.

The tibial nerve leaves the popliteal fossa under cover of the two heads of the gastrocnemius muscle and then courses deep (anterior) to the tendinous arch of the soleus with the popliteal artery to enter the posterior compartment of the leg, through which it continues inferiorly with the posterior tibial vessels. In the leg, the nerve lies deep to the soleus muscle and, for most of its course, on the surface of the tibialis posterior; however, in the lower third of the leg, it comes to lie against the posterior surface of the tibial shaft and becomes quite superficial, being covered only by the skin and fasciae and occasionally overlapped by the flexor hallucis longus. Its surface marking is a vertical line drawn down the midline of the leg from the inferior angle of the popliteal fossa to the midpoint between the calcaneal tendon and medial malleolus. At the medial aspect of the ankle, the relationship of the nerve to the posterior tibial vessels and flexor tendons can be remembered by the mnemonic "*T*om, *D*ick *A*nd *V*ery *N*ervous *H*arry," which stands for, from anterior to posterior, *T*ibialis posterior, flexor *D*igitorum longus, posterior tibial *A*rtery and *V*ein, tibial *N*erve, and flexor *H*allucis longus. The nerve terminates between the medial malleolus and the calcaneal tuberosity (heel) deep to the flexor retinaculum, by dividing into its terminal branches – the medial and lateral plantar nerves.

The *medial plantar nerve*, the larger terminal branch of the tibial nerve, originates deep to the flexor retinaculum and lies lateral to the medial plantar artery. The nerve travels deep to the abductor hallucis and then passes between it and the flexor digitorum brevis before giving off a medial proper digital nerve to the big toe (hallux) and dividing into three common plantar digital nerves. Cutaneous branches pierce the plantar aponeurosis to supply the skin on the medial aspect of the sole of the foot. Muscular branches supply the abductor hallucis, flexor hallucis brevis, flexor digitorum brevis, and the first lumbrical. Articular twigs supply the tarsal and metatarsal joints. The common plantar digital nerves further split into proper digital nerves, supplying the skin on the adjacent sides of the medial three and a half toes (similar to the distribution of the median nerve in the hand except for the second lumbrical).

The *lateral plantar nerve* travels forward and laterally from its origin beneath the flexor retinaculum, crossing the sole of the foot obliquely and lying medial to the lateral plantar artery. The nerve then courses anteriorly toward the base of the fifth metatarsal, between the flexor digitorum brevis and the flexor digitorum accessorius (quadratus plantae), terminating between the flexor digitorum brevis and abductor digiti minimi by splitting into its deep and superficial branches. Before dividing, it supplies the flexor digitorum accessorius and abductor digiti minimi and gives cutaneous branches that pierce the plantar fascia to supply the skin on the lateral aspect of the sole of the foot. The superficial branch further divides into two common plantar digital nerves which supply the flexor digiti minimi brevis and the two interossei in the fourth intermetatarsal space as well as the skin on the plantar aspect of the little toe and lateral half of the fourth toe. The deep branch accompanies the lateral plantar artery (as it swings medially to form the deep plantar arch) deep to the long flexor tendons and adductor hallucis, supplying the latter muscle as well as the second to fourth lumbricals and all the interossei (except those in the fourth intermetatarsal space supplied by the superficial branch). Its distribution is similar to that of the ulnar nerve in the hand, in that it supplies the majority of the intrinsic muscles of the foot.

Innervation	*Motor* – popliteus, gastrocnemius, soleus, plantaris, tibialis posterior, flexor digitorum longus and brevis, flexor hallucis longus and brevis, abductor hallucis, lumbricals, flexor accessorius (quadratus plantae), flexor digiti minimi, adductor hallucis, interossei, abductor digiti minimi
	Sensory – cutaneous to skin on posterior and lateral aspects of distal leg and sole of foot. Articular innervation to knee joint and joints of the foot

12.3.6 Common Peroneal (Fibular) Nerve

The *common peroneal (fibular or lateral popliteal) nerve* is about half the size of the tibial nerve and arises from the posterior branches of the anterior rami of the fourth and fifth lumbar and first and second sacral nerves (L4, L5, S1, and S2). After splitting off from the sciatic nerve (tibial component), it descends obliquely along the lateral border of the popliteal fossa toward the fibular head, medial to the biceps femoris, and between its tendon and the lateral head of the gastrocnemius. The nerve winds around the lateral aspect of the fibular neck (where it is very superficial and may easily be injured) deep to the peroneus longus muscle and gives off articular and cutaneous branches before dividing into its terminal superficial and deep peroneal nerves (Fig. 12.5).

Of the three articular branches, two course with the superior and inferior lateral genicular arteries to supply the posterolateral capsule of the knee joint, while the third (recurrent articular nerve) arises a little lower and runs with the anterior recurrent tibial artery to supply the anterolateral capsule of the knee joint and the proximal tibiofibular joint. The cutaneous branches, in the form of the sural communicating nerve (joins with the sural nerve from the tibial nerve) and the lateral sural nerve (lateral cutaneous nerve of the calf), supply the skin on the anterolateral and posterior aspects of the proximal leg.

The *deep peroneal (fibular, anterior tibial) nerve* arises from the common peroneal division between the fibular neck and the proximal portion of the peroneus longus and passes deep to the extensor digitorum longus to descend on the anterior aspect of the interosseous membrane, reaching the anterior tibial artery in the upper third of the leg. The nerve then courses inferiorly along the anterior aspect of the lower third of tibia just lateral to the anterior tibial artery (between the tibialis anterior medially and extensor hallucis longus laterally) before crossing the ankle under the extensor retinaculum and terminating as medial (cutaneous) and lateral (motor) branches. It supplies muscular branches to the tibialis anterior, extensor hallucis longus, and extensor digitorum longus (including the peroneus tertius) and an articular branch to the capsule of the ankle joint. The *medial terminal branch* runs along the dorsum of the foot, lateral to the dorsalis pedis artery, and connects with the medial branch of the superficial peroneal (fibular) nerve, terminating as dorsal digital nerves to adjacent sides of the hallux (big toe) and second toe (first web space). Its interosseous branch supplies the first dorsal interosseous muscle and the metatarsophalangeal joint of the big toe. The *lateral terminal branch* crosses the tarsus obliquely laterally deep to the extensor digitorum brevis, which it supplies. Its tiny interosseous branches supply the second dorsal interosseous muscle and the tarsal and metatarsophalangeal joints of the middle three toes.

The *superficial peroneal (fibular, musculocutaneous) nerve* also arises from the common peroneal bifurcation and descends along the anterior intermuscular septum. At first deep to the peroneus longus, it then courses anteroinferiorly between the peroneal (fibular) muscles (lateral compartment) and the extensor digitorum longus (anterior compartment) to pierce the deep fascia in the leg's distal third. Here, it becomes superficial and divides into medial and lateral branches. As it lies on the intermuscular septum between the lateral and anterior compartments, it sends muscular branches to the peroneus longus and brevis muscles (the peroneus tertius is supplied by the deep peroneal nerve) and cutaneous branches to the skin on the lateral aspect of the lower leg. The *medial branch* (*medial dorsal cutaneous nerve*) travels anterior to the ankle before dividing into two dorsal digital nerves, one supplying the skin on the medial aspect of the hallux (big, great toe) and the other the skin on the adjacent sides of the second and third toes (skin on the adjacent sides of the hallux and second toe is supplied by the deep peroneal nerve). It communicates with branches of the saphenous nerve and deep peroneal (fibular) nerves. The smaller *lateral branch* (intermediate dorsal cutaneous nerve) travels laterally across the dorsum of the foot and supplies the skin on the lateral aspect of the ankle before terminating as dorsal digital nerves supplying the skin on adjacent sides of the third, fourth, and fifth toes and communicating with the sural nerve.

Innervation	*Motor* – tibialis anterior, extensor hallucis longus, extensor digitorum longus and brevis, peroneus longus, brevis and tertius
	Sensory – articular innervation to the knee, ankle, and joints of the foot. Cutaneous to skin on upper anterolateral leg and dorsum of foot, dorsum and adjacent sides of all toes (except first web space)

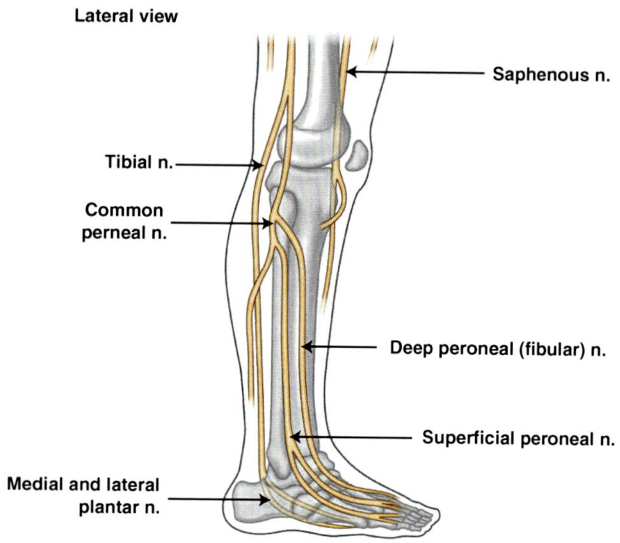

Fig. 12.5 Lower extremity nerves entering the leg. Terminal branches of the common peroneal nerve (deep and superficial peroneal nerves) enter the leg just distal to the fibular neck

12.3.7 Pudendal Nerve

The *pudendal nerve* is formed from the union of the anterior divisions of the second, third, and fourth anterior sacral rami (S2, S3, and S4) at the upper border of the sacrotuberous ligament. The nerve leaves the pelvic cavity together with the internal pudendal artery and vein through the greater sciatic foramen below the piriformis and between it and the coccygeus to enter the gluteal region. As the nerve transits through the gluteal region, it crosses the sacrospinous ligament posteriorly near its attachment to the ischial spine, lying superficial to the sacrospinous ligament but deep to the sacrotuberous ligament (an important landmark for the pudendal nerve block). At the level of the ischial spine, the internal pudendal vessels lie medial to the pudendal nerve. After crossing the sacrospinous ligament, the pudendal nerve (with the internal pudendal vessels) re-enters the pelvis (perineum) through the lesser sciatic foramen and courses anteriorly within the pudendal (Alcock's) canal on the medial aspect of the obturator internus along the lateral wall of the ischiorectal fossa (*the pudendal canal is formed from a split in the deep fascia over the obturator internus*). In the posterior part of the canal, it gives rise to the inferior rectal and perineal nerves and terminates anteriorly as the dorsal nerve of the penis (or clitoris).

The *inferior rectal nerve* pierces through the medial aspect of the pudendal canal and crosses the ischiorectal fossa obliquely from lateral to medial with the inferior rectal vessels to supply the external anal sphincter, the skin lining the lower part of the anal canal, and the skin around the anal verge. In females, it may supply sensory branches to the lower part of the vagina. It may sometimes arise directly from the sacral plexus. Its territory of supply overlaps with that of the perineal branch of the posterior femoral cutaneous and posterior scrotal (labial) nerves (see below).

The *perineal nerve* is the inferior and larger of the terminal branches of the pudendal nerve and arises from it in the posterior aspect of the pudendal canal. The nerve then courses forward beneath the internal pudendal artery in company with the perineal artery and divides into posterior scrotal (labial) and muscular branches. The *posterior scrotal (labial) nerves* pierce the perineal membrane (formerly called the inferior fascia of the urogenital diaphragm), course anteriorly in the lateral aspect of the urogenital triangle and supply the skin of the scrotum or labia majora, overlapping the territory of the perineal branch of the posterior femoral cutaneous and inferior rectal nerves. The posterior labial branches of the perineal nerve may also supply sensory innervation to the lower part of the vagina. The muscular branches are distributed to the adjacent superficial muscles of the perineum (e.g., superficial transverse perineal muscle) and the external anal sphincter. *Direct muscular branches* arising from the pudendal nerve itself supply the levator ani (pelvic diaphragm), external anal sphincter, superficial and deep transverse perineal muscles, sphincter urethrae, and the bulbospongiosus and ischiocavernosus muscles.

The *dorsal nerve of the penis* (*clitoris*), the terminal continuation of the pudendal nerve in males, courses forward above the internal pudendal artery along the medial aspect of the ischiopubic ramus deep to the perineal membrane. It supplies the corpus cavernosum, passes through the hiatus between the anterior aspect of the perineal membrane and pubic symphysis in company with the dorsal artery of the penis, and traverses through the suspensory ligament to enter the dorsal surface of the penis. The nerve ends in sensory branches in the glans penis. The corresponding nerve in females, the *dorsal nerve of the clitoris*, takes a similar course and ends in sensory branches in the glans clitoris although it is much smaller than in males.

12.3.8 Pelvic Splanchnic Nerves

Visceral branches of the sacral plexus, the *pelvic splanchnic nerves* (also known as the *nervi erigentes*), arise from the anterior rami of S2, S3, and S4 to provide parasympathetic innervation to the pelvic viscera via the superior and inferior hypogastric plexuses. In males, the pelvic splanchnic nerves play a critical role in maintaining erectile function, and damage to them (e.g., during prostatectomy or rectal surgery) may render the patient impotent.

Suggested Reading

Chapter 63: True pelvis, pelvic floor and perineum. In: Standring S, editor. Gray's anatomy. 40th ed. London: Churchill Livingstone; 2008. p. 1091–2.

Chapter 79: Pelvic girdle and lower limb: overview and surface anatomy. In: Standring S, editor. Gray's anatomy. 40th ed. London: Churchill Livingstone; 2008. p. 1336–40.

Chapter 80: Pelvic girdle, gluteal region and thigh. In: Standring S, editor. Gray's anatomy. 40th ed. London: Churchill Livingstone; 2008. p. 1384–5.

Schuenke M, Schulte E, Schumacher U. The nerves of the sacral plexus. In: Ross LM, Lamperti ED, editors. Thieme atlas of anatomy: general anatomy and musculoskeletal system. Stuttgart: Georg Thieme Verlag; 2006. p. 476–83.

Clinical Anatomy of the Trunk and Central Neuraxis

13

Anil H. Walji and Ban C.H. Tsui

Contents

A.H. Walji, MD, PhD
Division of Anatomy, Department of Surgery, Faculty of Medicine and Dentistry, University of Alberta, Edmonton, AB, Canada

B.C.H. Tsui, Dip Eng, BSc (Math), B Pharm, MSc, MD, FRCPC (✉)
Department of Anesthesiology and Pain Medicine,
Stollery Children's Hospital/University of Alberta Hospital,
2-150 Clinical Sciences Building, Edmonton,
AB T6G 2G3, Canada
e-mail: btsui@ualberta.ca

B.C.H. Tsui, S. Suresh (eds.), *Pediatric Atlas of Ultrasound- and Nerve Stimulation-Guided Regional Anesthesia*,
DOI 10.1007/978-0-387-79964-3_13

13.1 Spinal Nerves and the Vertebral Column

13.1.1 Origin of Spinal Nerves

Spinal nerves arise from the spinal cord and are part of the peripheral nervous system, along with the cranial and autonomic nerves and their ganglia. Spinal nerves supply somatic or body wall structures, in other words, structures derived embryologically from somites and somatic mesoderm. They also supply parietal membranes, namely, the parietal pleura, pericardium, and peritoneum, as well as the periosteum. There are 31 pairs of spinal nerves – 8 cervical (C1–C8), 12 thoracic (T1–12), 5 lumbar (L1–L5), 5 sacral (S1–S5), and 1 coccygeal (Co1). These spinal nerves are formed by the union of the ventral (anterior) and dorsal (posterior) spinal roots, each made up of smaller rootlets. The rootlets either converge to form the roots as they exit the cord if they are motor (efferent; ventral) or diverge from the roots as they enter the cord if they are sensory (afferent; dorsal). The dorsal roots bear sensory ganglia (dorsal root ganglia) containing the cell bodies of somatic and visceral sensory neurons.

Each typical spinal nerve is a mixed nerve containing somatic and visceral fibers, both efferent and afferent. The *motor (somatic efferent) fibers* supply skeletal muscle, while *sensory (somatic afferent) fibers* innervate skin and superficial fascia (subcutaneous tissues). The sensory fibers also supply receptors in joint capsules and ligaments, fasciae, and skeletal muscle (e.g., muscle spindles and Golgi tendon organs). In addition, all spinal nerves contain *sympathetic (visceral efferent) fibers* for supplying blood vessels, smooth muscle, and glands in the skin and blood vessels in skeletal muscle. The preganglionic sympathetic neurons arise from the lateral horn of the spinal gray matter (intermediolateral cell column) in the thoracic and upper two or three lumbar segments and synapse with postganglionic neurons in the *sympathetic trunk* (chain) at corresponding levels or track up and down the trunk to be distributed with spinal nerves at all levels. Some synapse with the postganglionics at higher or lower levels in the trunk to get into spinal nerves above T1 and below L2/3. Those destined for the head synapse mostly in the superior cervical ganglion. Finally, sacral spinal nerves from cord segments S2, S3, and S4 contain preganglionic *parasympathetic* fibers, which leave via the ventral rami of the sacral nerves and are destined for the pelvic viscera via pelvic plexuses and ganglia. These parasympathetic nerves are called the *pelvic splanchnic nerves* or the *nervi erigentes*. *Visceral afferent* fibers, carrying visceral sensation pain from the viscera, have their cell bodies in the spinal dorsal root ganglia with their peripheral processes passing through the sympathetic trunk via the rami communicantes without synapsing (without synapsing) and ending in the thoracic and abdominal viscera.

Soon after exiting the intervertebral (spinal) foramina, each spinal nerve in turn divides into a larger *ventral* and a smaller *dorsal* (*primary*) *ramus* (Fig. 13.1). The *ventral rami* course laterally and anteriorly to supply the muscles, subcutaneous tissues (superficial fascia), and skin of the neck, trunk, and upper and lower extremities. The *dorsal rami* course posteriorly and supply the paravertebral muscles, subcutaneous tissues, and skin of the back close to the midline. All dorsal rami are arranged and distributed segmentally, from C1 all the way down to coccyx 1 (Co1). The only ventral rami that are arranged and distributed segmentally are those of spinal nerves T1–T12. The ventral rami of T1–T11 are called the *intercostal nerves*, while the ventral ramus of T12 is the *subcostal nerve*. The intercostal nerves course through the 11 intercostal spaces beneath the intercostal vessels between the innermost and internal intercostal muscles, while the subcostal nerve runs along the posterior abdominal wall underneath the 12th pair of ribs. Ventral rami *not arranged segmentally* (C1 to C8 and L1 to Co1) fuse to form nerve plexuses. Thus, the neck, lower abdomen, pelvis, and extremities are supplied by nerve plexuses (cervical, brachial, lumbar, and sacral plexuses), while the thoracic and upper three quarters of the abdominal wall are supplied by the segmentally organized intercostal nerves.

It is important to realize that the first cervical (C1) nerve leaves the spinal cord and courses *above* the atlas (C1 vertebra); hence, the cervical nerves are numbered corresponding to the vertebrae inferior to them (e.g., the C6 nerve exits below C5 and above C6 vertebra; C8 nerve exits below C7 and above T1). From this point on, all the spinal nerves are named corresponding to the vertebral level above. For example, T3 and L4 spinal nerves exit below the T3 and L4 vertebrae, respectively.

13.1.2 Vertebral Column

This section reviews the developmental anatomy and growth of the vertebral column (spinal column or spine) and provides a basis for appreciating the improved visibility rendered when imaging the spine using ultrasound on the pediatric patient. It begins with the development of the vertebrae and vertebral column as a whole, followed by the growth and curves of the vertebral column and finally a brief description of the developmental anatomy of the thoracic and lumbar spine and sacrum.

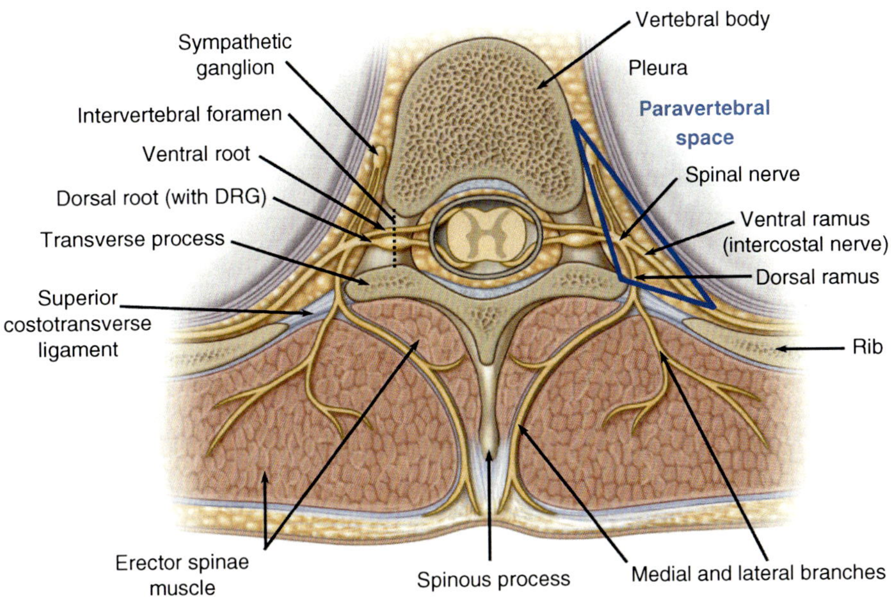

Fig. 13.1 Cross section of a thoracic vertebral segment with a simplified spinal nerve and paravertebral space shown (right side only). *DRG* dorsal root ganglion

13.2 Development of the Vertebral Column

As with most of the other bones of the human body, the development of the human vertebral column goes through three stages: mesenchymal (precartilaginous), chondrification (cartilaginous), and ossification (bony).

1. Mesenchymal (precartilaginous) stage
   During the fourth week of intrauterine life (IUL), sclerotomic mesenchymal cells of the somites (derived from the paraxial mesoderm) start to migrate toward the notochord which represents the primitive axial supporting structure. At this stage, the developing neural tube, notochord, and endoderm of the yolk sac are in close contact and are flanked by the paired dorsal aortae from which the *intersegmental arteries* branch off and course between the somites. In the thorax, these intersegmental arteries become the intercostal arteries; in the abdomen, they become the lumbar arteries. The mesenchymal tissue surrounding the notochord is subdivided by the intersegmental vessels into sclerotomic segments. The mesenchymal cells within the sclerotome become characterized by alternating regions of densely packed and loosely arranged cells between which an *intervertebral fissure* appears. This new segment forms the primitive vertebra consisting of a dense cranial zone separated by a loose caudal zone of cells by the intersegmental vessels.

   From the dense zone, three processes arise and extend dorsally, ventrally, and laterally. The dorsal extension is called the *neural process* and will form the vertebral neural arch. The ventral process will form the *centrum* (vertebral body), while the lateral process is related to the development of the vertebral *transverse process* and the attachment of the ribs. Therefore, the primordia of the definitive vertebrae are not formed from the mesenchymal cells of one somite but the recombination of the lesser and more condensed zones of mesenchyme derived from two adjacent somites. The intervertebral fissures fill with mesenchymal cells that migrate from the dense zone to form the *annulus fibrosus* of the intervertebral (IV) disk, whereas the notochord and inner cells of the annulus fibrosus degenerate to form the *nucleus pulposus*.
2. Chondrification (cartilaginous) stage
   During the sixth to seventh weeks of IUL, a pair of *chondrification centers* appears in each vertebral body followed by separate centers in each neural and transverse processes. The two centers in each vertebral body fuse at the end of the embryonic period (~9 weeks of IUL) to form a cartilaginous centrum or body. At the same time, the chondrification centers in the neural and transverse processes fuse with those in the centrum to form a cartilaginous model of the vertebra. The spinous and transverse processes arise from proliferation of chondrification centers in the vertebral neural arch and lateral process, respectively.
3. Ossification (bony) stage
   Ossification of the developing vertebrae commences during the embryonic period around the eighth to ninth weeks of IUL and is usually complete by the 25th year. Three *primary ossification centers* appear, one for the centrum and one for each half of the vertebral neural arch, followed by five *secondary (epiphyseal) ossification centers*. Centers for the vertebral arches appear classically first in the upper cervical vertebrae during the ninth to tenth weeks of IUL and then in successively lower vertebrae, reaching the lumbar vertebrae at around 12 weeks. Thus, at birth, each vertebra consists of three bony parts connected by cartilage. The vertebral neural arches usually fuse during the first 3–5 years of life, commencing in the lumbar region and progressing cranially. The vertebral arches articulate with the centrum at the cartilaginous neurocentral junctions (joints) or synchondroses, which permit the vertebral arches to grow and the vertebral canal to expand as the spinal cord enlarges. These neurocentral junctions disappear when the vertebral arches fuse with the centrum beginning in the cervical region during the third to sixth years of life. Until puberty, the superior and inferior surfaces of the bodies and tips of transverse and spinous processes are cartilaginous. Five *secondary centers of ossification* appear at the epiphyses of the vertebra around puberty: one for the tip of the spinous process, one each for the tips of the transverse processes and two annular ring-like epiphyses, one on the superior and one on the inferior rim of the vertebral body. The vertebral body is thus made up of two annular epiphyses with the mass of bone in between them which is derived from the centrum. It is important to point out that the adult vertebral body is not coextensive with the developmental centrum. Although the centrum will form the majority of the vertebral body, in the adult, the body includes parts of the neural arches posterolaterally. These secondary centers fuse with the rest of the vertebra around 25 years of age to form the definitive vertebra and the vertebral column. The atlas (C1), axis (C2), C7, sacrum, and coccyx are exceptions to this typical ossification pattern.

The majority of people have 7 cervical, 12 thoracic, 5 lumbar, 5 sacral (fused), and usually 4 (3 to 5) coccygeal (fused) vertebrae; however, about 2–3 % have one fewer or one or two additional vertebrae. When this occurs, there may be regional compensation (e.g., 11 thoracic and 6 lumbar vertebrae), so when determining the number of vertebrae, it is important to examine the entire vertebral column.

Growth and Curves of the Vertebral Column

The increase in length of the vertebral column is determined by the growth of its vertebral components. The various regions of the column and different parts of the vertebrae have differential rates of growth. The growth of the vertebral bodies begins in the thoracic and lumbar regions and extends craniocaudally. The lower part of the column grows faster than the upper as a functional prerequisite for providing better support. There are two periods of accelerated growth: the first between 2 and 7 years of age and the second between 9 and 15 years of age. The curves of the vertebral column become evident during the third month of IUL life. At first, there is only a slight curve, concave anteriorly, followed in the fifth month by the appearance of the sacrovertebral angle. Radiographic studies have shown, however, that 83 % of fetuses aged between 8 and 23 weeks already possess a cervical curve.

At birth, this embryonic anterior curvature is preserved in the thoracic and sacral regions. These areas of the column, concave anteriorly, are therefore referred to as the *primary curves*. The cervical curve is also present at birth although it becomes more accentuated when the baby starts supporting its head (around 3–4 months of life) and sitting upright (around 9 months of life). The lumbar curves appear later in response to the baby adopting the upright walking posture and walking unassisted (around 12 months of life). These are termed *secondary or compensatory curves* since they develop in response to biomechanical demands placed on the column and are convex anteriorly. Thus, the adult has four anteroposterior curves: cervical (secondary), thoracic (primary), lumbar (secondary), and sacrococcygeal or pelvic (primary), while the newborn has only three, cervical, thoracic, and sacral, the latter demarcated by the sacrovertebral angle. Between 3 and 9 months of life, the cervical curve becomes more marked in response to the biomechanical demands placed on it from the baby supporting its head and sitting upright, while after the first year, one sees the appearance of the lumbar curve in response to the need for supporting the baby's weight.

The cervical and lumbar curves in the adult are due mainly to the shapes of the intervertebral disks, while the thoracic curve is related more to the shapes of the thoracic vertebrae, which have a greater depth posteriorly. During intrauterine life, the vertebral column represents about three quarters of total body length, whereas at birth, it is reduced to two fifths due to the relatively rapid development of the lumbosacral region and lower extremities. This variation in the proportions of the vertebral column, head, trunk, and extremities causes the center of gravity of the body to shift caudally as the infant grows. In the newborn held in the upright erect posture, the center of gravity is at about the level of the xiphoid process and remains above the umbilicus throughout early childhood. At about 5–6 years, it is just below the umbilicus, and at around 13 years, it shifts to the level of the iliac crest. In the adult, the center of gravity lies at the level of the sacral promontory (the most forward projecting aspect of the upper edge of the first sacral vertebra).

13.2.1 Developmental Anatomy of the Thoracic and Lumbar Vertebral Column (Spine)

- At birth, the vertebrae of the thoracic and lumbar spine consist of three bony masses: a *centrum* anteriorly and two *vertebral neural arches* posteriorly, united by cartilage.
- Development of the *thoracic spine*:
  - The laminae typically unite in a caudo-cranial (upwards, T12 through T1) fashion, usually by the end of the first or beginning of the second year of life.
  - The centrum (body) fuses with the neural arches (neurocentral fusion), also in a caudal to cranial manner, generally by the end of the fifth year of life.
  - The transverse processes are present and prominent at birth; however, their tips, like the tips of the transverse processes, remain cartilaginous until puberty.
  - The three facets for articulation with the ribs at the costovertebral and costotransverse joints are present at birth.
  - The neurocentral and posterior synchondroses are not fused at birth; the posterior ones fuse within 2–3 months of postnatal life, and the neurocentral synchondroses close after 5–6 years of life.
- Development of the *lumbar spine*:
  - Fusion of the laminae of L1 through L4 occurs during the first year of life, with those of L5 fusing by 5 years of age.
  - Neurocentral fusion is generally complete by age 4.
  - Transverse processes begin to develop after the first year of life; however, their tips, like the tips of the spinous processes, are cartilaginous until puberty.
  - The lumbar secondary compensatory curve (through intervertebral disk modification) does not begin to develop until 6 or 8 months of age when the infant begins sitting upright and supporting its weight and becomes more apparent after the first year of life when the infant is able to adopt the upright posture and walk unassisted.
- The vertebral canal in young infants is quite small, with the thickness of the epidural space being as little as 1–2 mm.

- Secondary ossification centers in vertebral bodies and arches do not fuse with the rest of the vertebra until the early twenties, allowing continuing growth and development of the vertebral structures.
- In children, most vertebrae contain five secondary ossification centers (in the transverse and spinous processes as well as on the superior and inferior surfaces or rims of the vertebral bodies), which allow continual growth and remodeling of the vertebral column.
- In adults (early 20s), the vertebral column is essentially complete with the exception of fusion between the bodies of S1 and S2.
- In adults:
  - *The thoracic* vertebral bodies are of medium size and heart shaped (Fig. 13.1); vertebral (spinal) canals are small and nearly circular in shape; laminae are relatively small; spinous processes are long and oriented obliquely inferiorly (Figs. 13.2 and 13.3). Spinous processes overlap from T5–T8, the latter being the longest and most oblique, and their obliquity increases from T1–T9 then decreases in T10–T12. The transverse processes are relatively broad and robust for articulation with the ribs and generally face posterolaterally. The thoracic vertebrae are adapted mostly for articulation with the ribs and their role in movements of the chest wall during respiration; however, they also play a secondary role in supporting and transmitting the weight of the head and neck and the thorax to the lumbar segment of the column.
  - *The lumbar* vertebral bodies are large and kidney shaped; vertebral (spinal) canals are triangular in shape; laminae are thick; spinous processes are short and stout with a posterior (horizontal) orientation (Fig. 13.3); intervertebral disks are thickest with respect to the rest of the spine; within the lumbar spine itself, the disks are thicker anteriorly, contributing to the anterior lumbar curvature (lumbar lordosis). The transverse processes are long, slender, and directed laterally and are mostly for muscular attachments. The lumbar vertebrae are designed primarily for weight bearing and transmission, as reflected in the large size and robustness of their bodies, laminae, and IV disks.

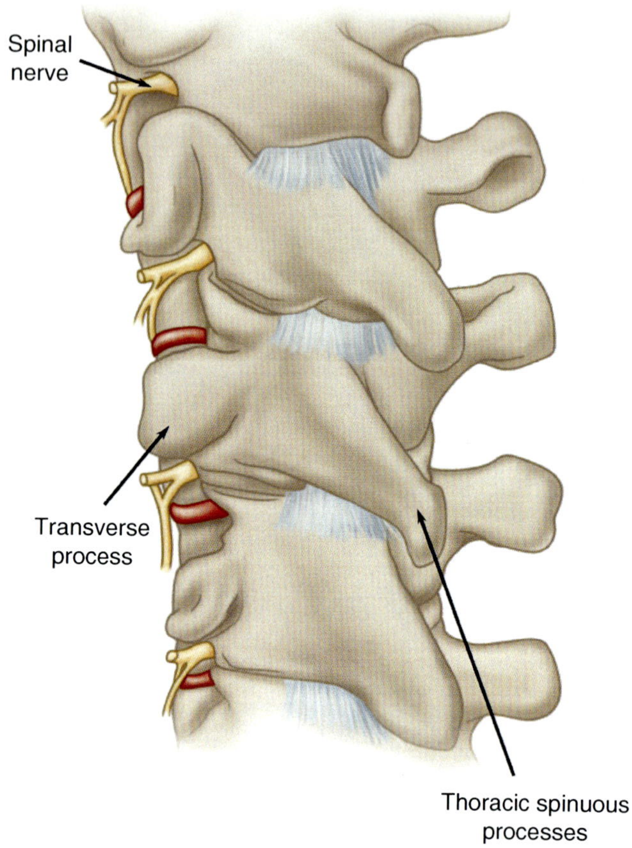

Fig. 13.2 Vertebrae of the thoracic spine, illustrating inferiorly oriented spinous processes

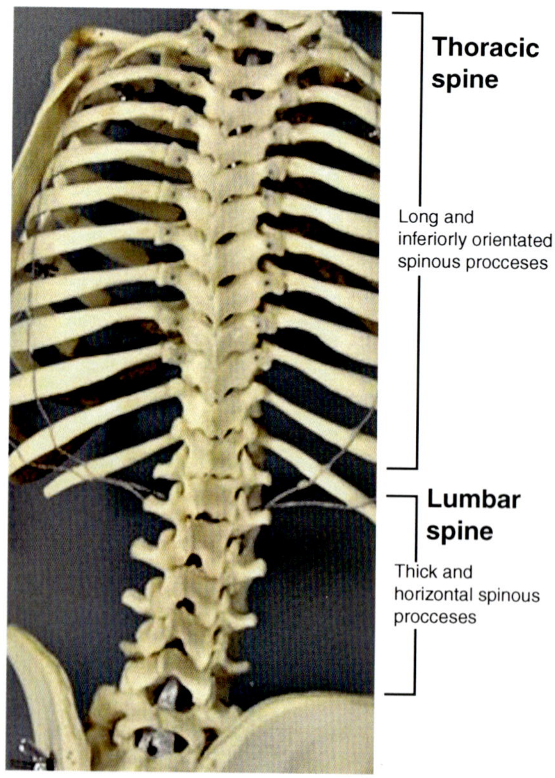

Fig. 13.3 Spinal column showing the thoracic and lumbar regions

13.2.2 Developmental Anatomy of the Sacrum

- In infancy and childhood, the sacrum is highly variable with respect to its shape and ossification and therefore also its visibility on ultrasound imaging (Fig. 13.4):
  - Like the lumbar spine, neonatal sacral vertebrae are composed of two half neural arches posteriorly and a centrum anteriorly.
  - S1 and S2 vertebrae contain lateral elements that will form the articular surfaces of the sacroiliac joints.
  - Compared to the lumbar spine, fusion and ossification are delayed in the sacrum; neurocentral fusion occurs between ages 2 and 6, and fusion of the neural arches to form spinous processes continues until age 15.
  - Ossification is a continual process that carries on until puberty with ventral fusion of S1–S2 occurring in the early 20s.
- Sacral vertebrae are oriented vertically until weight bearing around age 1.
- Beyond puberty, the *sacral hiatus* is an inferiorly placed opening into the caudal epidural space, below the fifth sacral vertebra and between it and its inferior "horns" or cornua (this is because the S5 laminae fail to fuse) (Fig. 13.4). In young infants, the sacral hiatus is generally lower, below the fifth sacral vertebra, and since there is much less ossification of the sacrum, ultrasound imaging in infants is generally rendered easier and generates superior image quality.
- The posterior sacrococcygeal ligament (membrane) has superficial and deep laminae and covers the sacral hiatus externally; this ligament requires penetration by the needle for epidural needle entry (see Fig. 13.5).

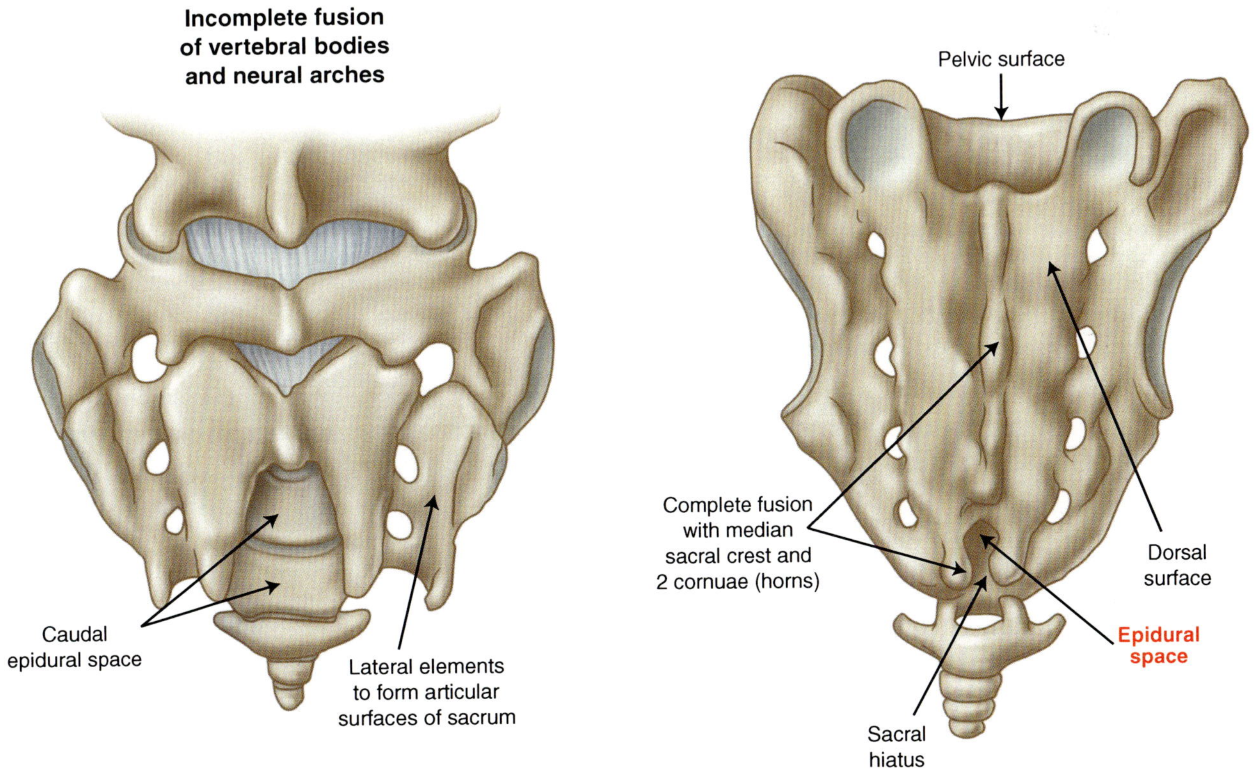

Fig. 13.4 Posterior view of infant (*left*) and adolescent (*right*) sacra, illustrating incomplete fusion of the sacral neural arches. Also shown is the incorporation of lateral elements which form the articular surfaces to form the sacroiliac joints

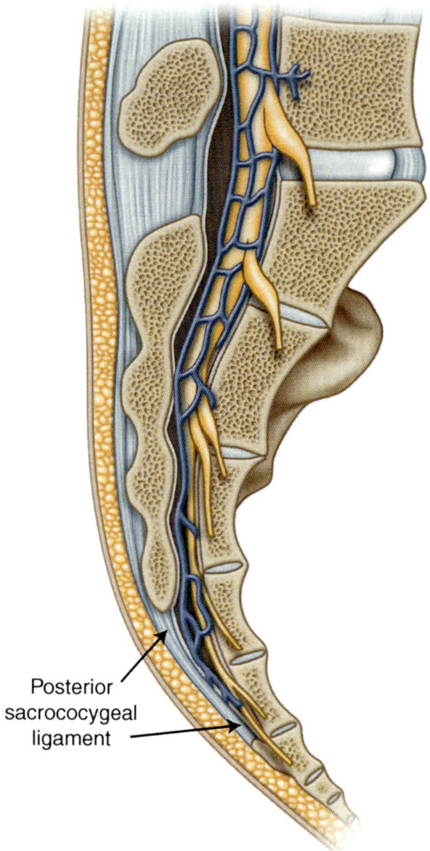

Fig. 13.5 The caudal epidural space. When performing epidural entry in this location, puncture of the posterior sacrococcygeal ligament minimizes the risk of potential needle trauma to the spinal cord

13.3 Costovertebral Articulations

The costovertebral articulations (Fig. 13.6) are relevant primarily for paravertebral and intercostal blockades, although practitioners will encounter these joints during ultrasound-guided epidurals as the imaging technique will incorporate these structures. The ribs articulate with the vertebral column through two synovial joints, one for the head of the rib (costovertebral) and the other for the tubercle (costotransverse):

- *Costovertebral joint:* the head of the rib articulates through a synovial joint with demi-facets on adjacent thoracic vertebral bodies and the corresponding intervertebral disk of the upper vertebral joint, e.g., 7th rib with bodies of T6, T7, and T6–T7 disk (except for the 1st and 10th–12th ribs, which articulate with a single vertebral facet through a simple synovial joint). The synovial joint cavities of the remaining costovertebral joints are bisected by an intra-articular ligament resulting in double synovial compartments. The joints are enclosed in fibrous capsules lined on the inside with synovial membrane and reinforced by capsular, radiate, and intra-articular ligaments.
- *Costotransverse joint:* articular facets on the tubercles of the ribs articulate through synovial joints with the transverse processes of the corresponding thoracic vertebrae (the 11th and 12th ribs lack this articulation since they do not possess tubercles). The joints are enclosed in thin fibrous capsules lined with synovial membrane and reinforced by ligaments. The ligaments are the superior and lateral costotransverse and the costotransverse ligament, the latter filling the interosseous gap (costotransverse foramen) between the neck of the rib and its adjacent vertebral transverse process. The primary purpose of these articulations is to facilitate movements of the ribs for respiratory excursions of the thorax.

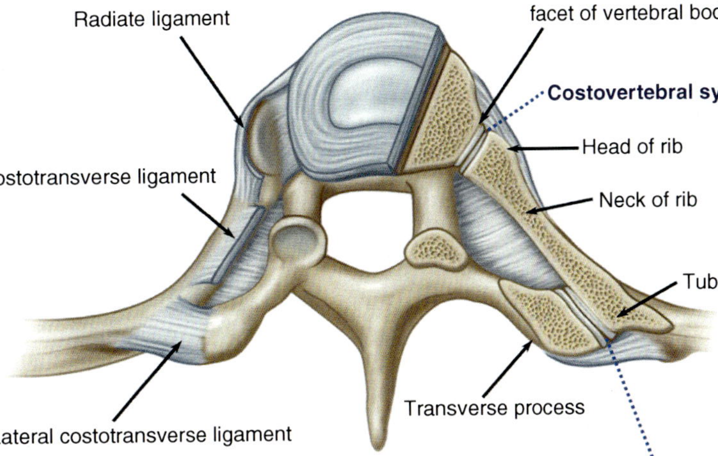

Fig. 13.6 Costovertebral articulations. *Left side*: costovertebral and costotransverse synovial joints, illustrating exterior surfaces with ligamentous coverings; *right side*: section through the synovial joints

13.4 Paravertebral Space

The paravertebral space is a bilateral wedge-shaped space on either side of the vertebral column and between the individual vertebrae, extending the column's entire length, through which the spinal nerves course after exiting from the intervertebral foramina. In the thoracic region, its boundaries are as follows (Fig. 13.1):

- Medially: vertebral body, intervertebral disk and foramen, and spinous process
- Anterolaterally: parietal pleura
- Posteriorly: costotransverse joint and the adjacent parts of the transverse process and the rib, approximately 2.5 cm (for adolescents) from the tip of the transverse process, often in a slightly caudal orientation

The paravertebral space communicates medially with the intervertebral foramen throughout the length of the column with the exception of the sacrum and coccyx. In the thoracic region, it is continuous laterally with the intercostal space, and adjacent levels of the paravertebral space communicate with each other. In the lumbar region, however, the paravertebral space is divided into segments by the attachments of the psoas major muscle.

13.5 Thoracic Spinal Nerves and Intercostal Nerves

- There are 12 pairs of thoracic spinal nerves: T1–T12.
- The intercostal nerves are the *ventral primary rami* of thoracic spinal nerves T1–T11.
- The ventral primary ramus of thoracic spinal nerve T12 is called the *subcostal nerve*, which courses beneath the 12th rib along the posterior abdominal wall.
- The thoracic spinal nerves arise from the thoracic segments of the cord from the union of dorsal and ventral roots and emerge from the *intervertebral (spinal)* foramina to course through the *paravertebral space* en route to the structures they supply in the thoracic and abdominal walls.
- The intervertebral foramina are found between adjoining neural arches near their junctions with the vertebral bodies, where adjacent *vertebral notches* on the pedicles of the vertebra above and below contribute to the formation of the foramen.
- As they course through the intervertebral foramina, the spinal nerves have clinically important relations with the boundaries of the foramina.
- Forming the complete perimeter of an intervertebral foramen, these boundaries are, *superiorly and inferiorly*, the vertebral notches of the pedicles of adjoining vertebrae; *anteriorly*, the posterolateral aspects of the adjacent vertebral bodies and intervening IV disk; and, *posteriorly*, the fibrous capsule of the synovial facet (zygapophyseal) joint between the superior and inferior articular processes of the vertebrae.
- Each spinal nerve, together with its spinal artery, a small venous plexus, and its own meningeal branch(es), traverses the intervertebral foramen.
- After exiting through the intervertebral foramen, each spinal nerve quickly divides into a small *dorsal (primary) ramus* (branch) to supply the paravertebral (paraspinal) muscles and skin of the back and a larger *ventral (primary) ramus* that swings around from posterolateral to anteromedial along the chest wall to supply the intercostal spaces, the adjacent thoracic wall, and the anterior abdominal wall (Fig. 13.1).
- The ventral (primary) rami of thoracic spinal nerves T1–T11 form the 11 pairs of *intercostal nerves* for the 11 intercostal spaces (see Fig. 11.6) and the *subcostal nerve* (T12), which courses just underneath the 12th rib.
- The intercostal nerves give off cutaneous branches at the lateral and anterior aspects of the thoracic and abdominal walls that supply the skin and superficial fascia (subcutaneous tissues) in these regions.
- Thoracic spinal nerves T2 through T12 (intercostal nerves and subcostal nerve) and lumbar spinal nerve L1

(iliohypogastric and ilioinguinal nerves) can be blocked for surgical intervention (Fig. 13.7).

Initially, the intercostal nerves course through the posterior aspects of the intercostal spaces, between the intercostal membrane and the parietal pleura, and then course laterally past the angles of their respective ribs between the innermost and internal intercostal muscles. Laterally, they give off both collateral branches (running adjacent to the nerve within the intercostal space) and lateral cutaneous branches, the latter of which divide into ventral and dorsal rami. The first intercostal nerve branches into two nerves; the first of which leaves the thorax near the neck of the first rib and contributes to the brachial plexus, while the second travels a path similar to those below it within the intercostal space. The lateral cutaneous branch of the second intercostal nerve is the *intercostobrachial nerve*, which pierces the second intercostal space and crosses the axilla to reach the medial and posterior aspects of the arm where it supplies the skin and subcutaneous tissues.

As the intercostal nerves travel laterally, anteriorly, and then medially to reach the anterior aspect of the thoracic wall, they contact the parietal pleura again before giving off the *anterior cutaneous nerves of the thorax*. The first to sixth intercostal nerves (T1–T6) proceed in their intercostal spaces between the innermost and internal intercostal muscles and beneath the intercostal vessels until they approach the sternum where they end as the *anterior cutaneous nerves of the thorax*. Intercostal nerves 7 (T7) through 11 (T11) and the subcostal nerve (T12) continue from their intercostal and subcostal spaces into the anterior abdominal wall, in which they supply and end as the *anterior cutaneous nerves of the abdomen* (T7–T12). As these nerves enter the anterolateral abdominal wall, they course in the plane between the transversus abdominis and internal oblique muscles, which corresponds to the plane between the innermost and internal intercostal muscles in the thorax. The tenth intercostal nerve, for example, the cutaneous branches of which supply the periumbilical skin, travels laterally between the transverse abdominis and internal oblique muscles; courses anteriorly and then medially around the abdominal wall; pierces the posterior rectus sheath; pierces through the rectus abdominis, supplying it; and then pierces the anterior rectus sheath to become the anterior cutaneous branch (Figs. 13.8, 13.9, and 13.10). Intercostal nerves T7 to T9 and T11 take a similar course through the anterior abdominal wall. They supply the muscles, skin, and subcutaneous tissues of the anterolateral abdominal walls, as well as the parietal peritoneum lining the abdominal walls. Cutaneous innervation to the anterolateral thoracic and abdominal walls by cutaneous branches of the intercostal nerves and subcostal nerve is organized segmentally (Fig. 13.7). Landmark dermatomes on the anterior thoracic and abdominal walls in the adult are the sternal angle (of Louis), T2; nipple, T4; xiphoid process, T7; umbilicus, T10; and suprapubic region, L1.

Innervation:	*Motor:* rectus abdominis; transversus abdominis; internal and external oblique; innermost, internal, and external intercostals; subcostales; transversus thoracis; serratus posterior (superior and inferior); and levatores costarum
	Sensory: skin and subcutaneous tissues on anterior and posterior thoracic and abdominal walls, parietal pleura, parietal peritoneum, skin and subcutaneous tissues on medial and posterior aspects of the arm (via brachial plexus and intercostobrachial nerve), and peripheral portions of the diaphragm

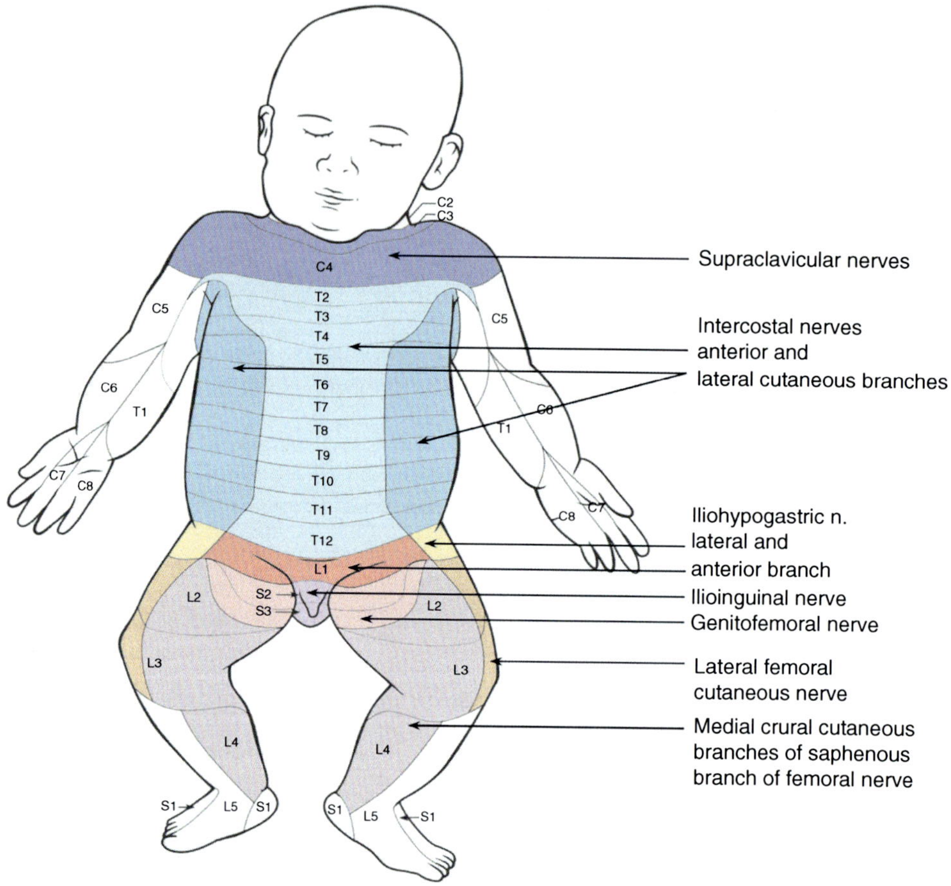

Fig. 13.7 Cutaneous innervation of the anterior trunk

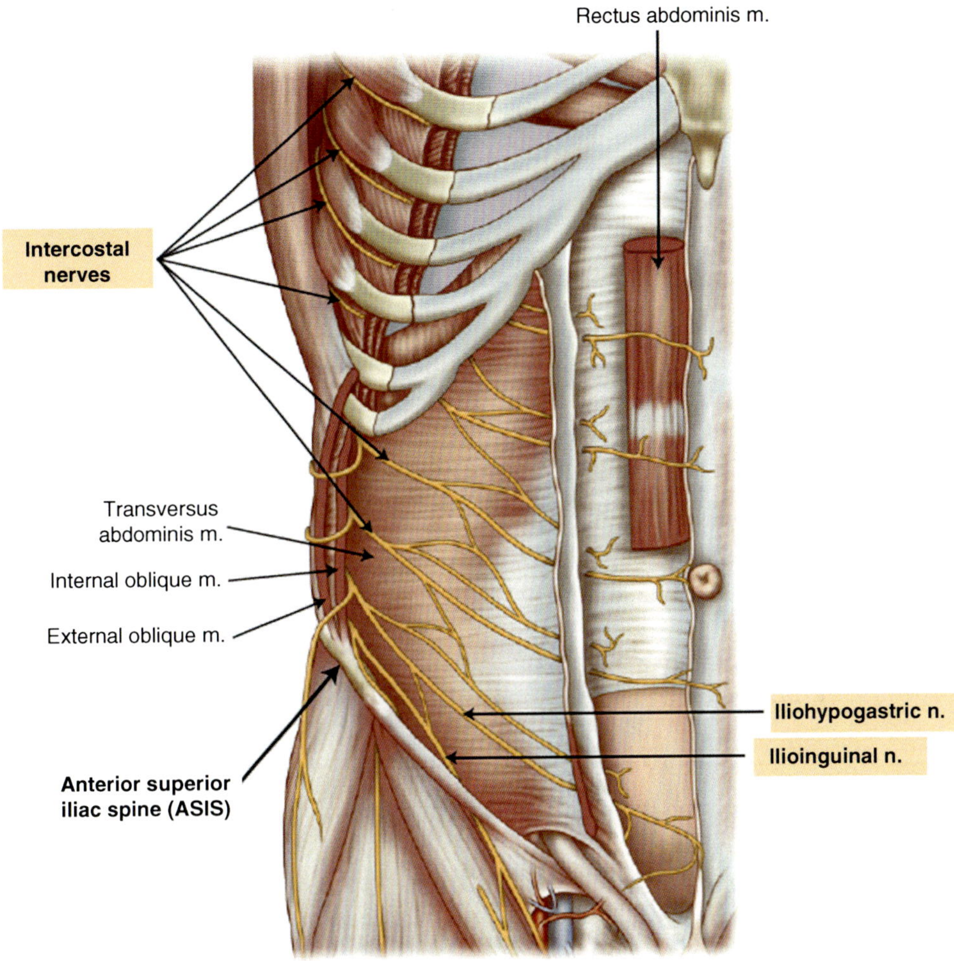

Fig. 13.8 Anterior view of the abdomen

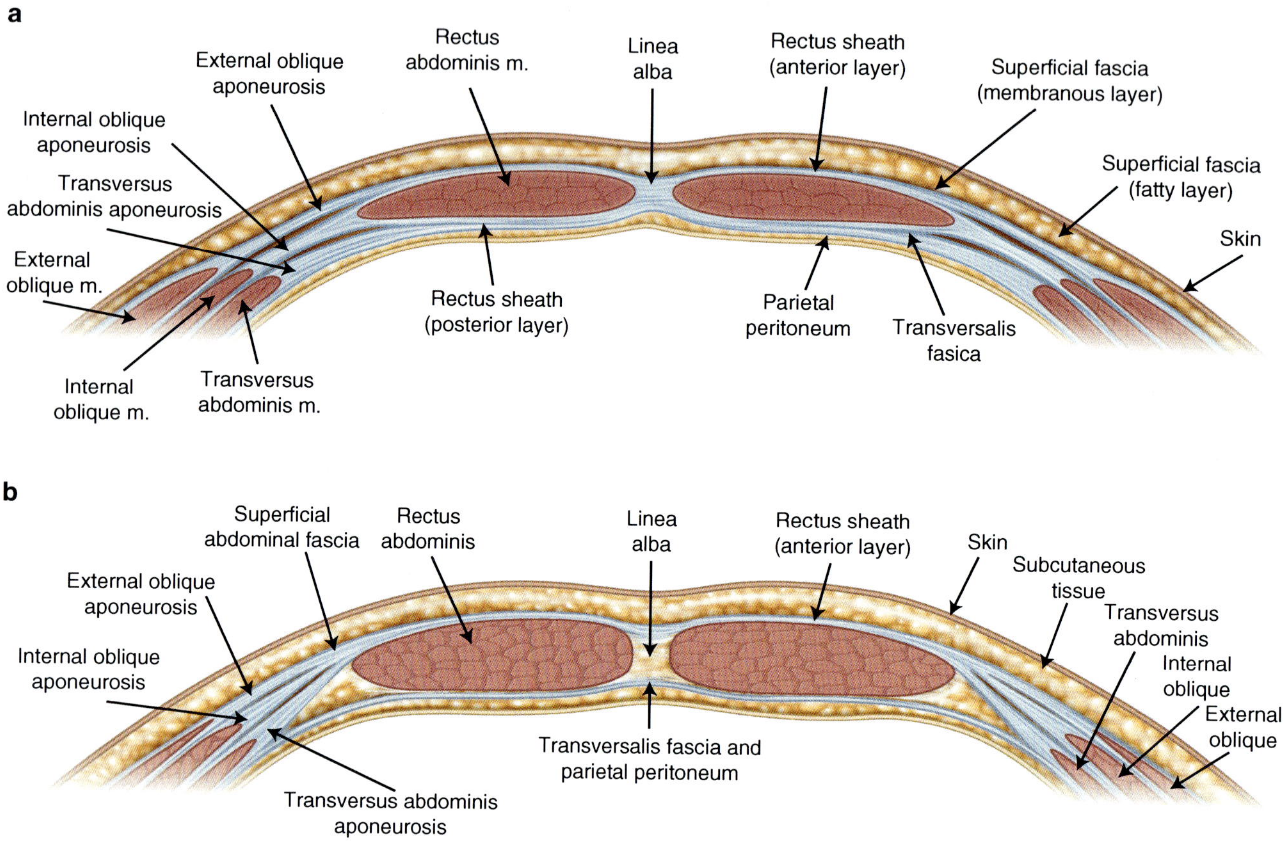

Fig. 13.9 Transverse view of the abdomen above (**a**) and below (**b**) the arcuate line of the abdomen (Douglas' line)

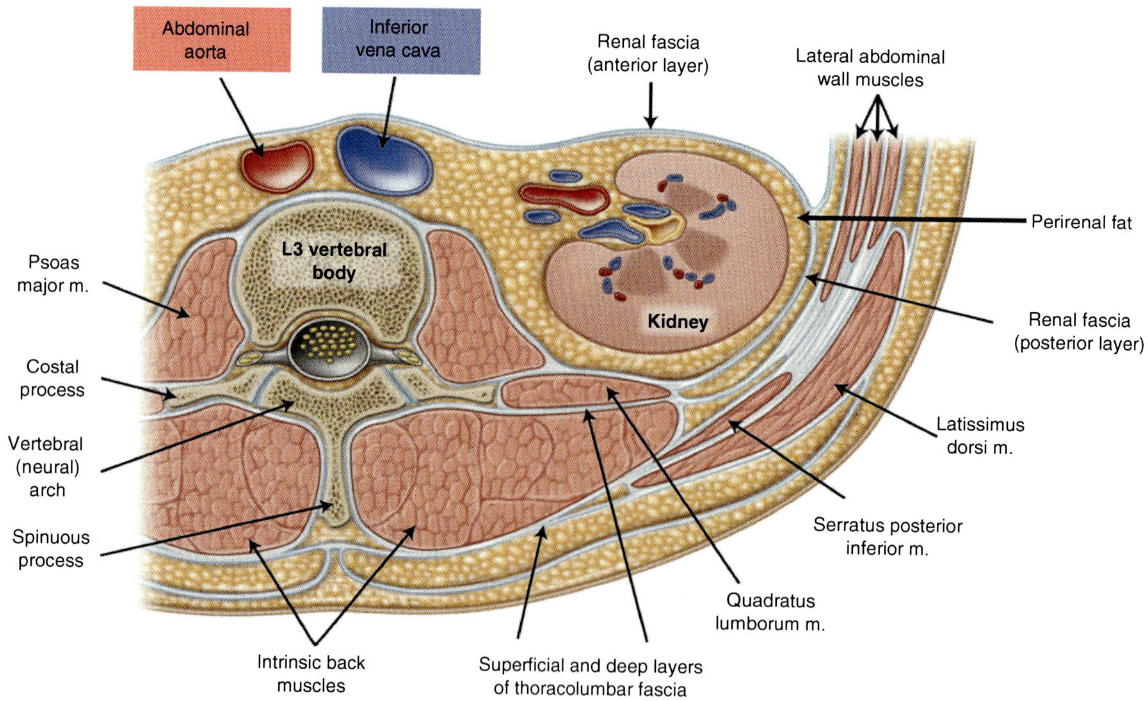

Fig. 13.10 Transverse view of the lumbar torso (L3 level)

13.6 Vertebral (Spinal) Canal

In order to safely and proficiently administer a spinal anesthetic in children, it is crucial to understand the anatomy of the vertebral (spinal) canal, including the level of termination of the spinal cord and dural sac, the relationship between vertebral levels and spinal cord segments, as well as the age-dependent variation in the volume of cerebrospinal fluid (CSF). This section reviews the gross and developmental anatomy of the vertebral column in order to provide a basis for appreciating the improved visibility when imaging the spine in the pediatric patient, followed by a brief segment explaining the relationship between vertebral levels and spinal cord segments.

The spinal cord and its nerve roots lie within the bony central canal of the vertebral column. The vertebral column consists of 7 cervical, 12 thoracic, 5 lumbar, 5 sacral, and 4 (3 to 5) coccygeal vertebrae. The developmental anatomy of the lumbar and sacral regions is of particular relevance to spinal anesthesia in infants and children.

- The vertebral (spinal) canal is the longitudinal, cylindrical space within the vertebral column created by successive vertebral foramina superimposed upon one another and extends from C1 vertebra to the bottom of the sacrum (sacral canal). Superiorly, it is continuous with the foramen magnum which transmits the spinomedullary junction. The vertebral canal houses the spinal cord with its blood vessels and surrounding meninges; the proximal portions of the spinal nerves within their dural sheaths, epidural fat, loose connective tissue, lymphatics, and small arterial branches; and the internal vertebral venous plexus. The latter five structures are found within the epidural space, a real space between the dura and the bony margins of the vertebral canal.
- The vertebral canal's anterior border is formed by posterior aspects of the vertebral bodies and the posterior longitudinal ligament; laterally, it is bordered by the pedicles, while posterolaterally and posteriorly, its boundaries are formed by the laminae, the ligamenta flava, and the posterior aspects of the vertebral neural arches, respectively.
- The lumbar segment of the vertebral (spinal) canal has been described as having a shape similar to that of an hourglass, with narrowing at the third and fourth lumbar levels. This feature is already present at age 3. Furthermore, the sagittal (anteroposterior) diameter of the vertebral canal does not differ significantly between the ages of 3–14 inclusive.
- The major structure within the vertebral canal is the spinal cord with its blood vessels, its cerebrospinal fluid, and its three meningeal coverings. The meninges are three concentric membranes surrounding the brain and spinal cord and providing support and protection to these delicate structures. The cranial and spinal meninges are continuous at the foramen magnum.

From superficial to deep, the three meninges surrounding the spinal cord are:

1. The *dura mater* (pachymeninx) which is the outermost fibrous and toughest layer of the meninges. Between the dura and the walls of the vertebral canal is the spinal epidural space, a real space containing epidural fat within loose connective tissue, lymphatics, small arterial vessels, and the internal vertebral venous plexus (see below).
2. The *arachnoid mater*, a much thinner and more delicate, mostly translucent spider web-like membrane which lines the inside of the dura and is separated from the next deep layer, the *pia mater*, by a real space, the *subarachnoid space*, through which it sends delicate trabeculae down to the pia mater. The spinal subarachnoid space contains cerebrospinal fluid (CSF) and the anterior and posterior spinal vessels. There is a potential *subdural space* within the vertebral canal since the dura and arachnoid are closely applied; however, accidental subdural penetration may occur during epidural injections.
3. The *pia mater*, the transparent innermost single-cell layered membrane tightly adherent to the surface of the spinal cord and inseparable from it. The pia mater intimately follows and dips into all the grooves and fissures on the surface of the cord. The arachnoid and pia together are sometimes referred to as the leptomeninges. Deep to the pia is a thick *subpial collagenous layer* which is continuous with the collagenous core of the *denticulate ligaments*. The latter, which are flat, triangular fibrous sheets on either side of the cord between the ventral and dorsal roots anchor the cord via their apices to the inside of the dura mater at regular intervals and provide it with structural support.

Intermediate layer: In addition to the three classically described layers of meninges surrounding the cord, there is an additional so-called intermediate layer of leptomeninges found just deep to the arachnoid but superficial to the pia and concentrated mostly around the posterior and anterior regions of the cord. This layer is perforated and lacelike in appearance and thickened focally to form the posterior, posterolateral, and anterior ligaments of the cord and provide it with additional support to that provided by the denticulate ligaments. Structurally, it is similar to the trabeculae crossing the cranial subarachnoid space and may play a role in dampening fluid waves in the CSF within the subarachnoid space.

13.6.1 Vertebral Levels, Spinal Nerve Roots, and Spinal Cord Segments

An appreciation of the clinical anatomy of the spinal cord as it relates to the vertebral column and the relationship between spinal cord segments and vertebral levels is important for the anesthesiologist. Since, due to differential growth rates, the spinal cord is shorter than the vertebral column, the more caudal spinal roots descend almost vertically for varying distances beyond the termination of the cord (conus medullaris) to reach their corresponding intervertebral foramina. As they do so, they form a divergent bundle of spinal roots resembling a horse's tail, the *cauda equina*, beyond the conus medullaris and surrounding the filum terminale. This sheaf of nerve roots is suspended within the cerebrospinal fluid in an expanded subarachnoid space, the lumbar cistern, the preferred site for performing a lumbar puncture.

With regard to the relationship between spinal cord segments and vertebral levels, the following estimation is helpful: at the cervical level, the tip of the vertebral spinous process corresponds to the succeeding spinal cord segment (i.e., the tip of the fifth cervical spine is opposite the sixth cervical spinal cord segment). At upper thoracic levels, this difference corresponds to two cord segments (i.e., the tip of the third thoracic spine is opposite the fifth thoracic cord segment); in the lower thoracic region, this difference increases to three segments (i.e., the tenth thoracic spine is opposite the first lumbar cord segment); the 12th thoracic spine lies opposite the first sacral cord segment; thus, there is a progressively increasing discrepancy between spinal cord segments and vertebral levels craniocaudally.

The adult spinal cord terminates in most cases at the level of the intervertebral disk between the first and second lumbar vertebrae (L1 and L2); however, there is some variation (see also Sect. 13.2.2). The neonatal spinal cord extends to the upper border of the third lumbar vertebra (L3), this level rising during the first 2 months after birth. There is marked variation however; the cord may terminate between L1–L3/4 at birth and between L1–L3 in children between the ages of 3 months to 15 years [1].

13.6.2 Spinal Nerves Above the Sacrum

- The *ventral* and *dorsal* roots (dorsal roots containing the dorsal root ganglia at this location) of the spinal nerves join as they leave the spinal cord, forming the mixed *spinal nerve*, which exits the vertebral canal through the intervertebral (spinal, neural) foramen.
- The ventral and dorsal roots as well as the proximal portions of the spinal nerves are enclosed within a sleeve of *dura mater*, which is an extension of the dura from that surrounding the cord. Deep to this sheath of dura mater is the arachnoid mater. The dural/arachnoid sleeve extends onto the spinal nerves for a short distance before blending with the epineurium surrounding the nerves.
- The *spinal epidural space* (Fig. 13.11) is a "real" space between the dura mater and the periosteum lining the vertebral (spinal) canal. This space is richly vascularized (internal vertebral venous plexus, small arterial branches, and lymphatics) and filled with epidural fat and loose connective tissue which surrounds the dura mater. It is bordered posteriorly by the *ligamentum flavum (interlaminar ligament)*, laterally by the pedicles, and anteriorly by the *posterior longitudinal ligament* which lies on posterior aspects of the vertebral bodies within the vertebral canal.
- *Gray* and *white rami communicantes* (Fig. 13.1) connect the spinal nerves to the sympathetic trunk (chain) ganglia to allow preganglionic sympathetic fibers leaving the spinal cord (T1–L2/3) to enter the trunk and leave it again to be distributed with spinal nerves at all levels.
- The spinal nerves divide into *ventral* and *dorsal (primary) rami* (Figs. 13.1 and 13.11); the dorsal rami supply the paravertebral muscles and skin near the midline of the back; the ventral rami of the thoracic spinal nerves form the intercostal and subcostal nerves (T1–T12) (Sect. 13.5) which supply the walls of the thorax and abdomen (including the parietal pleura and peritoneum). The remaining ventral rami (C1–T1 and L1–S3) form the cervical, brachial, lumbar, and sacral plexuses, which supply the muscles, skin, and subcutaneous tissues of the neck, lower trunk, and extremities.

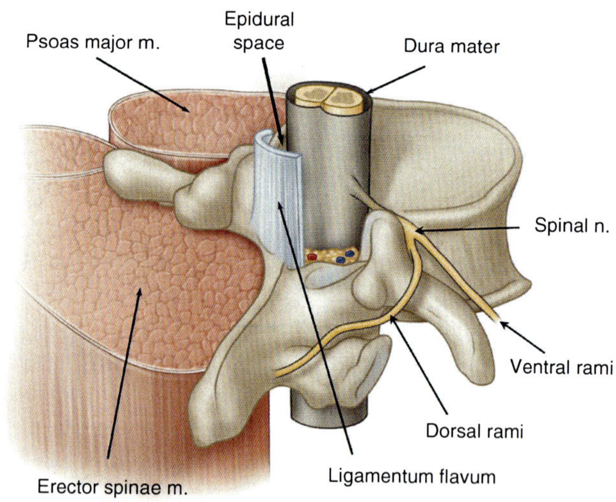

Fig. 13.11 The spinal epidural space

13.6.3 Termination of the Spinal Cord and Dural Sac

- The spinal cord occupies the upper two thirds of the vertebral canal. It begins at the superior border of the atlas vertebra (C1) and, in the average adult, ends at the *conus medullaris*, approximately at the level of the IV disk between the first and second lumbar vertebrae. Its level of termination varies somewhat between individuals and with posture, especially vertebral flexion, during which its position rises slightly. It may end as high as T12 or in some cases as low as the L2–L3 IV disk. There is some correlation between its level of termination and the length of the trunk, especially in females. The spinal cord appears to "decrease" in length significantly throughout prenatal and antenatal development, with the cord reaching as far down as S1 or 2 in the last few intrauterine months and as low as L2 or 3 at birth (Fig. 13.12). This apparent "decrease" is really the result of the greater rate of growth of the vertebral (spinal) column as compared to the cord and elongation of the lumbosacral region.
- The *dural sac* extends beyond this level, to approximately the second sacral vertebral level (S2); within the sac, the nerves forming the *cauda equina* run vertically from the conus medullaris in the lumbar section of the vertebral canal and within the sacral canal (between the posterior surface of the sacrum and the fused pedicles [intervertebral foramina in infants])
- The nerves forming the cauda equina are suspended within the cerebrospinal fluid occupying the subarachnoid lumbar cistern, which is the subarachnoid space below the conus medullaris and between it and the termination of the dural sac at S2. The arachnoid mater, lining the inside of the dura mater, also terminates at around the S2 before extending inferiorly with the *filum terminale*.
- The filum terminale is a filament of connective tissue about 20 cm long in the average adult that extends from the tip of the conus medullaris to the sacrum and coccyx. Its proximal or upper 15 cm or so, termed the *filum terminale internum* (internal filum terminale), is surrounded by extensions of the dura and arachnoid and reaches down to the posterior aspect of the second sacral vertebra (S2). Its distal or final 5 cm or so, termed the *filum terminale externum* (external filum terminale), fuses with the investing dura mater and attaches to the posterior aspect of the first coccygeal vertebral segment. The filum is continuous above with the pia lining the spinal cord. The central canal of the spinal cord continues into the filum terminale for a short distance (3 to 5 cm) although its patency is variable. The subarachnoid space surrounding the filum terminale internum is expanded to form the lumbar cistern, which contains the cauda equina and is the preferred site for obtaining a sample of CSF through a lumbar puncture.
- Despite the above classical description, a recent study suggests that the conus medullaris terminates most commonly at the level of the L1–L2 disk space and, in the absence of tethering, virtually never ends below the mid-body of L2.
  - The spinal cord and dural sac were traditionally thought to terminate at a more caudal level in neonates; however, ultrasonography and MRI scans have demonstrated that the location of the caudal displacement of the conus medullaris in tethered cord syndrome is similar in term infants and adults.
  - The dural sac in neonates and infants terminates more caudally at the level of S3 as compared to adults in whom it ends at S2.

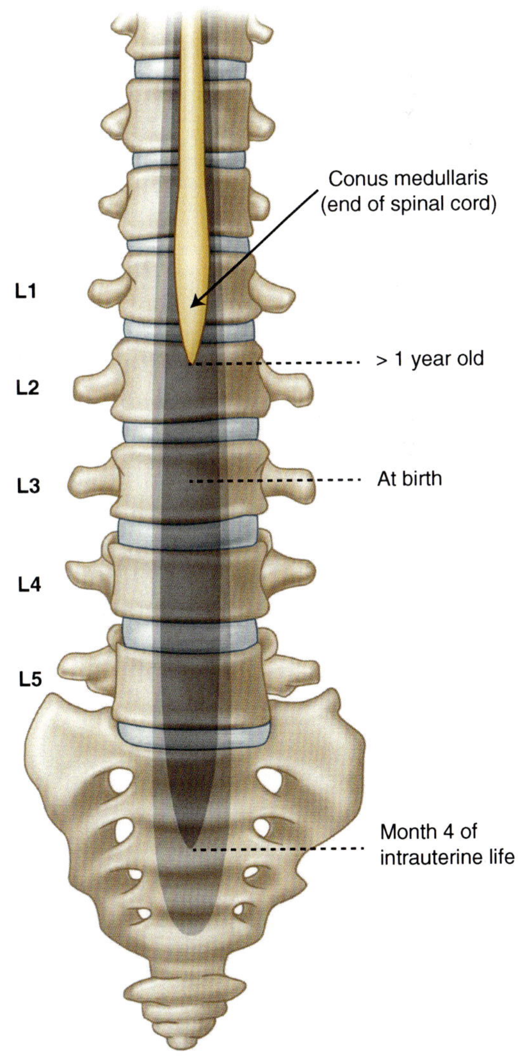

Fig. 13.12 Development of the spinal cord. The spinal cord appears to decrease in length significantly throughout early development due to the relatively faster growth of the vertebral column

13.6.4 CSF Volume

- CSF is produced from arterial blood by the choroid plexuses of the lateral, third, and fourth ventricles through a combined process of diffusion, pinocytosis, and active transfer.
- It is in a state of constant circulation through continuous production and reabsorption into the venous system, primarily through the arachnoid granulations in the superior sagittal sinus.
- While diffusion and the pressure gradient created within the CSF by virtue of its constant production and reabsorption are perhaps the major force causing the CSF to circulate, particularly around the cerebral hemispheres, its flow around the spinal cord is not that active and probably regulated to some extent by changes in body posture.
- Infants and neonates have a larger volume of CSF circulating on an ml/kg basis (neonates = 10 mL/kg; infants under 15 kg = 4 mL/kg; young children = 3 mL/kg) compared to adults (2 mL/kg). This fact may account for the higher dose of local anesthetic required per kilogram of body weight and shorter duration of action of spinal anesthesia in infants owing to the larger CSF volume in children.

Reference

1. Barson AJ. The vertebral level of termination of the spinal cord during normal and abnormal development. J Anat. 1970;106:489–97.

Suggested Reading

Cramer GD, Darby SA, editors. Clinical anatomy of the spine, spinal cord, and ANS. 3rd ed. St. Louis: Mosby; 2014.

Newell RLM. Spinal cord and spinal nerves: gross. In: Standring S, editor. Gray's anatomy. 40th ed. London: Churchill Livingstone, 2008; p. 749–61.

Clinical Anatomy of the Dermatomes and Innervation of the Joints

14

Anil H. Walji and Ban C.H. Tsui

Contents

A.H. Walji, MD, PhD
Division of Anatomy, Department of Surgery,
Faculty of Medicine and Dentistry, University of Alberta,
Edmonton, AB Canada

B.C.H. Tsui, Dip Eng, BSc (Math), B Pharm, MSc, MD, FRCPC (✉)
Department of Anesthesiology and Pain Medicine,
Stollery Children's Hospital/University of Alberta Hospital,
2-150 Clinical Sciences Building, Edmonton,
AB T6G 2G3, Canada
e-mail: btsui@ualberta.ca

B.C.H. Tsui, S. Suresh (eds.), *Pediatric Atlas of Ultrasound- and Nerve Stimulation-Guided Regional Anesthesia*,
DOI 10.1007/978-0-387-79964-3_14

14.1 Introduction

14.1.1 Dermatomes

With the exception of C1 (which does not have a sensory component), sensory fibers from the dorsal roots of the spinal nerves supply a specific segment or band of skin. This skin segment is termed a *dermatome*. For example, the C5-T1 spinal nerves provide cutaneous innervation to the upper extremity. There is considerable overlap between contiguous dermatomes, and adjacent dermatomes are generally arranged as consecutive horizontal bands on the surface of the axial skeleton and more or less vertical projections on the extremities. Anatomical knowledge of the respective dermatomes will help to block the appropriate skin segment during peripheral nerve blockade. Dermatomes are important particularly for peripheral nerve blockade. Clinically, fairly specific areas of regional anesthesia can be achieved based on the cutaneous innervation provided by the terminal nerves in that part of the body.

14.1.2 Myotomes

The ventral (motor) roots of the spinal cord provide motor innervation to the skeletal muscles by providing motor nerve fibers to the spinal nerves. A *myotome* is a block of skeletal muscle that is supplied segmentally by the ventral roots of a spinal nerve; movements of the extremities and trunk that are created by these myotomes can thus be classified segmentally (see segmental motor responses associated with nerve stimulation). In general, segmental innervation of the muscles can be fairly well differentiated. In addition to segmental (myotomal) distribution of innervation, there is also specific muscular distribution that is derived from the terminal nerves. Knowledge of this terminal nerve innervation becomes extremely important when blocking the brachial plexus branches at sites beyond the root level (e.g., during axillary block, it would be useful to use radial nerve motor responses to confirm posterior cord localization). Table 14.1 summarizes the origin of each terminal nerve and its objective movement upon electrical stimulation.

Table 14.1 Upper extremity (brachial plexus terminal motor nerves): origins and motor responses to nerve stimulation

Motion	Nerve	Cord	Division	Trunk	Root
Arm abduction	Suprascapular[a]			Upper	C5, C6
Arm abduction	Axillary	Posterior	Posterior	Upper	C5, C6
Elbow flexion	Musculocutaneous[b]	Lateral	Posterior	Upper	C5, C6
			Anterior		
Extension (dorsiflexion) of the elbow, wrist, hand, and fingers	Radial	Posterior	Posterior	Upper	C5, C6
			Posterior	Middle	C7
Latissimus dorsi twitch (shoulder shrug)	Thoracodorsal	Posterior	Posterior	Middle	C7
Forearm pronation and wrist flexion	Median (lateral head)	Lateral	Anterior	Upper	C5, C6
		Medial	Anterior and posterior	Middle	C7
			Anterior	Lower	C8, T1
Thumb flexion and opposition (flexion middle and ring finger)	Median	Medial	Anterior	Lower	C8, T1
Thumb flexion and opposition	Anterior interosseous	Medial	Anterior	Lower	C8, T1
Fifth finger flexion and opposition, ulnar deviation of the wrist	Ulnar	Medial	Anterior	Lower	C8, T1

[a]The suprascapular nerve may not be blocked during supraclavicular block if the needle is placed at the level of the divisions rather than the trunks. Also, infraclavicular block will not target the suprascapular nerve since this nerve leaves the plexus at the trunks

[b]The targets of brachial plexus block using the axillary approach are the terminal nerves of the upper extremity and branches at the cord level of the plexus. The musculocutaneous nerve may not be blocked if the injection fails to spread to the proximal location where it branches

14.1.3 Osteotomes

Osteotomes refer to specific regions of the bones throughout the extremities that are innerved by the terminal nerves (rather than by spinal segments as with dermatomes). The innervation of bones can be significantly different from that of the muscles and skin. A good knowledge of joint innervation is important for orthopedic surgery as well as other surgical specialties and neurology.

14.2 Innervation of the Upper Extremity

14.2.1 Dermatomes and Cutaneous Distribution of the Peripheral Nerves (Figs. 14.1, 14.2, 14.3, and 14.4)

Segmental Cutaneous Innervation of the Upper Extremity

- C3 and 4: upper shoulder region (supraclavicular nerves)
- C5: deltoid and lateral aspect of the arm
- C6: lateral arm, forearm, and thumb
- C7: the hand and middle three fingers
- C8: fifth finger and medial side of both the hand and lower forearm
- T1: medial side of the lower arm and upper forearm
- T2: medial side of the upper arm (intercostobrachial nerve)

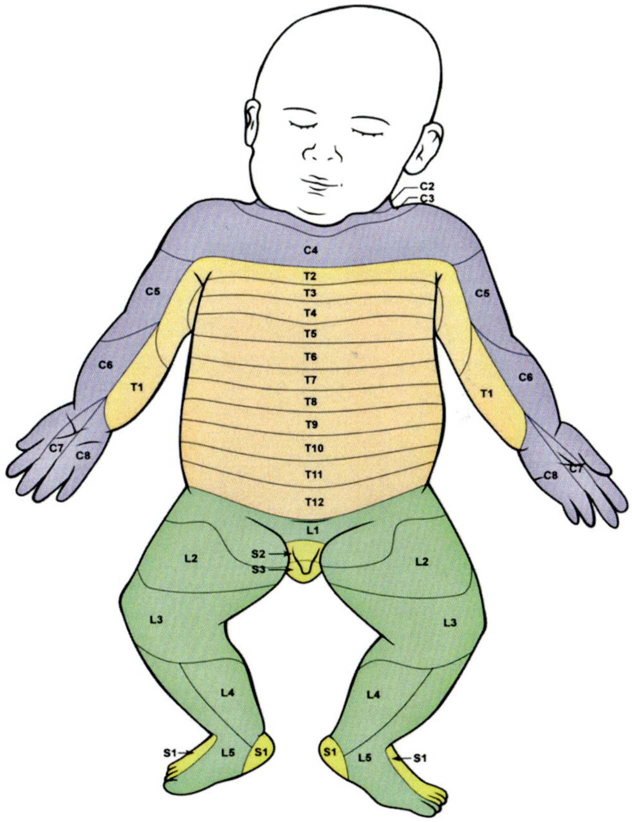

Fig. 14.1 Dermatomes; anterior view

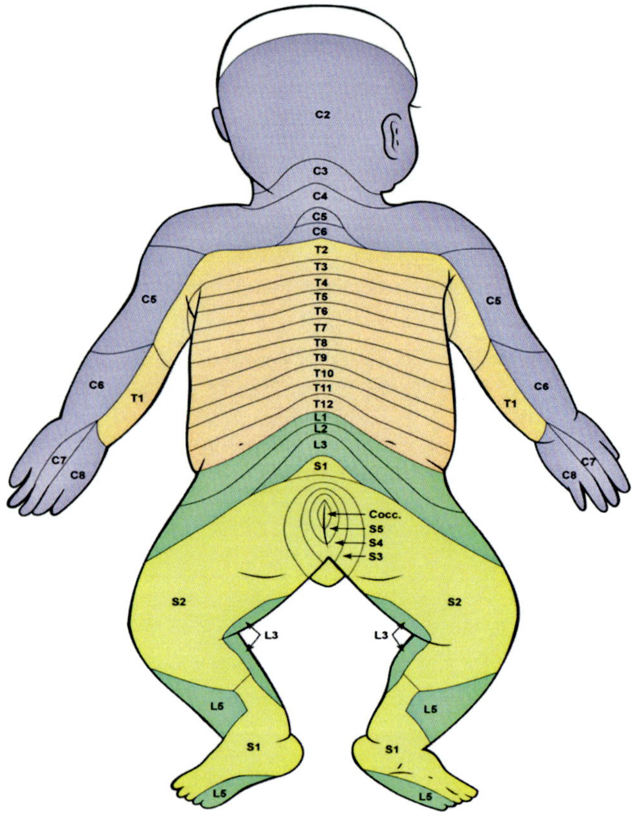

Fig. 14.2 Dermatomes; posterior view

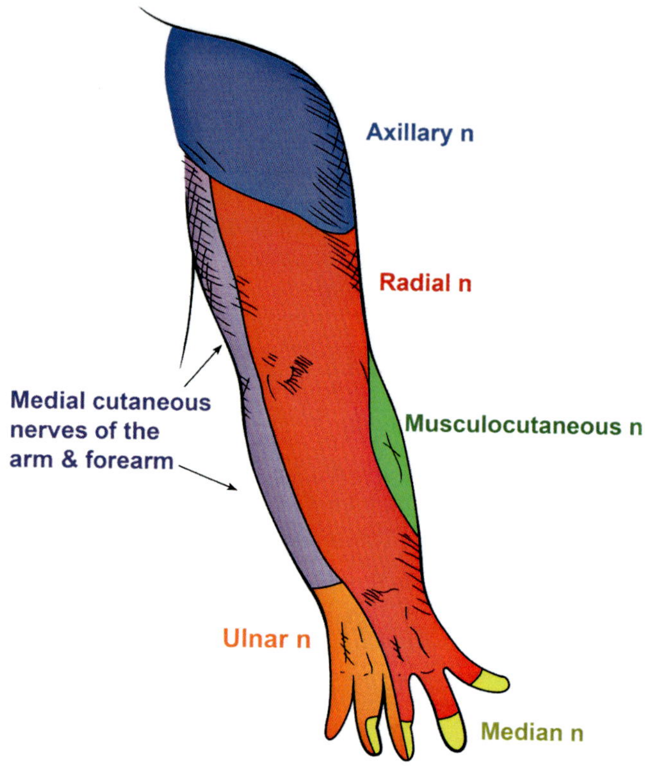

Fig. 14.4 Cutaneous distribution of the peripheral nerves of the upper extremity; posterior view

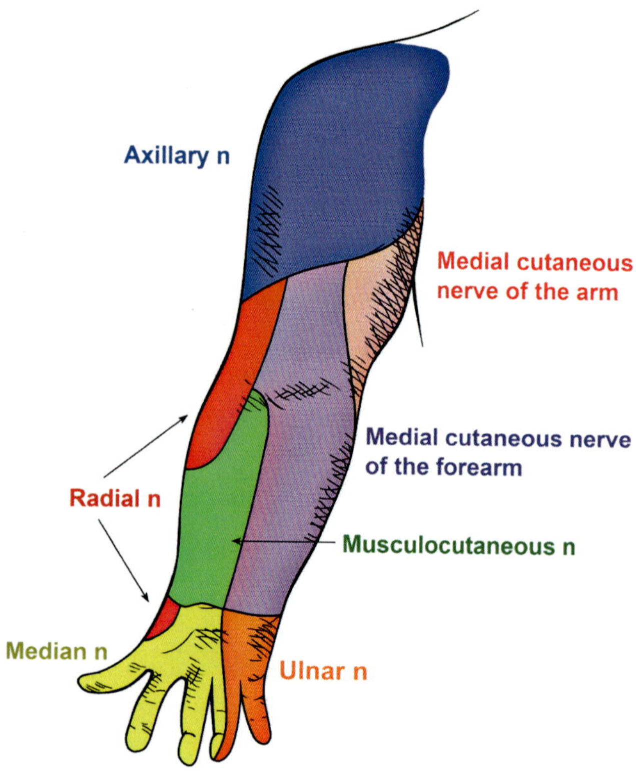

Fig. 14.3 Cutaneous distribution of the peripheral nerves of the upper extremity; anterior view

14.2.2 Myotomes

For clinical practice, it is important to understand that there is a specific distribution of innervation to skeletal muscles that is derived from the terminal nerves (Figs. 14.5 and 14.6). Table 14.1 summarizes the origin of each terminal nerve and its objective movement upon electrical stimulation.

Segmental Motor Responses Associated with Nerve Stimulation

- C5: lateral rotation and abduction of the arm at the shoulder joint
- C6: pronation and supination of the forearm
- C5 and 6: elbow flexion
- C6-8: medial rotation and adduction of the arm at the shoulder
- C6 and 7: elbow extension
- C6 and 7: wrist flexion and extension (long flexor and extensor muscles of the wrist)
- C7 and 8: digit flexion and extension (long flexors and extensors of the fingers), opposition of the thumb
- T1: intrinsic movements of the hand

Muscular Distribution of the Spinal Segments

- C5: rhomboids, supraspinatus, infraspinatus, anterior portion of deltoid, long head of biceps
- C6: teres major and minor, middle and posterior deltoid, short head of biceps, coracobrachialis, brachialis, brachioradialis, extensor carpi radialis longus and brevis, supinator, pronator teres
- C7: triceps, anconeus, extensor digitorum, extensor digiti minimi, extensor carpi ulnaris, abductor pollicis longus, extensor pollicis longus and brevis, extensor indicis, flexor carpi radialis
- C8: flexor digitorum superficialis and profundus, flexor carpi ulnaris, flexor pollicis longus, pronator quadratus, abductor and flexor pollicis brevis, opponens pollicis
- T1: flexor digitorum superficialis, abductor digiti minimi, adductor pollicis, flexor digiti minimi brevis, opponens digiti minimi, palmar and dorsal interossei, lumbricals

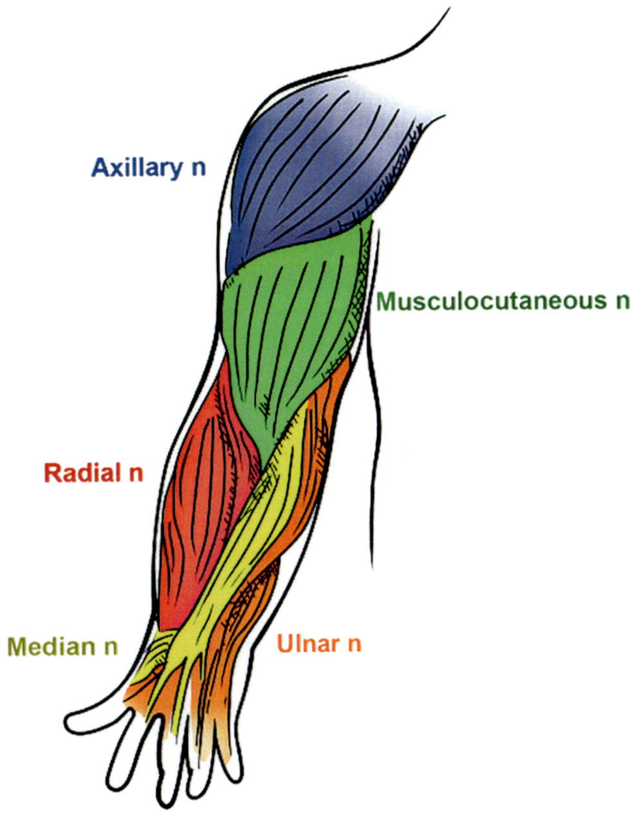

Fig. 14.5 Distribution of muscular innervations by the terminal nerves of the upper extremity; anterior view

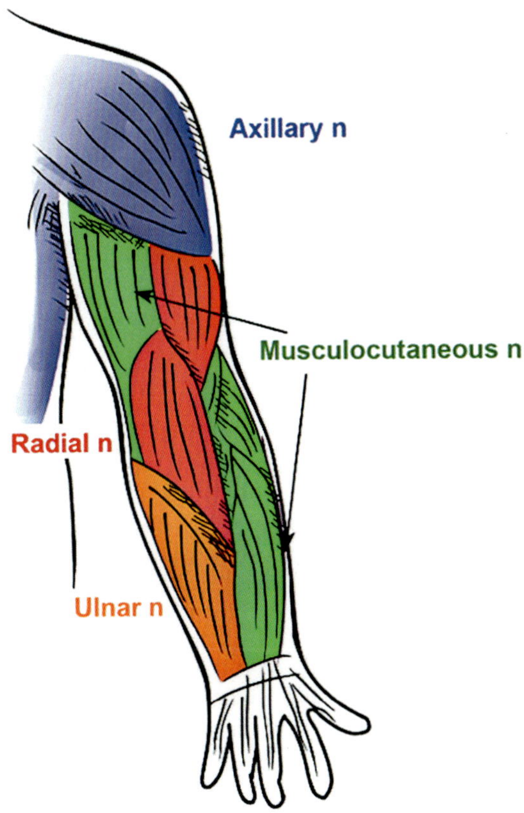

Fig. 14.6 Distribution of muscular innervations by the terminal nerves of the upper extremity; posterior view

14.2.3 Osteotomes

Terminal nerves, rather than spinal cord segments, distribute sensory innervation to specific regions of bones throughout the extremities. These terminal nerves also send articular branches to specific joints in the extremity. These regions of the bones, each supplied by a specific branch of a terminal nerve, are termed *osteotomes*; those for the upper extremity are summarized in Figs. 14.7 and 14.8.

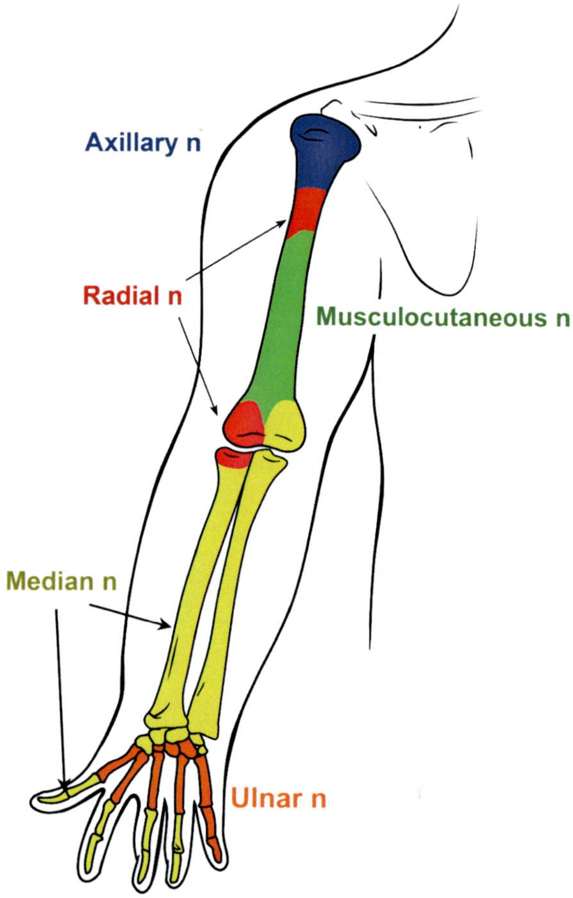

Fig. 14.7 Osteomes of the upper extremity; anterior view

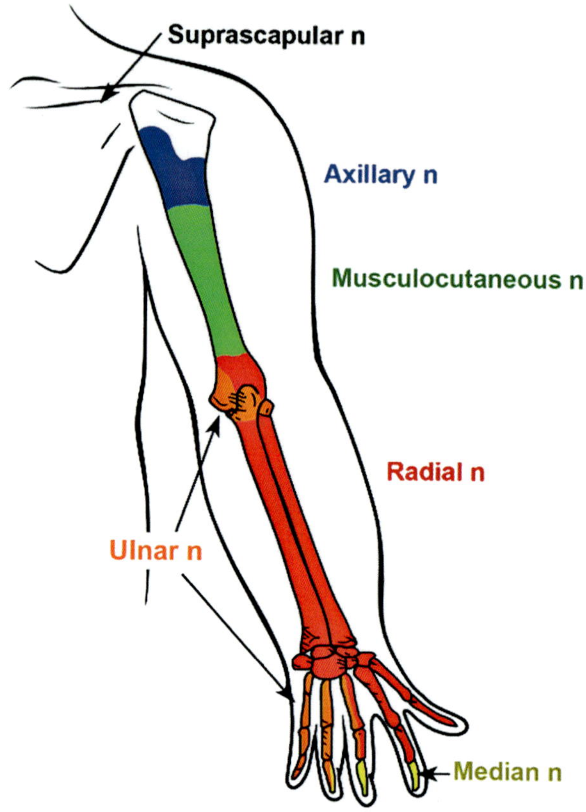

Fig. 14.8 Osteomes of the upper extremity; posterior view

14.2.4 Innervation of the Major Joints of the Upper Extremity

In general, the nerve supplying a joint also supplies the muscles which move the joint and the skin covering the articular attachments of those muscles (Hilton's law).

Table 14.2 outlines the innervation of the joints of the upper extremity joint innervation and associated motor responses associated with nerve stimulation during nerve block procedures.

Table 14.2 Innervation of the joints of the upper extremity joint innervation and motor responses associated with nerve stimulation

Joint	Nerve	Root	Motion
Shoulder			
Anterior and posterior	Suprascapular	C5, C6	Arm abduction
	Axillary	C5, C6	Arm abduction
Elbow			
Anterior	Musculocutaneous	C5, C6	Elbow flexion
	Radial	C5–C7	Extension of the elbow, wrist, and fingers
	Median	C5–T1	Thumb flexion and forearm pronation
Posterior	Radial	C5–C7	Extension of the elbow, wrist, and fingers
	Ulnar	C8, T1	Fifth finger flexion and opposition
Wrist	Radial (superficial)	C5–C7	Extension of the elbow, wrist, and fingers
	Median	C5–T1	Thumb flexion and forearm pronation
	Ulnar	C8, T1	Fifth finger flexion and opposition

14.2.4.1 Innervation of the Shoulder

The nerve supply to shoulder joint nerve supply is derived from the *axillary*, *suprascapular*, and *lateral pectoral* nerves, from branches arising from the posterior cord of the brachial plexus, possibly the radial nerve. Sympathetic innervation is derived directly from the stellate and perhaps from other lower cervical and/or upper thoracic sympathetic ganglia (Table 14.2). Recommended block(s) is/are shown in Fig. 14.9.

- Axillary nerve (articular branch): after leaving the posterior cord of the brachial plexus and descending laterally across the subscapularis muscle, the articular branch of the axillary nerve innervates mainly the inferior aspect of the joint capsule
  - A portion of the articular branch innervates the bicipital sulcus and forms anastomoses with fiber bundles from the posterior cord.
  - The branch leaves the plexus in proximity to where the axillary nerve forms and courses obliquely across the subscapularis muscle to reach the bicipital sulcus and inferior and superior aspects of the anterior surface of the joint capsule.
  - Terminal twigs course superiorly from the inferior aspect of the capsule to reach the anterior and posterior surfaces of the capsule.
    - Nerve fibers largely penetrate the fibrous layer of the capsule, while there is some penetration into the synovial layer and adjacent portions of the humerus.
    - Fibers which reach the posterior capsule join the lower articular branch of the suprascapular nerve; those coursing toward the anterior capsular surface jointly innervate this area with the branch from the posterior cord of the plexus.
- Lateral pectoral nerve: articular branches arise mainly from the lateral pectoral nerve.
  - Articular branch travels superior to the coracoid process to reach the acromioclavicular joint, with its terminal portion supplying the anterosuperior region of the shoulder joint capsule, as well as synovial tissue.
  - Sympathetic fibers which innervate the joint arise from both the stellate ganglion and the sympathetic trunk just superior to the stellate ganglion.
    - Fibers descend within the adventitia of the subclavian and axillary arteries to the point where the arteries enter the vascular area of the joint.
    - Fibers anastomose with the branch from the posterior cord of the brachial plexus.
    - Fibers also reach the region supplied by the lateral pectoral nerve.
- Suprascapular nerve: "upper" articular branch arises from the nerve as it courses through the supraspinous fossa, runs laterally to supply the periosteum of the coracoid process, the coracoacromial ligament, and the acromioclavicular joint, and finally reaches the superior aspect of the shoulder joint capsule.
  - After branching, fibers continue anteriorly to overlap with the areas supplied by the articular branch of the lateral pectoral nerve.
- Suprascapular nerve: "lower" articular branch leaves the nerve before its entrance into the infraspinous fossa and travels laterally to reach the posteroinferior region of the capsule deep to the infraspinatus and teres minor muscles.
  - Some fibers run inferiorly to reach the region innervated by the ascending fibers of the articular branch of the axillary nerve.

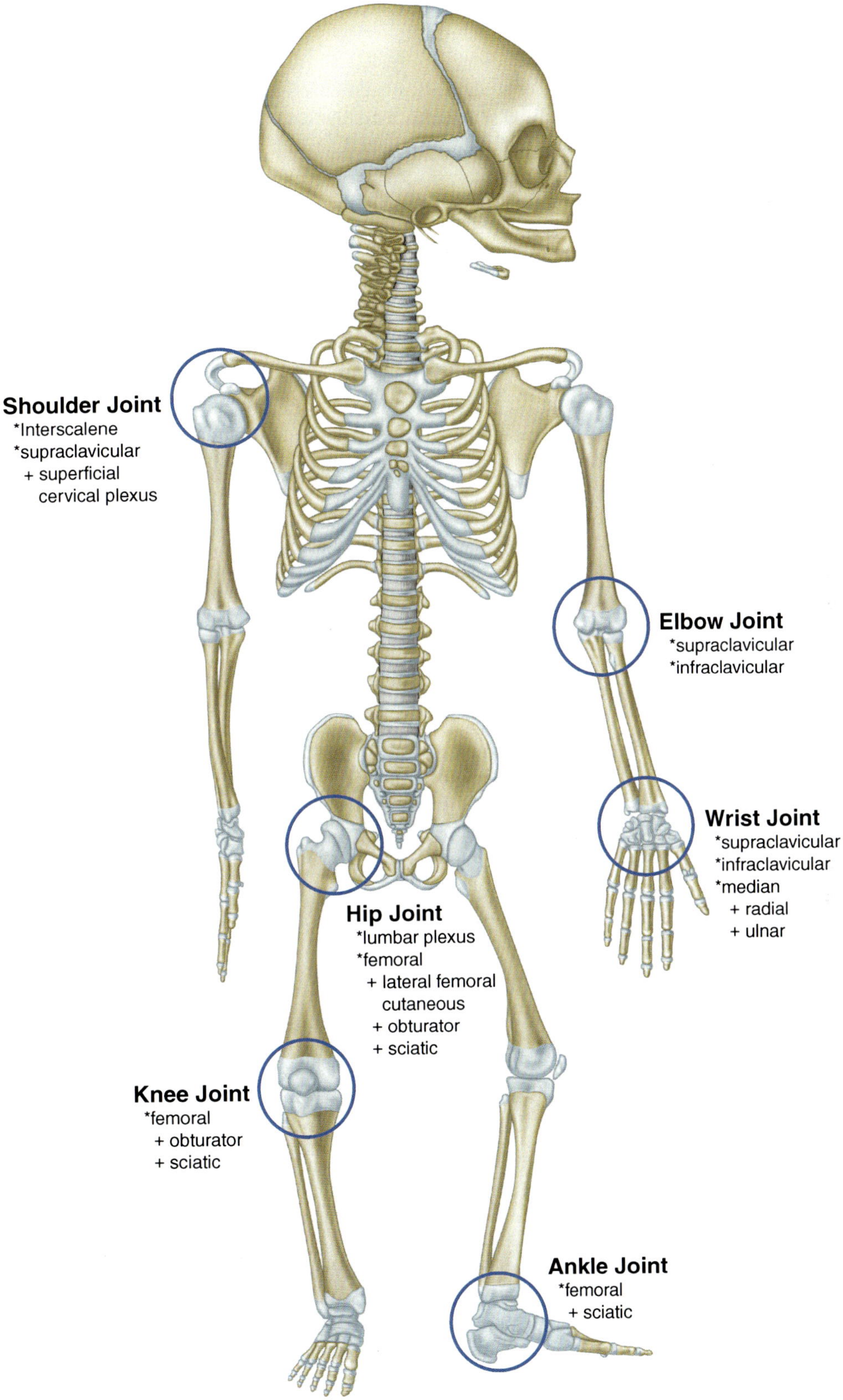

Fig. 14.9 Innervation of the major joints

14.2.4.2 Innervation of the Elbow

The elbow joint is supplied by the *musculocutaneous*, *median*, *ulnar*, and *radial* nerves; some of the articular branches course some distance within the upper arm musculature, while some are formed close to the elbow joint (Table 14.2; Fig. 14.9).

- Musculocutaneous nerve: articular branch arises from the nerve to the brachialis muscle.
  - After running along the medial aspect of this muscle, the nerve dives deep to supply the periosteum of the humerus and reach the anterior aspect of the joint capsule.
  - Nerve fibers run medially and laterally in the fibrous layer of the capsule; some reach the synovial tissue.
  - There may be anastomoses with the median (medially) and radial (laterally) nerves' articular branches.
- Median nerve: articular branches generally arise before the nerve passes between the heads of the pronator teres muscle and course somewhat recurrently to innervate the region of capsule near the medial epicondyle of the humerus.
  - A small branch of the nerve innervates the anterior capsule after coursing along the medial surface of the brachialis muscle; this branch anastomoses with a twig of the articular branch of the musculocutaneous nerve.
- Ulnar nerve: articular branches represented mainly by filaments forming as the nerve passes behind the medial epicondyle of the humerus.
  - Fibers supply the ulnar collateral ligament and reach the posteromedial region of the capsule; some ramify in the tissue forming the superior extension of the joint capsule.
- Radial nerve
  - The muscular branch supplying the anconeus muscle, formed proximally in the radial groove, runs within the lateral head of the triceps brachii muscle and provides filaments to the capsule lining the olecranon fossa (and perhaps to the posterolateral region of the capsule).
  - The ulnar collateral nerve (a branch of the radial nerve) also provides filaments to the capsule proximal to the olecranon process.
  - Fibers leaving the nerve after its entrance into the lateral intermuscular septum innervate the anterolateral region of the capsule (and radial collateral and annular ligaments).
  - As the nerve courses anterior to the elbow joint, a branch to the anterior region of the capsule anastomoses with articular fibers from the musculocutaneous nerve.

14.2.4.3 Innervation of the Wrist and Hand

While some joints of the wrist and hand receive sole innervation from one nerve, many receive innervation from multiple nerves, generally from those supplying the muscles that move that particular joint (Table 14.2; Fig. 14.9).

- *Ulnar* nerve: it supplies the wrist and hand through branches from the main nerve as well as through the digital nerves.
  - The dorsal branch of the ulnar nerve (before giving off digital branches) gives off branches which innervate the dorsal aspect of the joint between the triquetrum and pisiform, the lunate and hamate, the triquetrum and hamate, and the hamate and fourth metacarpal.
  - The deep branch of the ulnar nerve supplies the joints between the capitate and hamate, the capitate and second metacarpal, the capitate and third metacarpal, the hamate and fourth metacarpal, and the hamate and fifth metacarpal.
    - After innervating these joints at the bases of the metacarpals, long filaments are sent off to reach the metacarpophalangeal joints of the second, third, and fourth fingers.
    - The digital nerve branches supply the joint between the hamate and fifth metacarpal, the interphalangeal joints of the little finger on both medial and lateral sides, and the metacarpophalangeal joint of the fourth finger.
    - The dorsal and palmar digital nerves supply the metacarpophalangeal and interphalangeal joints of the fifth finger on medial and lateral sides and of the medial side of the fourth finger on the medial side.
- *Median* nerve: articular supply includes innervation from branches from the main nerve as well as through the digital nerves and the anterior interosseous nerve.
  - Before branching, the nerve supplies the radioscaphoid joint and the joints between the scaphoid and capitate and between the capitate and trapezoid.
  - The digital nerves innervate both sides of all joints of the first, second, and third fingers, as well as the lateral side of the joints of the fourth finger.
  - The anterior interosseous nerve supplies the distal radioulnar joint and sends branches to the radioscaphoid, radiolunate, and scaphoid-lunate joints.
- *Radial* nerve: superficial branch courses over the back of the hand and gives off many branches, including those to the radioscaphoid joint and to joints between the scaphoid and trapezium, the scaphoid and trapezoid,

the trapezium and first metacarpal, the trapezium and second metacarpal, and the trapezoid and second metacarpal.

- The dorsal digital nerves supply both sides of both joints of the thumb, both sides of the metacarpophalangeal and proximal interphalangeal joints of the second finger, and the lateral side of the metacarpophalangeal joint of the third finger.
- The dorsal digital nerve to the index finger provides a branch which runs deep to innervate the first and second metacarpals and has recurrent twigs which supply many of the carpal joints.
- The posterior interosseous nerve supplies the back of the carpus widely on its middle and medial aspects.

Innervation of the radiocarpal joint is provided by the anterior interosseous nerve (a branch of the median nerve) and posterior interosseous nerve (a branch of the radial nerve) interosseous nerves. Additional contributions are made by the median, radial, and ulnar nerves.

14.3 Innervation of the Lower Extremity

14.3.1 Dermatomes and Cutaneous Distribution of the Peripheral Nerves (Figs. 14.1, 14.2, 14.10, and 14.11)

Segmental Sensory Innervation (Dermatomes) of the Lower Limb

- L1: pelvic region (anterior) and upper medial thigh
- L2: upper and lateral aspects of the thigh
- L3: lower anterior medial aspect of the thigh and knee
- L4: anteromedial aspect of the leg and medial ankle
- L5: anterolateral aspect of the leg, medial aspect of the foot, medial aspect of the distal plantar surface of the foot, upper surface of the first to second/third toes
- S1: lateral side of the foot and sole and lateral three toes
- S2: posterior surface of the thigh and leg
- S3 and 4: the gluteal and perianal (posterior pelvic) region

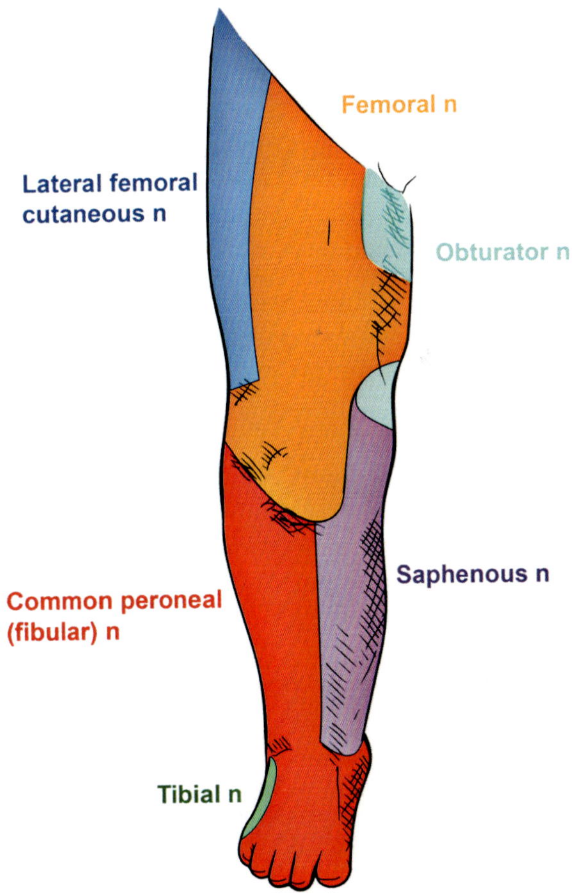

Fig. 14.10 Cutaneous distribution of the peripheral nerves of the lower extremity; anterior view

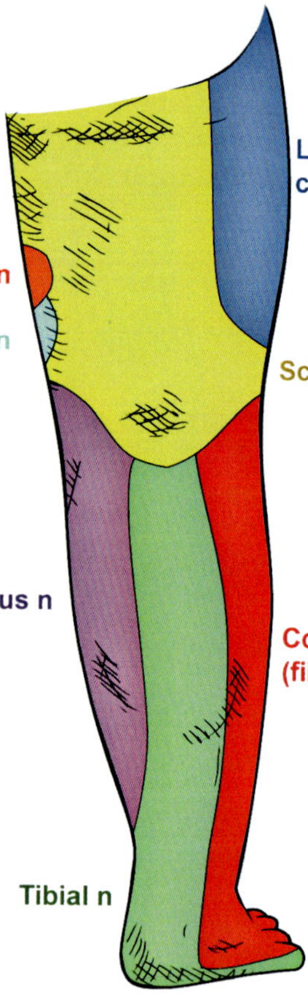

Fig. 14.11 Cutaneous distribution of the peripheral nerves of the lower extremity; posterior view

14.3.2 Myotomes

For clinical practice, it is important to understand that there is a specific distribution of innervation to skeletal muscles that is derived from the terminal nerves (Figs. 14.12 and 14.13). Tables 14.3 and 14.4 summarize the origin of each terminal motor nerve and its related movement; the segmental innervation of the lower extremity is depicted indirectly, through the origin of the terminal nerves.

Segmental Motor Responses Associated with Nerve Stimulation

- L2 and 3: flexion, adduction, and medial rotation of the hip
- L3 and 4: extension of the knee
- L4: foot inversion
- L4 and 5: dorsiflexion of the foot
- L5 and S1: extension, abduction, and lateral rotation of the hip and flexion of the knee
- L5 and S1: foot eversion
- S1 and 2: plantar flexion of the foot

Muscular Distribution of the Spinal Segments

- L2: psoas major, iliacus, gracilis, sartorius
- L3: adductor longus and brevis, rectus femoris
- L4: vastus lateralis and medialis, adductor magnus, tibialis anterior
- L5: tibialis anterior, extensor digitorum longus, extensor hallucis longus, peroneus (fibularis) tertius, extensor digitorum brevis, tibialis posterior, flexor digitorum longus, semimembranosus, semitendinosus, short head biceps femoris, tensor fasciae latae, gluteus medius, and minimus
- S1: peroneus (fibularis) longus and brevis, medial and lateral heads of gastrocnemius, soleus, biceps femoris, gluteus maximus, piriformis
- S2: abductor hallucis, abductor digiti minimi (quinti), interossei
- S2–4: external anal sphincter
- S4: bulbospongiosus (bulbocavernosus)

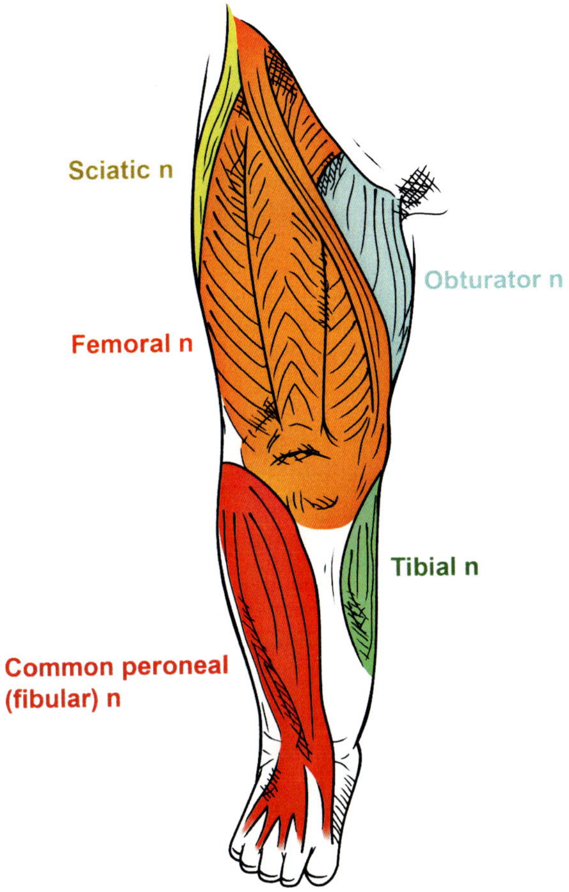

Fig. 14.12 Distribution of muscular innervations by the terminal nerves of the lower extremity; anterior view

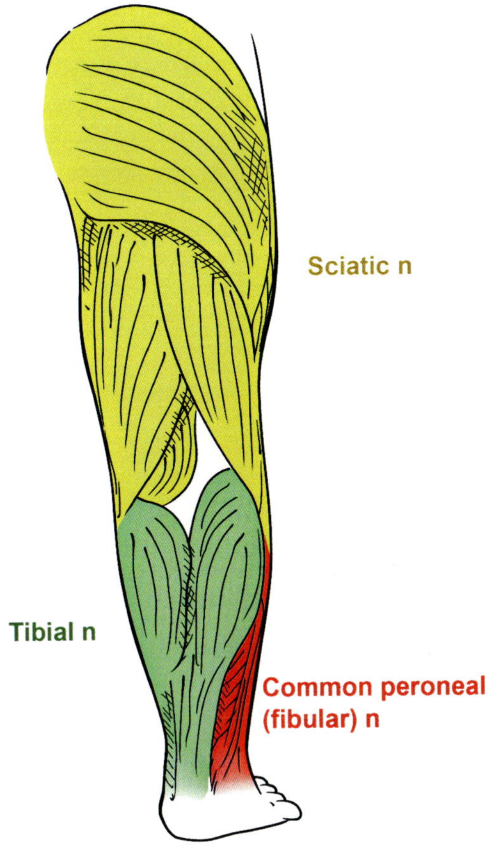

Fig. 14.13 Distribution of muscular innervations by the terminal nerves of the lower extremity; posterior view

Table 14.3 Lower extremity (lumbar plexus terminal motor nerves): origin and motor responses associated with nerve stimulation

Motion	Nerve	Division	Root
Adduction and flexion of the thigh	Obturator	Anterior	L2, L3, L4
Patellar twitch and knee extension	Femoral (*main nerve and its posterior branch*)	Posterior	L2, L3, L4
Thigh adduction only (pectineus)	Femoral (*anterior branch below inguinal ligament*)	Posterior	L2, L3, L4

Table 14.4 Lower extremity (sacral plexus terminal motor nerves): origin and motor responses associated with nerve stimulation

Motion	Nerve	Root
Anal sphincter	Pudendal[a]	S2, S3, S4
Gluteal twitch/thigh abduction (gluteus minimus and medius)	Superior gluteal[a]	L4, L5, S1
Gluteal twitch/thigh extension (gluteus maximus)	Inferior gluteal[b]	L5, S1, S2
Knee flexion and ankle plantar flexion	Tibial (above and below sciatic bifurcation)	L4, L5, S1, S2, S3
Ankle dorsiflexion	Common peroneal (fibular)	L4, L5, S1, S2
Ankle and toe extension	Deep peroneal (fibular)	L5, S1
Foot eversion (peroneus longus and brevis)	Superficial peroneal (fibular)	L5, S1
First toe abduction	Medial plantar	S1, S2
Fifth toe abduction	Lateral plantar	S1, S2, S3

[a]The pudendal and superior gluteal nerves will not be blocked with sciatic nerve block
[b]Only the posterior gluteal approach to sciatic nerve block will block the inferior gluteal nerve

14.3.3 Osteotomes

Terminal nerves, rather than spinal cord segments, distribute sensory innervation to specific regions of the bones throughout the extremities. These terminal nerves also send articular branches to specific joints in the extremity. These regions of the bones (*osteotomes*), each supplied by a specific branch of a terminal nerve, are summarized in Figs. 14.14 and 14.15.

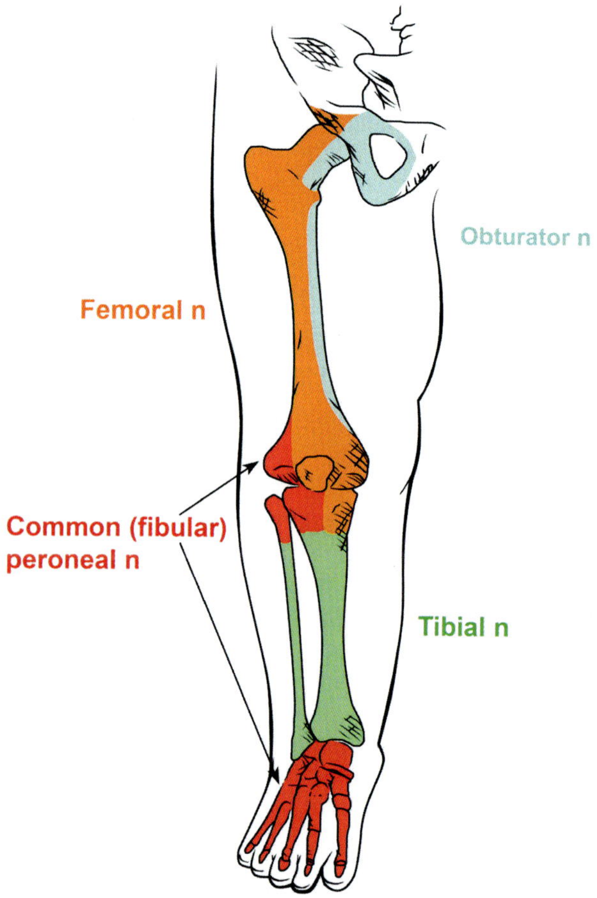

Fig. 14.14 Osteomes of the lower extremity; anterior view

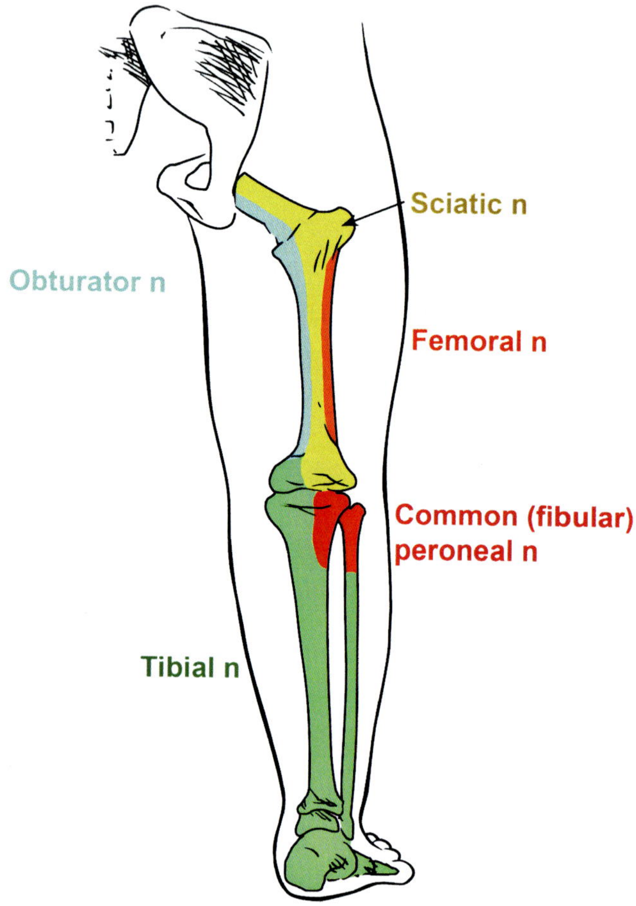

Fig. 14.15 Osteomes of the lower extremity; posterior view

14.3.4 Innervation of the Major Joints

Table 14.5 outlines the innervation of the joints of the lower extremity and associated motor responses resulting from nerve stimulation during nerve block procedures.

Table 14.5 Innervation of the joints of the lower extremity and motor responses associated with nerve stimulation

Joint	Nerve	Root	Motion
Hip			
Anterior	Femoral (nerve to rectus femoris)	L2–L4	Patellar twitch (thigh adduction if posterior division only)
	Obturator (anterior division)	L2–L4	Thigh adduction
Posterior	Sciatic (nerve to quadratus femoris)	L4, L5, S1	Gluteal twitch (quadratus femoris)
Knee			
Anterior	Femoral (articular branches)	L2–L4	Patellar twitch
	Tibial (articular branches)	L4, L5, S1, S2, S3	Knee and ankle flexion
	Common peroneal (fibular)	L4, L5, S1, S2	Ankle dorsiflexion
	Obturator	L2–L4	Thigh adduction
Posterior	Common peroneal (fibular)	L4, L5, S1, S2	Ankle dorsiflexion
	Tibial	L4, L5, S1, S2, S3	Knee and ankle flexion
Ankle	Tibial (above and below sciatic bifurcation)	L4, L5, S1, S2, S3	Knee flexion and ankle plantar flexion
	Common peroneal (fibular)	L4, L5, S1, S2	Ankle dorsiflexion
	Deep peroneal (fibular)	L5, S1	Ankle and toe extension
	Superficial peroneal (fibular)	L5, S1	Foot eversion (peroneus longus and brevis)
	Medial plantar	S1, S2	First toe abduction
	Lateral plantar	S1, S2, S3	Fifth toe abduction

14.3.4.1 Innervation of the Hip

Innervation of the hip is provided through articular branches from the femoral, obturator (and accessory obturator when present), and superior gluteal nerves, from the nerve to the quadratus femoris (the latter two from the sacral plexus) and possibly from the lumbar sympathetic ganglia (sympathetic supply) (Table 14.5; Fig. 14.9). Multiple blocks are needed (Fig. 14.9).

- *Femoral* nerve: articular branches arise from the common trunk of the nerve and/or from its muscular branches (nerves to rectus femoris, to vastus lateralis, and to pectineus).
  - When there are multiple articular branches, these often anastomose before reaching the joint capsule.
- Femoral nerve: terminal branches supply the iliofemoral ligament and the neighboring portion of the femur (along the intertrochanteric line).
  - The fibers which reach the capsule ramify in the fibrous layer, particularly the portion of the capsule which attaches to the femur.
  - Some of the terminal branches course posteriorly and superiorly.
- *Nerve to the pectineus*: articular branch courses along the medial edge of the iliopsoas muscle, then enters the anteromedial aspect of the capsule, and also innervates the neighboring region of the femur.
  - This region (including the pubofemoral ligament) is supplied by the nerve to the pectineus via an articular branch and, when present, also by a branch from the accessory obturator nerve.
- *Obturator* nerve: articular branches are given off within the obturator canal or distally from the anterior or posterior division of the obturator nerve; these branches travel laterally to supply the medial portion of the capsule and ramify in the fibrous layer of the capsule.
  - Some fibers reach the synovial tissue, and some course along the ligamentum teres (ligament of the head of the femur) to the acetabulum and femur.
- *Nerve to the quadratus femoris* descends on the ischium anterior to the sciatic nerve and innervates the ischiofemoral (ischiocapsular) ligament through one or two fine twigs.
- *Superior gluteal* nerve via the nerve's branch to the gluteus minimus muscle: twigs first innervate the fibrous layer of the superolateral region of the capsule then course anteriorly and inferiorly to reach the region supplied by the femoral nerve.
  - Sympathetic fibers from the lumbar ganglia may reach the capsule by accompanying the articular vessels.

14.3.4.2 Innervation of the Knee

Innervation of the knee joint is derived from the femoral, obturator, and sciatic (tibial, common peroneal [fibular], and recurrent peroneal [fibular]) nerves (Hilton's law) (Table 14.5; Fig. 14.9).

- *Femoral* nerve supplies the knee through articular branches of its saphenous branch as well as articular branches of its muscular branches to the vastus medialis, vastus intermedius, and vastus lateralis muscles.
  - *Saphenous* nerve: articular division arises at variable locations, often either from within the femoral triangle or just after the femoral artery passes through the adductor magnus muscle through the adductor hiatus, usually anastomoses with the articular fibers of the obturator nerve and nerve to the vastus medialis muscle.
    - Branch travels vertically, anterior to the tendon of the adductor magnus, and courses toward the anteromedial aspect of the joint capsule.
  - Articular branches from the femoral nerve supply the suprapatellar bursa, the patellar and femoral periosteum (via nerves to the vastus intermedius muscle), the anteromedial (saphenous nerve and nerve to vastus medialis) and anterolateral (nerve to vastus lateralis) aspects of the joint capsule, and the infrapatellar fat pad. Vascular branches supply the femoral artery and its branches.
- *Tibial* nerve: it is usually in the form of a large branch (although as many as five branches may exist), which arises either from the tibial portion of the sciatic nerve in the thigh (following closely with the sciatic nerve in its sheath) or from the tibial nerve within the popliteal fossa
  - The tibial nerve has several branches which form a dense plexus, with some fibers entering the adventitia of the popliteal vessels, some following the genicular vessels both medially and laterally, and most entering the fibrous layer of the joint capsule posteriorly and eventually the synovial tissue.
  - Branches or continuations of the nerve accompany the superior medial and inferior medial genicular arteries and bear the same names as the arteries. The superior medial genicular nerve supplies the periosteum and medial epicondyle while the inferior medial genicular nerve supplies the anterior portion of the capsule and the tibial periosteum.
  - Articular branches of the tibial nerve supply the posterior, medial, and lateral regions of the capsule, the infrapatellar fat pad, the tibial and perhaps fibular periosteum, and the superior tibiofibular joint.

- *Common peroneal* (fibular) nerve: articular branch arises either from the common peroneal portion of the sciatic nerve within the posterior mid-thigh or from the common peroneal (fibular) nerve within the popliteal fossa.
  - The branch joins either, or both, the superior or inferior lateral genicular arteries, is named accordingly, and supplies the anterolateral or lateral portions of the capsule, respectively.
  - The common peroneal (fibular) nerve supplies the anterolateral portion of the capsule, the infrapatellar fat pad, and the tibial periosteum.
- The anterolateral portion of the capsule is supplied jointly by the nerve to vastus medialis and common peroneal (fibular) nerve, with varying contributions depending on the distribution of each nerve.
  - The *recurrent common peroneal (fibular)* nerve supplies the anterolateral surface of the tibial periosteum, the tibial tuberosity, the infrapatellar fat pad, and the superior tibiofibular joint.
- *Obturator* nerve: anterior division frequently anastomoses with the articular branch of the saphenous nerve.
  - The division gives small twigs to the superior medial genicular artery (naming the terminal fibers as such), thus serving the same anteromedial aspect of the capsule as the saphenous and nerve to vastus medialis, before terminating by anastomosing with the branches of the tibial nerve thus forming the popliteal plexus and innervating the superior part of the posteromedial capsule.
  - Articular branches of the obturator nerve supply the superior part of the posteromedial capsule (as a portion of the popliteal plexus), the anteromedial portion of the capsule (as the superior medial genicular nerve, together with the saphenous nerve), and the infrapatellar fat pad.

14.3.4.3 **Innervation of the Ankle** (Table 14.5; Fig. 14.9)

- Superficial nerves at the ankle:
  - *Saphenous nerve*
    - The longest cutaneous branch from the femoral nerve which innervates the medial skin of the ankle
  - *Superficial peroneal (fibular) nerve*
    - Branches from the common peroneal (fibular) nerve and supplies the skin on the anterior aspect of the ankle
  - *Sural nerve*
    - Branches from the common peroneal (fibular) nerve and supplies skin on the lateral aspect of the ankle
- Deep nerves at the ankle:
  - *Deep peroneal* (fibular) (L5, S1): lies anterior to the tibia and interosseous membrane and lateral to the *anterior tibial artery and vein* at the ankle and is deep to and between the tendons of the *extensor hallucis longus and extensor digitorum longus* muscles, and beyond the extensor retinaculum, it branches into medial and lateral terminal branches.
    - The medial branch passes over the dorsum of the foot and supplies the first web space through two terminal digital branches.
    - The lateral branch traverses laterally and terminates as the second, third, and fourth dorsal interosseous nerves that supply the tarsal and metatarsophalangeal joints of the middle three toes.
  - *Tibial nerve (often called the posterior tibial nerve)* (S1–3): on the posterior aspect of the knee joint, it joins the posterior tibial artery and then runs deep until the lower third of the leg, where it emerges at the medial border of the calcaneal tendon (Achilles tendon).
    - Behind the medial malleolus, it lies beneath several layers of fascia and is separated from the Achilles tendon only by the tendon of the flexor hallucis longus muscle; the nerve is posteromedial to the *posterior tibial artery and vein*, which in turn are posteromedial to the tendons of the flexor digitorum longus and tibialis posterior muscles.
    - Just below the medial malleolus, the nerve divides into the *lateral* and *medial plantar* nerves.
    - The nerve innervates the ankle joint through its articular branches and, through its cutaneous branches, the skin over the medial malleolus, the inner aspect of the heel (including the skin over the Achilles tendon), and the dorsum of the foot (through the medial and lateral plantar nerves).

Suggested Reading

Bo WJ, Meschan I, Krueger WA. Basic atlas of cross-sectional anatomy: a clinical approach. Philadelphia: WB Saunders; 1980.

Ellis H, Feldman S, Harrop-Griffiths W, editors. Anatomy for anaesthetists. 8th ed. Hoboken: Wiley-Blackwell; 2004.

Gardner E. The innervation of the elbow joint. Anat Rec. 1948a;102:161–74.

Gardner E. The innervation of the knee joint. Anat Rec. 1948b; 101:109–30.

Garner E. The innervation of the hip joint. Anat Rec. 1948; 101:353–71.

Gray DJ, Gardner E. The innervation of the joints of the wrist and hand. Anat Rec. 1965;151:261–6.

Lee B. Atlas of surgical and sectional anatomy. Norwalk: Appleton-Century-Crofts; 1983.

Netter FH. Atlas of human anatomy. Summit: CIBA-GEIGY Corp.; 1989.

Part IV

Nerve Blocks of the Head and Neck

Trigeminal Nerve Blocks

15

Glenn Merritt and Ban C.H. Tsui

Contents

G. Merritt, MD
Department of Anesthesiology,
University of Colorado Hospital and Children's Hospital Colorado,
13123 East 16th Ave., Aurora, CO 80045, USA
e-mail: Merrittmd@aol.com

B.C.H. Tsui, Dip Eng, BSc (Math), B Pharm, MSc, MD, FRCPC (✉)
Department of Anesthesiology and Pain Medicine,
Stollery Children's Hospital/University of Alberta Hospital,
2-150 Clinical Sciences Building, Edmonton, AB T6G 2G3, Canada
e-mail: btsui@ualberta.ca

B.C.H. Tsui, S. Suresh (eds.), *Pediatric Atlas of Ultrasound- and Nerve Stimulation-Guided Regional Anesthesia*,
DOI 10.1007/978-0-387-79964-3_15

15.1 Indications

Blockade of the trigeminal nerve – the fifth cranial nerve – targets its three major branches (Fig. 9.1), the ophthalmic (V1, sensory), the maxillary (V2, sensory), and the mandibular (V3, sensory and motor to the muscles of mastication), and provides anesthesia to the anterior portion of the scalp, face, and much of the oral cavity. Some common clinical uses of trigeminal nerve block include (for a more comprehensive list, see Table 15.1):

- Ophthalmic nerve block (V1: supraorbital, supratrochlear):
  - Frontal craniotomies
  - Excision of scalp nevus
- Maxillary nerve block (V2: infraorbital, greater palatine):
  - Cleft palate surgery (maxillary, greater palatine, lesser palatine, nasopalatine)
  - Cleft lip surgery (infraorbital)
  - Nasal septum repair (infraorbital)
  - Endoscopic sinus surgery (infraorbital)
  - Surgical repair of soft tissue injury of the face (infraorbital)
- Mandibular nerve block (V3: mental)
  - Lower lip repair (mental)

Table 15.1 Indications for trigeminal nerve blocks in children

Nerve to be blocked	Indications
V1: Ophthalmic division	Frontal craniotomies Ventriculo-peritoneal shunt Dermoid cyst excision Pigmented nevus excision Ommaya reservoir placements in neonates Scalp lesions
V2: Maxillary division, including greater palatine nerve (GPN)	Cleft lip/palate repair Endoscopic sinus surgery Rhinoplasty Pulse dye laser for port wine stain removal Mole removal Transsphenoidal hypophysectomy Nasal tip reconstruction
V3: Mandibular division	Surgery involving the lower lip (e.g. hemangioma) Surgery involving the skin of the chin Trigeminal neuralgia in V3 Temporomandibular joint dysfunction

15.2 Block Techniques

The most comprehensive blockade of the trigeminal nerve targets the central ganglion. This block is usually performed by neurosurgeons under fluoroscopic guidance to treat disabling trigeminal neuralgia. Few anesthesiologists perform this technically difficult block, and it will not be described in detail here.

15.2.1 Superficial Transcutaneous Approach to Trigeminal Nerve Blocks: Supraorbital, Infraorbital, and Mental Nerve Block

The trigeminal block can be easily performed by injection of the three individual terminal superficial branches through a landmark-based approach using palpation of their respective foramina (Fig. 15.1). These bony landmarks are usually sufficient themselves for routine anesthetic purposes although ultrasound imaging may prove useful for locating them in some cases. An additional block of the supratrochlear nerve (terminal nerve of ophthalmic branch) is required if the field of anesthesia is to cross the midline of the forehead.

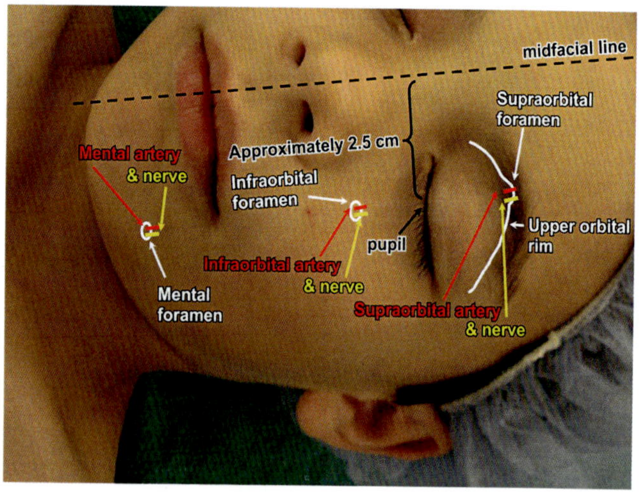

Fig. 15.1 Patient positioning and surface landmarks for superficial trigeminal nerve blocks in a 4-year-old child

15.2.1.1 Patient Positioning

- The patient is positioned lying supine.
- The patient's head may be placed to rest on a donut.

15.2.1.2 Landmarks and Surface Anatomy

- Each nerve is closely associated with a readily palpable foramen. Figure 15.2 illustrates the cross-sectional anatomy of each respective foramen, captured by Visible Human Visualization Software (VHVS) and MRI.
- The nerves are too superficial to visualize well with ultrasound. However, ultrasound can be used to identify the foramina by scanning sagittally in the medial to lateral direction [1]. The foramina create discontinuity in the hyperechoic line of the bone. The absence of hyperechogenic bony structure indicates the position of the foramen (Fig. 15.3). Using this method, the foramina can be landmarked and marked on the skin to facilitate easier identification of the needle insertion site. Color Doppler can also be used to verify the locations of the foramina by imaging the blood vessels associated with each foramen; however, these vessels are small and are often difficult to visualize.
  - All branches of the trigeminal nerve have been reported to lie in the same sagittal plane on each side of the face for adolescent and adult patients at a distance of approximately 2.5 cm lateral to the midsagittal line passing through the pupil [2]. Some reports indicate that accessory or double foramina may exist [3, 4], but unless one is attempting to enter the foramen while performing the nerve block, this should not affect clinical practice.
  - The supraorbital nerve enters the facial skeleton through the supraorbital foramen, which is located in the midsagittal plane at the level of the pupil. The supratrochlear nerve is located medial to the supraorbital foramen and can be found closer to the midfacial sagittal plane (Fig. 15.3a). The supraorbital notch is easily palpated at the medial upper angle of the orbit. Palpate the roof of the orbital rim starting from the midline. The more medial supratrochlear nerve is located at the upper internal angle of the orbital rim. Eipe et al. [5] describe their point of needle insertion as the intersection of a vertical line through the pupil of the eye and a horizontal line through the ala of the nose in their study of twenty children above 12 years of age.
  - The infraorbital notch (Fig. 15.3b) can be palpated easily along the floor of the orbital rim in children but can be difficult in the neonate due to the developing craniofacial skeletal configurations. If the foramen that exists inferior to the orbital rim cannot be palpated directly, it can be sought by gently probing with a small-gauge needle or found using surface landmarks as a guide. Alternatively, a simple mathematical formula can be utilized (distance from the midline = 21 mm + 0.5 × age (in years)) [2].
  - The mental nerve emerges from the mental foramen (Fig. 15.3c), which lies inferior to the outer lip at the level of the first premolar, midway between the upper and lower borders of the mandible [6].

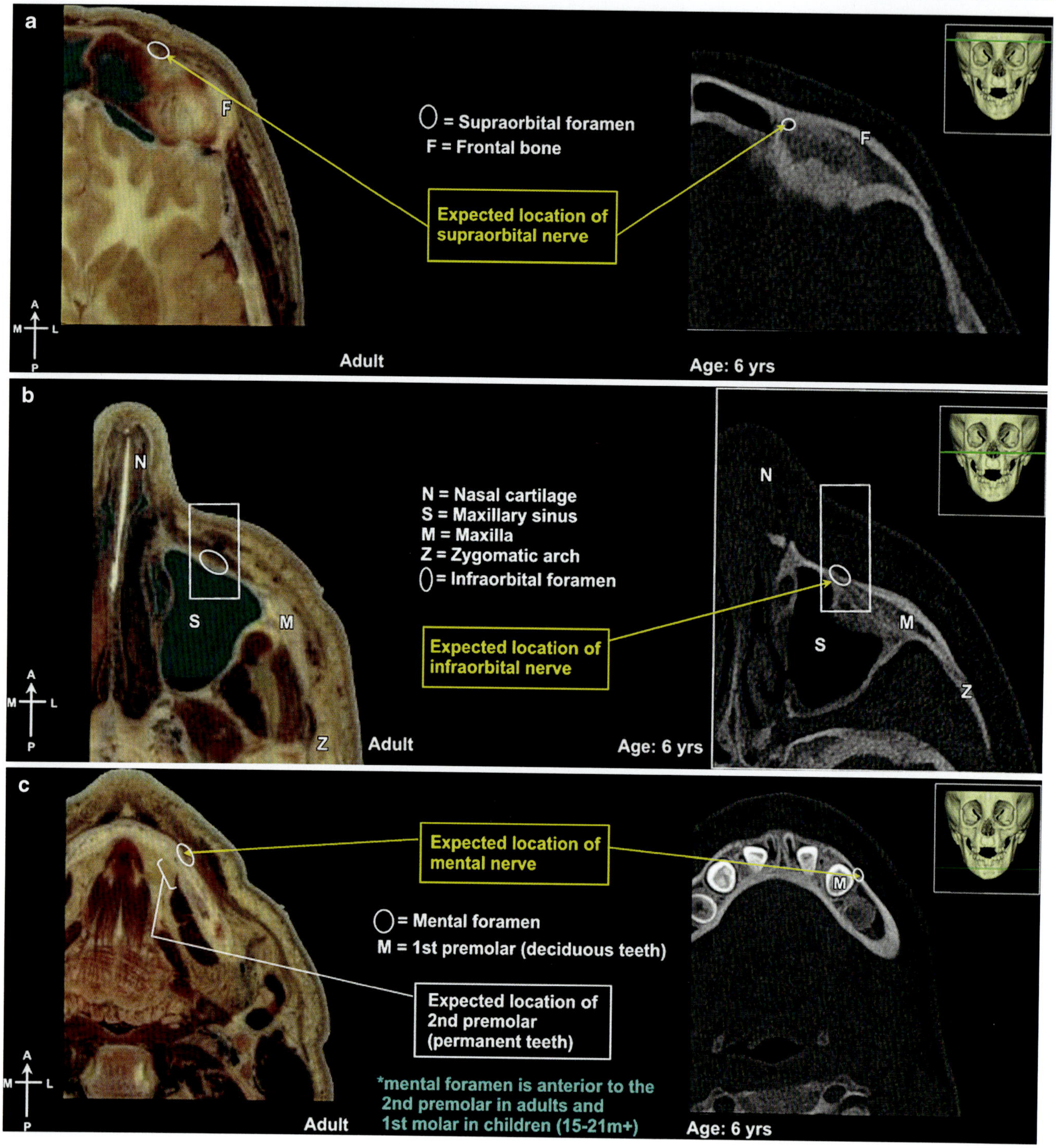

Fig. 15.2 VHVS and MRI of (**a**) supraorbital, (**b**) infraorbital, and (**c**) mental foramina

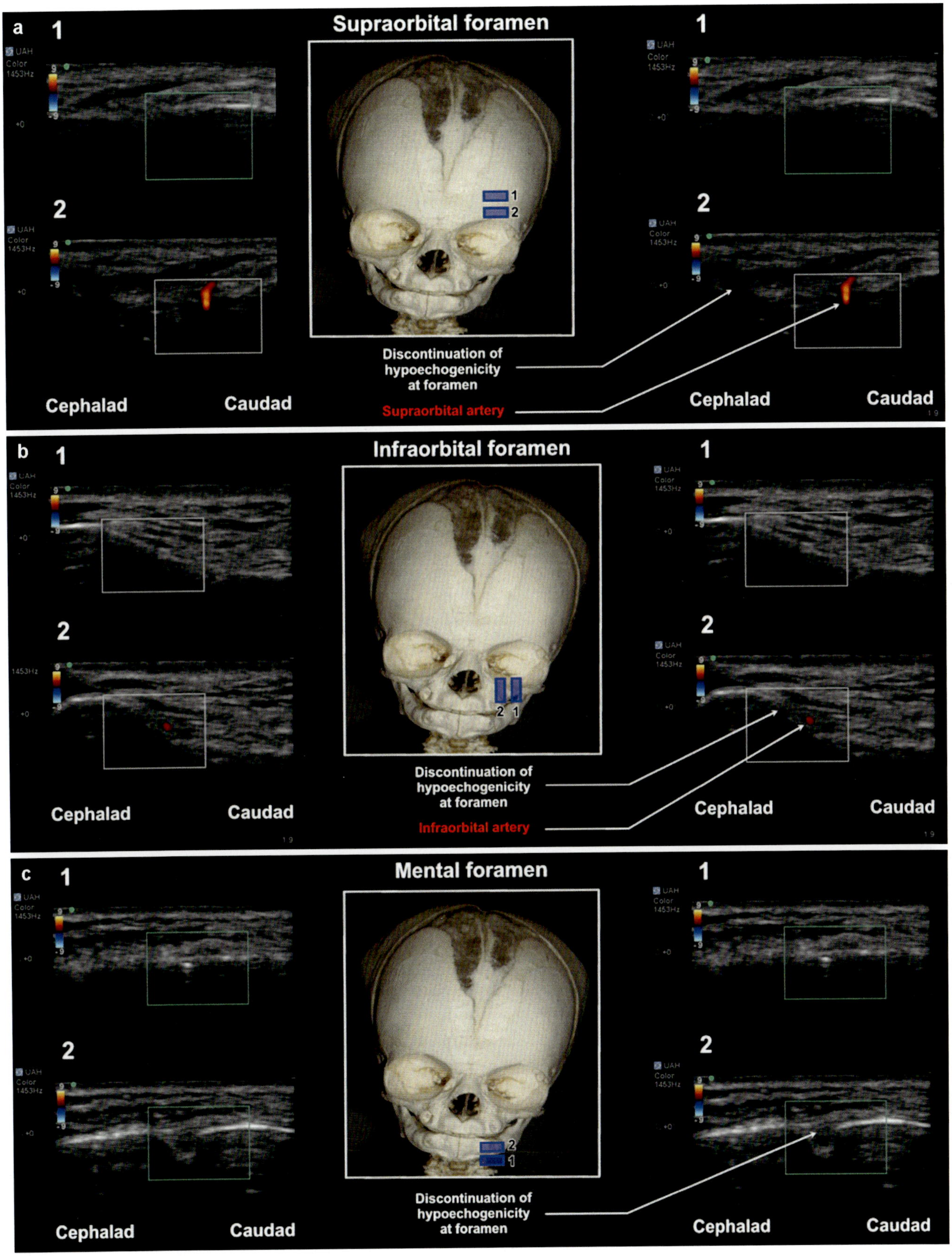

Fig. 15.3 Ultrasound images with color Doppler demonstrating discontinuity in the hyperechogenic line at the supraorbital (**a**), infraorbital (**b**), and mental (**c**) foramina. Ultrasound probe positioning is indicated by *blue bars* in the center panel: "1" represents starting position and "2" represents final position over the foramen

15.2.1.3 Considerations and Needle Insertion Technique (Infraorbital Nerve Block)

- Generally, short, 25G–30G hypodermic needles will be suitable for these blocks, provided that one is not trying to enter the foramen directly since this may require a larger needle for accurate placement. Longer needles are essential for:
  - Intraoral approaches to the infraorbital nerve in older children and adolescents (the infraorbital foramen may be located 2–3 cm away from the gingival sulcus)
  - Suprazygomatic maxillary nerve blocks in children of any age (depth of the pterygopalatine fossa from the superior junction of the zygoma and posterior orbital rim has been reported to be approximately 4 cm even in infants and young children)
  - Any approach to the pterygopalatine fossa from intra- or extraoral routes in children of all ages
- Most exiting foramina communicate directly with the inferior orbital fissure. Thus, when using techniques that require injection of local anesthetic into the foramen itself, orbital contents may be injured inadvertently if one is not conscious of the depths and anatomic characteristics of the various canals where the nerves exit the facial skeleton.
- Intraforaminal approaches are popular in many countries, but they have been reported to result in a higher incidence of paresthesia. Careful attention to injection pressure is critically important if the needle has entered the infraorbital canal itself. When placing the needle in these small foramina, the injection pressure must not be excessive, thereby minimizing trauma to the nerve. Intraforaminal approaches are not recommended for beginners since the basic approaches, when performed correctly, will provide excellent anesthesia and eliminate any risk of major complications.
- When determining the optimal technique for infraorbital nerve block, the choice of an extraoral percutaneous route or an intraoral route (see below) must be made. While many practitioners advocate one technique over the other, either approach is appropriate, provided that the practitioner understands the benefits and limitations of the various approaches:
  - The extraoral percutaneous approach is relatively simple, and a supervisor and surgical team can visualize the injection and confirm where both the needle and local anesthesia are being placed.
  - The intraoral approach has been reported to be less painful for the patient [7]. In our opinion, the ability to supervise accurate needle placement and exact area of local anesthetic placement may be limited to the individual performing the block, particularly in small infants with cleft lip and palate defects.
- Before the needle is introduced, the location and anatomic characteristics of the infraorbital foramen and the course of the exiting nerve branches should be studied. Understanding the shape and course of the foramen will help the practitioner decide how best to enter or, in most cases, avoid entering the foramen.
  - The infraorbital nerve travels from the foramen rotundum through the infraorbital canal and exits the facial skeleton through the infraorbital foramen. When examining the skull in the anterior plane, the infraorbital canal runs in a nasal-to-temporal direction; this directional information will help to plan entry or avoidance of the foramen.
  - If one plans on entering the foramen, then a nasal-temporal needle direction is recommended. For novice practitioners, a temporal-nasal needle direction will make it impossible to enter the canal. Any sagittally directed needle risks entering the foramen and should be avoided.
  - In infants, the infraorbital foramen will lie at the level of the nasal ala. The needle insertion point and location of the infraorbital foramen have been reported to be at the midpoint of a line drawn from the lateral orbital rim to the lateral corner of the mouth [8]. Due to the development of the craniofacial skeleton, a better surface landmark in older children is the intersection of a line drawn from the lateral orbital canthus to the nasal ala and another line passing sagittally through the medial edge (limbus) of the iris [9]. The foramen represents the initial point at which the infraorbital nerve starts to branch into its peripheral divisions.
- The branches of the infraorbital nerve include the inferior palpebral, external nasal, internal nasal, and superior labial branch (which has a medial and lateral division). Only 40 % of the time do the nerves exit as separate branches [10]; the other 60 % of the time, the nerves exit as a network. Regardless, it is critical to remember that all

the nerves travel in a lateral-to-medial direction toward the nasal ala. Successful nerve blockade is achieved when the local anesthesia spread matches these branching patterns. By understanding this principle, one can use visualization to determine when an adequate dose is achieved.

15.2.1.4 Needle Insertion Techniques: Infraorbital Nerve and Branches

- Mark the skin with landmarks: the easiest landmark to identify in almost all ages is a point at the intersection of a line passing through the orbit at the vertical level of the limbic sagittal line and a line drawn from the lateral edge of the orbit to the nasal ala rim. At this point, the infraorbital foramen may be palpated.
- Mark the foramen's location, and place the index finger of the hand contralateral to the side to be blocked on the superior aspect of the eyelid of the side to be blocked (e.g., left index finger on the child's right eyelid). This will enable the practitioner to hold the syringe like a pencil and perform accurate needle placement. Injection with the non-dominant hand requires practice but is worth the effort to improve accuracy.
- With the free hand's index finger, the patient's eye can be examined for abnormalities and to confirm that stage 2 anesthesia is not present. Following this, place the index finger below the orbit in the area of the infraorbital notch. Take care not to push the eye as this may cause a bradycardiac response.
- Lowering the eyelid and placing the finger on the inferior orbital rim can prevent local anesthetic from spreading in a superior direction, which is not necessary unless blockade of the inferior palpebral branch is needed for surgery. This will also help to prevent spread of local anesthetic to the loose soft tissues of the eye, which may lead to bruising and a black eye.
- The needle is inserted in a temporal-to-nasal direction, directly superior and lateral to the marked infraorbital foramen. Entering a small distance away from this mark will help ensure needle contact with the bone in the area of the foramen itself. The goal is to not enter the infraorbital foramen directly but to place the needle in proximity to the infraorbital foramen when contact with the maxilla occurs.
- Many authors describe backing the needle off the bone at this point. This is unnecessary but can be done if desired to decrease the risk of nerve injury. After aspiration of the syringe, inject enough local anesthetic to ensure spread to the nasal ala rim, thereby covering all nerve branching patterns. If local anesthetic tracks in any other direction, the block may not be accurate, and the needle should be repositioned.

Advanced Approaches

- Advanced extraoral approaches include modifying the above technique and using a needle insertion point either at the infraorbital rim in the area of the infraorbital notch itself or entry of the infraorbital foramen directly. These superiorly based techniques are best performed in older children or adolescents undergoing awake surgery and allow the block to be performed relatively rapidly using small volumes of local anesthetic. This approach can be performed with a smaller volume of a more concentrated local anesthetic solution and may work at volumes of 0.25–1 mL per side to achieve adequate anesthesia. By moving the needle to the area immediately below the foramen, the needle tip can be placed directly under the fascia surrounding the infraorbital nerve as it exits the foramen while using the maxilla as a backstop. When done accurately, local anesthetic will be injected at the under-surface of the foramen, providing consistent and reliable anesthesia. An added benefit is that a gentle and quick injection can gain a scared awake child's confidence.
- Entering the infraorbital foramen is another advanced technique and is best performed if one remembers to change the needle direction to nasal-temporal. The foramen is located 7–8 mm below the orbital rim in adults and older children. When entering from a percutaneous nasal ala approach, a longer needle may be required. Zide [11] suggests to place the needle in the center of an imaginary triangle formed by the nasal labial fold, the nasal ala fold, and the foramen. Using this technique, block success was 100 % in adults when 1 mL local anesthetic was placed directly in the foramen, and no cases of nerve injury were found. To date, no studies have been done in pediatric patients using this technique.

15.2.1.5 V1: Ophthalmic Branches

- The supraorbital and supratrochlear nerves are the terminal branches of V1 and can be blocked using one needle insertion with redirection (Fig. 15.4). After blocking the supraorbital nerve, the needle is withdrawn and redirected medially toward the supratrochlear foramen, where the supratrochlear nerve can be blocked.
- The external nasal branch of the anterior ethmoid nerve and infratrochlear nerve innervates portions of the nasal bridge and the skin of the nasal ala, apex, and vestibule of the nose. These terminal branches of V1 can be blocked by insertion of a needle at the junction of the cartilaginous and bony portion of the nose on both lateral edges.
  - This block is typically required for surgeries such as nasal fracture repair, rhinoplasty, and any cleft repair that involves the surgeon working on the tip of the nasal area.
  - Typically, 0.5–1 mL is deposited in a superficial area at this superior nasal area using a small-gauge needle. In the case of bilateral cleft lip repair, it is important to place additional local anesthesia at the base of the nasal septum to ensure coverage of the prolabial fold. Typically, this area is covered by infraorbital nerve block via a branch of the internal nasal branch. However, this branch may not exist secondary to the bilateral cleft palate. This block is extremely painful for the awake patient and should be performed following all other blocks.
- The mental canal angles medially and inferiorly; therefore, if the mental foramen cannot be palpated, subcutaneous injection can be performed above and lateral to the anticipated location of the mental foramen. This block can be performed intraorally or extraorally; anecdotal evidence suggests better success with the former approach, but no studies have been performed to confirm this.

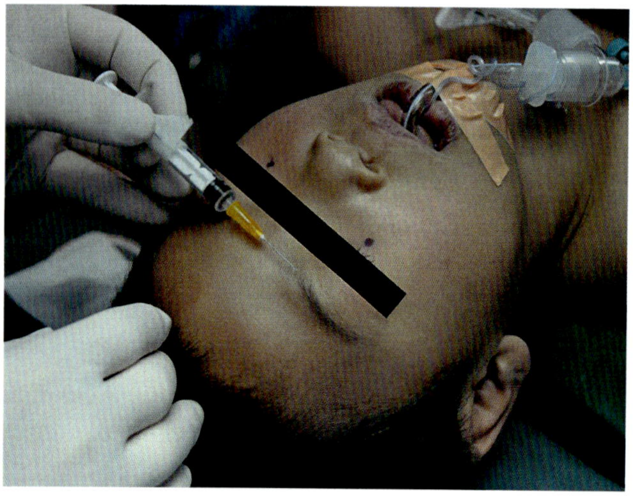

Fig. 15.4 Needle insertion for transcutaneous supraorbital nerve block

15.2.1.6 Local Anesthetic Application

- The choice of local anesthetic will depend on the purpose of the block and the duration of anesthesia required (e.g., 0.5–1 % lidocaine, 0.5–1 % mepivacaine for shorter procedures, and 0.2–0.5 % ropivacaine or bupivacaine for longer procedures). Textbooks will often quote the following doses for surgical anesthesia: 0.5–1.5 mL for infants, 2–3 mL for children, and 3–5 mL for adolescents. However, these volumes may be excessive, and in our experience, 1 mL or less is sufficient to block any infraorbital nerve provided the local anesthetic is placed accurately and one is attentive to adequate spread during block performance. Due to the vascularity of the face, epinephrine should always be used as an adjuvant to the local anesthetic to prolong duration of action. For diagnostic or therapeutic purposes, smaller volumes (0.5–1 mL) are recommended.
- After needle insertion, the appropriate local anesthetic dose (e.g., 1–2 mL of 0.5–1 % lidocaine, or 0.5–1 mL of 0.125–0.25 % bupivacaine, or 0.2 % ropivacaine with epinephrine (1:200,000)) is injected slowly after aspiration.
- Injection directly into the canals should be performed carefully to reduce the risk of neural injury.
- Ensure that the local anesthetic reaches all the relevant branches in order to achieve adequate anesthesia. While many practitioners commonly think that they are blocking the infraorbital nerve directly, it is important to remember that the nerve branches as soon as it exits the skull.
- Inaccurate placement of local anesthesia necessitates injection of larger volumes, which can be painful for awake and nonsedated patients. Inaccurate injection may also lead to partial blockade of maxillary nerve branches, which may fail to provide (1) adequate anesthesia to awake patients or (2) analgesia in the recovery room upon emergence.

Clinical Pearls

- The blocks should be followed by local compression to prevent hematoma formation.
- Intravascular injection is a rare but possible complication. Epinephrine (1:200,000) is a useful adjuvant that may help identify intravascular injection. Remember that the infraorbital artery lies in the middle of the nerve plexus, so aspiration of blood indicates that you are in the middle of the nerves. Repositioning the needle should lead to a successful block.
- With infraorbital blocks, the child may bite their lip due to numbness. Thus, parents need to be warned of this effect and that feeding may be affected.
- Skull nerve blocks can be used for craniotomy procedures and are also recommended to attenuate postoperative pain [12, 13]. The nerves blocked to achieve successful anesthesia for craniotomy include the supraorbital and supratrochlear nerves, the greater and lesser occipital nerves, the auriculotemporal nerves, and the greater auricular nerves. They can also be used for providing pain relief following minor surgical procedures on the forehead and scalp [14].
- Supraorbital nerve blocks have been associated with a high requirement for supplementation, perhaps due to the anatomic variation of the nerve. The nerve may exit the skull undivided or its medial and lateral branches may exit separately.

15.2.2 Intraoral Approach to Trigeminal Nerve Blocks: Infraorbital, Mental, and Greater Palatine Nerves

Trigeminal nerves can also be blocked via the intraoral approach.

15.2.2.1 Patient Positioning

- Supine with head resting on a donut.
- Greater palatine nerve: to keep the mouth open during blockade of the greater palatine nerve, a bite block or, more appropriate, a Dingman mouth retractor is required.

15.2.2.2 Landmarks and Surface Anatomy

- Infraorbital foramen: intraorally, locate the subsulcal groove at the level of the canine or first premolar (Fig. 15.5).
- Mental foramen: the buccal mucosa of the first premolar is identified (Fig. 15.6).
- Greater palatine foramen: in the intact palate, locate the greater palatine foramen medial and anterior to the first premolar in infants (Fig. 15.7) and second molar in adolescents. The nerve runs anterior to the foramen on the floor of the hard palate. In a patient with cleft palate, locate the greater palatine foramen by palpating the medial edge of the cleft palate. The end of the hard palate represents the level at which the greater palatine nerve exits the foramen and can be located consistently at this level. When palpating the medial bone edge, care must be taken to recognize the correct structures. Moving the finger randomly posterior risks palpating the hook of the hamulus rather than the true medial edge of the bone, which represents the level of the greater palatine foramen. Palpation of the hamulus will be too posterior, and injection here will result in ineffective anesthesia. To correct this, the finger should be moved toward the lateral edge of the palate, and a depression or groove will be felt, representing the foramen. This is the exit for the nerve and vascular pedicle that accompanies the nerve and supplies blood supply to the palatal tissues.

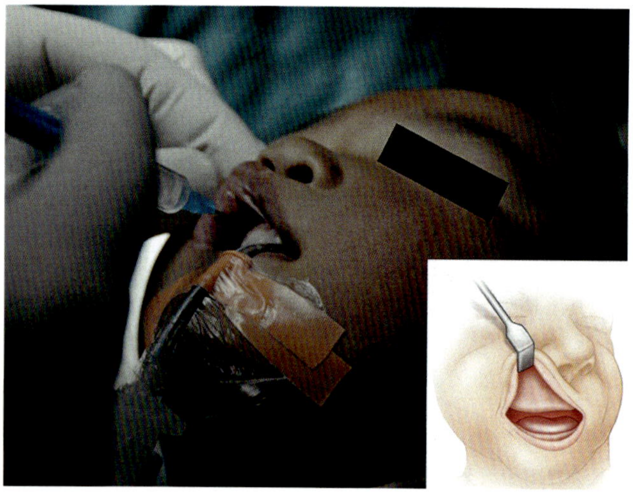

Fig. 15.5 Surface anatomy and needle insertion for intraoral infraorbital nerve block

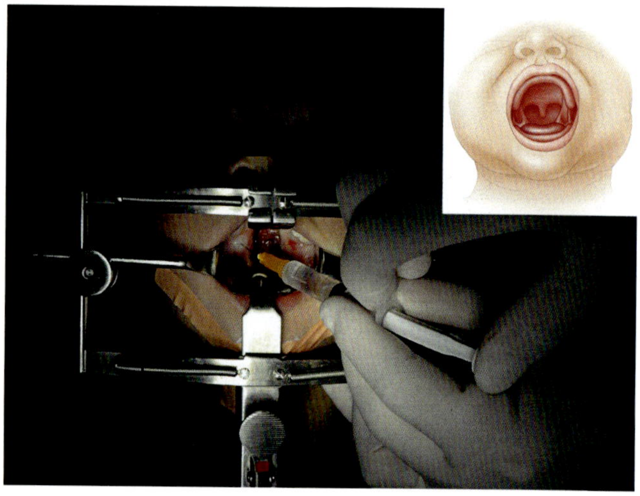

Fig. 15.7 Surface anatomy and needle direction for greater palatine nerve block

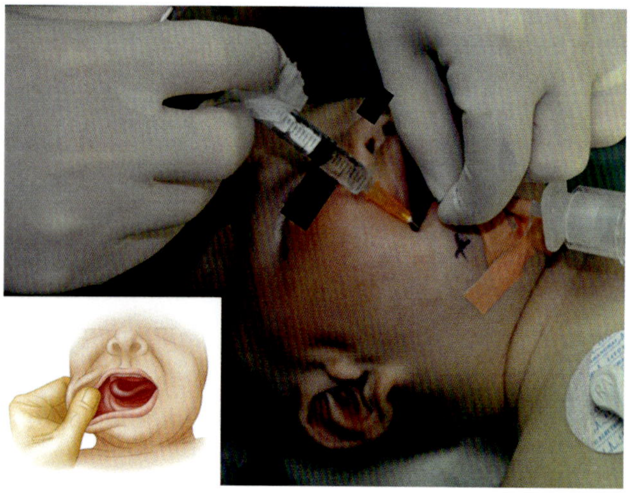

Fig. 15.6 Surface anatomy and needle direction for intraoral mental nerve block

15.2.2.3 Needle Insertion Technique

- Intraoral infraorbital nerve: evert the upper lip and, using a ≥45° angle, insert a 23G–27G needle into the buccal mucosa in the subsulcal groove (Fig. 15.5). A longer needle is needed to reach the level of the foramen. External palpation at the foramen will help to prevent the needle from entering the globe of the eye.
  - Lateral needle placement or local anesthetic spread risks partial blockade. Placing local anesthetic too far laterally on the maxilla may result in blockade of the middle or anterior superior alveolar nerves; in this case, only dental – not surgical – anesthesia may be achieved.
  - Inaccurate needle direction may make location of the foramen difficult since the needle is traveling in a sagittal or nasal-to-temporal direction from the buccal sulcus.
- Mental nerve: Evert the lower lip and insert a 25G–27G needle into the buccal mucosa between the canine and the first premolar (Fig. 15.6).
- Greater palatine nerve: for patients with an intact palate, insert a 25G–27G needle into the mucosa anterior to the greater palatine foramen (Fig. 15.7). For cleft palate repairs, several separate blocks will be needed since the greater palatine nerve is only one of the nerves that innervate the cleft palate. The nasopalatine nerve, which is a terminal branch of the maxillary nerve, innervates the anterior or primary palate and the front four teeth and will need to be blocked separately. The soft palate, which is supplied by the lesser palatine nerve and a plexus of nerves that arise from the glossopharyngeal plexus in the oral cavity, also requires a separate injection.
  - When blocking these nerves, it is critical that the mouth be opened as widely as possible with the assistance of some type of mouth retractor such as a Dingman retractor. Having a wide open view allows both the practitioner and surgeon to have a full view of needle placement and prevent injury to the vascular pedicle.
  - After locating the greater palatine foramen, the injection is performed in a cross-mouth technique, which will allow everyone involved in the operation to view needle insertion and local anesthetic spread.
  - Use of epinephrine as an adjunct is critical so that the blanching of mucosa can help determine optimum local anesthetic spread.
  - Performing the injection at the beginning of surgery allows local anesthetic spread to be followed without any confusion from the surgical injection, which is typically performed for palate hemostasis and dissection of soft tissues. Ideally, the injection is performed in a gentle, single-shot technique without hunting for the foramen directly.
  - Ideally, the needle will contact the bone of the palate in a periforaminal location. Typically, 0.5–1 mL local anesthesia is injected. Spread in the hard palate only indicates successful injection; if the soft palate tissues begin to dissect, then the needle may be too far posterior and may need to be repositioned slightly anterior.
  - After the greater palatine nerve is surrounded by local anesthetic, the needle is inserted in a posterior direction about 3–5 mm posterior from the original injection position. The soft tissues that make up the soft palate pedicle are expanded by an additional 0.5–1 mL of local anesthetic. The lesser palatine foramen is too difficult to locate clinically since it is very lateral on the palate and extremely small (Fig. 15.8). Since a plexus of nerves innervates the soft palate, spreading the local anesthetic through the soft palate tissues will ensure posterior spread to reach the lesser palatine foramen. Medial spread will help anesthetize the glossopharyngeal components and help to ensure complete palate anesthesia.

- The last nerve to block for palate anesthesia is the nasopalatine nerve (Fig. 15.8). It exits the nasopalatine foramen, which is located under the nasopalatine papilla in the front of the hard palate. The foramen is the entrance to a canal that travels in the direction of the tooth roots at a 45° angle.
  - A 25G–27G needle may be placed in this foramen; however, it is not uncommon to encounter difficulty entering the foramen, and some force may be required upon injection to ensure local anesthetic spread through the foramen.
  - If the cleft palate extends through the foramen, any injected local anesthesia will drip into the nasal vault and will not be effective. In this situation, it is possible to inject on both anterior surfaces of the palate to perform so-called partial palatal injections, which will anesthetize the anterior palate.
  - In some palate repairs, the vomer will also be used for the repair; additional local anesthesia should be placed here to ensure complete anesthesia of the surgical area.

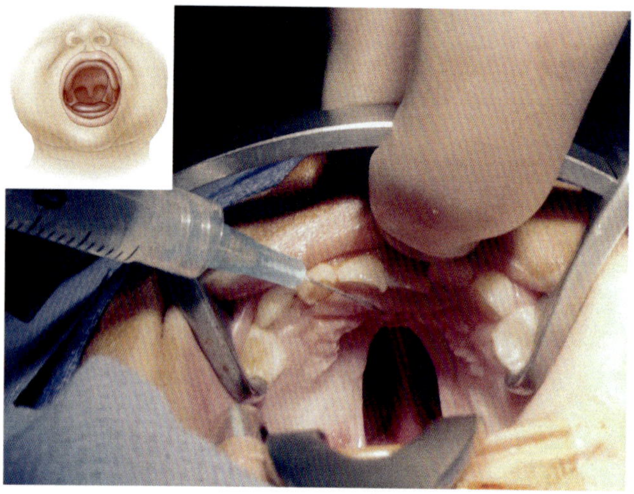

Fig. 15.8 Surface anatomy and needle direction for nasopalatine nerve block

15.2.2.4 Local Anesthetic Application

After aspiration, the appropriate local anesthetic dose (e.g., 1–2 mL of 0.5–1 % lidocaine, or 0.5–1 mL of 0.125–0.25 % bupivacaine, or 0.2 % ropivacaine with epinephrine 1:200,000) is slowly injected after aspiration.

15.2.3 Deep Trigeminal Nerve Blocks

Deep trigeminal nerve blocks are not commonly performed in the pediatric population; however, it is worth discussing the suprazygomatic maxillary nerve block, which has recently become popular for cleft palate repairs. These blocks have not been commonly performed, even in the adult population, most likely because of the deep insertion required to perform accurate nerve blockade and the potential for harm.

- Deep trigeminal blocks are required when the superficial block of the infraorbital nerve does not produce adequate anesthesia or when complete maxillary or mandibular anesthesia is required.
- Maxillary nerve block (often but not completely accurately referred to as sphenopalatine block) can be performed by a lateral approach to enter the sphenopalatine fissure. This can be achieved by approaching either above or below the zygomatic arch. Novice practitioners should exercise caution with this block since accurate needle placement requires insertion 3–4 cm deep into the skull base in a blind fashion. The recommended insertion point is at the junction of the superior zygoma and posterior orbit. The needle is inserted perpendicularly to contact the greater wing of the sphenoid at a depth of 2 cm. After bony contact, the needle is redirected 9° inferior and 20° anterior in the direction of the plane of the philtrum and is advanced 3–4 cm further to enter the pterygopalatine fossa (Fig. 15.9). A dose of 0.15 mL/kg is recommended after negative aspiration. The block is then repeated on the opposite side for complete maxillary nerve anesthesia.

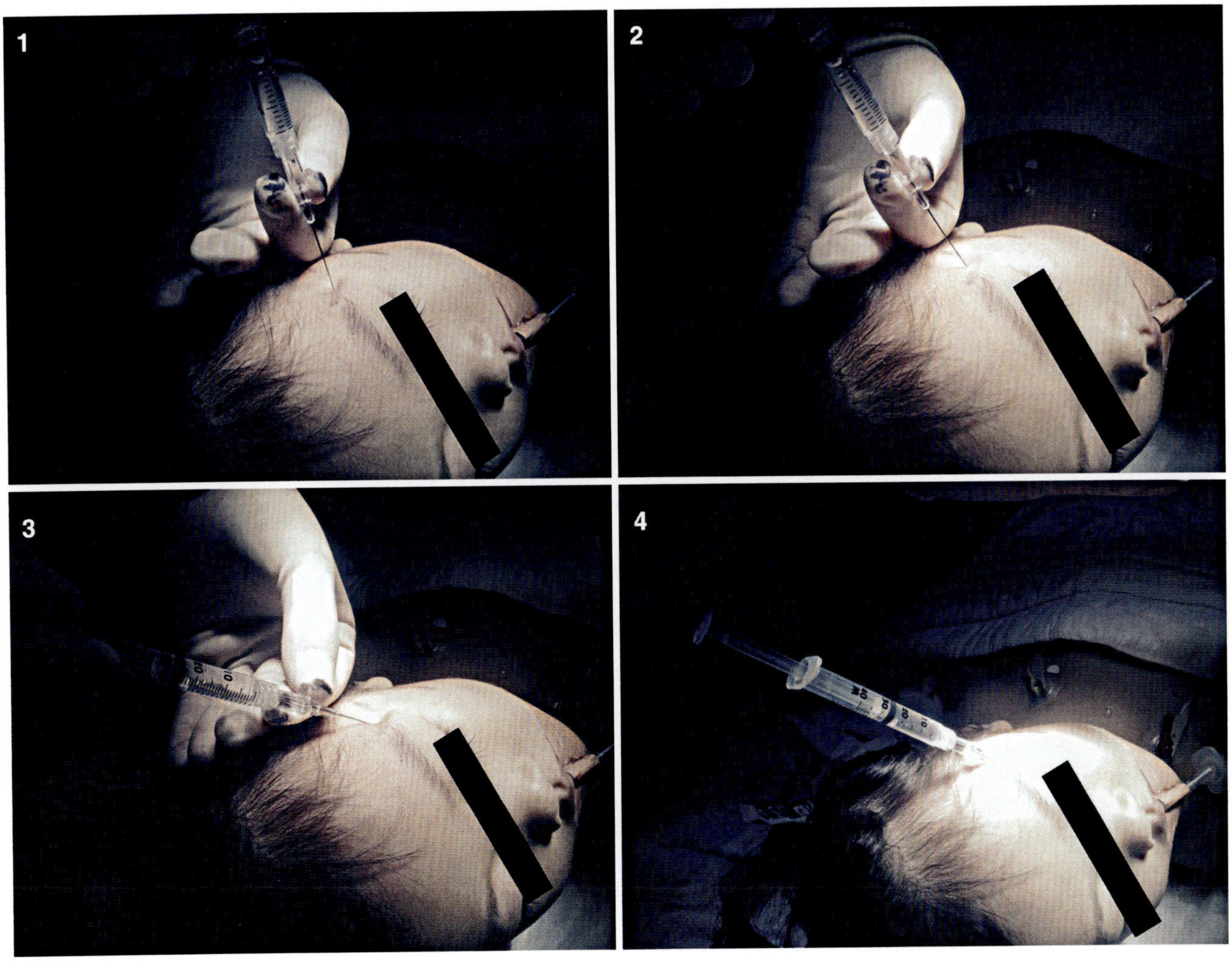

Fig. 15.9 Surface anatomy and needle direction for maxillary nerve block. (*1*) The needle is inserted perpendicularly to contact sphenoid; (*2*) the needle is redirected 9° inferior and then (*3*) 20° anterior; (*4*) the needle/syringe can hold its own position once the needle has entered the pterygopalatine fossa

The mandibular nerve can be blocked at the point where it leaves the cranium through the foramen ovale. The block can be done with an intraoral or extraoral approach through the intercondylar mandibular notch.

- When using an extraoral approach, place the needle through the notch in a perpendicular fashion, and contact the pterygoid plate. Measure the depth and move the needle posterior to walk off the pterygoid plate. The needle should be advanced no further than the depth of the pterygoid plate. While no pediatric studies exist to recommend accurate dosing, 1–3 mL of local anesthetic should achieve adequate anesthesia since the needle is close to the foramen ovale and skull base.

Due to the depth of these blocks (see Figs. 15.10 and 15.11), they should be performed by practitioners with related and adequate experience.

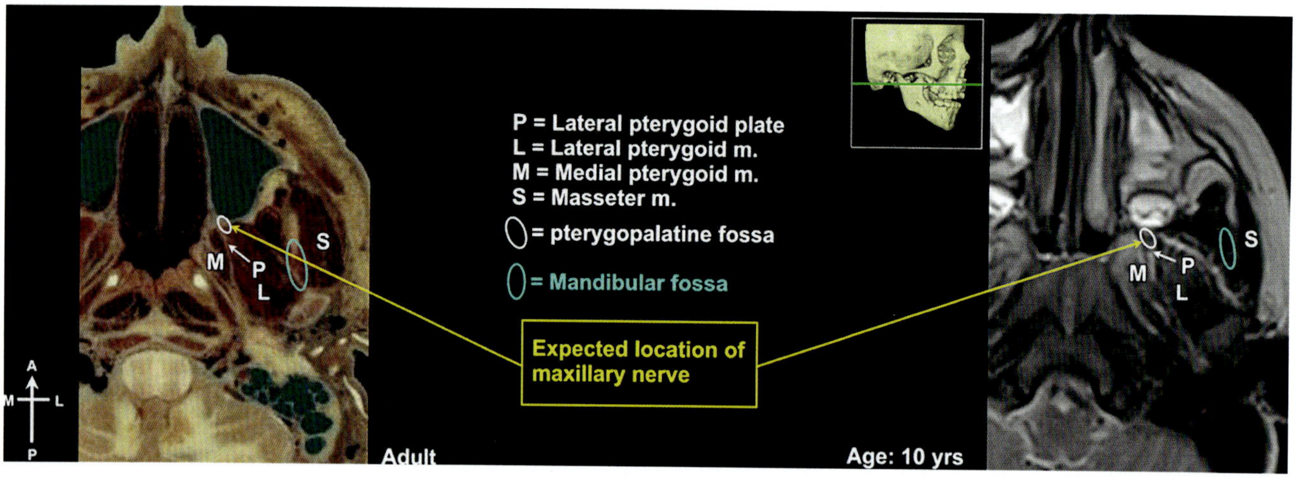

Fig. 15.10 VHVS and MRI images capturing the maxillary nerve during its course through the infraorbital groove and canal. This will be the location of a maxillary nerve block

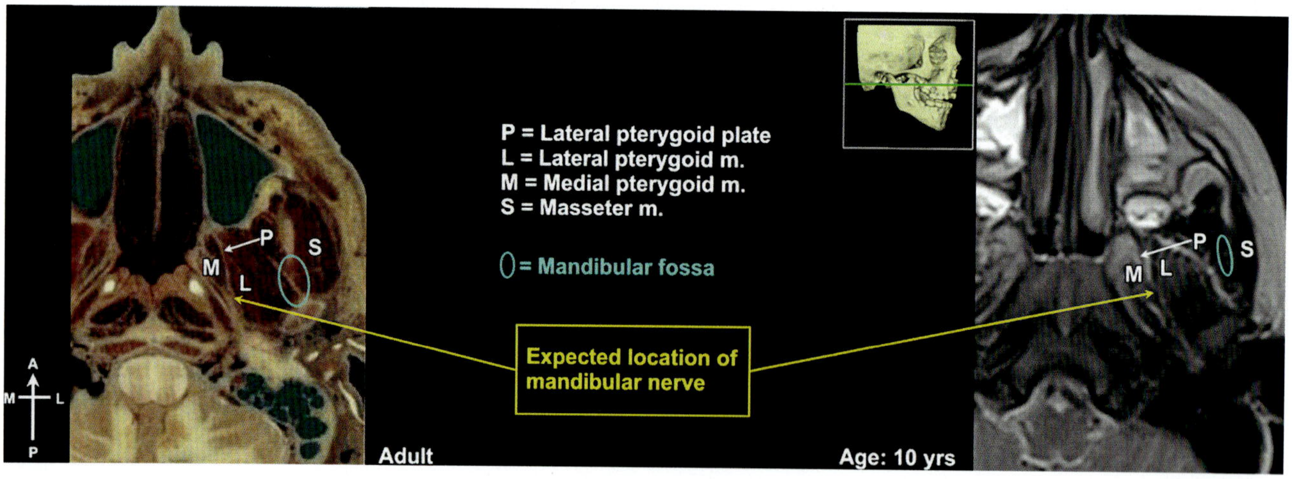

Fig. 15.11 VHVS and MRI of the mandibular nerve showing its position posterior to the maxillary nerve yet remaining medial to lateral pterygoid plate

15.3 Current Literature in Ultrasound-Guided Approaches

It has been reported that failure to achieve full anesthesia using traditional blocks of the trigeminal nerve is in the region of 22 % [15]. In pediatric patients, one reason for this may be that landmarks used to perform superficial trigeminal nerve blocks (particularly infraorbital) are absent or difficult to palpate in the neonate. Facial foramina can be localized accurately and reliably using ultrasound [1, 16], and this may provide an opportunity to improve success in these blocks. Tsui [1] described an ultrasound approach to locate the supraorbital, infraorbital, and mental foramina (see above). Identification of each foramen can be achieved using a high-resolution, short-footprint linear transducer; a disruption in the continuity of the bone will appear as scanning proceeds in a medial-to-lateral direction at the level of the foramina (Fig. 15.3). Color Doppler will prove useful to locate the respective artery within the foramen.

The effectiveness of trigeminal nerve block has been demonstrated in various studies. Ahuja et al. [17] showed a significant improvement in pain score in the infraorbital block group compared to normal saline infiltration in children scheduled for cleft lip repair. A double-blinded, randomized study also demonstrated a significant reduction in analgesia requirement and pain score in children who had an infraorbital nerve block compared to the conventional peri-incisional infiltration by the surgeon [18]. Recently, Mesnil et al. [19] observed the effectiveness of bilateral maxillary nerve blocks using a suprazygomatic approach, finding improved pain relief and a reduction in opioid consumption following cleft palate repair in infants. Furthermore, this approach minimizes the likelihood of entering the orbit and reduces the risk of vascular injury as the needle enters the infratemporal fossa and ultimately the sphenopalatine fossa in a superior-to-inferior direction. No significant difference was found in mandibular infiltration anesthesia and mandibular block for dental surgery in children [20]; however, in this study, mixed surgical cases with a relatively small sample size were investigated, which could introduce confounding factors.

The effectiveness of bilateral maxillary nerve blocks using a suprazygomatic approach with nerve stimulation [19] and ultrasound [21] has been reported. Using electrical stimulation, Mesnil et al. [19] showed that the disappearance of the temporal muscle twitch coincided with the needle's tip in the pterygopalatine fossa where local anesthetic was injected. More recently, this group successfully published a randomized, double-blind study evaluating an ultrasound-guided suprazygomatic maxillary nerve block [21]. They used a linear array probe located in the infrazygomatic area to allow out-of-plane visualization of the needle tip and local anesthetic spread in the pterygopalatine fossa. Both these approaches allowed improved pain relief and a reduction in opioid consumption following cleft palate repair in infants.

15.4 Case Study

Greater Palatine Nerve Block (Provided by S. Suresh)

A 5-month-old female infant, 6.5 kg in weight, with a past medical history of cleft lip and cleft palate and mother with cleft lip, presented for cleft palate surgery. Hemoglobin was measured at 9.8 g%. No preadmission medications were given. A greater palatine nerve block was administered; briefly, the mouth gag was placed by the surgeon, after which the greater palatine foramen was identified in the hard palate (this usually corresponds to the second molar in an older patient with dentition), and 0.5 mL 0.25 % bupivacaine was injected with a 27G needle into the area anterior to the greater palatine foramen bilaterally (cf. Fig. 15.7). Duration of surgery was 2 h, 35 min; block duration was 8–10 h. No ultrasound imaging considerations were necessary, and no additional opioid was needed in recovery. Patient outcome was excellent and resulted in early discharge from PACU.

References

1. Tsui BC. Ultrasound imaging to localize foramina for superficial trigeminal nerve block. Can J Anesth. 2009;56:704–6.
2. Suresh S, Voronov P, Curran J. Infraorbital nerve block in children: a computerized tomographic measurement of the location of the infraorbital foramen. Reg Anesth Pain Med. 2006;31:211–4.
3. Canan S, Asim OM, Okan B, Ozek C, Alper M. Anatomic variations of the infraorbital foramen. Ann Plast Surg. 1999;43:613–7.
4. Thakur G, Thomas S, Thayil SC, Nair PP. Accessory mental foramen: a rare anatomical finding. BMJ Case Rep. 2011; 2011; bcr0920103326.
5. Eipe N, Choudhrie A, Pillai AD, Choudhrie R. Regional anesthesia for cleft lip repair: a preliminary study. Cleft Palate Craniofac J. 2006;43:138–41.
6. Voronov P, Suresh S. Head and neck blocks in children. Curr Opin Anaesthesiol. 2008;21:317–22.
7. Lynch MT, Syverud SA, Schwab RA, Jenkins JM, Edlich R. Comparison of intraoral and percutaneous approaches for infraorbital nerve block. Acad Emerg Med. 1994;1:514–9.
8. Bosenberg AT, Kimble FW. Infraorbital nerve block in neonates for cleft lip repair: anatomical study and clinical application. Br J Anaesth. 1995;74:506–8.
9. Wilhelmi BJ, Mowlavi A, Neumeister MW, Blackwell SJ. Facial fracture approaches with landmark ratios to predict the location of the infraorbital and supraorbital nerves: an anatomic study. J Craniofac Surg. 2003;14:473–7.
10. Hu KS, Kwak HH, Song WC, Kang HJ, Kim HC, Fontaine C, Kim HJ. Branching patterns of the infraorbital nerve and topography within the infraorbital space. J Craniofac Surg. 2006;17:1111–5.
11. Zide BM, Swift R. How to block and tackle the face. Plast Reconstr Surg. 1998;101:840–51.
12. Suresh S, Bellig G. Regional anesthesia in a very low-birth-weight neonate for a neurosurgical procedure. Reg Anesth Pain Med. 2004;29:58–9.

13. Uejima T, Suresh S. Ommaya and McComb reservoir placement in infants: can this be done with regional anesthesia? Pediatr Anesth. 2008;18:909–11.
14. Suresh S, Wagner AM. Scalp excisions: getting "ahead" of pain. Pediatr Dermatol. 2001;18:74–6.
15. Pascal J, Charier D, Perret D, Navez M, Auboyer C, Molliex S. Peripheral blocks of trigeminal nerve for facial soft-tissue surgery: learning from failures. Eur J Anaesthesiol. 2005;22:480–2.
16. Hannan L, Reader A, Nist R, Beck M, Meyers WJ. The use of ultrasound for guiding needle placement for inferior alveolar nerve blocks. Oral Surg Oral Med Oral Pathol Oral Radiol Endod. 1999;87:658–65.
17. Ahuja S, Datta A, Krishna A, Bhattacharya A. Infra-orbital nerve block for relief of postoperative pain following cleft lip surgery in infants. Anaesthesia. 1994;49:441–4.
18. Prabhu KP, Wig J, Grewal S. Bilateral infraorbital nerve block is superior to peri-incisional infiltration for analgesia after repair of cleft lip. Scand J Plast Reconstr Surg Hand Surg. 1999;33:83–7.
19. Mesnil M, Dadure C, Captier G, Raux O, Rochette A, Canaud N, Sauter M, Capdevila X. A new approach for peri-operative analgesia of cleft palate repair in infants: the bilateral suprazygomatic maxillary nerve block. Pediatr Anesth. 2010;20:343–9.
20. Yassen GH. Evaluation of mandibular infiltration versus mandibular block anaesthesia in treating primary canines in children. Int J Paediatr Dent. 2010;20:43–9.
21. Sola C, Raux O, Savath L, Macq C, Capdevila X, Dadure C. Ultrasound guidance characteristics and efficiency of suprazygomatic maxillary nerve blocks in infants: a descriptive prospective study. Pediatr Anesth. 2012;22:841–6.

Suggested Reading

Belvis D, Voronov P, Suresh S. Head and neck blocks in children. Tech Reg Anesth Pain Manag. 2007;11(4):208–14.

Dalens B. Blocks of the head, neck, and face. In: Dalens B, editor. Regional anesthesia in infants, children, and adolescents. Philadelphia: Lippincott Williams & Wilkins; 1995. p. 398–401.

Suresh S, Polaner DM, Cote CJ. Regional Anesthesia. In: Cote CJ, Lerman J, Anderson BJ, Eds. 5th ed. Philadelphia: WB Saunders; 2013. p. 835–79.

Suresh S, Voronov P. Head and neck blocks in infants, children, adolescents. Pediatr Anesth. 2012;22:81–7.

Cervical Plexus Blocks

16

Ban C.H. Tsui

Contents

B.C.H. Tsui, Dip Eng, BSc (Math), B Pharm, MSc, MD, FRCPC
Department of Anesthesiology and Pain Medicine,
Stollery Children's Hospital/University of Alberta Hospital,
2-150 Clinical Sciences Building, Edmonton,
AB T6G 2G3, Canada
e-mail: btsui@ualberta.ca

B.C.H. Tsui, S. Suresh (eds.), *Pediatric Atlas of Ultrasound- and Nerve Stimulation-Guided Regional Anesthesia*,
DOI 10.1007/978-0-387-79964-3_16

16.1 Indications for Cervical Plexus Block

16.1.1 Indications for Superficial Cervical Plexus Block

- Carotid endarterectomy (with a deep cervical plexus block or infiltration)
- Surgical excision of lesions in the neck or "cape region" of the shoulder
- Surgical fixation of fractured clavicle
- To facilitate tunneling of interscalene brachial plexus catheters and as an adjunct to this block for total shoulder replacement

16.1.2 Indications for Combined Superficial and Deep Cervical Plexus Block

- Tympanomastoid surgery
- Otoplasty
- Cochlear implant
- Thyroidectomy
- Vocal cord surgery

16.2 Classic (Deep) Cervical Plexus Block

This block is not commonly used in young children. In addition to the depth of the block, it also has the potential for inadvertent phrenic nerve blockade, especially in young children, which may compromise their respiratory function. For this reason, bilateral deep cervical plexus block is considered contraindicated. Furthermore, the proximity of the deep cervical plexus to the vertebral and carotid arteries increases the risks of inadvertent vascular puncture and systemic absorption of local anesthetic (Fig. 16.1). A risk of spinal anesthesia is also present; therefore, high volumes of local anesthetic and high injection pressure should be avoided.

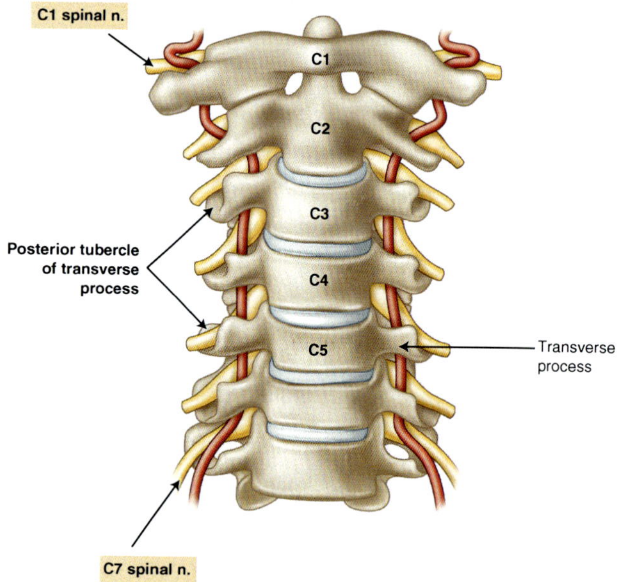

Fig. 16.1 Deep cervical plexus anatomy

16.2.1 Patient Positioning

- Supine with a small towel or pillow under the head, which is turned 45° to the contralateral side with slight neck extension

16.2.2 Landmarks and Surface Anatomy (Fig. 16.2)

- Landmarks include the posterior edge of the sternocleidomastoid muscle, the caudal portion of the mastoid process (see Clinical Pearls), the angle of the jaw, and the transverse processes of cervical vertebrae C2–C5.
- If no transverse processes can be palpated, the transverse process of C6 can be located at the level of the cricoid cartilage. A line is drawn from the mastoid process along the sternocleidomastoid muscle to the transverse process of C6. Each transverse process of C2–C5 is marked approximately 0.5–1 cm behind the line. The transverse process of C2 lies about 1–1.5 cm inferior to the mastoid process, depending on the age and size of the patient. Deep cervical plexus block is a variation of cervical paravertebral nerve block of C2–C4.

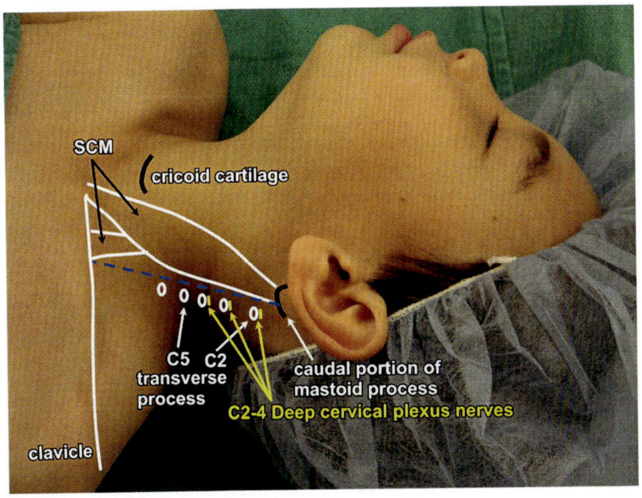

Fig. 16.2 Patient positioning and surface landmarks for a deep cervical plexus block. *SCM* sternocleidomastoid muscle

16.2.3 Needle Insertion Technique

- Three injections using a 22G–24G needle at the level of C2–C4 perpendicular to the horizontal plane and advanced slightly caudally and posteriorly (it is very important to avoid inadvertent intrathecal or epidural injection into the vertebral artery). The needle will typically contact the posterior tubercle of the transverse process (Fig. 16.1), upon which, the needle is withdrawn slightly, and the local anesthetic is injected after negative aspiration.

16.2.4 Nerve Localization and Local Anesthetic Application

- A nerve stimulator attached to an insulated needle can be used to localize the mixed spinal nerves. Correct position of the needle tip is confirmed when current intensity of 0.5 mA elicits a local neck muscle response [1].
- Concurrent use of ultrasound guidance is recommended to improve safety and efficacy of this block. The ultrasound image with corresponding MRI and VHVS images is shown in Figs. 16.3 and 16.4, where a selective deep cervical plexus block is performed in the groove between the longus capitis and scalenus medius.
  - After confirming contact with the transverse process, the needle is withdrawn slightly and a syringe is connected.
  - The dose of local anesthetic should be considered carefully, especially when multiple injections are performed. A dilute solution (0.5–1.0 % lidocaine [maximum dose 7 mg/kg] or 0.125–0.25 % bupivacaine [maximum dose 2 mg/kg]) with epinephrine (1:200,000 or 1:400,000) to detect inadvertent intravenous injection should be used. Generally, 1–3 mL of the solution is used at each injection site.

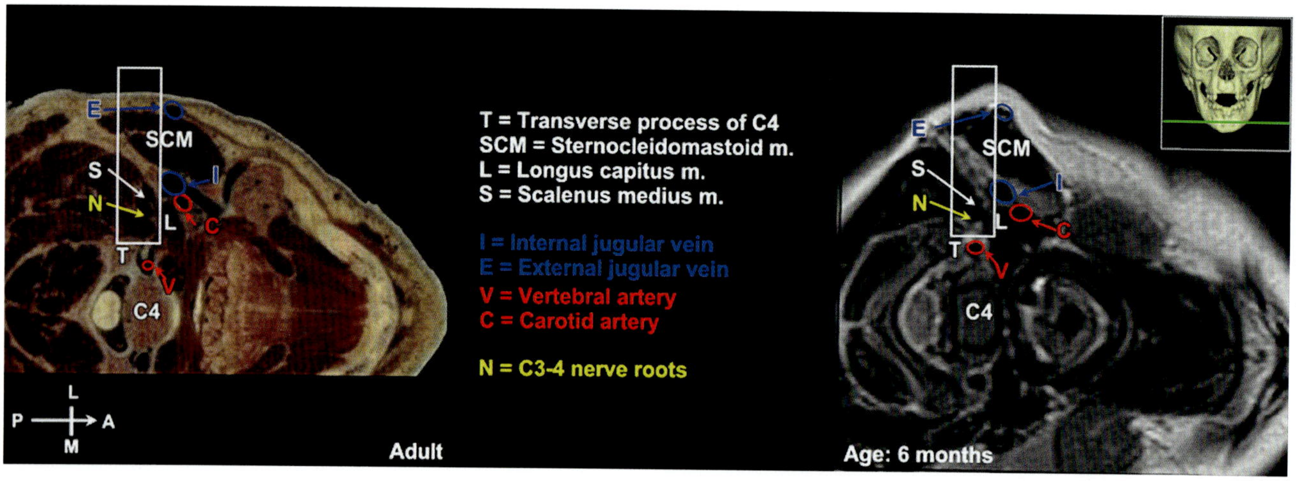

Fig. 16.3 VHVS and MRI images of the deep cervical plexus

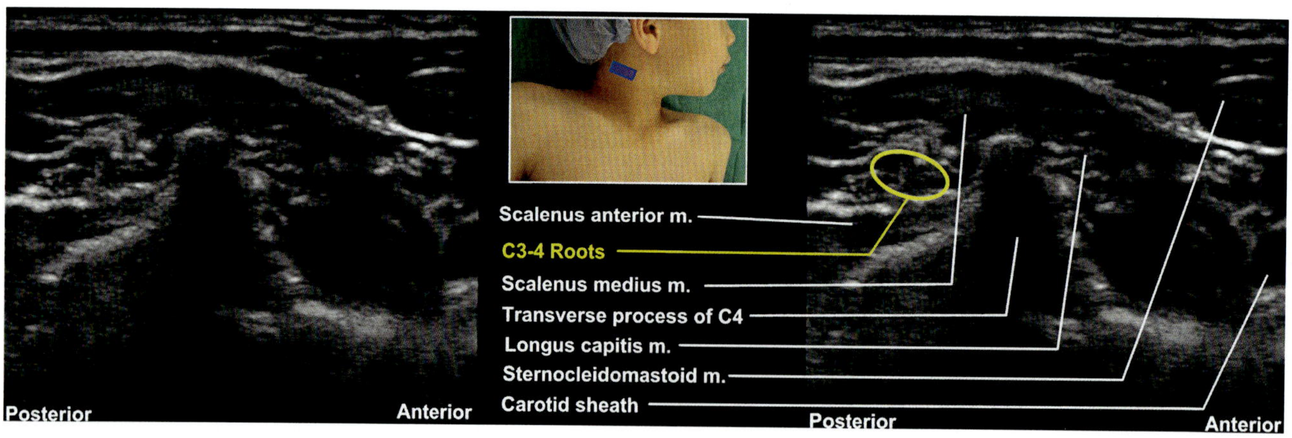

Fig. 16.4 Ultrasound image of the deep cervical plexus

Clinical Pearls

- At birth, the mastoid process only represents a small portion of the temporal bone. The mastoid width and depth increases rapidly up to the age of 7 years with no apparent gender dimorphism. The maximum size is apparent between years 11 and 19. This should be considered when palpating the attachment of the sternocleidomastoid muscle as a landmark for these blocks.
- The deep block may be performed by single injection at C3 or C4 as originally described by Winnie or by a standard three-injection technique.
- There are several life-threatening complications that may arise from deep cervical plexus block. A caudally directed needle is imperative; otherwise, injection into the vertebral artery (Fig. 16.5) may occur, potentially leading to convulsions, unconsciousness, and blindness. Subarachnoid or epidural injections are possible if the needle is advanced too far medially into the vertebral foramen. This is more likely in the cervical region because of the longer dural sleeves that accompany these nerve branches. Careful monitoring of the patient should continue for 60 min after the block has been performed.
- Phrenic nerve palsy leading to hemidiaphragmatic paresis is a common occurrence with this block; therefore, care must be taken in young children. Bilateral blocks are not recommended. Minimizing the volume of local anesthetic may limit blockade of the phrenic nerve.
- Other well-described side effects include Horner's syndrome (if the superior cervical or cervicothoracic ganglion is blocked), stellate ganglion block, and hoarseness due to recurrent laryngeal nerve block.
- The authors did not recommend performing the deep cervical plexus block unless it is strongly indicated.

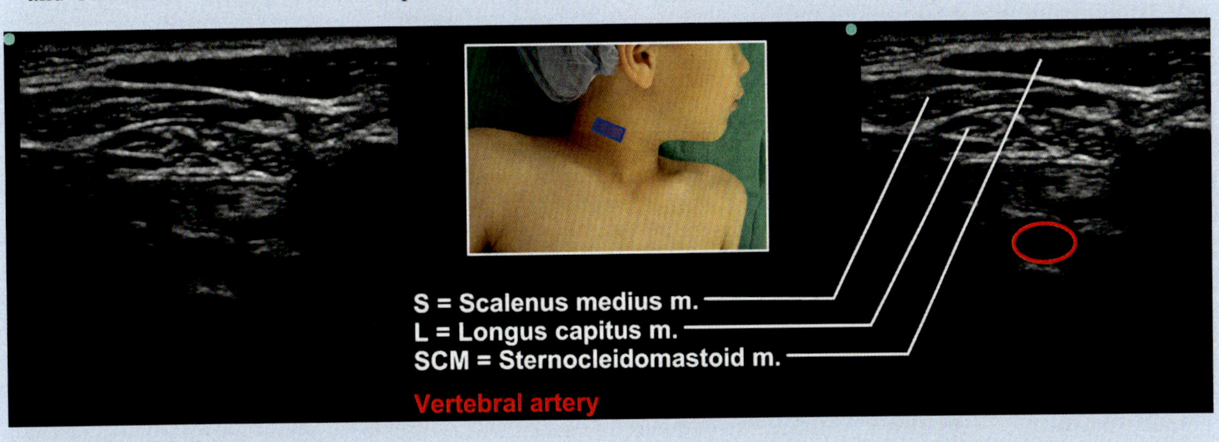

Fig. 16.5 Ultrasound image highlighting the close proximity of the vertebral artery to the deep cervical plexus

16.2.5 Current Literature for Deep Cervical Plexus Block

Zeidan described a nerve stimulator-guided deep cervical plexus block for carotid endarterectomy [1]. The transverse process is identified 1 cm posterior to the posterior border of the sternocleidomastoid. With a block needle connected to a nerve stimulator, the needle is inserted perpendicular to the skin, aiming slightly caudal at C2 level to elicit neck muscle contraction at a current intensity of 0.5 mA. Excellent results were reported with this technique; however, there was no description of the specific type of muscle response elicited to confirm correct placement of the needle versus direct muscle contraction from the stimulating needle itself. Data on pediatric patients are lacking.

A recent case series by Perisanidis et al. [2] assessed combined deep and intermediate cervical plexus block for oral and maxillofacial surgery in adults. Under ultrasound guidance, the authors injected 15 mL ropivacaine 0.75 % between the sternocleidomastoid and levator of the scapula muscles; after which, the needle was advanced to a position between the levator of the scapula and cervical transverse process, where another injection of 15 mL ropivacaine 0.75 % was done. All blocks were successful with no need for supplementary analgesics in the 24 h post-block period. Obviously, this dosage is too high for the pediatric population.

There have been reports of successful cervical plexus blocks to provide surgical anesthesia for lymph node biopsy and excision of thyroid nodules in adolescents using a single injection at the level of C3 [3]. When reviewing the literature describing ultrasound imaging techniques of deep cervical block in adults, the two most useful sonographic landmarks appear to be the groove between the longus capitis and scalenus medius [4] and the sulcus between the anterior and posterior tubercles of the transverse processes and posterior to the vertebral artery [5, 6].

16.3 Ultrasound-Guided Superficial Cervical Plexus Block

This block aims to anesthetize the four branches of the superficial cervical plexus, namely, the lesser occipital nerve, the great auricular nerve, the anterior or transverse cervical nerve, and the supraclavicular nerve (Fig. 16.6). These are all branches from the anterior primary rami of the C1–C4 nerve roots. Superficial cervical plexus block provides anesthesia to the ipsilateral occipital region, some of the ear, the anterior and posterior triangles of the neck, and the upper back, shoulder, and upper pectoral regions.

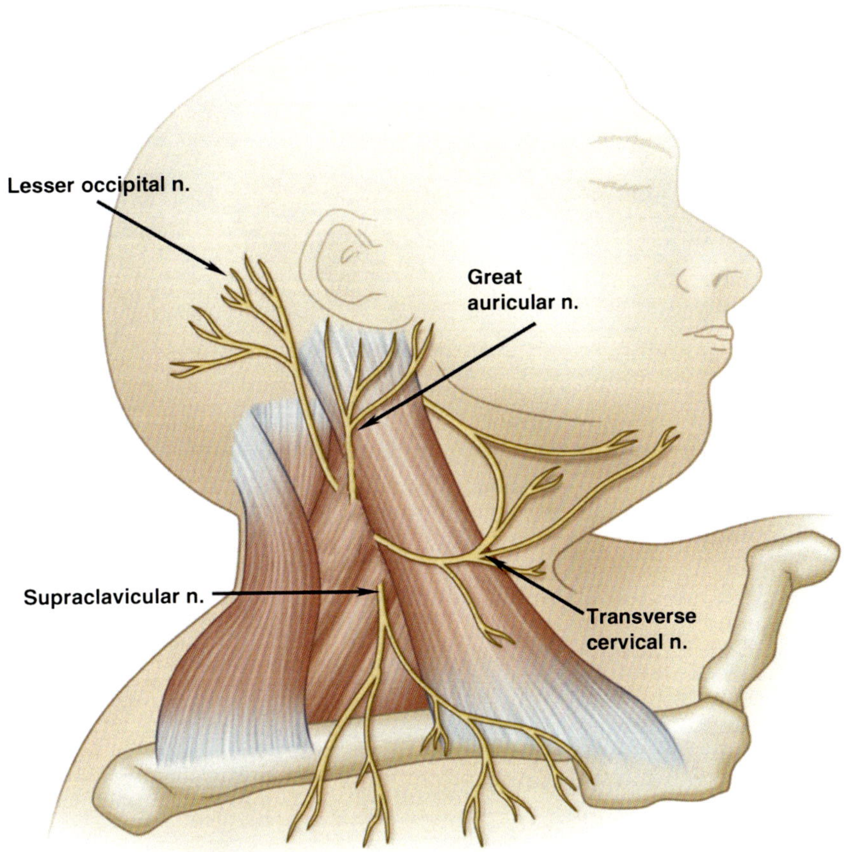

Fig. 16.6 Superficial cervical plexus anatomy

16.3.1 Patient Positioning

- The patient may be supine with the head turned 45° to the opposite side or lateral decubitus with the side to be blocked uppermost. Alternatively, the patient may be more comfortable with the head of the bed raised to 30° with the head turned or semilateral.

16.3.2 Landmarks and Surface Anatomy (Fig. 16.7)

- A horizontal line is drawn laterally from the cricoid cartilage (at the level of C6) to bisect a line drawn along the posterior border of the clavicular head of the sternocleidomastoid muscle (generally, this intersection is at the lower-third to midpoint of this muscle).

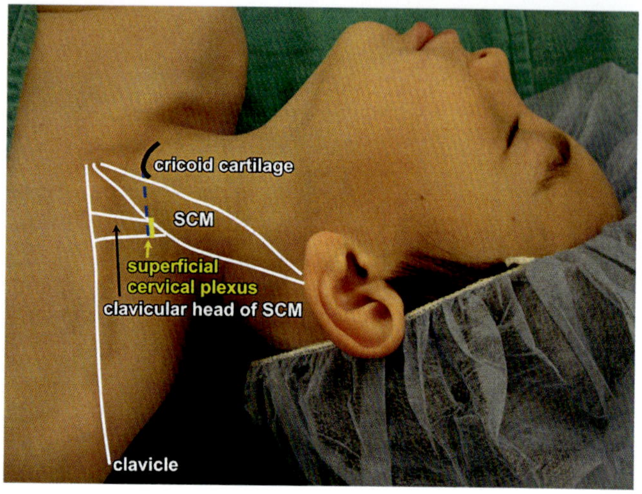

Fig. 16.7 Patient positioning and surface landmarks for a superficial cervical plexus block. *SCM* sternocleidomastoid muscle

16.3.3 Scanning Technique

- A linear (6–15 MHz) transducer is placed in a transverse location at the midpoint of the posterior border of the sternocleidomastoid muscle.
- The required depth is usually 2–4 cm for adolescents.
- Identify the fascial plane between the superficial cervical fascia, which invests the sternocleidomastoid muscle, and the deep cervical fascia, which invests the scalene muscles, deep cervical muscles, and the phrenic nerve.

16.3.4 Sonographic Appearance

- The nerve fibers may be visible with careful scanning and will be easier to see following local anesthetic injection; however, it is not necessary to identify them.
- The target for injection is the fascial plane between the superficial cervical fascia on the deep surface of the sternocleidomastoid muscle and the deep cervical fascia on the superficial surface of the anterior and middle scalene muscles (Figs. 16.8, 16.9, and 16.10).
- The interscalene brachial plexus lies deep to the deep cervical fascia at this point.
- The phrenic nerve can be difficult to visualize and lies deep cervical fascia on the surface of the anterior scalene muscle.
- The carotid sheath containing the carotid artery, internal jugular vein, and vagus nerve may also be visible deeper in the image.

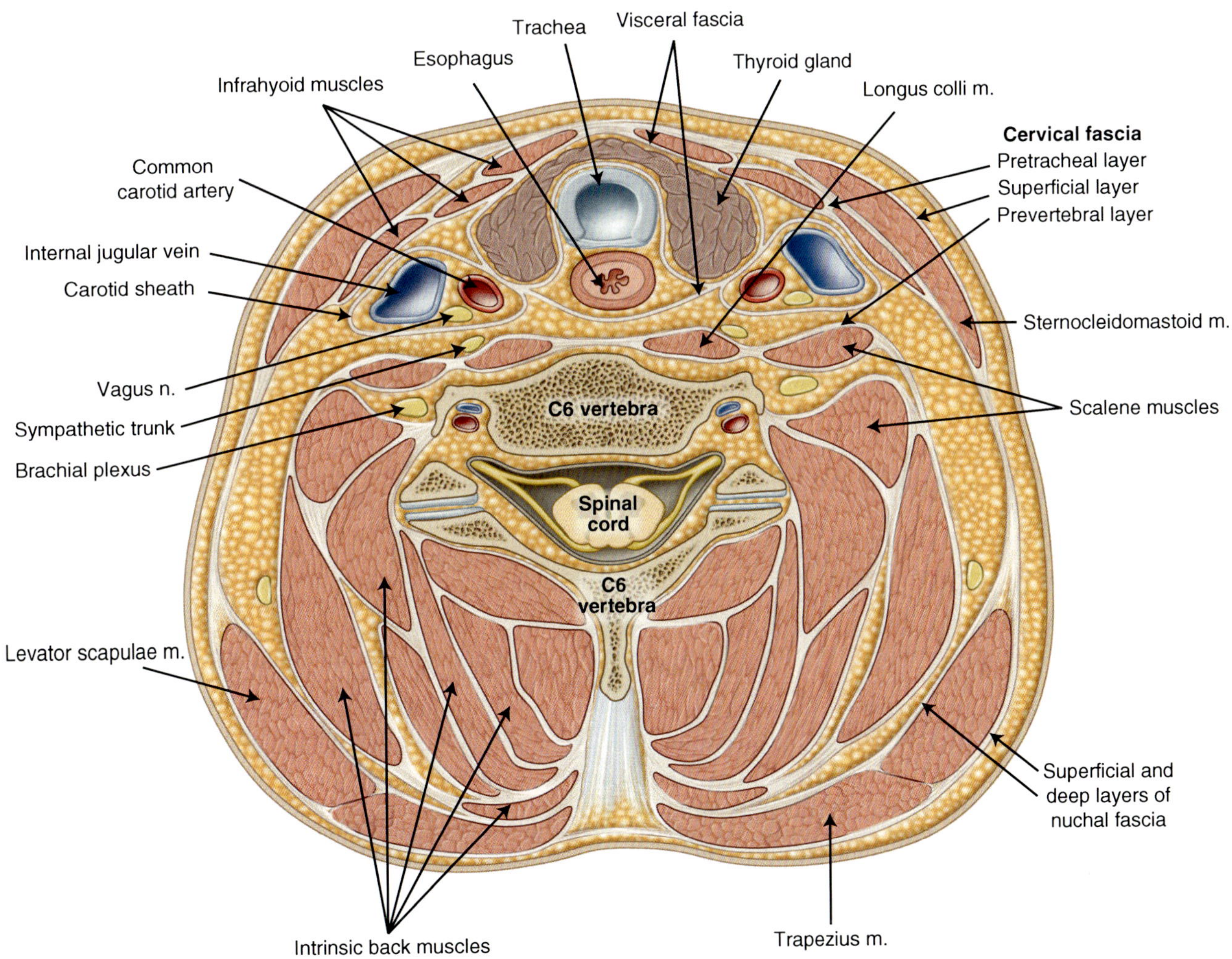

Fig. 16.8 Cross-section at C6 showing location of cervical fasciae

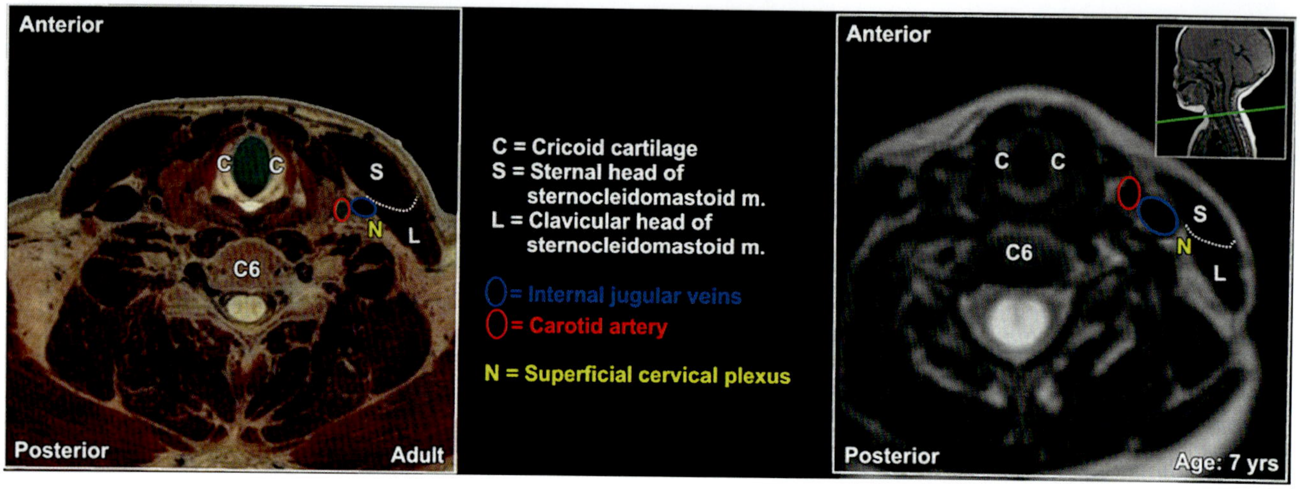

Fig. 16.9 VHVS and MRI images of the superficial cervical plexus

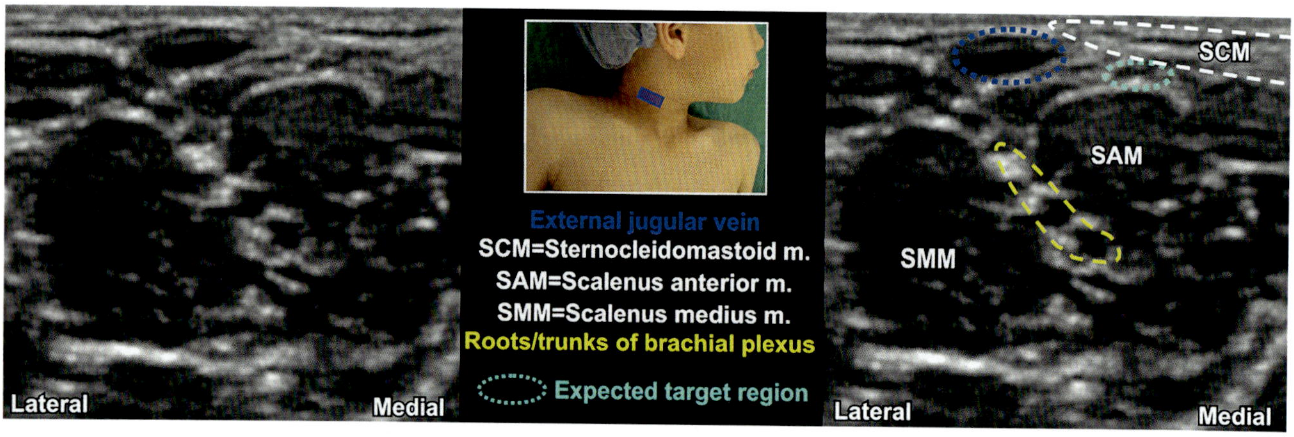

Fig. 16.10 Ultrasound image of the superficial cervical plexus

16.3.5 Needle Insertion Technique (Fig. 16.11)

- An injection of 1 mL lidocaine at the block needle insertion site will aid patient comfort when performed awake.
- Use a 2–3 cm, 22–27G bevel-tipped nerve block needle.
- An in-plane (IP) approach from lateral to medial should allow continuous visualization of the complete length of the needle, especially the tip, due to the superficial nature of the block and the flat angle of the needle.
- A "pop" may be felt as the needle penetrates the superficial cervical fascia.
- The tip of the needle should be just below and 0.5 cm medial to the middle of the posterior border of the sternocleidomastoid muscle and deep to the superficial cervical fascia during local anesthetic injection.

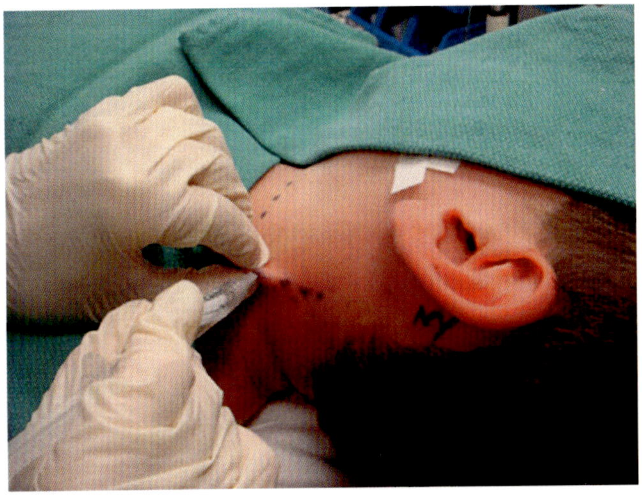

Fig. 16.11 Needle insertion for superficial cervical plexus block

16.3.6 Local Anesthetic Application

- Performing a test dose with D5W is recommended prior to local anesthetic application to visualize the spread and confirm needle tip localization.
- 0.1–0.2 mL/kg of local anesthetic (e.g., 0.25 % bupivacaine) should provide adequate spread.
- Correct needle position will separate the sternocleidomastoid and scalene muscles as well as ensure spreading of local anesthetic superiorly and inferiorly.
- After some space has been created by hydrodissection, the needle can be advanced slightly medially to enhance the local anesthetic spread.
- If intramuscular injection into the sternocleidomastoid or scalene muscles occurs, the needle will need to be repositioned into the correct plane.

16.3.7 Current Literature for Superficial Cervical Block

There is a paucity of evidence on the use of superficial cervical plexus blocks in children. Brownlow et al. [6] reported the use of a superficial cervical plexus block combined with mild sedation in a child with an anterior mediastinal mass who successfully underwent a diagnostic cervical node biopsy.

Clinical Pearls

- Complications associated with the superficial cervical plexus block include phrenic nerve paralysis leading to diaphragmatic dysfunction, vagus nerve block with resultant recurrent nerve paralysis, inadvertent intravascular injection, or inadvertent deep cervical plexus block.
- Hematoma and deep plexus block, with associated Horner's syndrome, are also possible following superficial cervical plexus block.

16.4 Great Auricular Nerve Blocks

Blocking the great auricular nerve can provide postoperative analgesia facilitating early discharge or omitting the need for hospital admissions. This is a superficial block, and ultrasound is not usually indicated. However, risks such as intravascular injection, hematoma, and injecting too far into the deep cervical plexus or vascular structures should be recognized.

Indications This is a branch of the superficial cervical plexus (Fig. 16.6) providing sensory innervations to the pinna and the postauricular region. Common indications of great auricular nerve block include:

- Tympanomastoid surgery
- Cochlear implant
- Craniotomies
- Otoplasty (with lesser occipital nerve)

Less common indications:

- Brachial cleft cyst excision
- Thyroidectomy
- Parathyroidectomy
- Clavicular fracture reduction
- Thyroplasty

16.4.1 Patient Positioning

- Supine with head turned to the contralateral side.

16.4.2 Landmarks and Surface Anatomy (Fig. 16.12)

- The cricoid cartilage (C6) is identified, and a line is drawn from it to the posterior border of the sternal head of sternocleidomastoid muscle (Fig. 16.6). In some patients, the external jugular vein may cross the neck at the point in which the cervical plexus wraps around the belly of the sternocleidomastoid muscle. Landmarks include the cricoid cartilage (level of C6), the posterior border of the sternocleidomastoid muscle, and in some children, the external jugular vein.

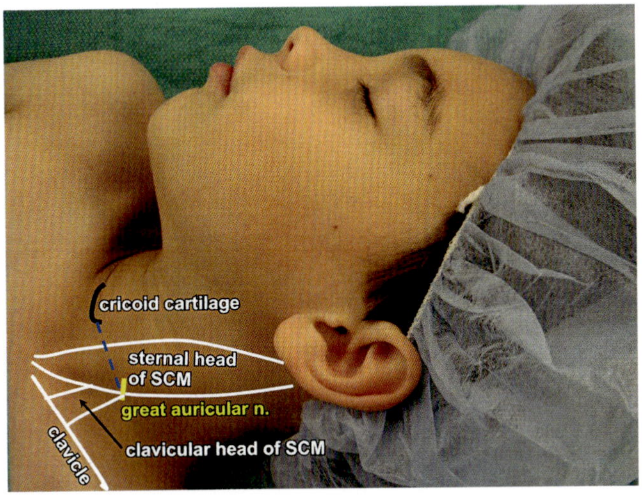

Fig. 16.12 Patient positioning and surface landmarks for great auricular nerve blocks. *SCM* sternocleidomastoid muscle

16.4.3 Needle Insertion Technique

- Using an acute angle to facilitate a superficial subcutaneous insertion, a 27G needle is advanced cephalad along the posterior border of the sternocleidomastoid muscle.

16.4.4 Nerve Localization and Local Anesthetic Application

- After negative aspiration, local anesthetic (e.g., 2–3 mL of 0.25 % bupivacaine with 1:200,000 of epinephrine) is injected in incremental doses to form a small subcutaneous wheal.

16.4.5 Current Literature for Great Auricular Nerve Block

Two randomized, double-blinded studies have demonstrated that the great auricular nerve block provides the same degree of pain relief as intravenous morphine with lower incidence of vomiting [7, 8]. However, the use of this block as a preemptive analgesic measure did not show any benefit in terms of quality or duration of postoperative analgesia in children undergoing tympanomastoid surgery [8].

Clinical Pearls

- Care should be taken to avoid intravascular injection and deep cervical nerve block.
- There is also a potential for phrenic nerve blockade.

16.5 Case Study

Superficial Cervical Plexus Block (*Provided by S. Suresh*)

A 12-year-old male, 17.5 kg in weight, presented for cochlear implant placement. The patient had undergone a hearing test and had a past history of sensorineural deafness. A tympanomastoidectomy, lasting 3 h, 25 min, was performed. A landmark-based superficial cervical plexus block was performed at the posterior border of the sternocleidomastoid and at the level of the cricoid cartilage (see Fig. 16.11). A subcutaneous injection was completed with the needle pointed cephalad. A 27G needle was used, and 2 mL 0.25 % bupivacaine was injected; duration of the block was 12 h. An additional 0.5 mg of morphine was given for pain and postoperative recovery was excellent with no PONV.

References

1. Zeidan A, Hayek F. Correspondence: nerve stimulator-guided cervical plexus block for carotid endarterectomy. Anesthesia. 2007;62:299–300.
2. Perisanidis C, Saranteas T, Kostopanagiotou G. Ultrasound-guided combined intermediate and deep cervical plexus nerve block for regional anesthesia in oral and maxillofacial surgery. Dentomaxillofac Radiol. 2013;42:29945724.
3. Tobias JD. Cervical plexus block in adolescents. J Clin Anesth. 1999;11:606–8.
4. Soeding P, Eizenberg N. Review article: anatomical considerations for ultrasound guidance for regional anesthesia of the neck and upper limb. Can J Anesth. 2009;56:518–33.
5. Sandeman DJ, Griffiths MJ, Lennox AF. Ultrasound guided deep cervical plexus block. Anaesth Intensive Care. 2006;34:240–4.
6. Brownlow RC, Berman J, Brown Jr RE. Superficial cervical block for cervical node biopsy in a child with a large mediastinal mass. J Ark Med Soc. 1994;90:378–9.
7. Suresh S, Barcelona SL, Young NM, et al. Postoperative pain relief in children undergoing tympanomastoid surgery: is a regional block better than opioids? Anesth Analg. 2002;94:859–62.
8. Suresh S, Barcelona SL, Young NM, et al. Does a preemptive block of the great auricular nerve improve postoperative analgesia in children undergoing tympanomastoid surgery? Anesth Analg. 2004;98:330–3.

Suggested Reading

Belvis D, Voronov P, Suresh S. Head and neck blocks in children. Tech Reg Anesth Pain Manag. 2007;11(4):208–14.

Dalens B. Blocks of nerves supplying the head and neck. In: Dalens B, editor. Pediatric regional anesthesia. Boca Raton: CRC; 1990. p. 465–8.

Dalens B. Blocks of the head, face, and neck. In: Dalens B, editor. Regional anesthesia in infants, children, and adolescents. Philadelphia: Lippincott Williams & Wilkins; 1995. p. 440–5.

Suresh S, Voronov P. Head and neck blocks in infants, children, adolescents. Pediatr Anesth. 2012;22(1):81–7.

Occipital Nerve Blocks

17

Ban C.H. Tsui

Contents

B.C.H. Tsui, Dip Eng, BSc (Math), B Pharm, MSc, MD, FRCPC
Department of Anesthesiology and Pain Medicine,
Stollery Children's Hospital/University of Alberta Hospital,
2-150 Clinical Sciences Building, Edmonton,
AB T6G 2G3, Canada
e-mail: btsui@ualberta.ca

B.C.H. Tsui, S. Suresh (eds.), *Pediatric Atlas of Ultrasound- and Nerve Stimulation-Guided Regional Anesthesia*,
DOI 10.1007/978-0-387-79964-3_17

17.1 Indications

Anesthetizing the greater occipital nerve provides analgesia for:

- Occipital craniotomy
- Shunt revision
- Diagnosis and treatment of occipital neuralgia and cervicogenic headaches.

Combined lesser occipital and great auricular nerve blocks are indicated for postoperative analgesia for:

- Otoplasty

17.2 Block Techniques

The greater occipital nerve lies medial to the occipital artery which forms a reference point [1] for both ultrasound guidance (not shown here) and the landmark technique when performing these blocks (Figs. 17.1 and 17.2). Since the nerve can be relatively easily located medially to the palpable occipital artery along the superior nuchal line, a simple landmark approach with careful and frequent aspiration between injections is often sufficient. However, an ultrasound-guided approach has been described [2].

17.2.1 Patient Positioning

- Supine with head turned to the contralateral direction.
- The head can be tilted forward slightly to expose the prominent nuchal ridge of bone at the posterior base of the skull.
- Can be completed with the patient prone in preparation for surgical position.

Fig. 17.1 Occipital nerve anatomy

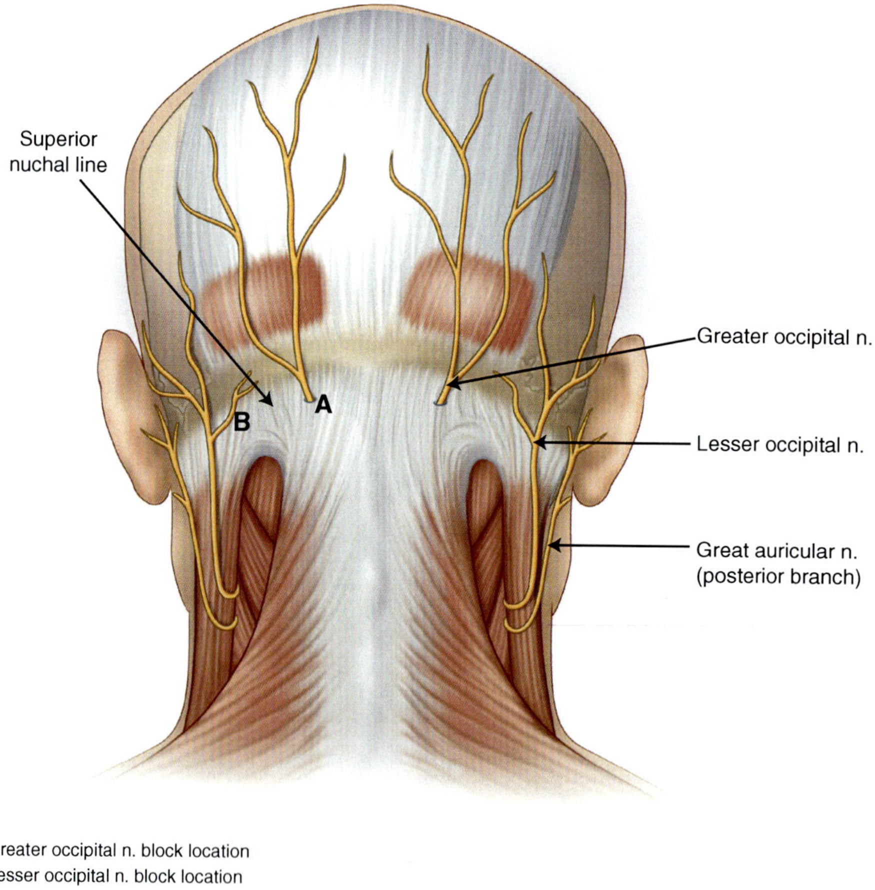

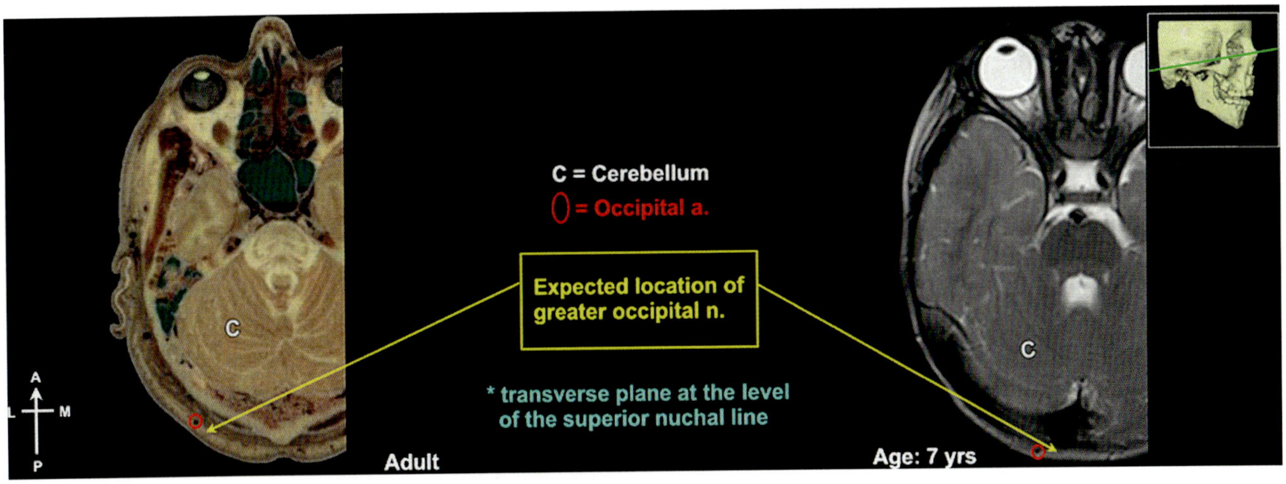

Fig. 17.2 VHVS and MRI images capturing the expected location of the greater occipital nerve

17.2.2 Landmarks and Surface Anatomy (Fig. 17.3)

- Greater occipital nerve: The nerve is typically located lateral (1–2 cm) and inferior (1–2 cm) to the external occipital protuberance. In adults, it is found one-third of the distance from the external occipital protuberance to the mastoid process [1], which will typically locate the lateral border of the insertion of the erector muscles of the neck. Alternatively, the nerve can be located directly medial to the easily palpated occipital artery.
- Lesser occipital nerve: This nerve is located lateral to the greater occipital nerve (approximately 2.5 cm in adolescent patients), along the inferior nuchal line.

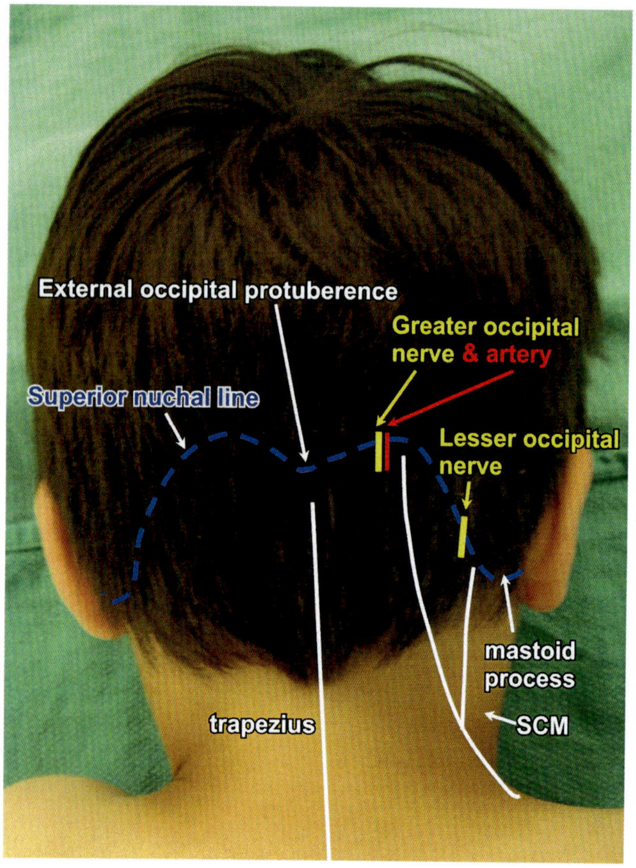

Fig. 17.3 Surface landmarks for greater and lesser occipital nerve blocks. *SCM* sternocleidomastoid muscle

17.2.3 Needle Insertion Technique (Figs. 17.4 and 17.5)

- A short, fine intradermal needle (e.g., 2–3 cm, 25G–27G) is introduced with a slight cranial angulation at each mark to the depth of the skull itself. Generally, the greater occipital nerve is the primary target, but if more anterior anesthesia of the scalp is required, the lesser occipital nerve branches are also blocked by advancing the needle subcutaneously from this point in an anterior direction toward the mastoid process.

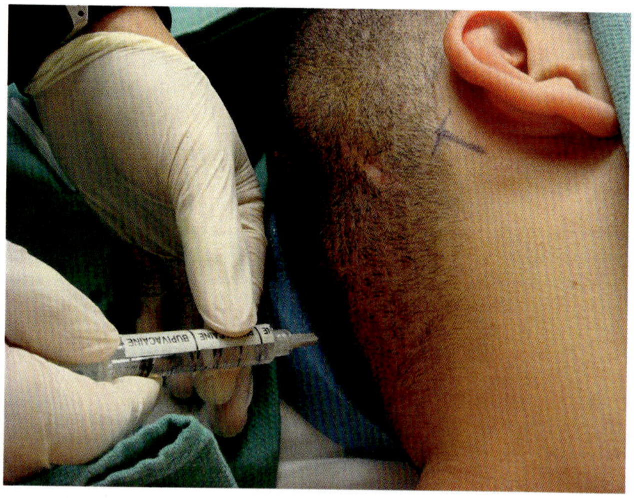

Fig. 17.4 Surface anatomy and needle insertion for greater occipital nerve block

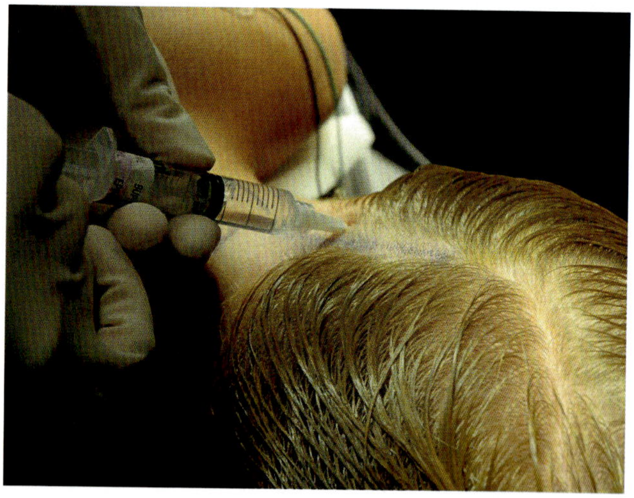

Fig. 17.5 Surface anatomy and needle direction for lesser occipital nerve block

17.2.4 Local Anesthetic Application

- After slight withdrawal after bone contact, local anesthetic is injected (e.g., 0.5–1 mL of 0.5–1 % lidocaine for diagnostic procedures or 2–3 mL of 0.125–0.25 % bupivacaine with epinephrine 1:400,000 for therapeutic procedures) after aspiration.
- A fanlike injection can be used, with gentle massage of the area to allow adequate spread of local anesthetic.
- For lesser occipital nerve anesthesia, a band of anesthetic solution can be deposited along the line between skin entry and the mastoid process using 2–3 mL of local anesthetic.

Clinical Pearl
Complications with this technique are rare. Care must be taken not to advance the needle anteriorly under the skull, as the foramen magnum might be entered unintentionally with a long needle. Local hematoma may be produced with superficial injection, but this is only a temporary problem.

17.3 Current Literature in Ultrasound-Guided Approaches

A recent cadaveric study compared two techniques of ultrasound guidance for greater occipital nerve block, using both the traditional block site and a selective approach at a proximal location where the nerve curls around the lower border of the obliquus capitis inferior muscle after emerging below the posterior arch of the atlas [2]. A transverse midline orientation is initially used to identify the external occipital protuberance. A caudal scan is used to identify the spinous process of C2 by its bifid appearance. A lateral rotation of the transducer is used to locate the obliquus capitis inferior muscle. The nerve is identified during its cranial course where it lies superficial to the muscle. Reported success of the simulated block, defined by spread of dye to the nerve, was 80 % using the traditional landmarks compared to 100 % with the new selective technique. The selectivity of this block may be important in certain circumstances, for instance, in diagnosing occipital neuralgia. However, for most anesthesia purposes, the traditional block site is suitable.

17.4 Case Study

Occipital Nerve Block (*Provided by A. Sawardekar*)
A previously healthy 34-month-old boy, 16 kg in weight, presented to the emergency room with new onset of headache and blurred vision. A CT scan and MRI of the brain revealed a posterior fossa tumor. A posterior fossa craniotomy and tumor resection (glioma) was scheduled. A bilateral occipital nerve block was administered using a landmark approach with 22G needle and 3 mL 0.25 % bupivacaine injected into each side. Duration of the surgery was 280 min, and block duration was 12 h. No additional analgesics were needed. The patient received two additional doses of oral acetaminophen during the 24-h period following surgery.

References

1. Becser N, Bovim G, Sjaastad O. Extracranial nerves in the posterior part of the head. Anatomic variations and their possible clinical significance. Spine. 1998;23:1435–41.
2. Greher M, Moriggl B, Curatolo M, et al. Sonographic visualization and ultrasound-guided blockade of the greater occipital nerve: a comparison of two selective techniques confirmed by anatomical dissection. Br J Anaesth. 2010;104:637–42.

Suggested Reading

Belvis D, Voronov P, Suresh S. Head and neck blocks in children. Tech Reg Anesth Pain Manag. 2007;11(4):208–14.
Suresh S, Polaner DM, Cote CJ. Regional Anesthesia. In: Cote CJ, Lerman J, Anderson BJ, Eds. 5th ed. Philadelphia: WB Saunders; 2013. p. 835–79.
Suresh S, Voronov P. Head and neck blocks in infants, children, adolescents. Pediatr Anesth. 2012;22(1):81–7.

18 Blockade of the Auricular Branch of the Vagus Nerve (Nerve of Arnold)

Ban C.H. Tsui

Contents

B.C.H. Tsui, Dip Eng, BSc (Math), B Pharm, MSc, MD, FRCPC
Department of Anesthesiology and Pain Medicine,
Stollery Children's Hospital/University of Alberta Hospital,
2-150 Clinical Sciences Building, Edmonton,
AB T6G 2G3, Canada
e-mail: btsui@ualberta.ca

B.C.H. Tsui, S. Suresh (eds.), *Pediatric Atlas of Ultrasound- and Nerve Stimulation-Guided Regional Anesthesia*,
DOI 10.1007/978-0-387-79964-3_18

18.1 Indications

Blockade of the nerve of Arnold can be used in children undergoing myringotomy and tube placement, tympanostomy, and paper patch myringoplasty.

18.2 Block Technique

Since the nerve can be easy to block at the tragus of the ear and the injection is superficial in nature, a simple landmark-based approach is commonly used and is described here.

18.2.1 Patient Positioning

- Supine with the head turned to the contralateral side.

18.2.2 Landmarks and Surface Anatomy (Figs. 18.1 and 18.2)

- The tragus of the ear is identified and pulled forward.

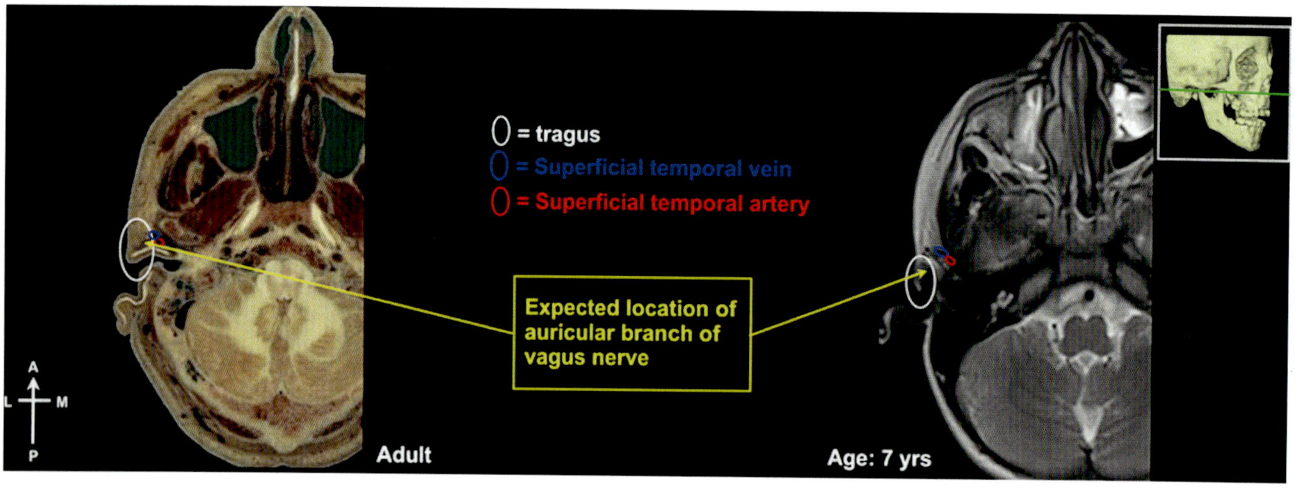

Fig. 18.1 VHVS and MRI images of the expected location of the auricular branch of the vagus nerve (nerve of Arnold)

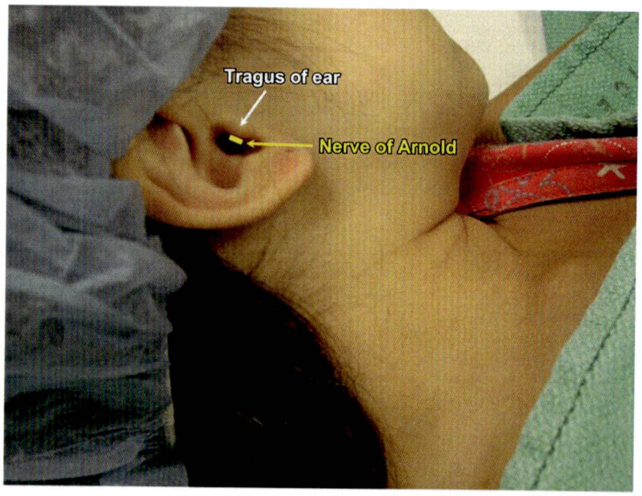

Fig. 18.2 Patient positioning and surface landmarks for nerve of Arnold block

18.2.3 Needle Insertion Technique

- A 30G needle is inserted into the posterior tragus, approximately 45° to the horizontal (Fig. 18.3).

18.2.4 Local Anesthetic Application

- Inject local anesthetic solution (e.g., 0.2–0.3 mL of 0.25 % bupivacaine with epinephrine 1: 200,000 or 0.2–0.3 mL of 2 % lidocaine with epinephrine 1: 200,000) after aspiration.

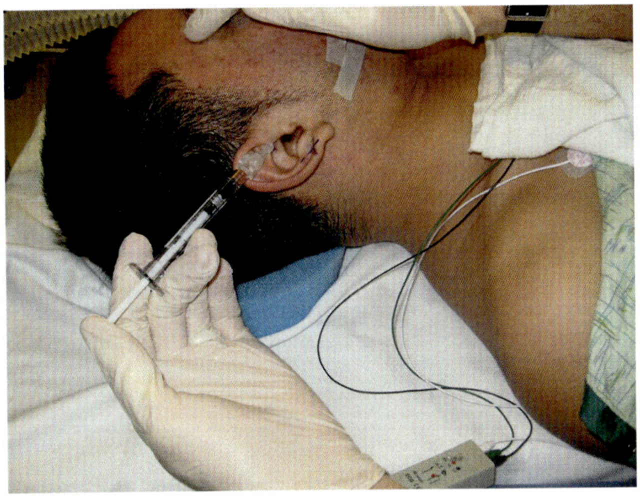

Fig. 18.3 Surface anatomy and needle direction for nerve of Arnold block

18.3 Current Literature in Ultrasound-Guided Approaches

This novel regional technique was investigated in a randomized, double-blinded study comparing children receiving the nerve of Arnold block or intranasal fentanyl for myringotomy. No difference was found in postoperative pain relief, amount of rescue analgesics used, nausea and vomiting, or time to discharge between groups [1].

18.4 Case Study

Nerve of Arnold Block (*Provided by S. Suresh*)

A 16-year-old male, weighing 59.3 kg, with a past medical history of hearing loss, was diagnosed with bilateral otitis media and long-standing bilateral tympanic membrane perforations based on an audiogram and binocular microscopy. The patient was scheduled for tympanoplasty. A nerve of Arnold block was performed with a 27G needle and an injection of 0.3 mL 2 % lidocaine (see Fig. 18.3). Surgery lasted two and a half hours; block duration was 3.5 h. The patient rated his pain as 3/10 20 min postoperatively and 0/10 at discharge. Ketorolac (Toradol) injection (30 mg) was provided for postoperative analgesia.

Reference

1. Voronov P, Tobin MJ, Billings K, et al. Postoperative pain relief in infants undergoing myringotomy and tube placement: comparison of a novel regional anesthetic block to intranasal fentanyl-a pilot analysis. Ped Anesth. 2008;18:1196–201.

Suggested Reading

Belvis D, Voronov P, Suresh S. Head and neck blocks in children. Tech Reg Anesth Pain Manag. 2007;11(4):208–14.

Suresh S, Voronov P. Head and neck blocks in infants, children, adolescents. Pediatr Anesth. 2012;22(1):86–7.

Part V

Nerve Blocks Above the Clavicle

Interscalene Brachial Plexus Block

19

Ban C.H. Tsui

Contents

B.C.H. Tsui, Dip Eng, BSc (Math), B Pharm, MSc, MD, FRCPC
Department of Anesthesiology and Pain Medicine,
Stollery Children's Hospital/University of Alberta Hospital,
2-150 Clinical Sciences Building, Edmonton,
AB T6G 2G3, Canada
e-mail: btsui@ualberta.ca

B.C.H. Tsui, S. Suresh (eds.), *Pediatric Atlas of Ultrasound- and Nerve Stimulation-Guided Regional Anesthesia*,
DOI 10.1007/978-0-387-79964-3_19

19.1 Indications

The interscalene approach to brachial plexus blockade targets the roots and proximal trunks of the plexus between the anterior and middle scalene muscles at the level of the sixth cervical vertebra (C6) (see Figs. 10.1 and 10.2) and provides anesthesia to the upper arm including the shoulder. While the interscalene approach may fail to anesthetize the distal roots of the plexus, it consistently anesthetizes the axillary and musculocutaneous nerves, which are frequently missed when performing an axillary block.

Indications

- Shoulder and humerus surgery

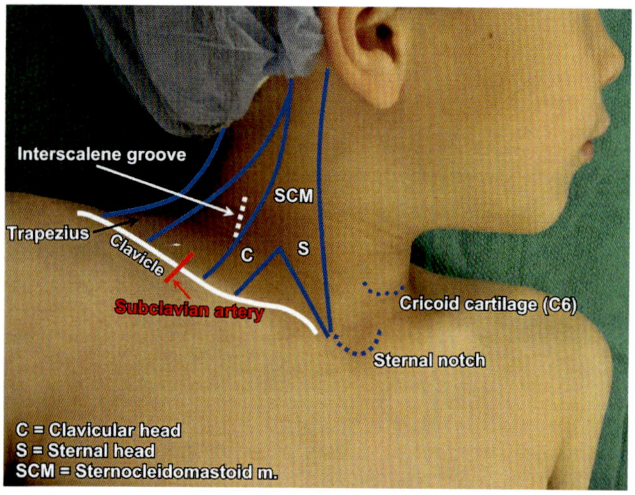

Fig. 19.1 Patient positioning and surface landmarks for interscalene brachial plexus block

19.2 Surface Anatomy (Fig. 19.1)

19.2.1 Patient Positioning

The patient lies supine with the head rotated approximately 45° to the nonoperative side after general anesthesia has been induced. Surface landmarks include:

- Clavicular head of the sternocleidomastoid muscle:
  - The lateral border of the sternocleidomastoid muscle marks the location of the anterior scalene muscle. This portion of the sternocleidomastoid muscle can be accentuated by asking the child to reach in the direction of the ipsilateral knee before induction of general anesthesia.
- Interscalene groove:
  - The groove is located between the anterior and middle scalene muscles approximately 1 cm above the separation of the sternal and clavicular heads of the sternocleidomastoid muscle. The anterior scalene muscle lies immediately behind the lateral border of the clavicular head of the sternocleidomastoid muscle at the level of the cricoid cartilage (C6). The groove is made more pronounced by asking older children to raise the head or take a deep breath while awake.
- Chassaignac's tubercle:
  - The anterior tubercle on the C6 vertebra is located at the intersection of the interscalene groove with the transverse plane of the cricoid cartilage. This landmark is more applicable in adolescents (whose vertebrae are better developed).

When using the interscalene approach, the point of needle insertion is at the level of C6 within the interscalene groove. For the parascalene approach, a line is drawn between the midpoint of the clavicle and the transverse process of C6. The needle insertion site is two-thirds of the way down this line, near the external jugular vein.

19.3 Nerve Stimulation Technique (Tables 14.1 and 19.1)

Table 19.1 Responses and recommended needle adjustments for use during nerve stimulation at the interscalene level

Correct response to nerve stimulation
Twitches elicited from the upper and middle trunks (pectoralis, deltoid, biceps brachii muscles) and middle and lower trunks (triceps, forearm or hand muscles) with current intensity of at least 0.4 mA (0.1–0.3 ms) verify stimulation of the brachial plexus
Other common responses and needle adjustments
Muscle twitch from electrical stimulation
Neck (anterior scalene or sternocleidomastoid)
Explanation: needle usually anteromedial to plexus
Needle adjustment: withdraw needle to subcutaneous tissue and reinsert in a 10–20° more posterior angle
Diaphragm (phrenic nerve)
Explanation: needle plane is too anterior
Needle adjustment: withdraw needle to subcutaneous tissue and reinsert in a 15° more posterior angle
Scapula (thoracodorsal nerve to serratus anterior muscle)
Explanation: needle tip is too posterior and deep to brachial plexus
Needle adjustment: withdraw to subcutaneous tissue and reinsert in a more anterior plane
Trapezius (accessory nerve)
Explanation: needle tip too posterior to plexus
Needle adjustment: withdraw to subcutaneous tissue and reinsert in a more anterior plane
Bone contact
Needle stops a depth of 1–2 cm (transverse process of cervical vertebrae or first rib), without twitches
Explanation: needle shaft angle is too posterior and touching anterior tubercles
Needle adjustment: withdraw to subcutaneous tissue and reinsert in a 15° more anterior angle
Vascular puncture
Most commonly carotid artery puncture; seen as arterial blood aspiration
Explanation: needle angle and tip anterior to plexus
Needle adjustment: withdraw completely for pressure treatment and reinsert tip 1–2 cm posterior
Alternative explanation: vertebral artery puncture. Especially a risk in OOP technique or when *there is difficulty with needle tip visualization* in either plane
Needle adjustment: needle tip is too medial, must be withdrawn and reinserted laterally

19.3.1 Needle Insertion

A flowchart illustrating the needle insertion site and procedures is shown in Fig. 19.2.

- A 22G–25G, 30–35 mm (depending on the age and size of the child), short-beveled needle is inserted at an acute angle relative to the skin surface and directed medially, posteriorly, and caudally.
- In children, the compact arrangement of anatomical structures within the neck may warrant a modified, angled needle insertion (as compared to the perpendicular orientation often used in adults) in order to prevent inadvertent puncture of the vertebral artery or epidural/subarachnoid space [1].

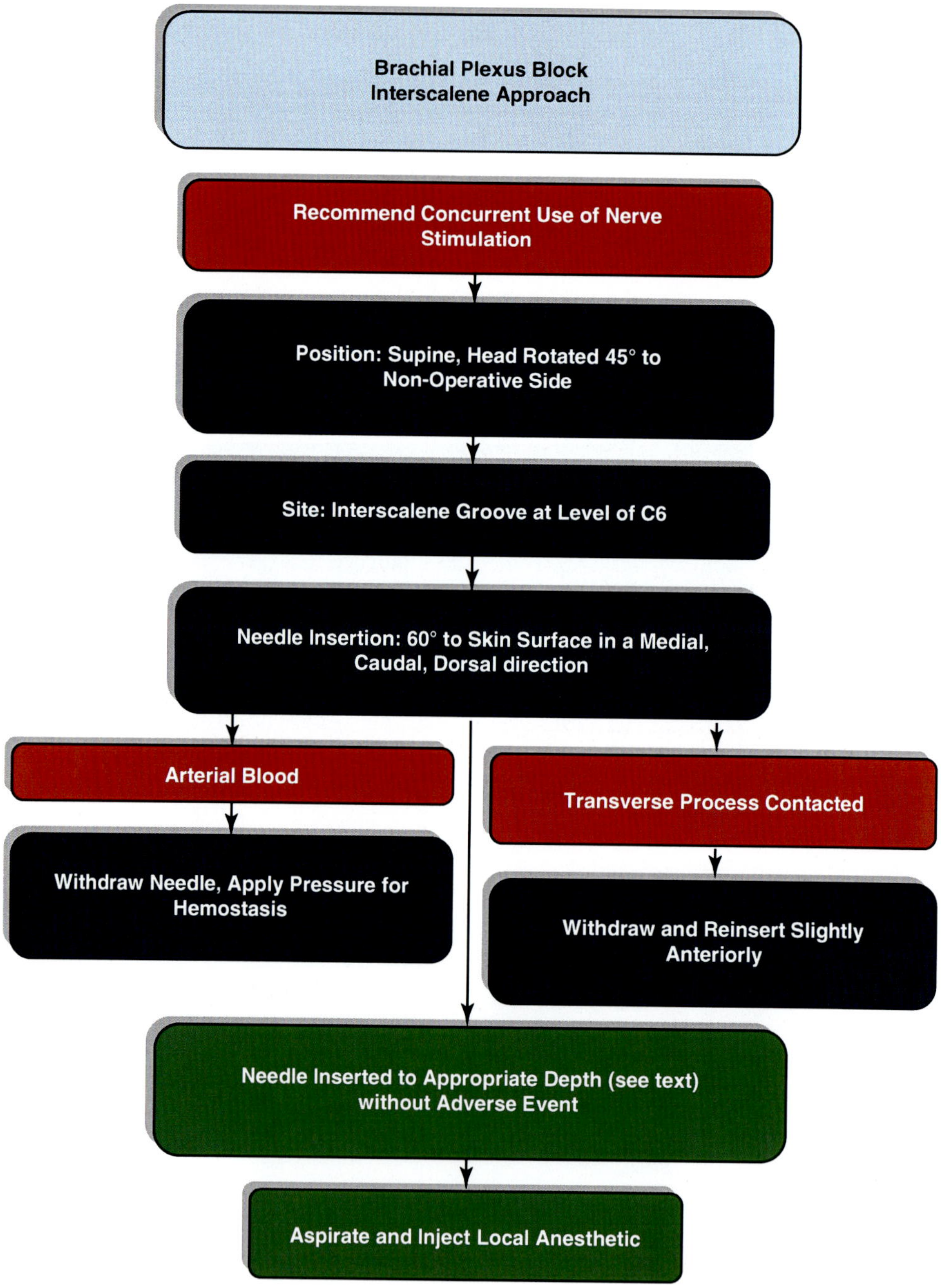

Fig. 19.2 Flowchart of needle insertion and procedures for an interscalene brachial plexus block

Clinical Pearl

- Needle insertion below C6 has been described (including the parascalene approach described by Dalens et al. [2]); both approaches are successful.
- For the parascalene approach, a line is drawn between the midpoint of the clavicle and the transverse process of C6 (Chassaignac's tubercle). The needle is inserted perpendicular to the skin two-thirds of the way down this line near the external jugular vein.

19.3.2 Current Application and Appropriate Responses

Figure 19.3 illustrates the procedure for employing nerve stimulation techniques for interscalene brachial plexus block.

- Applying an initial current of 0.8–1.0 mA (2 Hz, 0.1–0.3 msec) is sufficient for stimulation of the plexus.
- After obtaining the appropriate motor response, the current is reduced to aim for a threshold current of 0.4 mA (0.1–0.2 msec).
- Motor response cessation at currents less than 0.2 mA indicates the needle is probably intraneural.
- Twitches elicited from the upper and middle trunks (pectoralis, deltoid, biceps brachii muscles) and lower trunks (triceps, forearm, and hand muscles) verify stimulation of the brachial plexus.

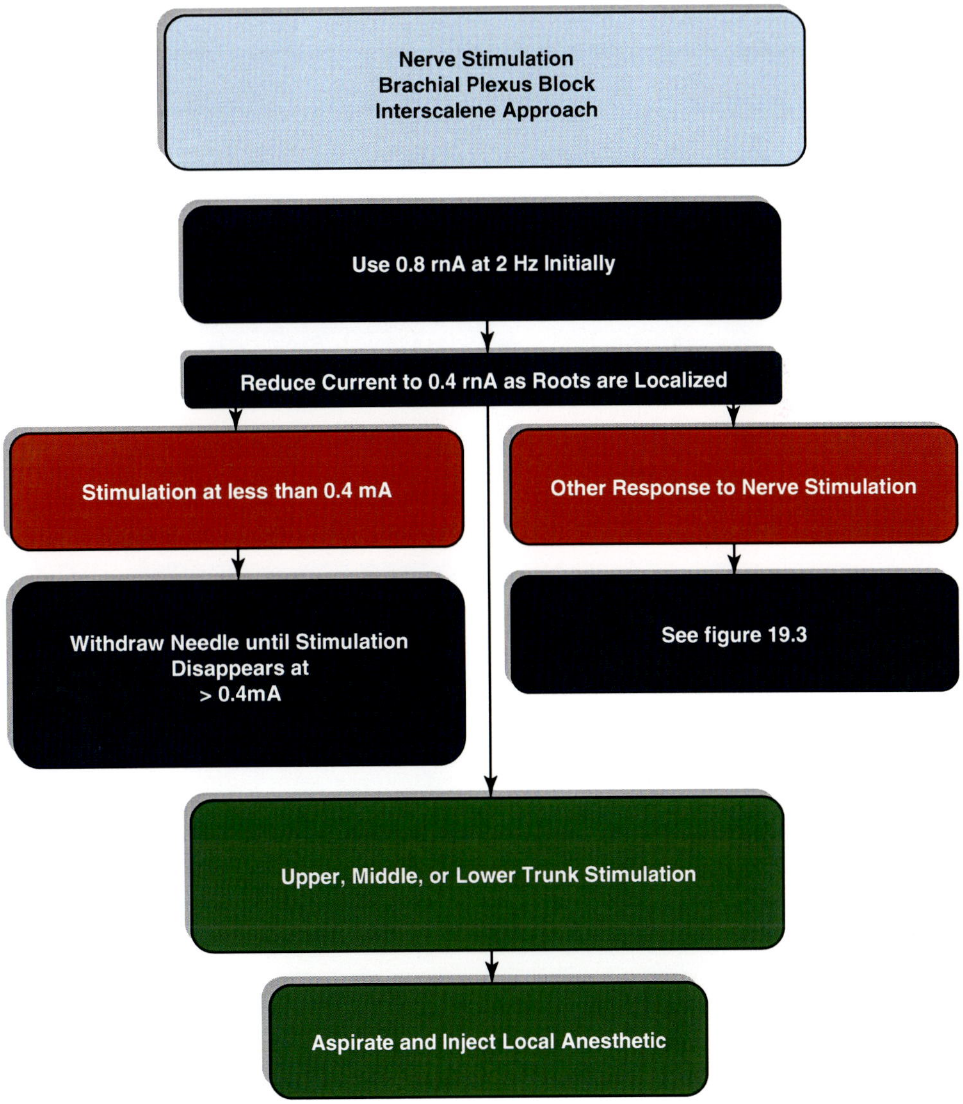

Fig. 19.3 Flowchart of procedure for employing nerve stimulation techniques for interscalene brachial plexus block

19.3.3 Modifications to Inappropriate Responses

An algorithm of modifications to inappropriate responses to nerve stimulation is shown in Fig. 19.4.

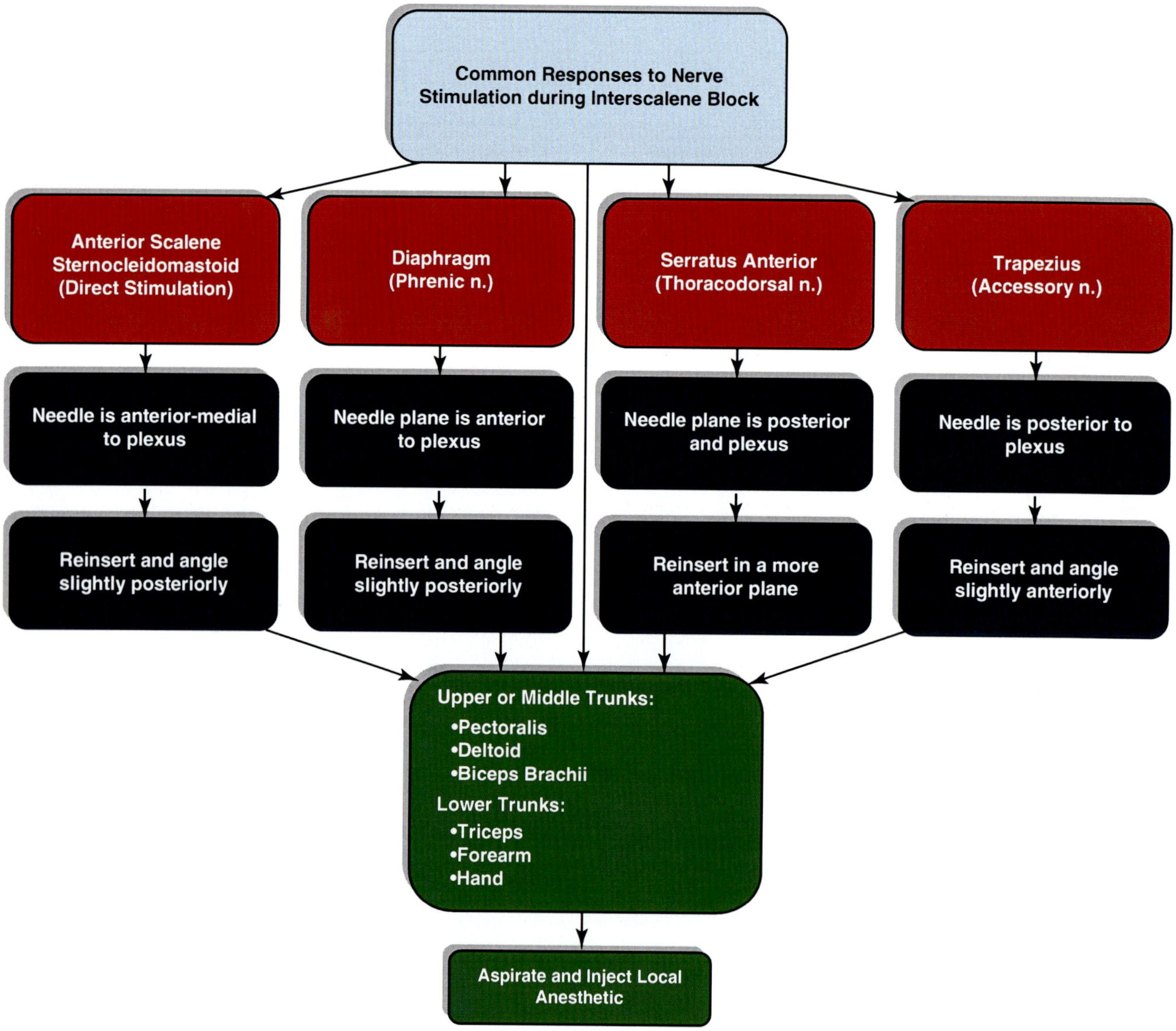

Fig. 19.4 Flowchart of modifications to inappropriate responses to nerve stimulation during interscalene block

19.4 Ultrasound-Guided Technique

For a summary of ultrasound-guided interscalene block techniques, see Fig. 19.5. Major anatomical structures in the brachial plexus as captured by MRI and VHVS images are shown with the corresponding ultrasound image in Fig. 19.6.

The roots of the plexus are clearly visible in the ultrasound image with corresponding cadaveric and MRI images. Table 19.2 summarizes particular imaging considerations in pediatric populations. Patient positioning and anatomical landmarks are the same for ultrasound techniques as they are for landmark and nerve stimulation techniques. If nerve stimulation is employed in conjunction with ultrasound imaging, the previous section can be referred to for appropriate responses and modifications.

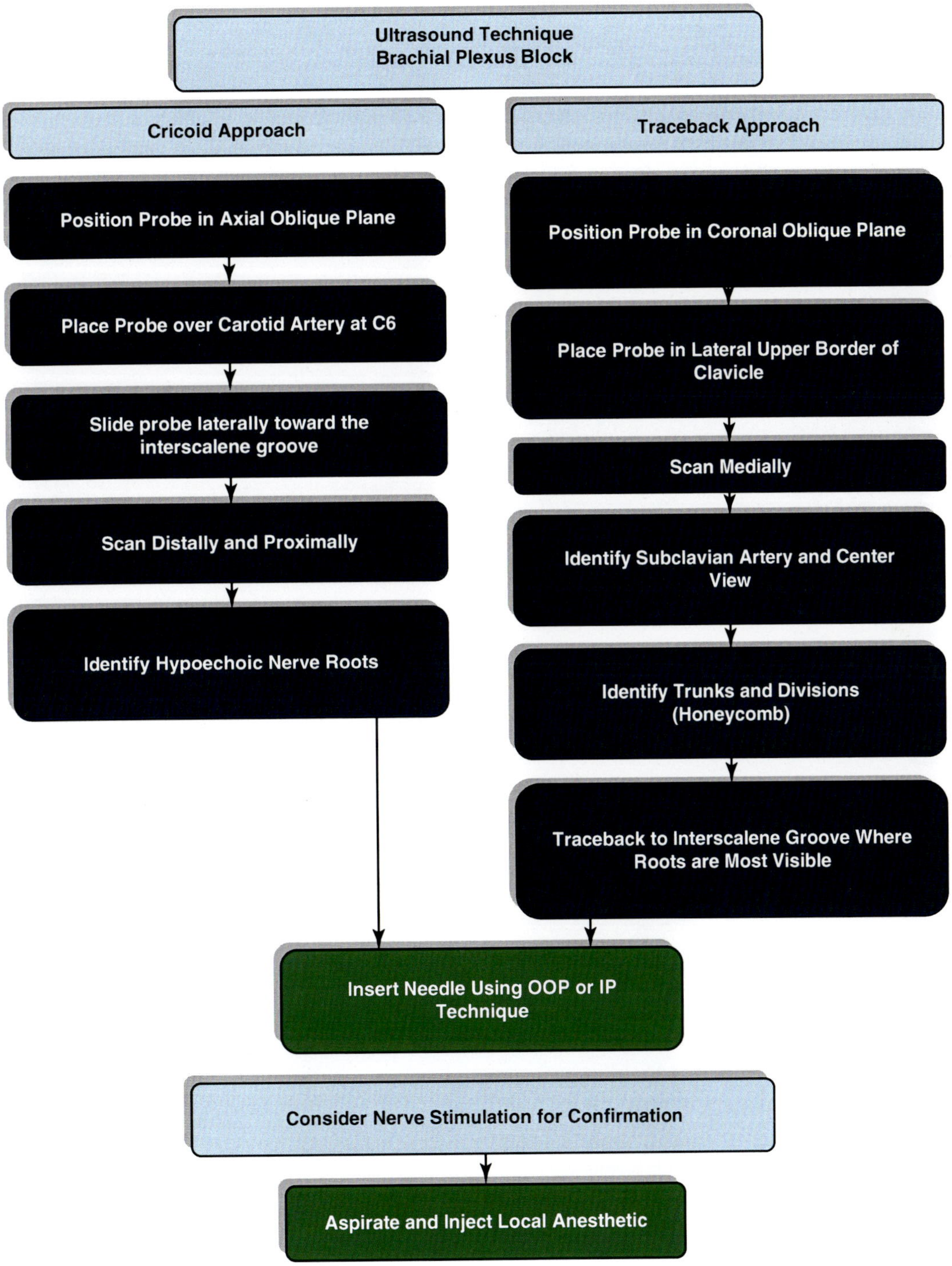

Fig. 19.5 Flowchart of ultrasound-guided techniques in interscalene blocks

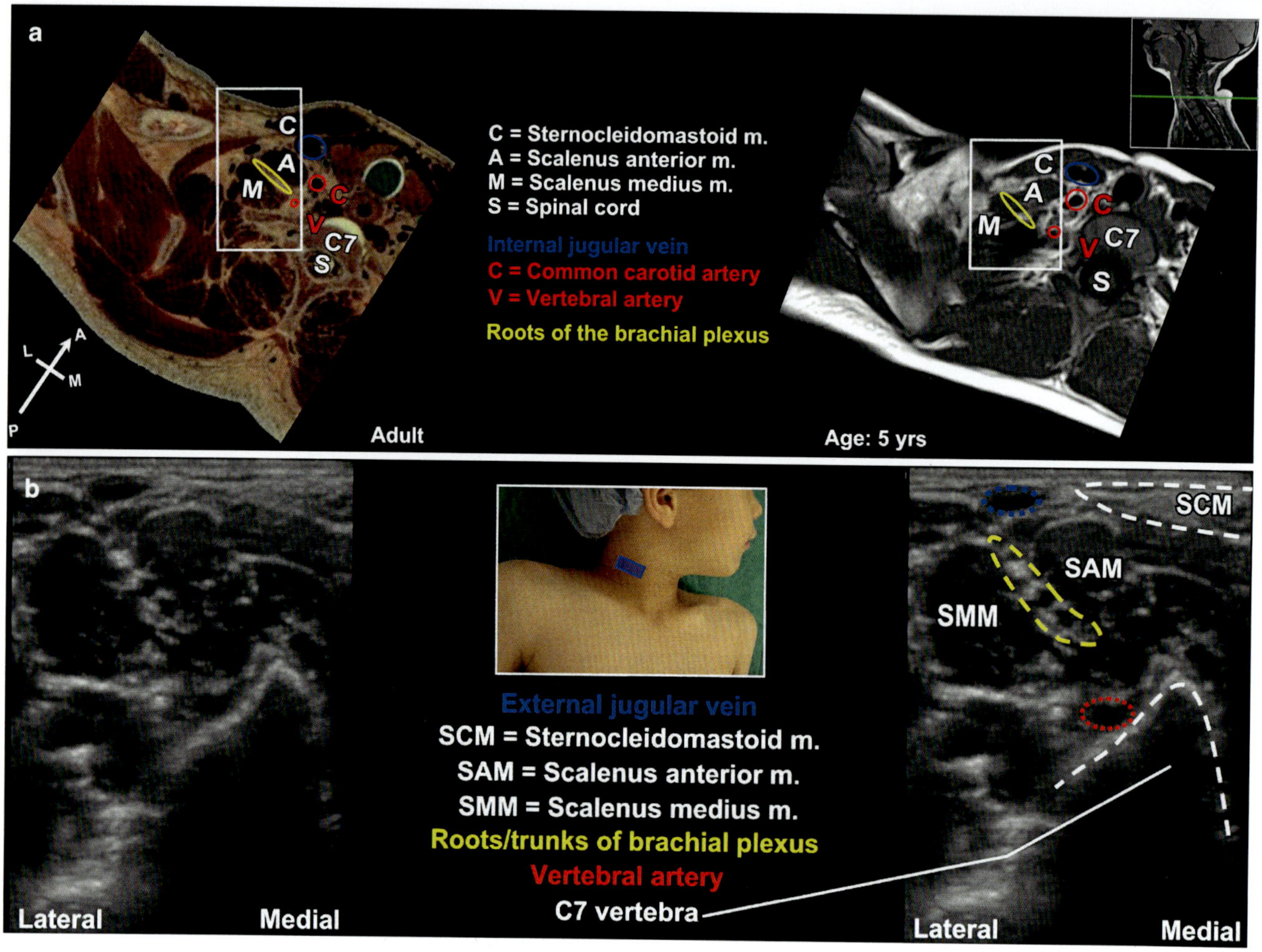

Fig. 19.6 (**a**) VHVS and MRI images of anatomical structures in the brachial plexus. (**b**) Ultrasound image of the brachial plexus at the interscalene groove

Table 19.2 Anatomical and imaging considerations for interscalene block

Pediatric patients	Adult patients
• The proximity of vascular structures and the brachial plexus increases the risk of vascular puncture, especially of the vertebral artery	• There is a relatively greater distance between the vascular and neural structures
• The interscalene groove is not always at the lateral border of the sternocleidomastoid muscle; it can be situated medially or laterally. Therefore, the "traceback" technique is recommended for localization (see text)	• The interscalene groove is usually located at the lateral border of the sternocleidomastoid muscle
• All roots of the brachial plexus can be visualized with ultrasonography, especially in small children	• C5 to C7 roots can be easily identified using ultrasonography, whereas C8 to T1 roots are rarely visible
• Roots of the brachial plexus are situated relatively superficially at the level of the interscalene block; in very young children, these roots may be only a few millimeters beneath the skin	• Roots of the brachial plexus are situated relatively deeply
• A parascalene approach to the brachial plexus has been described, which may reduce the risk of vascular injection and sparing the adjacent nerves (i.e., phrenic), pleura, epidural/spinal spaces, and spinal cord in pediatric patients when compared to the landmark technique of interscalene and supraclavicular block	• The parascalene approach can also be used safely in adults. However, with ultrasound guidance, pertinent structures could be avoided and a smaller volume of local anesthetic can be used. This may spare the phrenic nerve

19.4.1 Preparing the Site

Prepare the needle insertion site and skin surface with an antiseptic solution.

Prepare the ultrasound probe surface by applying a sterile adhesive dressing to it prior to needling as discussed in Chap. 4.

19.4.2 Scanning Technique

A high-frequency (10–5 MHz) hockey stick or linear transducer (13–6 MHz) is recommended to delineate the complex arrangements of the superficial structures in this region.

- The use of color Doppler ultrasound can be of great assistance to confirm the location of the carotid artery and internal jugular vein (for the cricoid cartilage approach) or the subclavian artery (for the traceback approach).

Two scanning techniques for interscalene brachial plexus imaging are described below:

19.4.2.1 Cricoid Cartilage Approach

- With the probe in an axial oblique plane, begin the scan in the interscalene groove at the level of the cricoid cartilage (C6), and move the probe proximally and distally.
- Note the apparent change in size of the anterior scalene muscle, from smaller proximally above C6 to larger distally. Also note the hypoechoic nerve roots as they emerge from the intervertebral foramina.
- It may be difficult to visualize the neural structures in young children using this approach due to the variability of the location of the brachial plexus. It may be beneficial to scan the neck inferiorly to the supraclavicular region to identify the nerve structures, which appear as a cluster of hypoechoic structures and resemble a "bunch of grapes" (see traceback approach below).

19.4.2.2 Traceback Approach (Fig. 19.7)

- The probe is positioned in a coronal oblique plane at the midpoint to medial aspect of the upper border of the clavicle.
- The pulsating subclavian artery becomes visible. (The probe may have to be moved laterally while maintaining contact with the clavicle.) Doppler ultrasound can greatly assist with identification of this structure.
- The probe is adjusted to place the subclavian artery in the center of the image. The brachial plexus (trunks/divisions) can be seen in short axis as a tightly enclosed cluster (i.e., a honeycomb-like arrangement), superior and lateral to the subclavian artery.
- The image can be optimized by tilting the probe anteriorly or posteriorly.
- The scanning angle is maintained as the plexus is traced in a cephalad direction along the interscalene groove to the level of the cricoid cartilage (C6) to reveal a transverse view of the neural structures located deep to the sternocleidomastoid muscle between the anterior and middle scalene muscles.

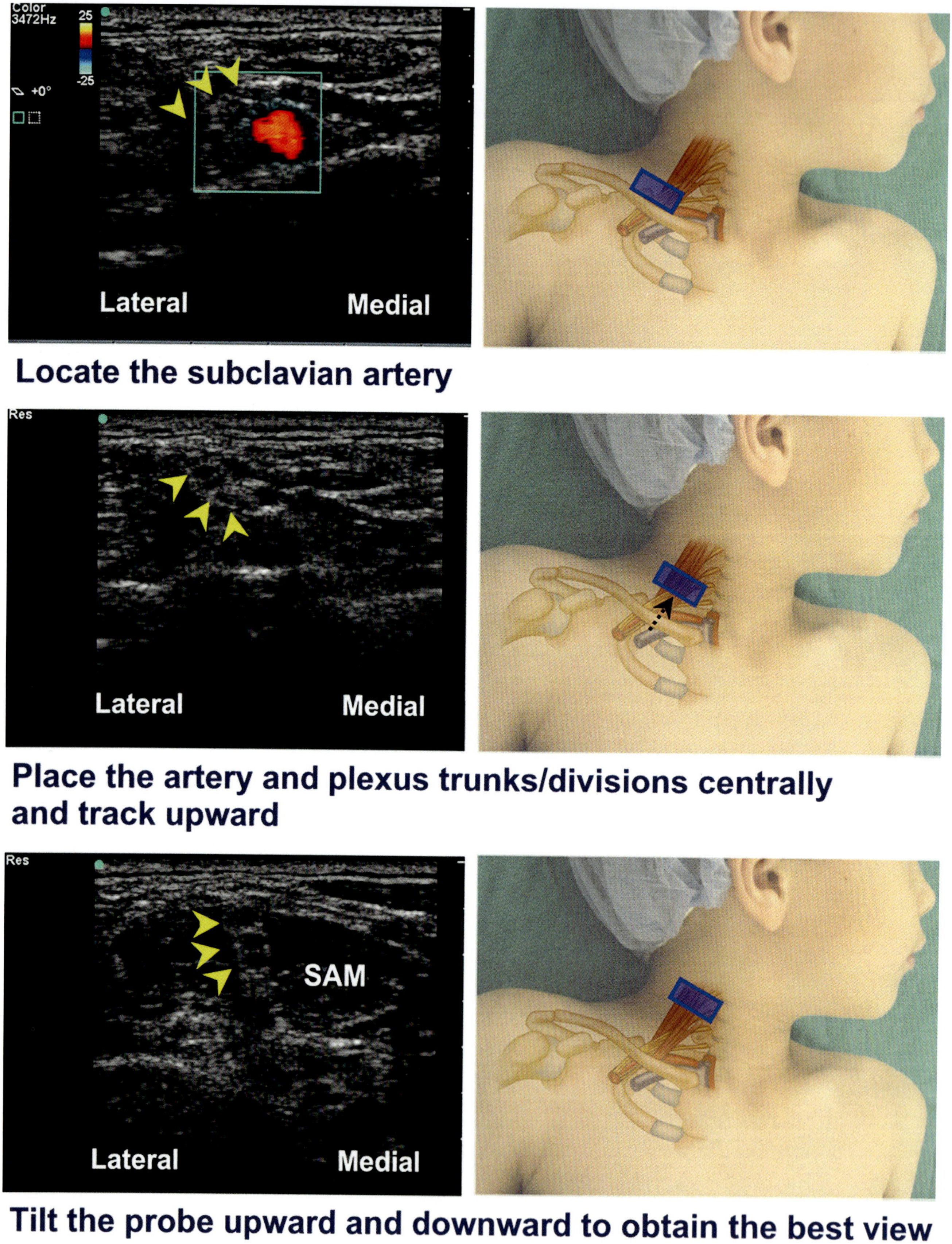

Fig. 19.7 Ultrasound traceback approach for interscalene block

19.4.3 Sonographic Appearance

- At the level of the cricoid cartilage and deep to the sternocleidomastoid muscle:
  - The common carotid artery is the pulsatile structure which appears circular while the internal jugular vein, superior and lateral to the artery, appears flatter in shape and is easily compressible; both are anechoic structures.
  - The nerve/plexus structures are located posterolateral to the vessels.
- At the interscalene groove in the short-axis view (Fig. 19.6):
  - If using a traceback approach, the cluster or "honeycomb" image will become multiple distinct round or oval hypoechoic structures as the probe is traced cephalad.
  - The sternocleidomastoid muscle is triangular and superficial overlying the internal jugular vein and common carotid artery. The structures are clearly discernible; the anechoic vessels appear dark and the artery appears pulsatile.
  - Lateral to the vessels and posterior to the sternocleidomastoid muscle lies the anterior scalene muscle. More posterolaterally, the middle and posterior scalene muscles appear as a single mass.
  - In a sagittal oblique section, brachial plexus *roots and/or trunks* are visualized most commonly as three (this number varies depending on the scan level) round or oval-shaped hypoechoic structures, sometimes with internal punctate echoes.
  - Scanning proximally and distally to capture a view of the most distal structures (C8/T1 roots or lower trunk) is useful since it will improve the chance of providing blockade of the entire plexus.
  - If the ultrasound field of view is large:
    - The hypoechoic C6 transverse process may be seen with an acoustic shadow effect beyond the level of the common carotid artery and directly medial to the middle scalene muscle (if visible at this high position in the neck).
    - The vertebral artery and vein may be seen deep to the plexus and anterior to the C6 transverse process. Occasionally, the vertebral vessels may only be seen at the C7 level, as they are located inside the transverse process at and above C6.

19.4.4 Needle Insertion

- Begin with local anesthetic infiltration of the skin.
- Use a 22G–25G, 30–35 mm short-beveled insulated block needle.
- In-plane (IP; long axis) approach (Fig. 19.8):
  - With the probe aligned to view the plexus in short axis, the needle is inserted from lateral to medial through the middle scalene muscle into the interscalene groove.
- Out-of-plane (OOP; short axis) approach (Fig. 19.9):
  - Although the OOP approach is described here, the IP approach is preferred to reduce the risk of complications with this block technique.
  - The probe should be placed with the brachial plexus centered in the middle of the ultrasound screen to ensure that needle insertion at the probe's midline will result in accurate needle placement.
  - With the clinician standing cephalad or caudad to the probe, determine the needle puncture site at a location cranial to the probe (in short axis to the plexus) and at a distance equal to the depth of the middle root.
  - Angle the needle incrementally in a stepwise fashion as follows:
    - Start with an angle of 10° to localize the needle tip as a bright dot on the ultrasound display. Withdraw the needle to the point where the needle tip disappears from view
    - Reinsert the needle caudally in a "walk-down" manner until the required depth is achieved and the needle tip is seen in proximity to the nerves.
    - If the initial puncture site is the same distance from the probe as the nerve target is from the skin, the approximate final angle of insertion (as calculated with simple trigonometry) will be 45°.
- For both IP and OOP approaches, scanning prior to needling will determine the angle, required trajectory distance, and vertical depth of needle penetration.
- A maximum depth should be less than 1–2 cm, even in mature teenage adolescents. A report described the roots of the brachial plexus as 0.4 cm deep in a 7-year-old child under ultrasound imaging [3].

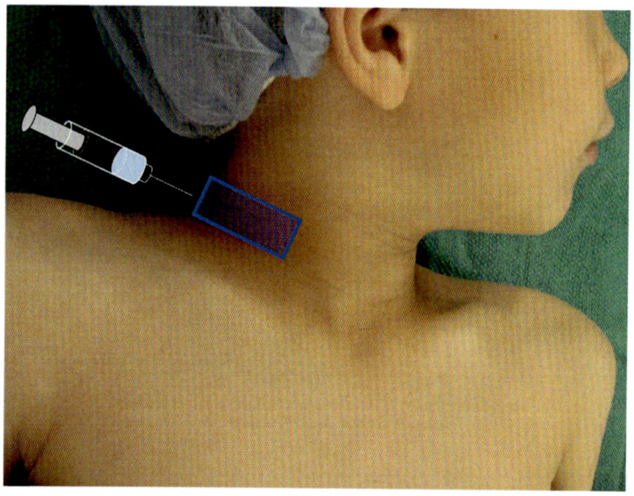

Fig. 19.8 In-plane needling technique for ultrasound-guided interscalene block. *Blue rectangle* indicates ultrasound probe footprint

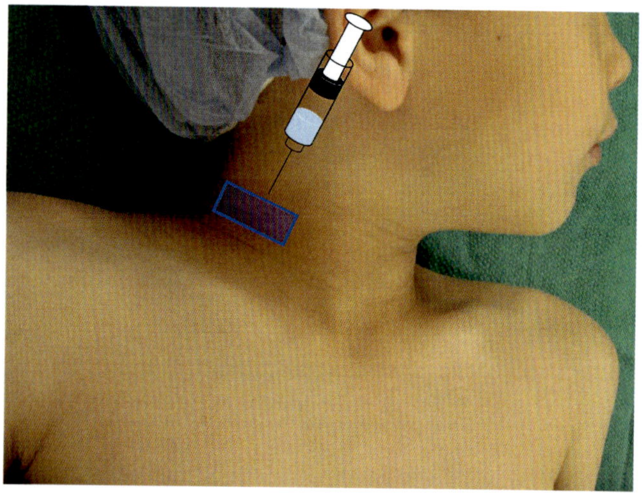

Fig. 19.9 Out-of-plane needling technique for ultrasound-guided interscalene block. *Blue rectangle* indicates ultrasound probe footprint

19.5 Local Anesthetic Application

- The authors typically use a 0.25 % bupivacaine solution at a 0.2–0.3 mL/kg without exceeding the maximum dose of 2 mg/kg.
- Different duration times of analgesic block were shown to be independent of the type and concentration of local anesthetic used (0.125–0.25 % bupivacaine or 0.1–0.2 % ropivacaine) in children who underwent shoulder arthroscopy. The duration of sensory block averaged 15±4.5 h [4].
- Epinephrine may be added at 1:200,000, although it is recommended to also note changes in the ST segment or T wave on the ECG for reliable indication of intravascular injection.

19.5.1 Clinical Pearls: Interscalene Block

- Nerve stimulation is recommended to confirm the identity of the nerve structures prior to the injection of local anesthetic.
- Performing a test dose with D5W is recommended prior to local anesthetic application to visualize the spread and confirm nerve localization. Flush the syringe and injection tubing adequately prior to this test, as residual air bubbles will cause sonographic artifacts that may reduce the image quality for subsequent local anesthetic injection. Deposit local anesthetic in the midst of the neural structures so that it spreads to surround the nerves circumferentially.
- Local anesthetic distention in this compartment is seen as a hypoechoic fluid expansion resulting in separation of the brachial plexus from its sheath.
- It is important to confirm a negative aspiration of blood and CSF prior to injection of local anesthetic since the brachial plexus at this location is in proximity to the vessels and subarachnoid space.
- In adults, it has been shown that a bolus injection of normal saline through an already-sited interscalene catheter is sufficient to reverse inadvertent phrenic nerve block and restore diaphragm function (see Sect. 8.4.2.1).

19.6 Current Literature in Ultrasound-Guided Approaches

A recent recommendation by the ASRA Practice Advisory on Neurologic Complications in Regional Anesthesia and Pain Medicine stated that interscalene block should not be performed in anesthetized or deeply sedated patients [5]. However, as DeVera et al. [6] stated in their correspondence, there is minimal advantage to performing interscalene blocks in children, who are unable to provide feedback of paresthesia. It is safer to perform interscalene blocks (and other peripheral nerve blocks) in anesthetized or deeply sedated children since they will not be a moving target. DeVera et al. reported their record of safety during the first 5 years, in which 1,657 upper- and lower-extremity peripheral nerve blocks were performed in children under general anesthesia as young as 2 months of age. Furthemore, a recent report from the Pediatric Regional Anesthesia Network (PRAN) concluded that placement of interscalene blocks in children under general anesthesia is no less safe than placement in awake adults [7].

There has been a paucity of literature on ultrasound-guided interscalene blocks. van Geffen et al. [3] reported an interesting case of a 7-year-old child with femur-fibula-ulna (FFU) syndrome with hypoplasia of the humerus. She had undergone a fistula resection of the proximal rudiment of the humerus at 3 years of age. She was scheduled for resection of a painful exostosis on the 2-cm-long humerus rudiment. Interscalene block under ultrasound guidance was performed using a high-frequency (10–5 MHz) linear probe. The roots of the brachial plexus were identified and 8 mL of 0.75 % ropivacaine was used, which provided 20 h of analgesia postoperatively. This case demonstrated the importance of ultrasound imaging for a peripheral nerve block, especially where nerve localization would have been difficult due to the absence of the musculature for motor response from nerve stimulation.

Recently, Fredrickson et al. [8] reported a case of an 11-year-old child with Erb's palsy who underwent extensive derotation humeral osteotomy for severe contracture deformity that was limiting external shoulder rotation. An interscalene catheter was inserted using ultrasound guidance as well as nerve stimulation (the stimulation threshold was 0.46 mA) with an OOP approach under general anesthesia. A bolus of 8 mL of 0.5 % ropivacaine was injected via the catheter, followed postoperatively by ropivacaine 0.2 % at 2 mL/h with on-demand boluses of 4 mL every 30 min to a maximum of 30 mL per 4 h. The child reported excellent postoperative analgesia without any opioid requirement, and the catheter was removed on postoperative day 2.

Another recent case report described the use of ultrasound-guided interscalene block for repair of a fractured lateral humeral condyle [9]. The patient, a 17-month-old child, was a poor candidate for general anesthesia due to an upper respiratory infection and drug-induced hepatitis. Together with 20 μg fentanyl and 50 mg thiopental sodium, the interscalene block – performed with a 25 mm, 24G needle and 1.5 mL 0.5 % ropivacaine – was sufficient for surgical anesthesia. No additional sedative or analgesic was needed, and the patient's postoperative pain was well-controlled.

19.7 Case Study

Interscalene Brachial Plexus Block (*Contributed by A. Sawardekar*)

A 13-year-old male, 65 kg, presented with a 6-week history of left upper arm pain. An MRI of the left arm revealed a mass of the left proximal humerus. An open biopsy and curettage of the mass was scheduled, and the patient received an ultrasound-guided interscalene brachial plexus block for the procedure. The block was administered in plane with a 22G needle and a 13–6 MHz linear high-frequency probe (see Fig. 19.10); 13 mL of 0.25 % bupivacaine was injected. Surgery lasted 120 min, and block duration was 8 h. No additional analgesics were required. The patient was discharged home after 2 h in the recovery room and was given instructions to take oral hydrocodone once sensation had returned to the operative extremity.

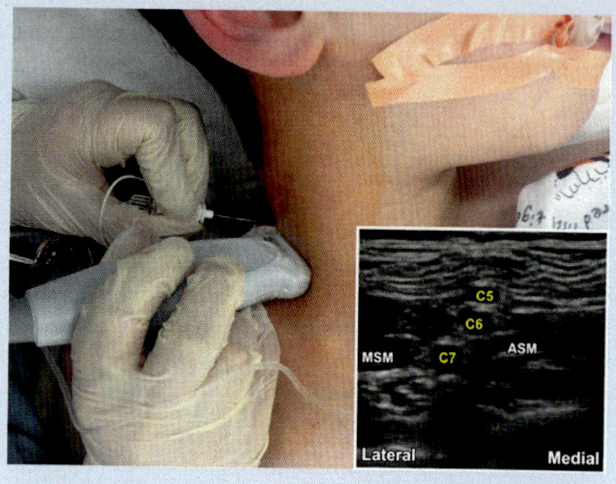

Fig. 19.10 Ultrasound-guided interscalene block. *MSM* middle scalene muscle, *ASM* anterior scalene muscle. See Case Study for details

References

1. Marhofer P. Upper extremity peripheral blocks. Tech Reg Anesth Pain Manag. 2007;11:215–21.
2. Dalens B, Vanneuville G, Tanguy A. A new parascalene approach to the brachial plexus in children: comparison with the supraclavicular approach. Anesth Analg. 1987;66:1264–71.
3. van Geffen GJ, Tielens L, Gielen M. Ultrasound-guided interscalene brachial plexus block in a child with femur fibula ulna syndrome. Pediatr Anesth. 2006;16:330–2.
4. Ganesh A, Wells L, Ganley T, et al. Interscalene brachial plexus block for post-operative analgesia following shoulder arthroscopy in children and adolescents. Acta Anaesthesiol Scand. 2008;52: 162–3.
5. Neal JM, Bernards CM, Hadzic A, et al. ASRA practice advisory on neurologic complications in regional anesthesia and pain medicine. Reg Anesth Pain Med. 2008;33:404–15.
6. Devera HV, Furukawa KT, Scavone JA, et al. Interscalene blocks in anesthetized pediatric patients. Reg Anesth Pain Med. 2009; 34:603–4.
7. Taenzer A, Walker BJ, Bosenberg AT, et al. Interscalene brachial plexus blocks under general anesthesia in children: is this safe practice? A report from the Pediatric Regional Anesthesia Network (PRAN). Reg Anesth Pain Med 2014;39:502–5.
8. Fredrickson MJ. Ultrasound-assisted interscalene catheter placement in a child. Anaesth Intensive Care. 2007;35:807–8.
9. Lee JH, Kim YR, Yu HK, et al. Ultrasound-guided interscalene brachial plexus block in a pediatric patient with acute hepatitis -a case report-. Korean J Anesthesiol. 2012;62:568–70.

Suggested Reading

Neal JM, Gerancher JC, Hebl JR, Ilfeld BM, McCartney CJ, Franco CD, Hogan QH. Upper extremity regional anesthesia: essentials of our current understanding. Reg Anesth Pain Med. 2009;34:134–70.

Suresh S, Polaner DM, Cote CJ. Regional Anesthesia. In: Cote CJ, Lerman J, Anderson BJ, Eds. 5th ed. Philadelphia: WB Saunders; 2013. p. 835–79.

Tsui BC. Interscalene block. In: Tsui BC, editor. Atlas of ultrasound and nerve stimulation-guided regional anesthesia. New York: Springer; 2007. p. 63–74.

Supraclavicular Brachial Plexus Block

20

Ban C.H. Tsui

Contents

B.C.H. Tsui, Dip Eng, BSc (Math), B Pharm, MSc, MD, FRCPC
Department of Anesthesiology and Pain Medicine,
Stollery Children's Hospital/University of Alberta Hospital,
2-150 Clinical Sciences Building, Edmonton,
AB T6G 2G3, Canada
e-mail: btsui@ualberta.ca

B.C.H. Tsui, S. Suresh (eds.), *Pediatric Atlas of Ultrasound- and Nerve Stimulation-Guided Regional Anesthesia*,
DOI 10.1007/978-0-387-79964-3_20

20.1 Indications

The supraclavicular approach to brachial plexus blockade targets the trunks and/or divisions of the brachial plexus where they lay cephaloposterior to the subclavian artery above the mid-clavicle and first rib (see Figs. 10.1 and 10.2).

Indications

- Hand, forearm, and elbow surgery

20.2 Surface Anatomy (Fig. 20.1)

The patient is positioned supine with the head turned approximately 45° to the contralateral side after general anesthesia has been induced. The operative arm extends down the patient's side, parallel to the body. If necessary, the arm can be pulled down gently towards the knee. A comfortable ergonomic position should be planned to improve block performance. The block may be completed while positioned lateral to the side to be blocked at the level of the upper arm or at the head of the table looking towards the patient's feet. Surface landmarks include:

- Clavicle: the needle insertion site is approximately at the midpoint of the clavicle.
- Subclavian artery pulsation: this serves as the principal landmark; the plexus is located immediately posterolateral to the subclavian artery.

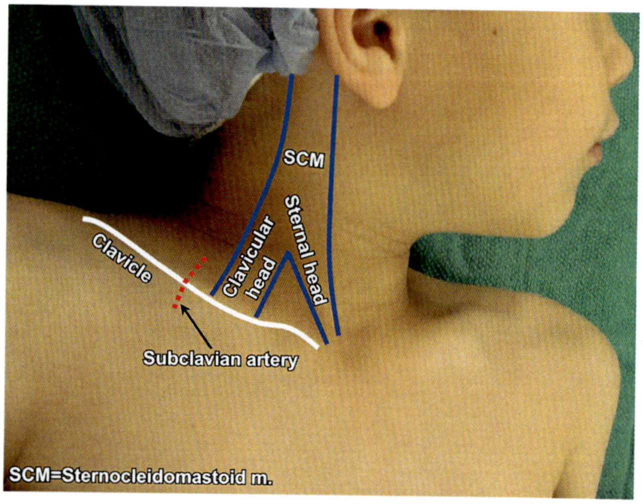

Fig. 20.1 Patient positioning and surface landmarks for supraclavicular block of the brachial plexus

20.3 Nerve Stimulation Technique (Tables 14.1 and 20.1)

Nerve stimulation responses can be useful to minimize the risk of intraneural injection and to confirm proximity of the needle to the target trunk. Because of the high risk of pneumothorax and vascular puncture during supraclavicular blockade, the authors strongly recommend an ultrasound-guided approach. See "Ultrasound-Guided Technique" below for a description of anatomical landmark identification, patient positioning, and needle insertion technique.

Table 20.1 Responses and needle adjustments for use with nerve stimulation at the supraclavicular level

Correct response to nerve stimulation
The correct responses are similar to those observed when using the interscalene approach. At this location, the brachial plexus is starting to divide from trunks into anterior and posterior divisions. Twitches of pectoralis, deltoid, biceps (upper trunk), triceps (upper/middle trunk), forearm (upper/middle trunk), and hand (lower trunk) muscles with current intensity of 0.4 mA (0.1–0.3 ms) are acceptable. Distal responses (hand or wrist flexion or extension) are best to confirm needle placement within the fascia
Other common responses and needle adjustments
Muscle twitch from electrical stimulation
Diaphragm (phrenic nerve)
Explanation: unlikely as the needle plane is too anterior
Needle adjustment: withdraw needle to the subcutaneous tissue and reinsert in a 15° more posterior angle
Vascular puncture
Subclavian artery puncture: indicated with arterial blood withdrawal
Explanation: needle tip is deep to the plexus
Needle adjustment: withdraw completely for pressure treatment and reinsert carefully while observing the needle tip at all times using in-plane approach
Bone contact
Needle stops at a depth of 3 cm (first rib)
Explanation: needle is inserted too deep and well beyond the plexus. However, this scenario is unlikely with ultrasound guidance, unless tip of the needle is not visualized (needle not properly aligned with the ultrasound beam)
Needle adjustment: withdraw to subcutaneous tissue and reinsert
Pleural contact
Needle tip seen beyond the white line (first rib) and a pocket is observed to form beyond the bright line
Explanation: needle is inserted too deep, traversed the plexus and subclavian artery, and has entered the pleural space. However, it is unlikely with US-guided technique
Needle adjustment: withdraw needle to subcutaneous tissue and reinsert if there is a strong clinical indication

20.3.1 Needle Insertion

Depth of insertion depends on age and weight of the patient. It is a nonlinear relationship, i.e., for a 10 kg child, the depth of insertion is about 10 mm. For every 10 kg increase in weight, the depth of insertion increases 3 mm until the child reaches 50 kg. After that, advance 1 mm for every 10 kg increase in weight. The maximum depth should not exceed 35 mm (see Table 20.2).

Table 20.2 Weight-dependent depth of needle insertion for supraclavicular brachial plexus block

Patient weight (kg)	Recommended depth of needle insertion (mm)
10	10
20	13
30	16
40	19
50	22
60	23
70	24

20.3.2 Current Application and Appropriate Responses

Figure 20.2 illustrates the procedure for employing nerve stimulation techniques for supraclavicular nerve block.

- An initial current of 0.8 mA (2 Hz, 0.1–0.3 ms) is sufficient for stimulation of the plexus. After obtaining the appropriate motor response, the current is reduced to aim for a threshold current of 0.4 mA (0.1–0.2 ms). Motor response cessation at currents greater than 0.4 mA or less than or equal to 0.2 mA indicates that the needle may either be too distant from the nerve or may have breached the epineurium, respectively.
- As the trunks of the brachial plexus begin to divide at this block location, twitches of the pectoralis deltoid, biceps (upper trunk), triceps (upper/middle trunk), forearm (upper middle trunk), and hand (lower trunk) muscles may be elicited, depending on the needle location.
- Obtaining a distal response in the hand or wrist indicates optimal needle placement for a successful block.
- In children, the spread of anesthetic solution may be greater than for adults since the fascia is less adherent to the nerve trunks. This increases the likelihood of a successful block with any motor response.

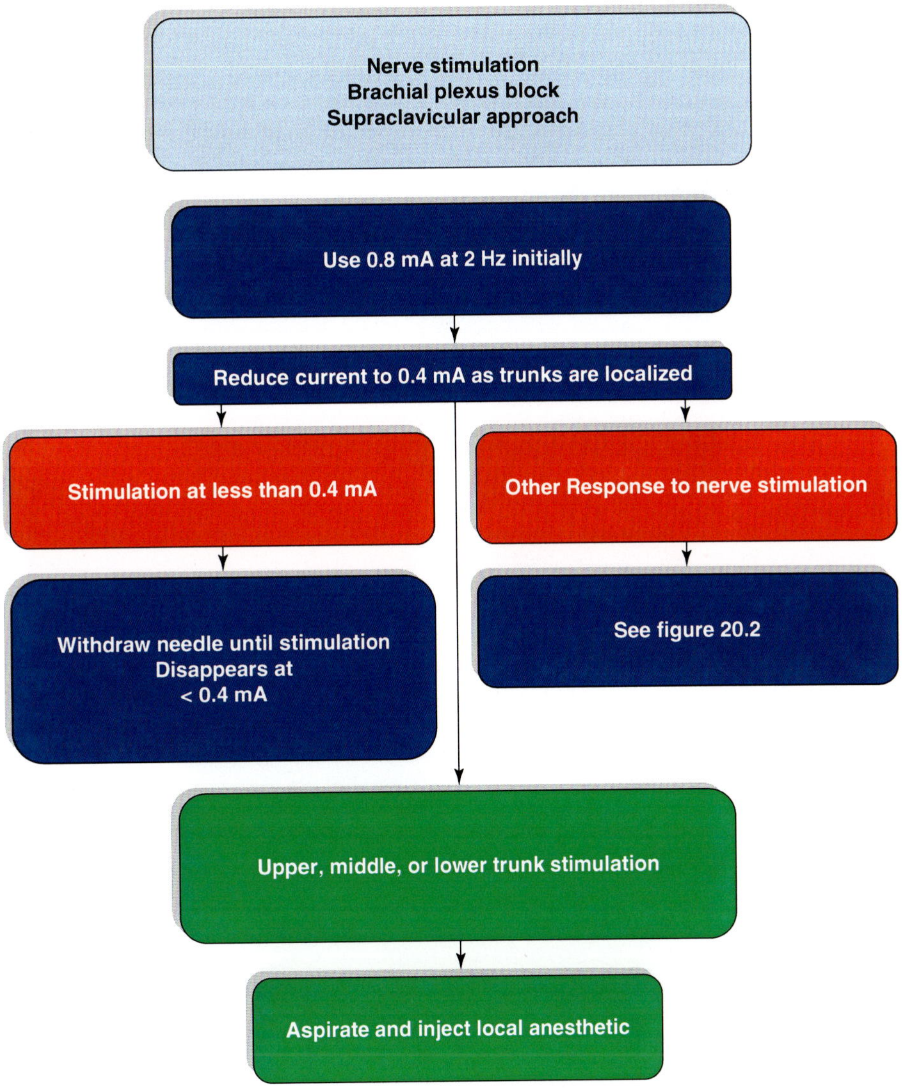

Fig. 20.2 Flowchart of the procedure for employing nerve stimulation techniques for supraclavicular nerve block

20.3.3 Modifications to Inappropriate Responses

An algorithm of modifications to inappropriate responses to nerve stimulation is shown in Fig. 20.3.

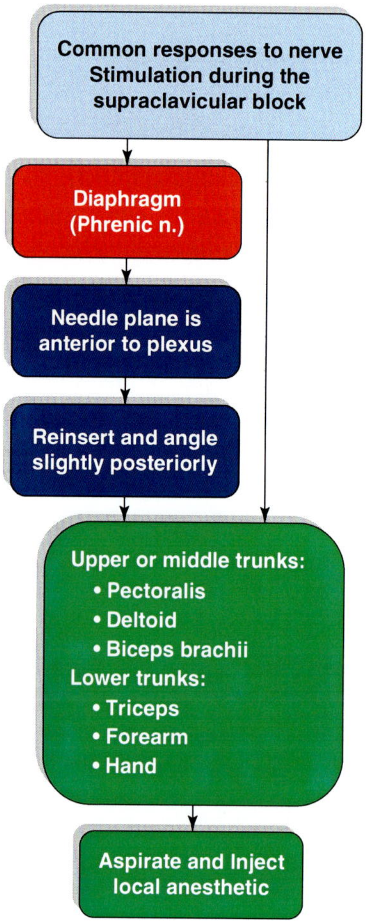

Fig. 20.3 Flowchart of modifications to inappropriate responses to nerve stimulation during supraclavicular brachial plexus block

20.4 Ultrasound-Guided Technique

For a summary of ultrasound guidance techniques in supraclavicular blocks, see Fig. 20.4.

Major anatomical structures in the brachial plexus as captured by MRI and VHVS images are shown with the corresponding ultrasound image in Fig. 20.5a.

Prepare the needle insertion site and skin surface with an antiseptic solution. Prepare the ultrasound probe surface by applying a sterile adhesive dressing to it prior to needling, as discussed in Chap. 4.

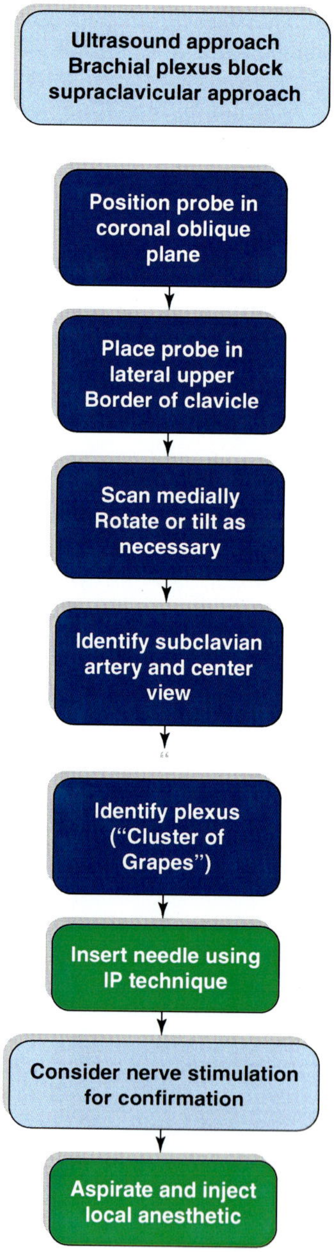

Fig. 20.4 Flowchart of ultrasound-guided techniques in supraclavicular blocks

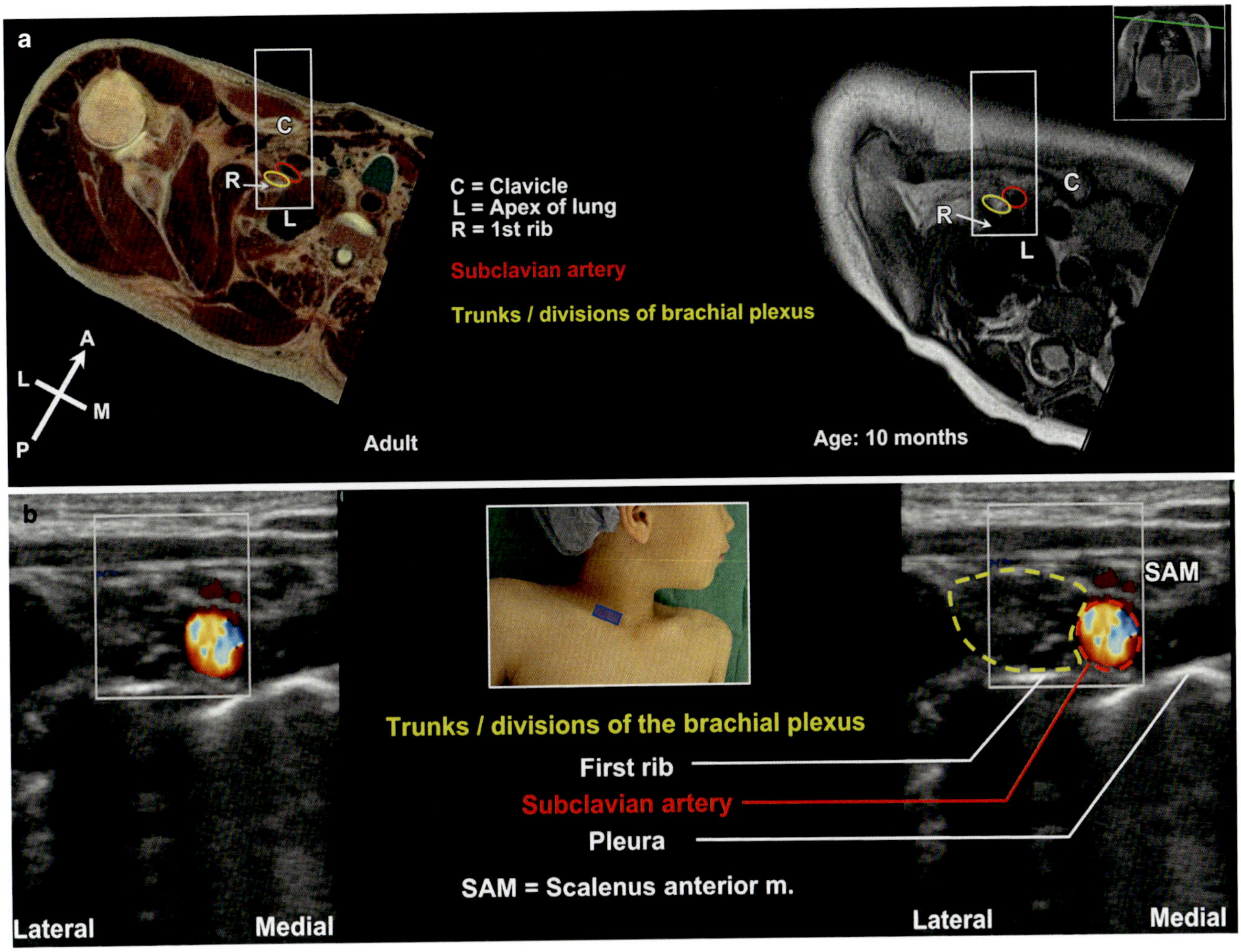

Fig. 20.5 (**a**) VHVS and MRI images of anatomical structures in the brachial plexus at a supraclavicular section. (**b**) Ultrasound image of the brachial plexus at the supraclavicular level

20.4.1 Scanning Technique

The required depth of penetration is usually less than 1 cm for children and 1–2 cm for teenagers.

- The major challenge with ultrasound imaging in this region is the presence of a bony prominence (clavicle) and curved soft tissue contour that can interfere with imaging of the brachial plexus in short-axis view.
- Typically, a high-frequency hockey stick probe is used for small children. A curved array probe with a small footprint is extremely useful in compact areas and for patients in whom the brachial plexus is at a greater depth (older and/or obese children). The small footprint allows unrestrained needle movement around the probe, and the low to moderate frequency improves visualization of deeper structures.

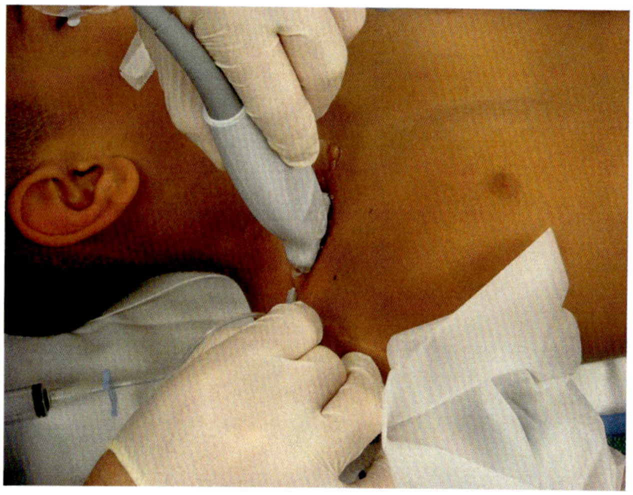

Fig. 20.6 Scanning technique for supraclavicular brachial plexus block

- Generally, the nerve structures are most visible when the angle of incidence is 90° to the ultrasound beam.
- Failure to maintain either good skin-probe contact or a 90° beam-to-nerve incidence angle can result in an anisotropy effect and alter the appearance of the plexus (see Chap. 3).
- The probe is first placed in a coronal oblique plane at the lateral end of the upper border of the clavicle. It is then moved medially until an image of the subclavian artery appears on screen. The subclavian artery is characterized by its pulsatile property and can be confirmed with color Doppler (Fig. 20.5b). Some dorsal and ventral rotation of the probe may be necessary to improve image clarity. This scanning technique is illustrated in Fig. 20.6.
- With the subclavian artery in the middle of the screen, the plexus can be viewed superior and lateral to the artery above the first rib.

20.4.2 Sonographic Appearance

Figure 20.5b illustrates the sonographic anatomy of a young child. Table 20.3 summarizes imaging considerations in the pediatric population.

- The subclavian artery is anechoic, hypodense, pulsatile, and round; its identity can be confirmed by color Doppler.
- The trunks/divisions of the brachial plexus can be found superior and lateral to the subclavian artery in the ultrasound image plane. They appear as a cluster of at least three (more as the probe is traced distally) hypoechoic structures similar to a "bunch of grapes."
- The fascicular linings/sheaths of the brachial plexus trunks are hyperechoic, outlining the "grape-like" structures.
- The first rib lies deep to the artery and appears as a hyperechoic linear structure with a hypoechoic bony shadow underneath.
- The lung pleura appear as a hyperechoic line accompanied by a hyperechoic shadow due to air artifacts underneath.
- Inferomedial to the smaller subclavian artery is the anechoic, oval-to-round subclavian vein; the anterior scalene muscle lies between the artery and vein.

Table 20.3 Anatomical and imaging considerations for supraclavicular block

Pediatric patients	Adult patients
• The trunks of the brachial plexus can become divisions at this level, but the tight space makes neural ultrasound imaging and needling more challenging	• The trunks of the brachial plexus can also become divisions at this level; however, more available space allows for clear visualization of neural structures using ultrasonography
• The brachial plexus at the level of the supraclavicular block is situated superficially and in proximity to the pleura. This increases the risk of pleural puncture and pneumothorax	• The roots of the brachial plexus are situated more deeply, and there is a greater distance between the roots and the pleura

20.4.3 Needle Insertion

- Infiltrate the skin with local anesthetic.
- A 30 mm, 21G–23G insulated needle is suitable for this block.
- *We consider the out-of-plane technique dangerous for supraclavicular block and do not recommend this approach.*
- Perform an in-plane (IP) needling technique using a small footprint curved (Fig. 20.7) or hockey stick probe:
  - The needle is inserted immediately above the clavicle in a lateral-to-medial direction and with a slightly cephalad angulation to avoid the lung. The authors find that a medial-to-lateral direction is often limited by the compact space.
  - Visualization of the needle tip at all times using an IP approach can minimize the occurrence of pneumothorax and vascular puncture. The IP approach with lateral-to-medial needle insertion ensures needle-nerve contact before the subclavian artery is approached, thereby reducing the risk of inadvertent vascular puncture.
  - Directing the needle towards the thorax during this approach increases the risk of pleural puncture. Vigilant identification of the pleura is required throughout the procedure in addition to constant visualization and awareness of the needle tip.

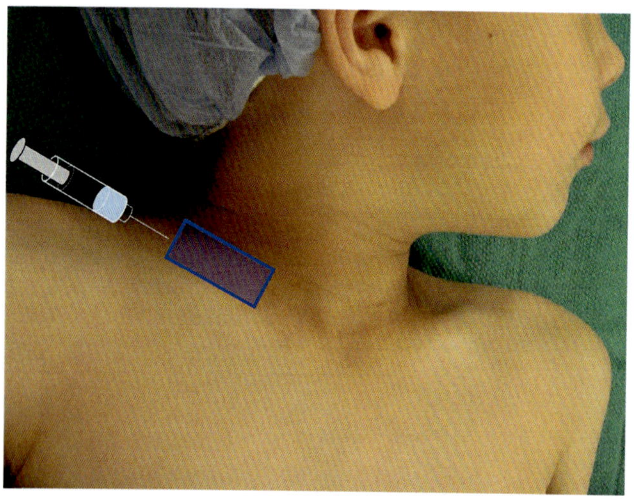

Fig. 20.7 In-plane needling technique for supraclavicular block. *Blue rectangle* indicates ultrasound probe footprint

20.5 Local Anesthetic Application

- Blockade at this level can be achieved with volumes of local anesthetic as low as 0.15–0.2 mL/kg. Recommended local anesthetics are 0.25 % bupivacaine, 0.5 % bupivacaine, 0.2 % ropivacaine, or 2 % lidocaine.
- *Ultrasound Considerations*:
  - Performing a test dose with D5W is recommended prior to local anesthetic application to visualize the spread and confirm nerve localization.
  - In our experience, it is best to deposit local anesthetic next to the nerve structures in the supraclavicular window immediately lateral to the subclavian artery on top of the first rib. Injection in this location will often lift the nerve structures superiorly and away from the first rib and subclavian artery.
  - The hypoechoic spread of local anesthetic appears to surround the nerves on the ultrasound screen.
  - If the spread of anesthetic seems inadequate for the whole plexus, reposition the needle prior to further injection.

20.6 Current Literature in Ultrasound-Guided Approaches

Ultrasound-guided supraclavicular block has been described primarily in the adult literature, although there have been several reports published in the pediatric literature. Using a technique similar to the one described for adults, De Jose Maria and colleagues randomized 80 children to receive supraclavicular or infraclavicular brachial plexus blocks [1]. Supraclavicular blocks used a needle (short beveled, 22G–25G, 35–50 mm) aligned IP to a high-frequency probe placed in the coronal oblique plane once the brachial plexus trunks/divisions (forming a cluster of hypoechoic nodules) were visualized lateral to the subclavian artery (hypoechoic and pulsatile) and close to the underlying first rib (hyperechoic and curvilinear). The authors directed the needle from lateral to medial in order to approach the plexus lateral to the artery and prevent direct contact of the plexus. A linear probe with a 35 mm footprint was used, although other smaller footprint linear or curvilinear probes may be appropriate for some cases due to the reduced contact area and array characteristics [2].

In the report described above, De Jose Maria et al. [1] compared the success rate, complications, and block performance times of the blocks in children scheduled for upper limb surgery. Light general anesthesia was provided to all patients. In addition to the above outcomes, the block duration and volumes of ropivacaine 0.5 % used were recorded for the supraclavicular approach. Both block approaches were effective (with failure defined as any amount of supplemental analgesia required during surgery or within the first 4 h after the block), and neither was associated with complications. Patients requiring supplemental analgesia intraoperatively had block failure of the radial (one with infraclavicular block) and ulnar (two from both groups) nerves. Two patients receiving infraclavicular block had accidental puncture of their axillary artery. The supraclavicular block was faster to perform (9 versus 13 min; 95 % confidence interval for this difference was 2–6 min and was statistically significant). The sensory and motor blocks using the supraclavicular approach lasted 6.5 and 5 h, respectively. Approximately 6 mL of ropivacaine was used.

Steinfeldt et al. [3] described a case where a supraclavicular brachial plexus Angiocath™ (BD Medical, Sandy, UT, USA) was inserted under ultrasound guidance. This procedure was performed in a 7-year-old child prior to emergence of general anesthesia for humeral osteotomy and pinning. This approach facilitated postoperative testing of the peripheral nerves prior to injection of local anesthetic (5 mL of 0.25 % bupivacaine) for postoperative analgesia.

A unique case of bilateral supraclavicular block combined with caudal anesthesia was described by Vermeylen et al. [4]. In this case, a 2-year-old boy required amputation of all four extremities following pneumococcal sepsis. After administering the caudal block, ultrasound-guided supraclavicular blocks were performed on each side using 2.5 mL ropivacaine (5 mg/mL) per side. The ability to visualize spread of the local anesthetic allowed the authors to use a minimal dose, avoiding toxicity. Postoperative pain relief was excellent.

Yang et al. [5] described a series of four cases in which pediatric patients received supraclavicular brachial plexus blocks for upper extremity surgery. In all cases, the block was successful and provided adequate anesthesia and analgesia. Two of the patients received perineural catheters to manage postoperative pain; no adverse events involving the catheters were reported.

Visualization of the needle tip and its relation to the plexus should reduce associated complications and increase significantly the use of supraclavicular block. Indeed, the rapid onset of this block offers the most reliable blockade of the brachial plexus for analgesia and anesthesia of the entire upper extremity, to the degree that it is referred to as a "spinal for the upper extremity" at our facility.

Clinical Pearls: Supraclavicular Block

- If anesthesia of the lower trunk is needed for hand surgery, it is advisable to inject local anesthetic immediately next to the inferior portion of the nerve cluster, close to the first rib.
- Some experts recommend deferring this block until the operator reaches reasonable competency in other ultrasound-guided nerve blocks. In practice, we often find it easier to perform a low interscalene block instead of a true supraclavicular block, with a similar clinical result.
- The risk of pneumothorax may be reduced by avoiding overinflation of the lung or by temporarily reducing positive pressure ventilation if the patient is intubated.

20.7 Case Study

Supraclavicular Brachial Plexus Block (Provided by S. Suresh)

A 5-year-old female patient, 20.4 kg, presented for closed reduction percutaneous pinning of the left elbow. After induction of general anesthesia, the patient received an elbow X-ray and X-ray with fluoroscopy in the OR. An ultrasound-guided supraclavicular nerve block was administered with a 20G needle (see Fig. 20.8); 3.5 mL 0.25 % bupivacaine with epinephrine 1:200,000 was given for postoperative analgesia. Block duration was 6–12 h, and surgery lasted for 2 h and 8 min. Pain reporting following surgery was 0/10 (FLACC scale) at PACU admission and 0/10 (FLACC scale) at PACU discharge.

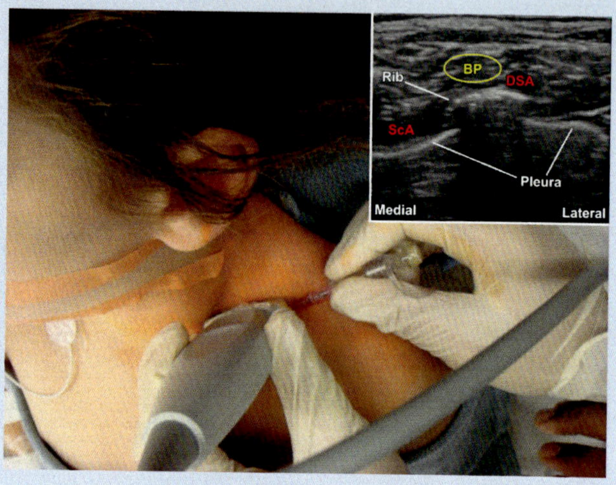

Fig. 20.8 Ultrasound-guided supraclavicular brachial plexus block. *BP* brachial plexus, *DSA* dorsal scapular artery, *ScA* subclavian artery (See Case Study for details)

References

1. De Jose MB, Banus E, Navarro EM, et al. Ultrasound-guided supraclavicular vs infraclavicular brachial plexus blocks in children. Pediatr Anesth. 2008;18:838–44.
2. Tsui BC, Twomey C, Finucane BT. Visualization of the brachial plexus in the supraclavicular region using a curved ultrasound probe with a sterile transparent dressing. Reg Anesth Pain Med. 2006;31:182–4.
3. Steinfeldt J, Robison T, Przybylo HJ. Placement of an US-guided supraclavicular block postoperatively in children: can we make this easy? Pediatr Anesth. 2010;20:780–1.
4. Vermeylen K, Berghmans J, Van de Velde M. Ultrasound as guidance for a combined bilateral supraclavicular and caudal block, in order to reduce the total anaesthetic dose in a two year old child after a pneumococcal sepsis. Acta Anaesthesiol Belg. 2011;62:151–5.
5. Yang CW, Cho CK, Kwon HU, et al. Ultrasound-guided supraclavicular brachial plexus block in pediatric patients -a report of four cases. Korean J Anesthesiol. 2010;59(Suppl):S90–4.

Suggested Reading

Karmakar MK, Kwok WH. Ultrasound-guided regional anesthesia. In: Cote CJ, Lerman J, Todres ID, editors. A practice of anesthesia for infants and children. 4th ed. Philadelphia: WB Saunders; 2009. p. 924.

Neal JM, Gerancher JC, Hebl JR, Ilfeld BM, McCartney CJ, Franco CD, Hogan QH. Upper extremity regional anesthesia: essentials of our current understanding. Reg Anesth Pain Med. 2009;34:134–70.

Tsui BC. Supraclavicular block. In: Tsui BC, editor. Atlas of ultrasound and nerve stimulation-guided regional anesthesia. New York: Springer; 2007. p. 75–85.

Part VI

Nerve Blocks Below the Clavicle

Infraclavicular Brachial Plexus Block

21

Ban C.H. Tsui

Contents

B.C.H. Tsui, Dip Eng, BSc (Math), B Pharm, MSc, MD, FRCPC
Department of Anesthesiology and Pain Medicine,
Stollery Children's Hospital/University of Alberta Hospital,
2-150 Clinical Sciences Building, Edmonton,
AB T6G 2G3, Canada
e-mail: btsui@ualberta.ca

B.C.H. Tsui, S. Suresh (eds.), *Pediatric Atlas of Ultrasound- and Nerve Stimulation-Guided Regional Anesthesia*,
DOI 10.1007/978-0-387-79964-3_21

21.1 Indications

Infraclavicular nerve blocks target the cords of the brachial plexus where they surround the axillary artery (see Fig. 10.1). These blocks are suitable for upper arm, elbow, forearm, and hand surgery. Blocks in awake or mildly sedated children have been described, although the practice of undertaking this block once the child is anesthetized is more common.

Indications

- Surgery of the upper arm including the proximal humerus, elbow, forearm, and hand.

21.2 Surface Anatomy (Fig. 21.1)

Preferably, the patient is positioned supine with a pillow under the shoulder. The arm is adducted and the elbow flexed at 90° with the hand resting on the abdomen. If the patient is awake, the arm may rest at the patient's side if this will avoid discomfort. Surface landmarks include:

- Cephalad
  - Clavicle
- Medially
  - Sternal notch and sternoclavicular joint
  - Medial end of the clavicle
- Laterally
  - Anterior aspect of the acromion: palpate the clavicle and move laterally to the acromioclavicular joint. The acromion can be differentiated from the humerus through passive movement of the arm.
  - Coracoid process: medial and inferior to the acromioclavicular joint, which can be palpated just medial to the head of the humerus.

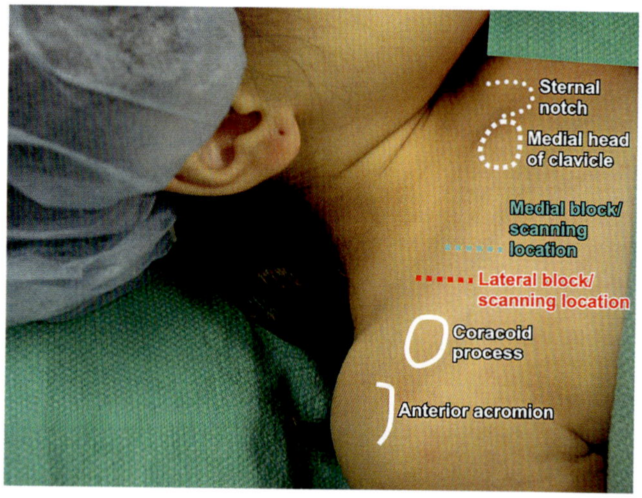

Fig. 21.1 Patient positioning and surface landmarks for infraclavicular brachial plexus block

21.3 Nerve Stimulation Technique (Table 14.1)

21.3.1 Needle Insertion (Figs. 21.2 and 21.3)

- Clean the skin with antiseptic solution, and drape the patient to ensure sterility.
- Infiltrate the skin with local anesthetic (e.g., 0.5 mL of 1 % lidocaine).
- The point of needle insertion depends on the age of the patient, but is approximately 0.5–1 cm inferior to the coracoid process.
- Insert a 30–50 mm, 21–24G insulated needle in a vertical direction while applying nerve stimulation.
- If the needle encounters a bone (rib), the needle has been placed too deep to the plexus. Withdraw the needle to the subcutaneous tissue and reinsert. See Table 21.1 for responses and recommended needle adjustments when using nerve stimulation for infraclavicular block.
- Blood aspiration indicates axillary artery/vein puncture. If this occurs, carefully reinsert the needle after complete withdrawal.
- An initial current of 0.8 mA (frequency 2 Hz, pulse width 0.1 msec) is sufficient for stimulation of the plexus. The current is then reduced to aim for a threshold current of 0.4 mA while maintaining the appropriate motor response.
- A distal motor response of hand or wrist flexion or extension is ideal.
- Ultrasound guidance will help reduce the incidence of both bone contact and vessel puncture.

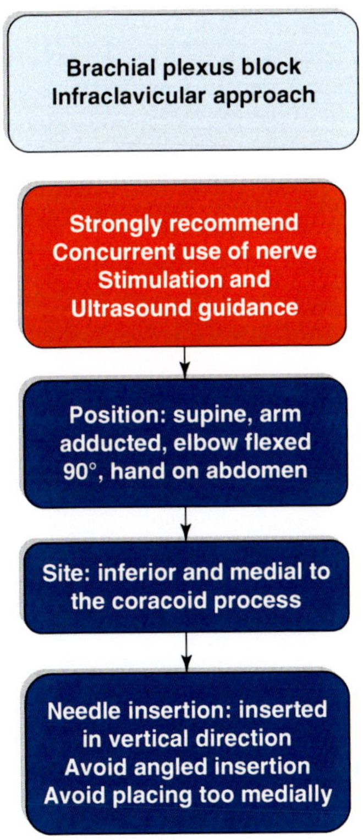

Fig. 21.2 Flow chart of the procedures and needle insertion site for an infraclavicular block of the brachial plexus

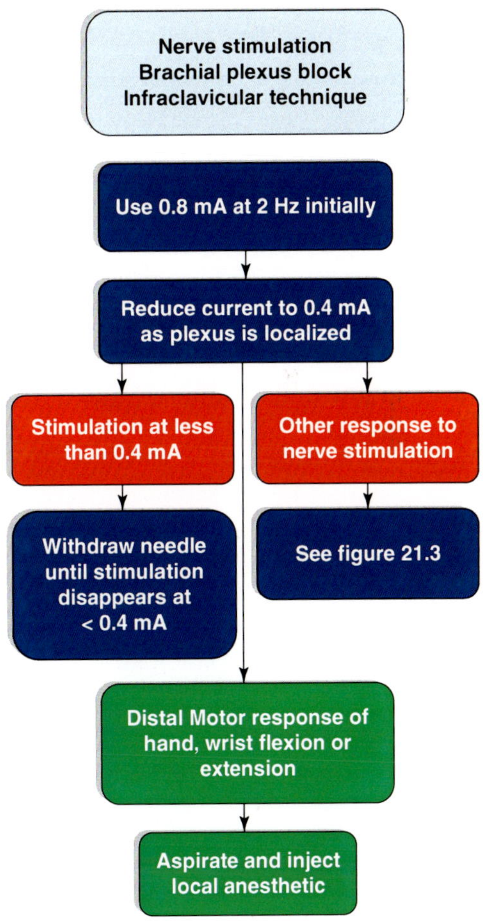

Fig. 21.3 Flowchart of the procedure for employing nerve stimulation techniques for infraclavicular nerve block

Table 21.1 Responses and recommended needle adjustments for use during nerve stimulation at the infraclavicular location

Correct response from nerve stimulation
Distal responses (hand or wrist flexion or extension) are best for surgery of the elbow and below
Other common responses and needle adjustments
Muscle twitches from electrical stimulation
Pectoralis (adduction of arm)
Explanation: needle tip is too shallow
Needle adjustment: advance needle deeper
Deltoid (axillary nerve stimulation)
Explanation: needle tip is too inferior
Needle adjustment: withdraw needle to subcutaneous tissue and reinsert slightly more superiorly
Biceps (musculocutaneous nerve)
Explanation: needle tip is too superior
Needle adjustment: withdraw needle to subcutaneous tissue and reinsert slightly more inferiorly
Vascular puncture
Cephalic vein (seen as blood withdrawal when needle appears to be placed superficially)
Explanation: cephalic vein is superficial to the plexus and the subclavian artery and vein
Needle adjustment: withdraw needle and redirect carefully while observing the needle tip at all times using in-plane approach
Subclavian or axillary artery/vein puncture (seen as blood aspiration)[a]
Explanation: artery and vein are next to the plexus
Needle adjustment: withdraw needle completely for pressure treatment and reinsert carefully while observing the needle tip at all times using in-plane approach; if the blood is venous, the needle tip is likely too caudal
Bone contact
Needle stops at rib
Explanation: needle is inserted too deep and has passed the plexus and subclavian artery. However, it is unlikely with ultrasound-guided technique
Needle adjustment: withdraw needle to subcutaneous tissue and reinsert
Pleural – more risk with medial locations of needle insertion
Needle observed to pass beyond the white line (rib), with a pocket forming
Explanation: needle is inserted too deep, has passed the plexus and subclavian artery, and is entering into the pleural space. However, it is unlikely with US-guided technique
Needle adjustment: withdraw to subcutaneous tissue and reinsert

[a]Subclavian vessels when needle insertion is at a more medial location; axillary vessels when block is performed at a more lateral location

21.3.2 Modifications to Inappropriate Responses

See Fig. 21.4.

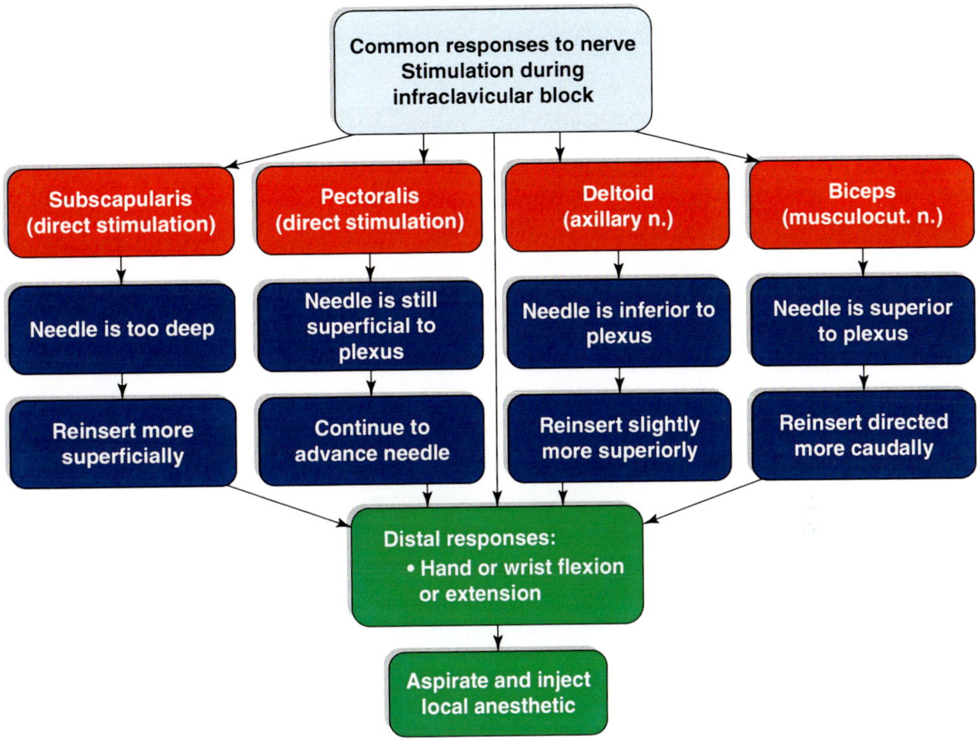

Fig. 21.4 Flowchart of modifications to inappropriate responses to nerve stimulation during infraclavicular brachial plexus block

21.4 Ultrasound-Guided Technique (Fig. 21.5)

It is common to perform an infraclavicular brachial plexus block with the patient's elbow flexed and the hand resting on the abdomen or with the arm resting at the patient's side. However, it may be more advantageous to position the patient with the elbow flexed and the arm abducted and externally rotated when completing the block under ultrasound guidance. This maneuver can render the cords taut and bring them to a more superficial location, thus accentuating their ultrasonographic appearance. Stretching the cords also brings the nerves closer around the axillary artery, which may facilitate local anesthetic spread around the nerves.

The location of the needle puncture will be where the brachial plexus cords, axillary vessels, and pleura are visualized best. It is ideal to make small probe adjustments (i.e., superior-inferior or medial-lateral) with the goal to have a well-defined cross section of the axillary artery. Blocks below the clavicle are associated with complications (Table 21.2); therefore, knowledge of the anatomical details of this region is crucial to perform this block correctly (Fig. 21.6a) and to avoid adverse events. Similar to the nerve stimulation technique, a lateral approach decreases the risk of pleural puncture, although a more medial location will allow higher resolution of the structures (Fig. 21.6b). If using a medial puncture site, ensure to maintain a view of the pleura and needle tip on the ultrasound screen at all times.

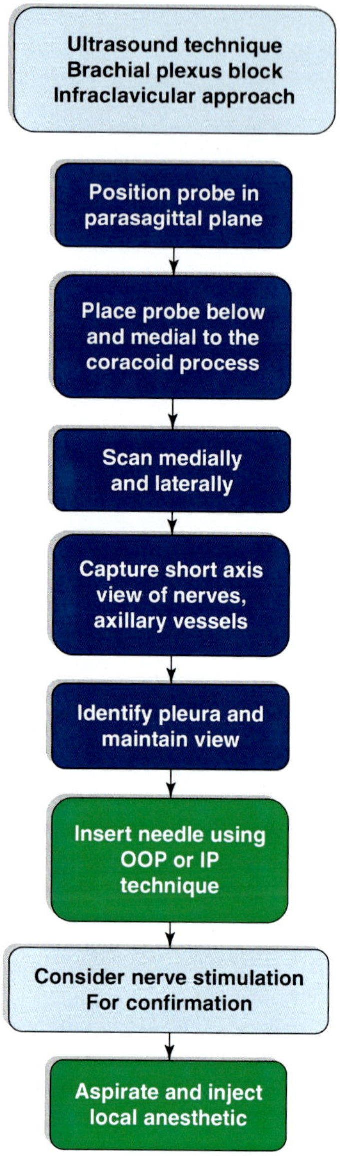

Fig. 21.5 Flowchart of ultrasound-guided techniques for infraclavicular nerve block

Table 21.2 Complications of nerve blocks below the clavicle

1. Hematoma
Intravascular injection: arterial or venous
Avoid multiple needle insertions
Apply form pressure over the needle insertion site after needle withdrawal
2. Pneumothorax
Needle too medial, near the cupola of the lung
Pay attention to the site and angle of needle insertion
If using ultrasound, keep the lungs in view to avoid trauma to the pleura
3. Nerve injury
From intraneural injections
Use a nerve stimulator to confirm needle position. Withdraw needle when there is nerve stimulation at <0.4 mA to avoid intraneural injection
Avoid high pressure during administration of injectates. See Chap. 1 for compressed air injection technique

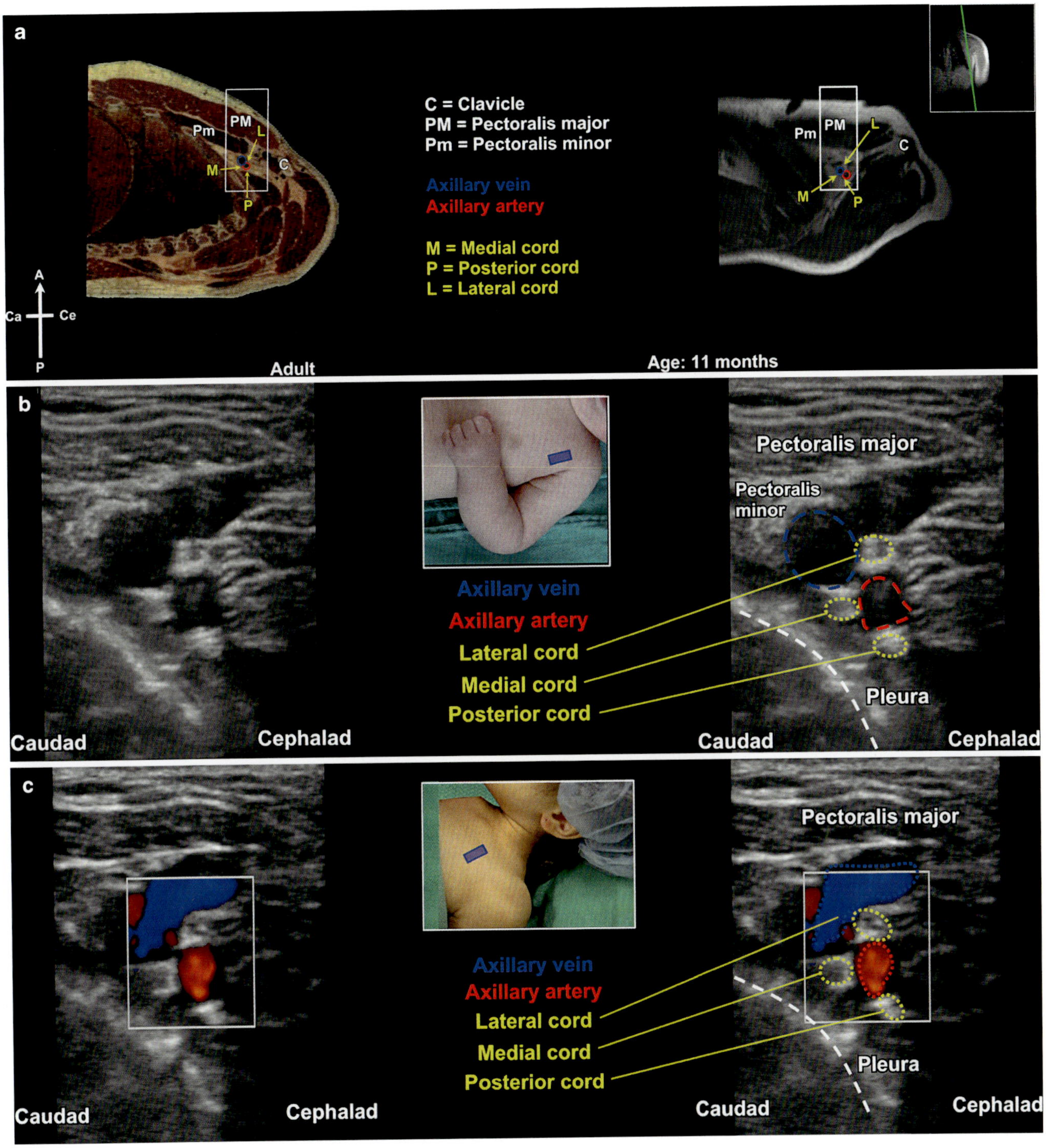

Fig. 21.6 (**a**) VHVS and MRI images of anatomical structures in the brachial plexus at an infraclavicular section. (**b**) Ultrasound image of the brachial plexus at the infraclavicular level at a lateral scanning location. (**c**) Ultrasound image of the brachial plexus at the infraclavicular level at a medial scanning location

21.4.1 Preparing the Site

Prepare the needle insertion site and skin surface with an antiseptic solution. A sterile adhesive dressing should be applied to the ultrasound probe prior to needling.

21.4.2 Scanning Technique (Fig. 21.5)

A small footprint linear array transducer (7–13 MHz frequency) will provide good visualization in young children. A curved array transducer (7–4 MHz frequency) will provide a wider field of view and improved definition to allow better imaging of the neurovascular structures in older or larger children when the plexus is found at a depth >4 cm.

The required depth of penetration is usually within 2–3 cm at a lateral location inferior to the coracoid process. This can be shallower or deeper depending on the size of the pectoralis muscle layers.

Below and slightly medial to the coracoid process, position the probe in a parasagittal plane, and move the probe medially and laterally to capture the best possible short axis view of the nerve structures and axillary vessels. The artery is often the first identifiable structure.

When the neurovascular structures are poorly visualized, the probe can be directed medially towards the midpoint of the clavicle. At this level, the cords can be found posterolateral to the subclavian artery. It is important to identify the pleural cavity and maintain it within view throughout the procedure especially with a more medial block approach.

As vascular puncture and pneumothorax are the most likely complications of this block, it is advisable to use color Doppler to identify the axillary artery and vein and the cephalic vein, particularly if the neural structure is in doubt.

21.4.3 Sonographic Appearance

In the parasagittal plane at the lateral coracoid infraclavicular region (immediately medial and inferior to the coracoid process), using a linear probe (Fig. 21.6b):

- The coracoid process is the most cephalad structure and appears hypoechoic with an associated hypoechoic bony shadow.
- The pectoralis major and minor muscles are separated by a hyperechoic lining, which is the perimysium.
- The pectoralis minor muscle is superficial to the axillary neurovascular bundle. Within this bundle the large axillary vein lies medial and caudad to the artery and the cords of the plexus surround the artery (lateral cord cephalad, posterior cord deep, and medial cord caudad).
- The lateral and posterior cords of the plexus are often readily visualized as hyperechoic oval structures.
- The medial cord may not be readily identified because it lies between the axillary artery and vein and can sometimes be posterior or even slightly cephalad to the axillary artery.
- The pleura will appear as a hypoechoic cavity outlined by a sloping hyperechoic line and is often located in very close proximity to the neurovascular structures.
- The deep aspect of the image may show an underlying rib (2nd or 3rd).

In the parasagittal plane at a more medial location – the midpoint of the line between anterior acromion and jugular notch (Fig. 21.6c):

- The cords of the plexus are seen as round hypoechoic nodules, lying cephalad and lateral to the subclavian artery.
- The subclavian vein lies anteromedial, and the cephalic vein lies superficial to subclavian artery. The veins may be hard to visualize or may appear irregularly shaped and less hypoechoic than the artery.
- The pleural cavity is found inferior and posterior to the hyperechoic first rib. The pleural cavity may appear hyperechoic due to an air artifact.
- Because the plexus and vessels are superficial and immediately anterior to the pleura, it is important to maintain a good view of the pleura and needle tip throughout the procedure.

21.4.4 Needle Insertion

- A 30–50 mm, 21G–24G insulated needle should be used if performing nerve stimulation. Both in-plane (IP) and out-of-plane (OOP) approaches are appropriate for ultrasound-guided infraclavicular block. If a more medial block location is used, an IP technique is preferable. This will allow the needle tip to be tracked continually to help avoid pleural puncture. Conversely, OOP needling has a reduced needle path length which may reduce the discomfort if the block is being performed on a conscious child.
- When using an IP approach (Fig. 21.7), introduce the block needle cephalad to the probe and advance it caudally at approximately a 45–60° angle to the skin. At the lateral block location, after passing through the pectoral muscles, the needle will first contact the lateral cord. It is best to advance the needle deeper so that it is posterior to the axillary artery and therefore able to contact the posterior cord. Local anesthetic infiltration at this point will often create a U-shaped spread around the axillary artery. However, pulling the needle tip back and completing a second injection anterior to the axillary artery will usually ensure a good distribution of local anesthetic surrounding all three cords.
- For an OOP approach (Fig. 21.8), insert the needle at the midpoint of the probe, angling it from medial to lateral. The distance from the probe that the needle is inserted will depend on the insertion angle of the needle and the distance from the probe to the target structure. We recommend using a 45° angle of insertion so that the insertion point of the needle will be the same distance from the probe as the depth of the plexus, forming a right-angled triangle with the plexus, probe, and needle insertion point. Additionally, the use of an incremental needling technique, such as the "walk down" approach, will enable careful tracking of the needle tip position.

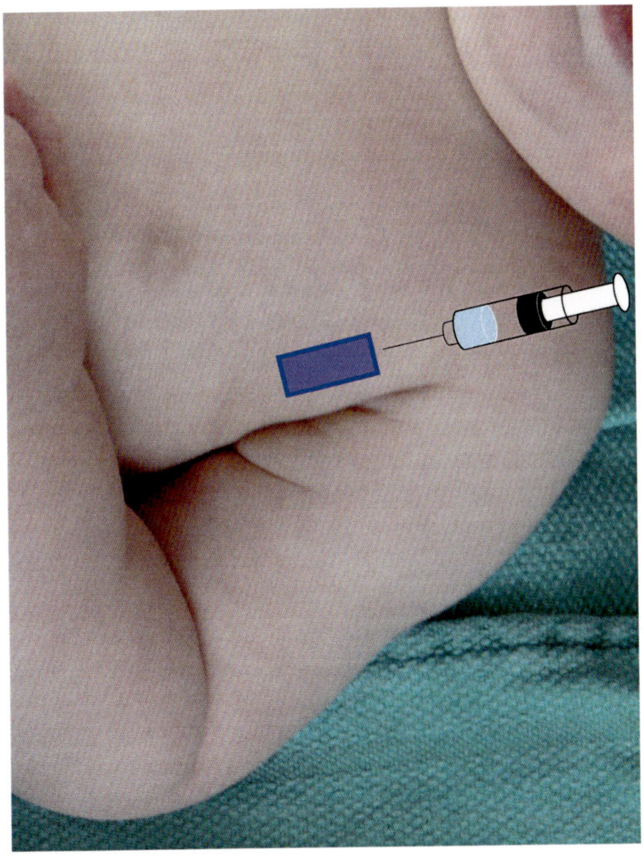

Fig. 21.7 In-plane needling technique for ultrasound-guided infraclavicular brachial plexus block. *Blue rectangle* indicates probe footprint

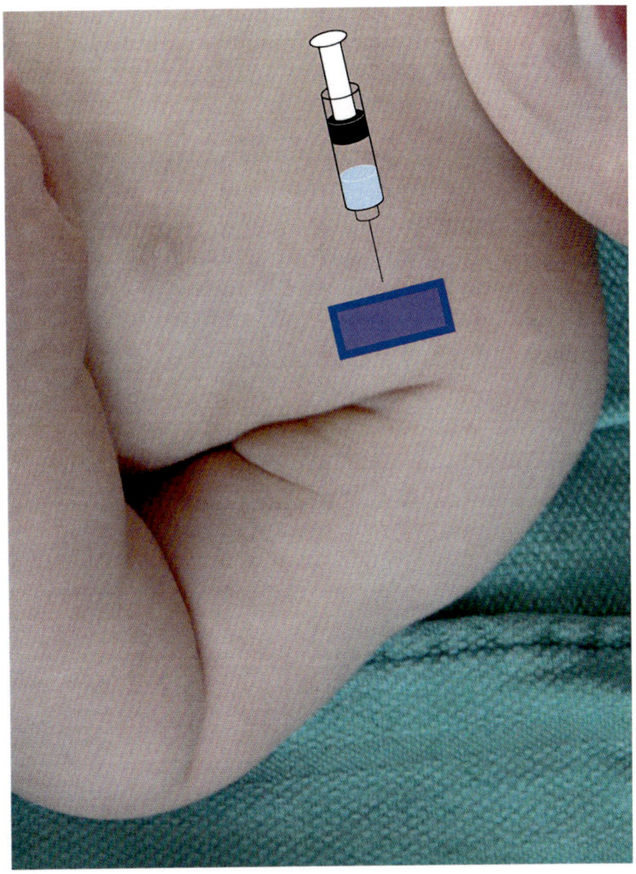

Fig. 21.8 Out-of-plane needling technique for ultrasound-guided infraclavicular brachial plexus block. *Blue rectangle* indicates probe footprint

21.5 Local Anesthetic Application

We recommend using nerve stimulation for confirmation prior to local anesthetic injection. Injecting an initial test dose of D5W is recommended prior to local anesthetic application to visualize the spread and confirm nerve localization.

For an infraclavicular block, 0.5 mL/kg of 0.2–0.5 % ropivacaine or 0.25–0.5 % bupivacaine can be used, although in very small children, the concentration may need to be adjusted to obtain an adequate volume to achieve the block (minimum of 5 mL).

A hypoechoic fluid collection is often observed, accentuating the imaging of adjacent nerve structures.

Local anesthetic deposited posterior to the axillary artery with cephalad and caudad spreading seems to result in consistent surgical anesthesia in the hand when performing the block in the lateral position. If local anesthetic does not surround all the cords, stop halfway through and reposition the needle prior to applying the remaining injectate. If a circumferential spread is not achieved despite repositioning, consider pulling the needle tip back and completing a second injection anterior to the axillary artery as described above.

21.6 Current Literature in Ultrasound-Guided Approaches

Marhofer et al. [1] described their use of ultrasound-guided lateral infraclavicular block for surgical anesthesia in children. The patients were placed supine with their arm adducted, elbow flexed, and forearm placed on their abdomen. A linear probe was placed transversely below the clavicle to capture an image of the brachial plexus. The authors reported successful visualization of the plexus in all 40 patients studied. The needle was inserted OOP, 1 cm from the inferior aspect of the probe, and directed slightly cranially towards the lateral border of the plexus. Local anesthetic spread was viewed surrounding the plexus. Compared to the conventional nerve stimulation technique, the authors found ultrasound to be superior in terms of (1) visual analogue scores (VAS) during block performance, (2) sensory onset times (mean onset times were 9 versus 15 min), (3) longer duration of sensory block (384 versus 310 min), and (4) better sensory and motor block scores 10 min after block insertion in patients that were assessed. Ultrasound guidance also improves success rates for infraclavicular block in pediatric patients, as demonstrated in a recent clinical trial comparing two groups of patients receiving either an ultrasound-guided block or a nerve stimulation-guided block [2].

The faster onset and longer duration of the blocks has been attributed to ultrasound aiding in more accurate deposition of the local anesthetic to the brachial plexus. At 30 min, all blocks, whether placed by ultrasound or nerve stimulation, were successful, and general anesthesia was not required in any of the patients. There was no difference in the VAS 30 min after the block or during surgery.

De Jose Maria et al. [3] recently compared the efficacy of ultrasound-guided infraclavicular and supraclavicular blocks. For the infraclavicular block, these authors placed the probe below the clavicle, either parallel to the clavicle or using a slightly parasagittal plane, depending on the visibility of the plexus. A medium frequency probe (thus allowing greater visualization of deeper structures) was used in some of the older children in order to improve the visibility of the pleura and vessels. In contrast to Marhofer et al. [1], the needle was placed immediately cephalad to the probe and the probe was held in a transverse orientation, therefore effectively using an OOP approach. Both groups used a fairly steep angle of needle insertion. The needle was redirected when necessary to ensure the cords were adequately surrounded by local anesthetic solution, and the spread of local anesthetic was monitored during performance of the block.

It is important to note that there is a great deal of individual anatomical variation in the location of the cords around the artery. At this location, the nerve structures appear hyperechoic, rather than hypoechoic as seen in a more cephalad position, probably due to an increase in the number of fascicles and amount of hyperechoic connective tissue. The cervical pleura is situated closest to the brachial plexus cords at medial locations within the infraclavicular fossa; thus, when performing an infraclavicular block on children, a more lateral puncture site is recommended. Ultrasound imaging offers visualization of the related anatomy and the approaching needle. This is particularly useful in children to help avoid multiple punctures and because some anatomical landmarks (i.e., the coracoid process) are underdeveloped, making landmark-based techniques difficult in children. Similar to the supraclavicular approach, an IP needle alignment may provide superior outcomes with this block, since viewing the needle tip and shaft at all times will help to ensure that the vessels and cervical pleura are not punctured.

The advantages of continuous infusions using an infraclavicular approach over an axillary or supraclavicular approach in children and adults have been described in the literature. Advantages cited include the ease of placing, stabilizing, and securing a catheter that passes through major and minor pectoralis muscles [4, 5].

Loland et al. [6] reported the successful use of brachial plexus perineural infusion when caring for pediatric patients following near-amputation of the dominant hand. An ultrasound-guided infraclavicular brachial plexus catheter was installed in the recovery room after reconstructive surgery, and a continuous infusion of 0.2 % ropivacaine was maintained for 24 days. The authors concluded that in pediatric upper extremity limb salvage, perineural local anesthetic infusion prolonged the benefits of brachial plexus blockade further into the postoperative period.

Clinical Pearls: Infraclavicular Block

- Place the linear probe medial to the coracoid process and inferior to the clavicle.
- After recognizing the axillary artery, look for the cords of the brachial plexus surrounding the artery.
- Place the needle using an IP approach, with the tip of the needle aimed towards the posterior cord.
- In small children, it can be difficult to undertake an IP approach from above the ultrasound probe as there is often not enough space between the clavicle and the probe. In this case, either an OOP approach or the approach described by Marhofer et al. [1], with the needle insertion caudad to the ultrasound sound probe, is appropriate.
- Avoid using a medially positioned ultrasound probe and needling technique due to proximity to the pleura.

21.7 Case Study

Infraclavicular Block (Provided by S. Suresh)

An 8-year-old female patient, 50.3 kg, with no medical or relevant family history presented for open reduction and fixation of the right small finger following proximal phalanx and distal intraarticular fracture based on X-ray of the finger 4 days prior to surgery. The patient received an ultrasound-guided infraclavicular block, performed with a 22G needle and 10 mL 0.25 % bupivacaine with 1:200,000 epinephrine (see Fig. 21.9). Block duration was 6–12 h; duration of surgery was 1 h and 42 min. Pain reporting in recovery was 5/10 (FACES) 10 min following surgery and 0/10 (FACES) 1 h following surgery. Postoperative analgesia consisted of ketorolac injection (24 mg) and morphine (Duramorph) injection 1 mg with a total of three doses given.

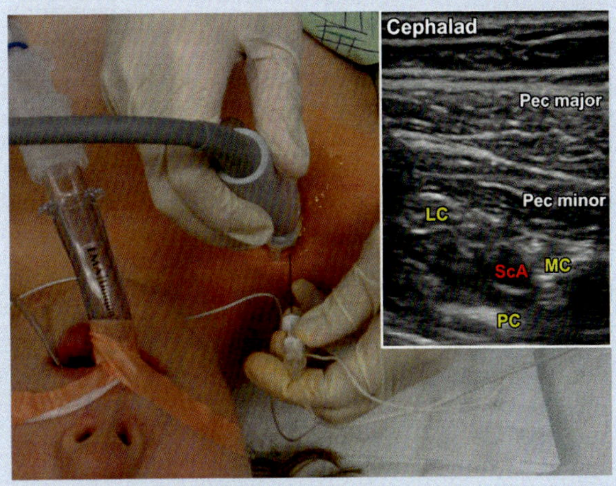

Fig. 21.9 Ultrasound-guided infraclavicular brachial plexus block. *Pec major* pectoralis major, *pec minor* pectoralis minor, *LC* lateral cord of brachial plexus, *MC* medial cord, *PC* posterior cord, *ScA* subclavian artery. See Case Study for details

References

1. Marhofer P, Sitzwohl C, Greher M, Kapral S. Ultrasound guidance for infraclavicular brachial plexus anesthesia in children. Anaesthesia. 2004;59:642–6.
2. Ponde VC, Diwan S. Does ultrasound guidance improve the success rate of infraclavicular brachial plexus block when compared with nerve stimulation in children with radial club hands? Anesth Analg. 2009;108:1967–70.
3. De Jose MB, Banus E, Navarro EM, et al. Ultrasound-guided supraclavicular vs infraclavicular brachial plexus blocks in children. Pediatr Anesth. 2008;18:838–44.
4. Dadure C, Raux O, Troncin R, et al. Continuous infraclavicular brachial plexus block for acute pain management in children. Anesth Analg. 2003;97:691–3.
5. Ponde VC. Continuous infraclavicular brachial plexus block: a modified technique to better secure catheter position in infants and children. Anesth Analg. 2008;106:94–6, table.
6. Loland VJ, Ilfeld BM, Abrams RA, Mariano ER. Ultrasound-guided perineural catheter and local anesthetic infusion in the perioperative management of pediatric limb salvage: a case report. Pediatr Anesth. 2009;19:905–7.

Suggested Reading

Karmakar MK, Kwok WH. Ultrasound-guided regional anesthesia. In: Cote CJ, Lerman J, Todres ID, editors. A practice of anesthesia for infants and children. 4th ed. Philadelphia: WB Saunders; 2009. p. 924–5.

Neal J, Gerancher JC, Hebl J, Ilfeld B, McCartney C, Franco C, Hogan Q. Upper extremity regional anesthesia: essentials of our current understanding. Reg Anesth Pain Med. 2009;34:134–70.

Tsui BC. Infraclavicular block. In: Tsui BC, editor. Atlas of ultrasound and nerve stimulation-guided regional anesthesia. New York: Springer; 2007. p. 87–98.

Axillary Block of the Brachial Plexus

22

Ban C.H. Tsui

Contents

B.C.H. Tsui, Dip Eng, BSc (Math), B Pharm, MSc, MD, FRCPC
Department of Anesthesiology and Pain Medicine,
Stollery Children's Hospital/University of Alberta Hospital,
2-150 Clinical Sciences Building, Edmonton,
AB T6G 2G3, Canada
e-mail: btsui@ualberta.ca

B.C.H. Tsui, S. Suresh (eds.), *Pediatric Atlas of Ultrasound- and Nerve Stimulation-Guided Regional Anesthesia*,
DOI 10.1007/978-0-387-79964-3_22

22.1 Indications

The ulnar, median, radial, and musculocutaneous nerves are the primary targets of an axillary block. The ulnar, median, and radial nerves surround and follow the axillary artery from the apex of the axilla along the humerus. The musculocutaneous nerve often leaves the plexus via the lateral cord, proximal to the axillary apex, and needs to be blocked separately.

Indications

- Surgery of the elbow, forearm, wrist, or hand

22.2 Surface Anatomy (Fig. 22.1)

The patient is positioned supine with the arm abducted 70–80° and externally rotated, the elbow flexed at 90°, and the dorsum of the hand facing the table. Surface landmarks include:

- Anterior axillary fold
  - Formed by the pectoralis major muscle
  - Palpating the axillary artery just deep to the insertion of this muscle will identify the optimal site of needle insertion if attempting to block the musculocutaneous nerve.
- Posterior axillary fold
  - Formed by the latissimus dorsi and teres major muscles.
  - The lower part of the axillary artery can be palpated anterior to this fold on the medial side of the arm; trace this pulse to a proximal location for an optimal block for targeting all the nerves.
- Bicipital sulcus or groove
  - A groove between the tendons of the biceps and triceps brachii muscles

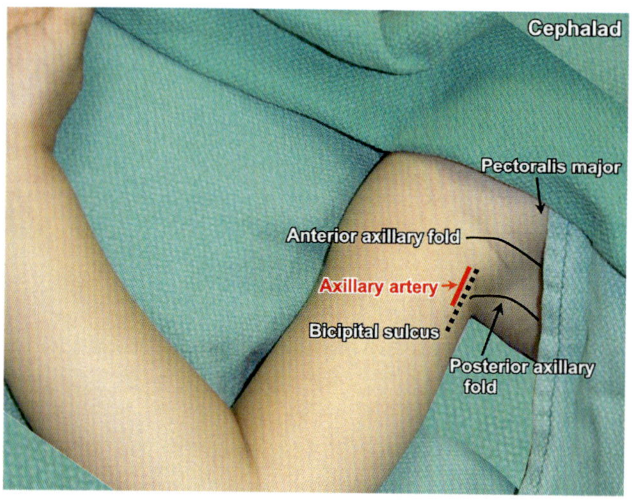

Fig. 22.1 Patient positioning and surface landmarks for axillary block of the brachial plexus

22.3 Nerve Stimulation Technique (Figs. 22.2 and 22.3; Tables 14.1 and 22.1)

- A 30–50 mm, 22–24G insulated needle is typically introduced at the upper border of the axillary artery in a direction towards the midpoint of the clavicle using approximately a 45° angle to the skin and directing the needle medially, dorsally, and caudally. A perpendicular needle direction may also be used, with the needle directed towards the upper border of the artery and the humerus.
- A "pop," indicating loss of resistance, is felt as the needle penetrates the axillary sheath surrounding the plexus.
- Applying an initial current of 0.8–1.0 mA (2 Hz, 0.1 ms) is sufficient for stimulation of the plexus. The current is reduced to aim for a threshold current of 0.4 mA (0.1 ms) while obtaining the appropriate motor response.
- A distal motor response in the hand is ideal, although forearm twitches may be used.
- Bone contact indicates that the needle has advanced to the humerus and that the needle should be withdrawn.
- Arterial blood in the tubing indicates axillary artery puncture, and the needle should be withdrawn slightly; venous blood (axillary vein) necessitates withdrawing and redirecting the needle more laterally or superiorly.
- For the separate block of the musculocutaneous nerve, elbow flexion is the desired motor response.
- The musculocutaneous nerve is usually found between the biceps and coracobrachialis muscles (Fig. 22.6a). In order to block the nerve, a separate needle puncture within the belly of the coracobrachialis muscle is performed. After grasping the belly of the muscle, use the same needle insertion site as for the axillary block, and direct the needle towards the interior of the muscle.
- If a tourniquet is required for the surgery, the intercostobrachial nerve should be anesthetized using a small ring of local anesthetic at the upper aspect of the arm. Alternatively, a small amount of local anesthetic solution can be injected during the withdrawal of the needle.

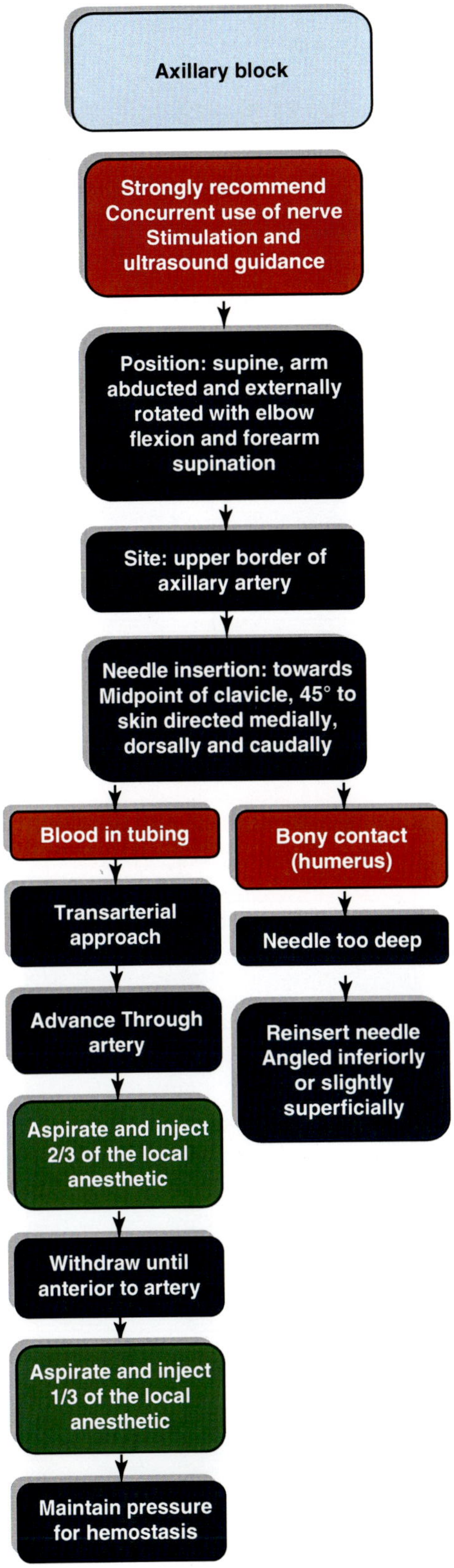

Fig. 22.2 Flowchart of procedures and needle insertion site for axillary brachial plexus block

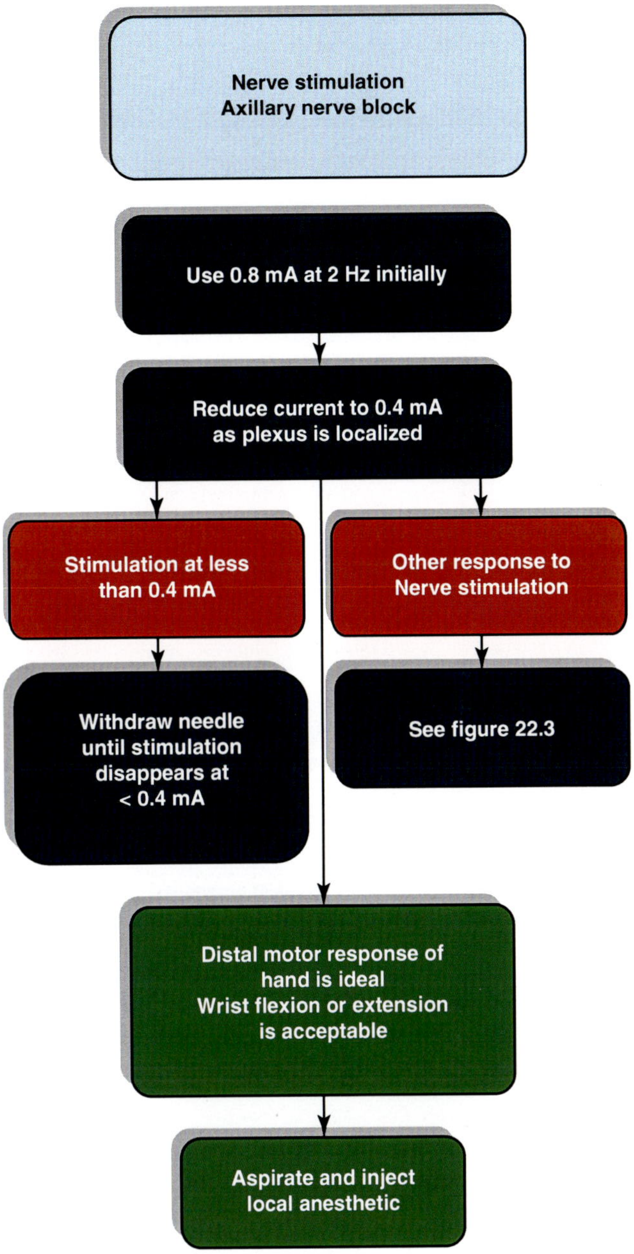

Fig. 22.3 Flowchart of the procedure for employing nerve stimulation techniques for axillary brachial plexus block

Table 22.1 Responses and recommended needle adjustments for nerve stimulation-guided axillary brachial plexus block

Correct response from nerve stimulation
Hand twitch with approximately 0.4 mA (median, radial or ulnar nerve)
For a higher success rate, multiple injections at each nerve are recommended:
Median nerve (C5–C8, T1; flexion of middle, index fingers, and thumb and pronation and flexion of wrist), ***ulnar*** nerve (C7–8,T1; flexion of ring and little fingers and ulnar deviation of wrist), ***radial*** nerve (C5–8, T1; extension of fingers and wrist)
Other common responses and needle adjustments
Muscle twitches from electrical stimulation
Upper arm (local twitches from biceps or triceps)
Explanation: needle angle is too superior or inferior
Needle adjustment: withdraw completely and redirect accordingly
Vascular puncture
Axillary artery with arterial blood in tubing
Explanation: needle in lumen of axillary artery
Needle adjustment: inject 2/3 of the local anesthetic posterior to the artery and 1/3 anterior to the artery
Axillary venous blood in tubing
Explanation: needle in lumen of axillary vein
Needle adjustment: redirect slightly more laterally or superiorly
Paresthesia without motor response
Needle has contacted brachial plexus
Explanation: stimulator, needle, or electrode malfunctioning
Needle adjustment: none if typical distribution of paresthesia (inject); reinsert if atypical
Bone contact
Humerus (2–3 cm deep)
Explanation: needle has advanced beyond plexus, too deep
Needle adjustment: withdraw to subcutaneous tissue and reinsert with an angle 20–30° more superior or inferior

22.3.1 Modifications to Inappropriate Responses

See Fig. 22.4

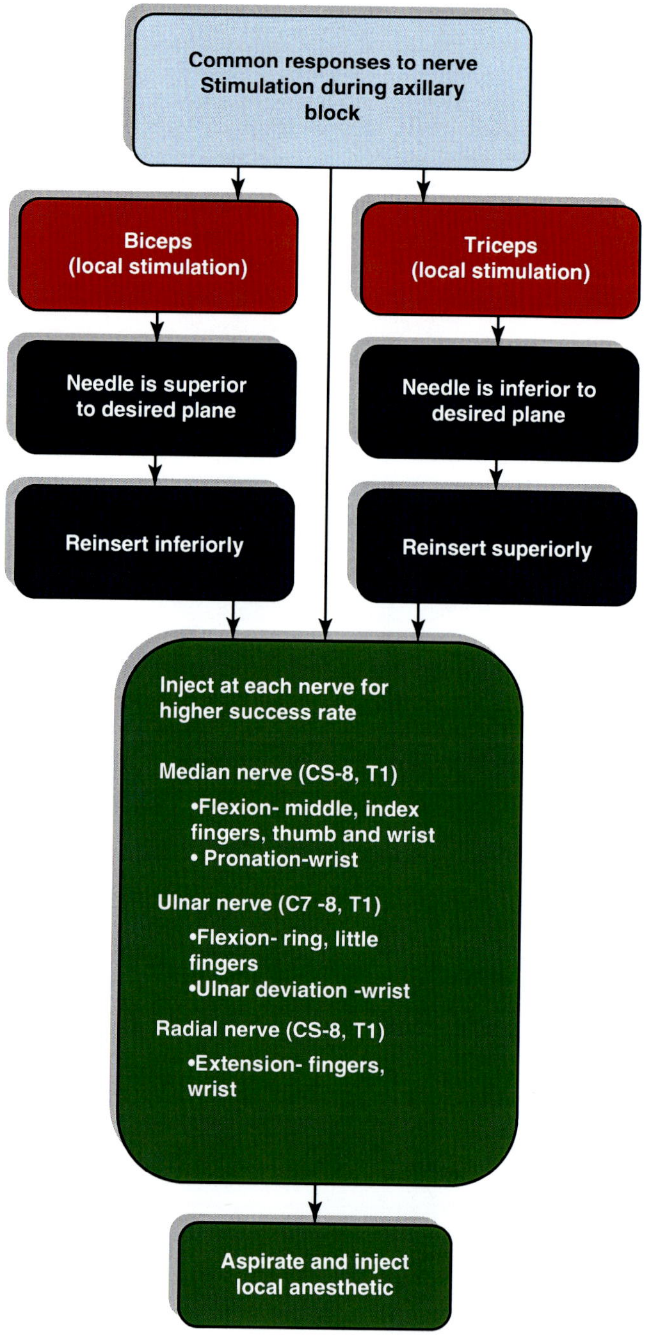

Fig. 22.4 Flowchart of modifications to inappropriate responses to nerve stimulation during axillary brachial plexus block

22.4 Ultrasound-Guided Technique (Fig. 22.5)

The terminal nerves of the brachial plexus at the axillary level are shown in the MRI image and ultrasound image (Fig. 22.6).

22.4.1 Preparing the Site

- Prepare the needle insertion site and skin surface with an antiseptic solution.
- Prepare the ultrasound probe surface by applying a sterile adhesive dressing to it prior to needling.

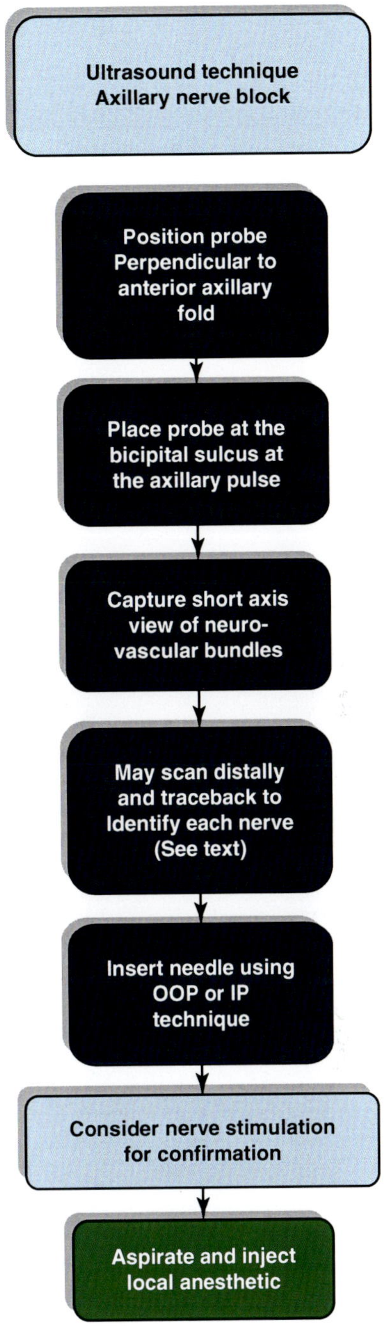

Fig. 22.5 Flowchart of ultrasound-guided techniques in axillary brachial plexus block

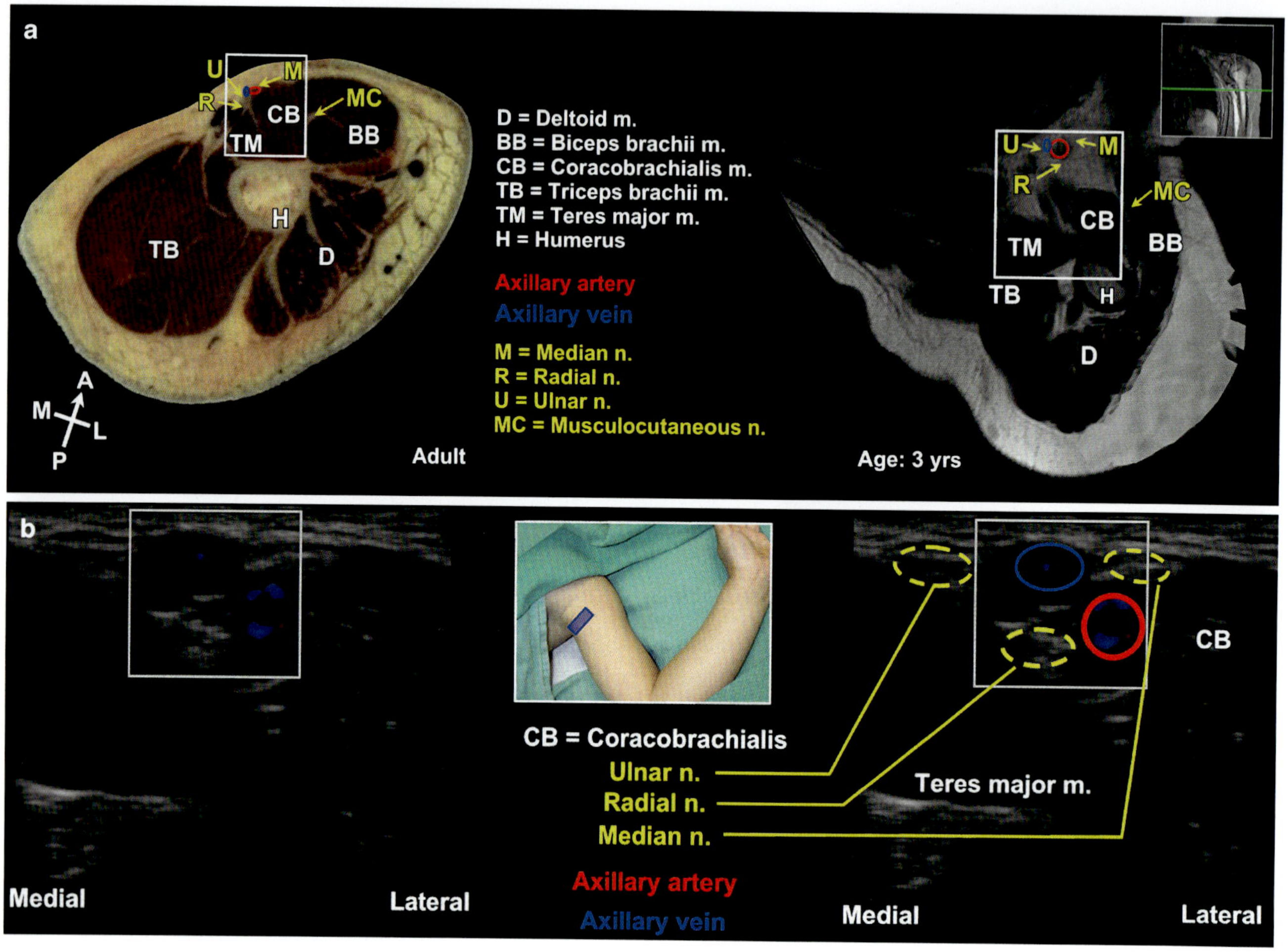

Fig. 22.6 (**a**) VHVS and MRI images of anatomical structures in the brachial plexus at the axilla. (**b**) Ultrasound image of the brachial plexus at the axilla

22.4.2 Scanning Technique

- The patient is positioned with the arm abducted at 80–90°, externally rotated and flexed at the elbow.
- High-frequency (10–15 MHz) linear probes are generally recommended for imaging as the nerves are found superficially (1–2 cm) below the skin.
- Small footprint probes are most useful for young or small children.
- The probe is positioned in a transverse plane perpendicular to the axis of the humerus at the level of the bicipital sulcus and over the location of the palpable axillary artery. This should offer a transverse or short-axis view of the neurovascular bundle (Fig. 22.6b).
- An initial scan should identify the axillary artery and vein. Subsequent adjustments should be made to view all the terminal nerves.
- Distal scanning along the course of each nerve is suggested to accurately identify each terminal nerve:
  - The radial nerve starts its course posterior to the axillary artery and travels deeper to the posterior aspect of the humerus towards the radial groove of the humerus (adjacent to the deltoid tuberosity).
  - The median nerve lies superior (lateral in the image) to the axillary artery in the axilla. The nerve, while moving to the medial aspect, follows closely the axillary/brachial artery towards the cubital fossa.
  - The ulnar nerve lies medial and inferior (superficial and medial in the image) to the axillary artery in the axilla and travels medially in the arm to reach the ulnar nerve sulcus behind the medial epicondyle of the humerus.
- Color Doppler should be used to confirm the location of the artery and is able to distinguish the artery from small nerves that appear to be pulsating on ultrasound.
- The most proximal location at the apex of the axilla may be the best for viewing all the terminal branches of the brachial plexus.

22.4.3 Sonographic Appearance

- In a transverse cross section, using a high-frequency, small footprint ("hockey stick") probe (Fig. 22.6b), coracobrachialis muscles are seen on the right superior aspect. The deeper teres major muscle is seen inferior to the neurovascular bundle.
- The anechoic and circular axillary artery lies in the middle and is adjacent to both the biceps and coracobrachialis muscles.
- The compressible anechoic axillary vein (two may be present) lies superficial (although there are many variants) between the median and ulnar nerves.
- The axillary artery runs deep to the vein and is surrounded by the nerves.
- The nerves appear round to oval in short axis with a honeycomb-like appearance of hypoechoic neutral structures surrounded by hyperechoic connective tissue (epineurium) rims.
- The median nerve is often located superior to the artery, lying between the artery and biceps brachii muscle.
- The ulnar nerve is usually located inferior and superficial to the artery.
- The radial nerve lies deep/posterior to the artery at the midline.
- Clockwise around the axillary artery, the nerves are arranged median, ulnar, and radial, but there are many variations.
- The musculocutaneous nerve is commonly located in the hyperechoic plane between the biceps and coracobrachialis muscles (see above) and varies significantly in its appearance: proximally, it may appear round-oval, and distally, it may be triangular. Occasionally, it may also appear flat.

22.4.4 Needle Insertion

While a single-injection technique has been shown to be successful in children (perhaps due to minimal septae within the sheath), the use of ultrasound may improve success if injections are performed after the needle is directed towards each nerve. The technique used will depend on the state of the patient (level of sedation and comfort) and visibility of the nerves.

- Use a 30–50 mm, 22–24G insulated needle if using nerve stimulation.
- Both in-plane (IP) and out-of-plane (OOP) needle approaches can be used for axillary block.
- An OOP approach is similar to the traditional blind procedure with the needle distal and perpendicular to the probe placed in transverse axis to the nerves (Fig. 22.7). Place the needle 1 cm from the probe at a 30–45° angle from the skin and align the needle insertion site with the neurovascular bundle target.
- The IP approach involves inserting the needle at an acute angle (20–30°) to the skin in a superior-to-inferior direction (Fig. 22.8). The block needle is initially directed posteriorly and deep to the median nerve and axillary artery to locate the radial nerve. We recommend the initial injection of local anesthetic at this location to minimize distortion of the image from the spread of hypoechoic local anesthetic solution. Next, retract the needle and inject local anesthetic around the median nerve, followed by injection around the ulnar nerve which is most superficial. It is important to note that the relative location of the nerves can be variable.
- For intercostobrachial and medial cutaneous nerve blocks, subcutaneous injections should be performed on the medial surface of the upper arm all the way from the biceps brachii to the triceps brachii muscles.
- For musculocutaneous nerve blocks, often the best results will be from infraclavicular blockade; however, the nerve may also be blocked in a separate injection during the axillary approach, either above the artery into the body of the coracobrachialis (with elbow flexion as nerve stimulation response) or at a mid-humeral location.

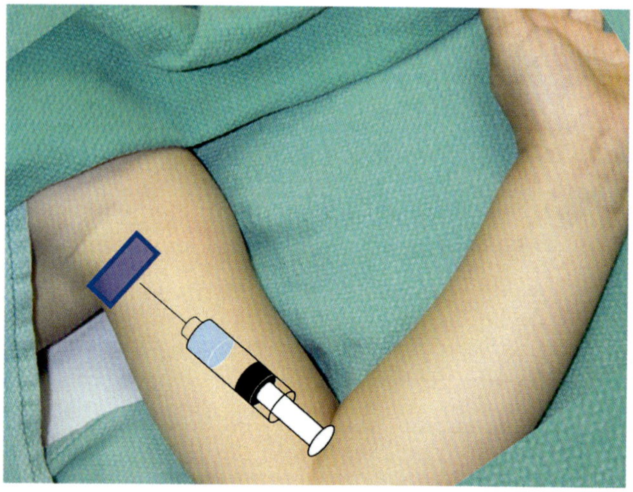

Fig. 22.7 Out-of-plane needling technique for ultrasound-guided axillary brachial plexus block. *Blue rectangle* indicates probe footprint

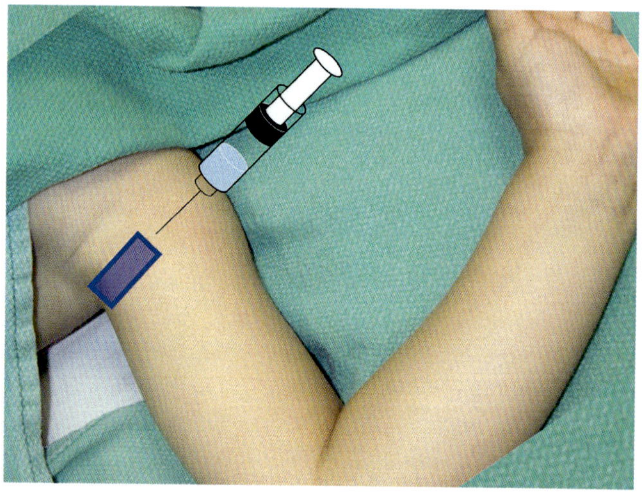

Fig. 22.8 In-plane needling technique for ultrasound-guided axillary brachial plexus block. *Blue rectangle* indicates probe footprint

22.5 Local Anesthetic Application

- Tracing the nerves distally or proximally along their known path may be adequate in some cases to identify the individual nerve branch (see "Scanning"). Nevertheless, it is recommended to identify each nerve separately through the use of electrical stimulation to improve block performance.
- Performing a test dose with D5W is recommended prior to local anesthetic application to visualize the spread and confirm nerve localization.
- The dose of local anesthetic is 0.2–0.3 mL/kg 0.25–0.5 % bupivacaine, ropivacaine, or levobupivacaine. For the musculocutaneous nerve, inject 0.5–1 mL of local anesthetic solution deep to the fascia.
- A proper injection is indicated by fluid spread completely around the nerve structure and nerve movement away from the needle tip. Improper injection (e.g., injection outside the sheath) is indicated by a partial asymmetrical fluid expansion not immediately adjacent to the nerve structure.
- Nerve visualization often becomes more difficult after local anesthetic injection.

22.6 Current Literature in Ultrasound-Guided Approaches

In adults, while multiple-injection techniques seem to be superior to those using single or double injections, the success rate of axillary block using single-injection technique in children seems to be similar to that of the multiple-injection technique. Nevertheless, rates of success are still moderate at 70–80 % [1], and to ensure adequate circumferential spread of local anesthetic around each of the individual nerves, multiple injections and needle redirections are commonly required. Various strategies have been used to improve success rates (e.g., pressure applied distally and/or transarterial approaches to more effectively block the posterior cord), although they appear to have limited benefits in children.

Two case reports describe the use of axillary block for anesthesia for pseudosyndactyly repair in recessive dystrophic epidermolysis bullosa patients. Englbrecht et al. [2] administered an ultrasound-guided axillary block by targeting each of the ulnar, median, radial, and musculocutaneous nerves, in that order, with 3 mL mepivacaine 1 % and 2 mL bupivacaine 0.18 % using a 24G SonoPlex NanoLine needle. General anesthesia was not given, and pain control was effective during and after surgery.

Boschin et al. [3] performed bilateral axillary brachial plexus block in a 3-year-old who presented for surgery to repair pseudosyndactyly of all fingers. Both hands were repaired during the same surgery, and the axillary blocks were administered before each side was operated on. Blocks were performed under ultrasound guidance; a 24G needle was inserted using an in-plane approach, and 7.5 mL ropivacaine 0.25 % was injected in each side. There were no issues with pain control following surgery.

A recent study by Elnour et al. [4] compared ultrasound- and nerve stimulation-guided axillary block in patients undergoing forearm and hand surgery. They demonstrated higher (but not significantly) block success, shorter block performance time, and increased block duration in the ultrasound group.

Three expert reviews have been recently published which describe axillary block as performed by the respective authors [5–7]. This block should be performed with a similar technique to that used in adults, using IP needle alignment with a high-frequency probe placed transversely to the humerus and using multiple injections to surround all the terminal nerves of the plexus. Multiple punctures may be necessary to anesthetize all the relevant nerves for many surgical procedures (i.e., brachial cutaneous, medial antebrachial, and possibly musculocutaneous nerves will require separate blockade).

Clinical Pearls: Axillary Block

- Place a hockey stick probe or a linear small footprint probe in the axilla as proximal as possible.
- The needle is directed from superior to inferior using an in-plane approach.
- The structures are superficial and can usually be easily identified. The radial nerve is occasionally challenging to locate.
- Color Doppler can be used to recognize the vascular structures.
- Local anesthetic should be injected to surround each of the terminal nerves.

22.7 Case Study

Axillary Block (Provided by S. Suresh)

A female infant with Apert syndrome, 15 months of age and weighing 11.9 kg, was presented for right-hand thumb-index and middle-ring complex syndactyly reconstruction with a full-thickness skin graft from the right antecubital fossa, as well as endoscopic release of bilateral coronal sutures, bilateral supraorbital release, and craniofacial reconstruction. Diagnosis was based on bilateral X-rays of the hands (two views) and CT/CTA with contrast of the bilateral upper extremity. For syndactyly repair, an ultrasound-guided, in-plane axillary block was performed using a 22G needle and 6 mL 0.25% bupivacaine (see Fig. 22.9). Block duration was 6–12 h. Postoperative analgesia consisted of hydrocodone-acetaminophen (Lortab) 2.5–167 mg/5 mL solution 1.2 mg, given 5 h after surgery.

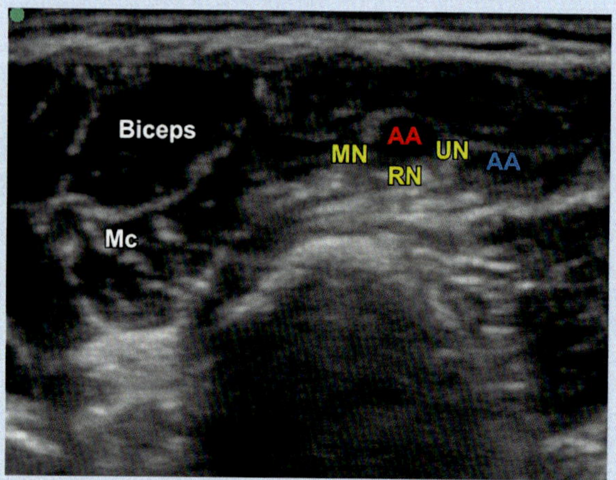

Fig. 22.9 Ultrasound-guided axillary brachial plexus block. *Mc* musculocutaneous nerve, *MN* median nerve, *RN* radial nerve, *UN* ulnar nerve, *AA* axillary artery, *AV* axillary vein. See "Case Study" for details

References

1. Carre P, Joly A, Cluzel FB, et al. Axillary block in children: single or multiple injection? Pediatr Anesth. 2000;10:35–9.
2. Englbrecht JS, Langer M, Hahnenkamp K, Ellger B. Ultrasound-guided axillary plexus block in a child with dystrophic epidermolysis bullosa. Anaesth Intensive Care. 2010;38:1101–5.
3. Boschin M, Ellger B, van den Heuvel I, et al. Bilateral ultrasound-guided axillary plexus anesthesia in a child with dystrophic epidermolysis bullosa. Pediatr Anesth. 2012;22:504–6.
4. Elnour HA, Hana MG, Rizk SN, Soaaida S. Ultrasound guided axillary brachial plexus block in pediatric surgical patients. Egypt J Anesth. 2009;25:281–90.
5. Marhofer P. Upper extremity peripheral blocks. Tech Reg Anesth Pain Manag. 2007;11:215–21.
6. Rapp H, Grau T. Ultrasound-guided regional anesthesia in pediatric patients. Tech Reg Anesth Pain Manag. 2004;8:179–98.
7. Roberts S. Ultrasonographic guidance in pediatric regional anesthesia. Part 2: techniques. Pediatr Anesth. 2006;16:1112–24.

Suggested Reading

Dalens B. Infraclavicular brachial plexus blocks. In: Dalens BJ, editor. Pediatric regional anesthesia. Boca Raton: CRC Press; 1990. p. 247–51.

Karmakar MK, Kwok WH. Ultrasound-Guided Regional Anesthesia. In: Cote CJ, Lerman J, Anderson BJ, Eds. 5th ed. Philadelphia: WB Saunders; 2013. p. 880–908.

Mather SJ. Upper limb blocks. In: Peutrell JM, Mather SJ, editors. Regional anaesthesia for babies and children. Oxford: Oxford University Press; 1997. p. 101–5.

Tsui BC. Axillary block. In: Tsui BC, editor. Atlas of ultrasound and nerve stimulation-guided regional anesthesia. New York: Springer; 2007. p. 99–107.

Terminal Nerve Blocks of the Upper Extremity

23

Ban C.H. Tsui

Contents

B.C.H. Tsui, Dip Eng, BSc (Math), B Pharm, MSc, MD, FRCPC
Department of Anesthesiology and Pain Medicine,
Stollery Children's Hospital/University of Alberta Hospital,
2-150 Clinical Sciences Building,
Edmonton, AB T6G 2G3, Canada
e-mail: btsui@ualberta.ca

B.C.H. Tsui, S. Suresh (eds.), *Pediatric Atlas of Ultrasound- and Nerve Stimulation-Guided Regional Anesthesia*,
DOI 10.1007/978-0-387-79964-3_23

23.1 Median Nerve Block

- The median nerve innervates muscles which produce flexion and opposition of the thumb, middle, and index fingers, as well as pronation and flexion of the wrist. The nerve carries fibers from all roots and trunks of the brachial plexus.
- At the level of the axilla, the nerve initially lies superior to the axillary artery and then descends along the medial aspect of the arm, lateral to the brachial artery (continuation of the axillary artery). It then crosses the artery, usually anteriorly, at the midpoint of the humerus at the insertion of the coracobrachialis muscle.
- The nerve crosses the elbow, lying medially on the brachialis muscle and just medial to the brachial artery and vein (all of these medial to the biceps brachii tendon). The cross-sectional view at the antecubital fossa seen in Fig. 10.8 illustrates its relationship to the artery, vein, and adjacent musculature.
- Passing deep to the bicipital aponeurosis and median cubital vein, the nerve divides between the two heads of the pronator teres muscle, giving off the anterior interosseous nerve, which supplies the flexor pollicis longus and pronator quadratus muscles and the lateral half of the flexor digitorum profundus muscle.
- Distal to the antecubital fossa, cutaneous sensory branches emerge and supply the palm, the palmar aspects of the first three digits, and the lateral half of the fourth digit (there may be some variation in overlap of cutaneous innervation from the ulnar nerve of the medial one and a half digits).
- At the most distal skin crease of the wrist, the median nerve lies near the midline, passes deep to the flexor retinaculum, and divides into medial and lateral branches.
- Through its innervation of the lateral two lumbricals, it mediates flexion of the metacarpophalangeal joints and extension of the interphalangeal joints of digits two and three.
- The median nerve supplies the thenar muscles, the lateral two lumbricals, and all the muscles in the anterior compartment of the forearm except the flexor carpi ulnaris and the medial half of the flexor digitorum profundus, which are supplied by the ulnar nerve.

23.1.1 Surface Anatomy (Fig. 23.1)

The patient is placed supine with the arm abducted slightly, the elbow flexed approximately 30°, and the forearm resting on an arm board. Surface landmarks include:

- Medial
  - Medial epicondyle of the humerus
- Lateral
  - Brachial artery pulse: immediately medial to the biceps brachii tendon.
  - Biceps brachii tendon: lateral to the brachial artery and median nerve, it may be best palpated with slight elbow flexion.

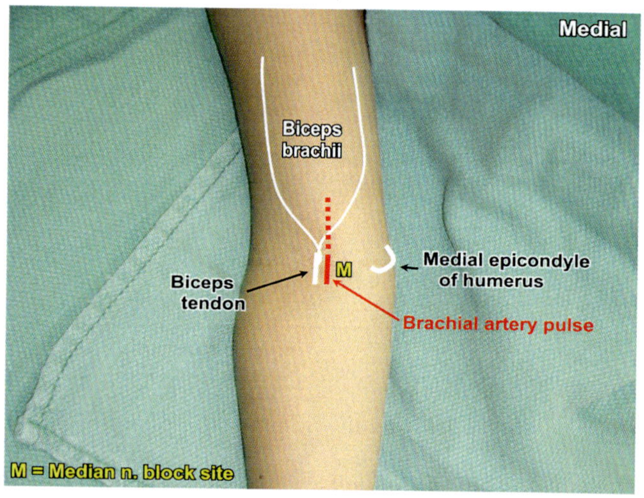

Fig. 23.1 Surface anatomy and landmarks for median nerve block

23.1.2 Nerve Stimulation Technique (Table 14.1)

- The median nerve is superficially located at the elbow, and a short needle (3–4 cm at most) with a short bevel should be used for the blocks.
- Complete elbow extension should be avoided to reduce the chance of elbow joint penetration.
- Insert the needle perpendicular to the skin immediately medial to the pulse of the brachial artery.
- Twitches will be seen in the lateral three digits (flexion of the thumb, index, or middle finger), although wrist flexion or forearm pronation can also indicate adequate nerve localization.

23.1.3 Ultrasound-Guided Technique

Refer to the VHVS and ultrasound images for the relevant anatomy (Fig. 23.2).

23.1.3.1 Scanning Technique

- High-frequency (10+ MHz) probes should be used for visualizing the median nerve in children.
- Place the probe in the axial plane with the center of the probe just medial to the biceps tendon in order to capture a transverse view of the nerve (medially) and adjacent brachial artery (laterally).
- Both the nerve and artery lie quite superficial, and the nerve can be larger than the artery at this location.
- Color Doppler may be used to confirm the identity of the artery and of the nerve on its medial aspect.

23.1.3.2 Sonographic Appearance

The nerve appears oval/peanut-shaped and lies medial to the artery, which is often circular and smaller than the nerve (Fig. 23.2b).

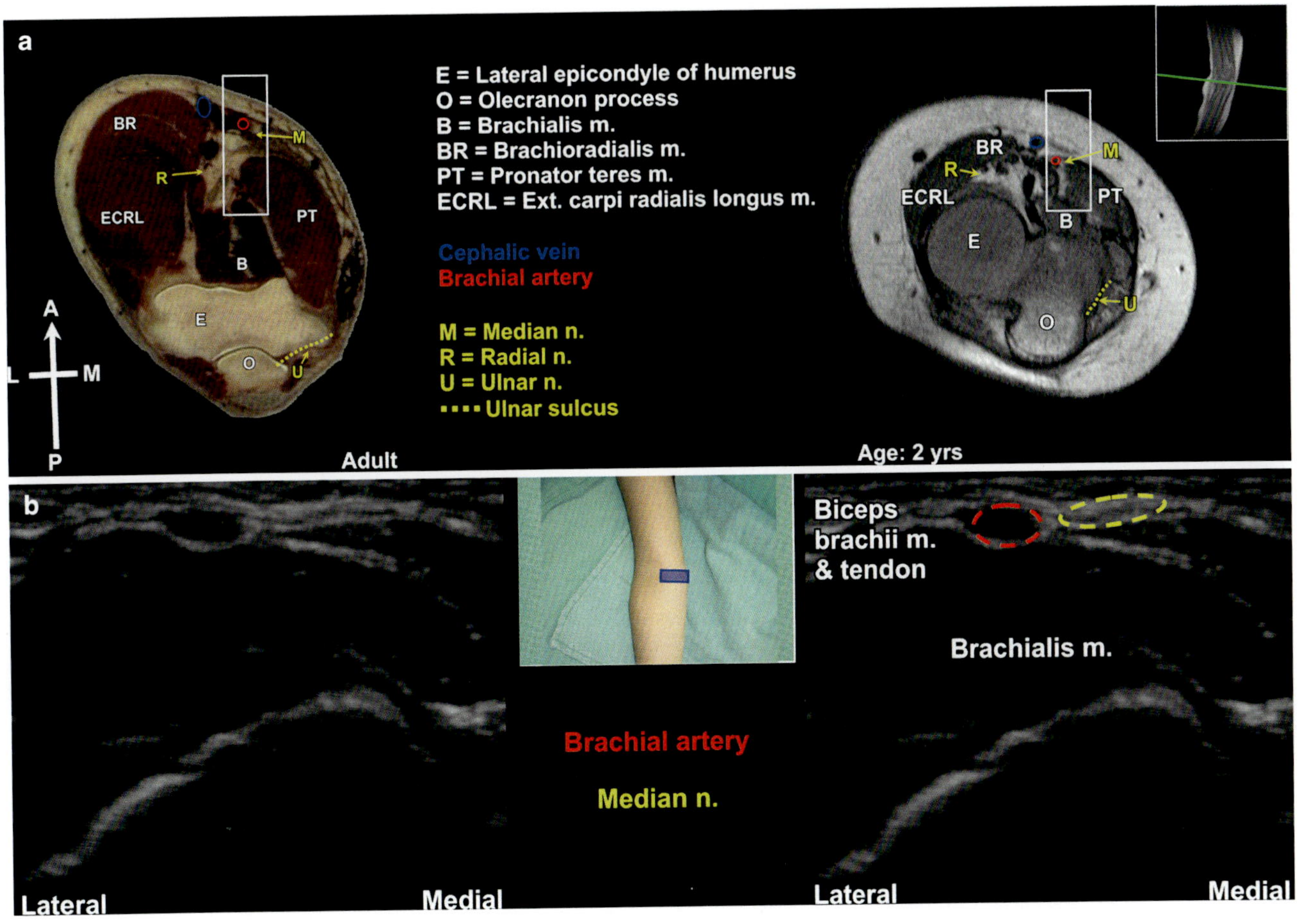

Fig. 23.2 (a) VHVS and MRI images at the antecubital fossa. (b) Ultrasound image of the median nerve at the antecubital fossa

23.1.3.3 Needle Insertion

- An in-plane (IP) or out-of-plane (OOP) approach may be used to block the median nerve at the level of the elbow.
- For the IP approach (Fig. 23.3), insert the needle medial to the median nerve in order to avoid the brachial artery. The needle will be perpendicular to the median nerve, and the goal will be to inject local anesthetic around the nerve. This approach may cause more discomfort in an awake patient due to a longer needle path compared to the OOP technique.
- For the OOP approach (Fig. 23.4), position the nerve at the center of the ultrasound screen, and insert the needle in cross section to the transversely placed probe in a cephalad direction.
- Place the needle initially at a small distance (e.g., 1 cm) from the probe in order to view the needle tip once the needle has reached the nerve.

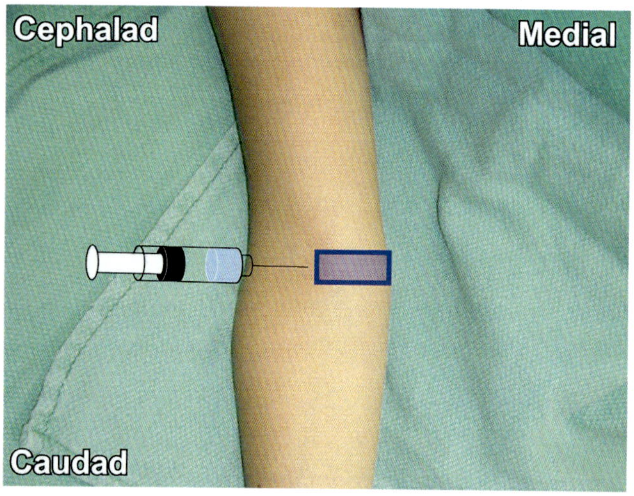

Fig. 23.3 In-plane needling approach for ultrasound-guided median nerve block. *Blue rectangle* indicates probe footprint

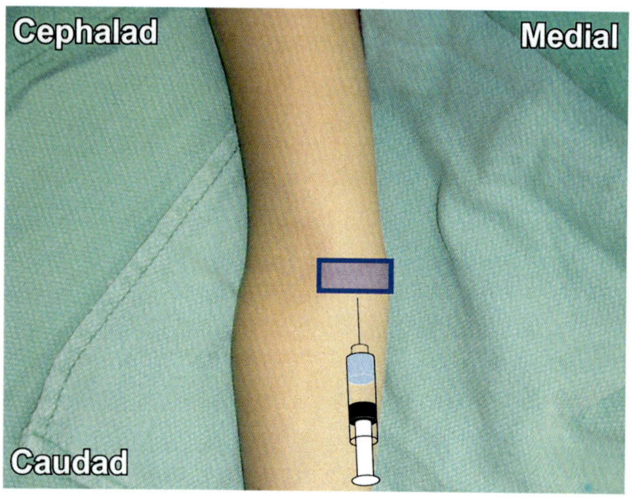

Fig. 23.4 Out-of-plane needling approach for ultrasound-guided median nerve block. *Blue rectangle* indicates probe footprint

23.1.4 Local Anesthetic Application

- The median nerve can be blocked using a 3–4 cm needle, insulated if using nerve stimulation, with 2–3 mL of 0.25–0.5 % ropivacaine.
- Performing a test dose with D5W is recommended prior to local anesthetic application to visualize the spread and confirm nerve localization.
- Aim to spread approximately 1–3 mL of local anesthetic around the nerve in a circular fashion in order to avoid nerve contact but obtain a complete block.
- The local anesthetic injection will appear as an expansion of hypoechogenicity surrounding the nerve.

23.1.5 Case Study

Median Nerve Block at the Elbow

(Contributed by A. Spencer)

A 12-year-old girl, 44 kg in weight, presented for hand surgery. An X-ray showed a mildly displaced intra-articular fracture of the distal portion of the proximal phalanx of the left thumb without involvement of the epiphyseal growth plate. The patient required an open reduction and internal fixation of the proximal phalanx and underwent a general anesthetic combined with an ultrasound-guided median nerve and radial nerve block at the elbow. Both blocks were performed with a 40 mm, 22G needle using an in-plane approach (see Figs. 23.5 and 23.10). Four mL of 0.5 % bupivacaine was used for each block; block duration was 6–12 and 8–12 h for the median and radial nerve blocks, respectively. The duration of surgery was 1 h, 10 min. Pain reporting was 0/10 at both 30 and 60 min post-op with sensory block noted in the median and radial territories. Postoperative analgesia consisted of acetaminophen 500 mg po q4h prn and ibuprofen 400 mg po q6h prn.

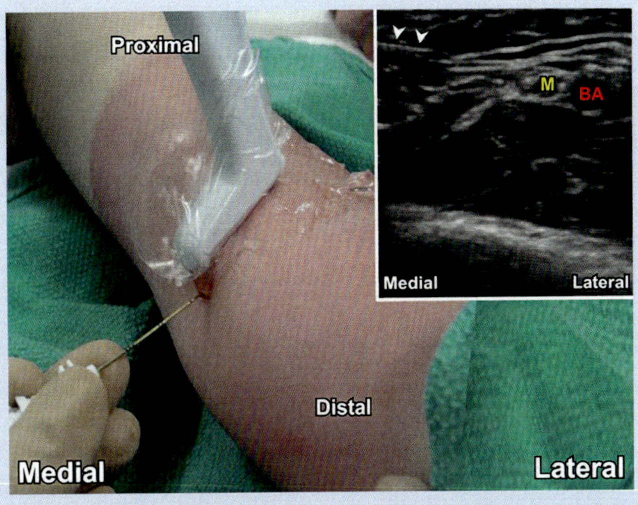

Fig. 23.5 Ultrasound-guided median nerve block. *M* median nerve, *BA* brachial artery, *arrowheads* indicate needle position (see Case Study for details)

23.2 Radial Nerve Block

- The radial nerve innervates muscles which produce extension (dorsiflexion) of the wrist and digits. The nerve carries fibers from the upper and middle trunks, the posterior division, and the posterior cord of the brachial plexus and emerges from the posterior aspect of the plexus.
- The nerve's origin lies posterior to the second and third parts of the axillary artery, and it descends within the axilla across the subscapularis, teres major, and latissimus dorsi muscles (the nerve lies on the insertion of this latter muscle).
- It then passes between the medial and lateral heads of the triceps brachii muscle and descends obliquely across the posterior aspect of the humerus along the spiral (radial) groove at the level of the deltoid muscle insertion (Fig. 10.11). It travels posterior and medial to the deep brachial artery of the arm at this location.
- The nerve reaches the lateral margin of the humerus above the elbow before crossing over the lateral epicondyle and entering the anterior compartment of the arm in a deep groove between the brachialis and brachioradialis muscles proximally and the extensor carpi radialis longus muscle distally.
- In front of the lateral epicondyle of the humerus, the nerve divides and continues as the superficial radial (sensory) and the deep posterior interosseous (motor) nerves.
- The radial nerve supplies the posterior compartments of the arm and forearm, including the skin and subcutaneous tissues. It also supplies the skin on the posterior aspect of the hand laterally near the base of the thumb and the dorsal aspect of the index finger and the lateral half of the ring finger up to the distal interphalangeal crease.

23.2.1 Surface Anatomy (Fig. 23.6)

The patient is placed supine with the arm abducted slightly, the elbow flexed approximately 30°, and the forearm resting on an arm board. Surface landmarks include:

- Deltoid tuberosity: internal rotation of the arm accentuates the posterior deltoid region and enables the deltoid muscle to be traced to its point of insertion on the tuberosity. The spiral groove lies just distal to the tuberosity.
- Lateral epicondyle of the humerus: palpate from proximal to distal along the lateral aspect of the humerus toward the elbow, and feel the curvature of the lateral supracondylar crest proximal to the epicondyle.
- Biceps brachii muscle: palpate the lateral border of the distal muscle belly. The radial nerve lies deep and lateral to this portion of the muscle.

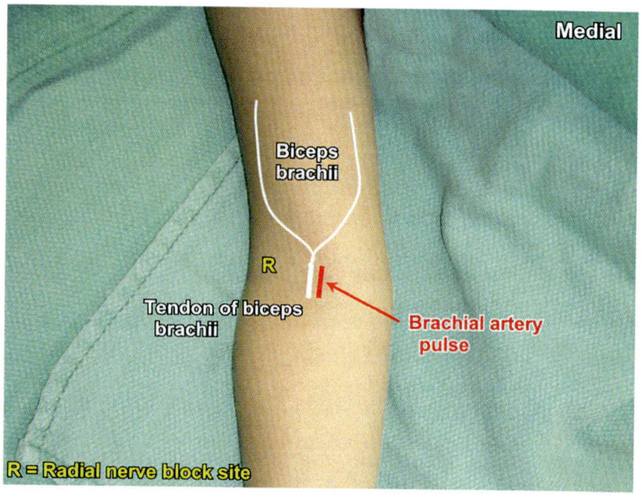

Fig. 23.6 Surface anatomy and landmarks for radial nerve block

23.2.2 Nerve Stimulation Technique

- The nerves are all superficially located at the elbow, and a short needle (3–4 cm) with a short bevel should be used for all blocks.
- Complete elbow extension should be avoided to reduce the chance of elbow joint penetration.
- The point of puncture is on a line joining the epicondyles, at the location between the biceps brachii tendon and the brachioradialis muscle. Insert the needle using a 30–60° angle horizontally, directed cephalad.
- Needle contact to the humerus indicates that the needle is too deep, while deep insertion without bone contact indicates that the needle has passed the anterior aspect of the arm, lateral to the humerus, without contacting the nerve.
- Twitches will appear on the radial aspect of the operative hand; extension (dorsiflexion) of the wrist and digits is the specific motor response.

23.2.3 Ultrasound-Guided Technique

23.2.3.1 Scanning Technique

- High-frequency (10–15 MHz) probes should be used in children due to the short distance from the skin to the nerve.
- Place the probe in the axial plane at the lateral aspect of the distal upper arm (1–2 cm above the elbow joint at the level of the supracondylar ridge of the humerus), lateral to the biceps tendon, and medial to the upper aspect of the brachioradialis muscle. Locate the round radial nerve before its division to deep and superficial branches. To confirm the nerve's identity, it can be traced distally to and past the elbow, where the branches appear as two adjacent hyperechoic "bubbles."
- Alternatively, the nerve can be traced proximally to where it descends obliquely across the posterior aspect of the humerus along the spiral (radial) groove at the level of the deltoid insertion. The nerve lies posteromedial to the deep brachial artery at the posterior humeral location. Color Doppler can be valuable in localizing the nerve (Fig. 23.7).
- It may be useful to first locate the nerve at the posterior humeral location with subsequent tracing laterally and anterior to the elbow location.

23.2.3.2 Sonographic Appearance

- The nerve lies sandwiched between the brachialis and brachioradialis muscles, near the lateral curvature of the rectangular-appearing humerus.
- Above the elbow, the nerve is usually oval-round, while at its point of division, it becomes flattened, containing two hypoechoic areas.
- At the posterior humeral location, the deep brachial artery (of similar size to the nerve) lies anterolateral to the oval nerve; both appear to rest on the oval-shaped humerus (Fig. 23.7b).
- Note that most experts prefer to place the block at a more distal location (i.e., antecubital) (Figs. 23.7c & d).

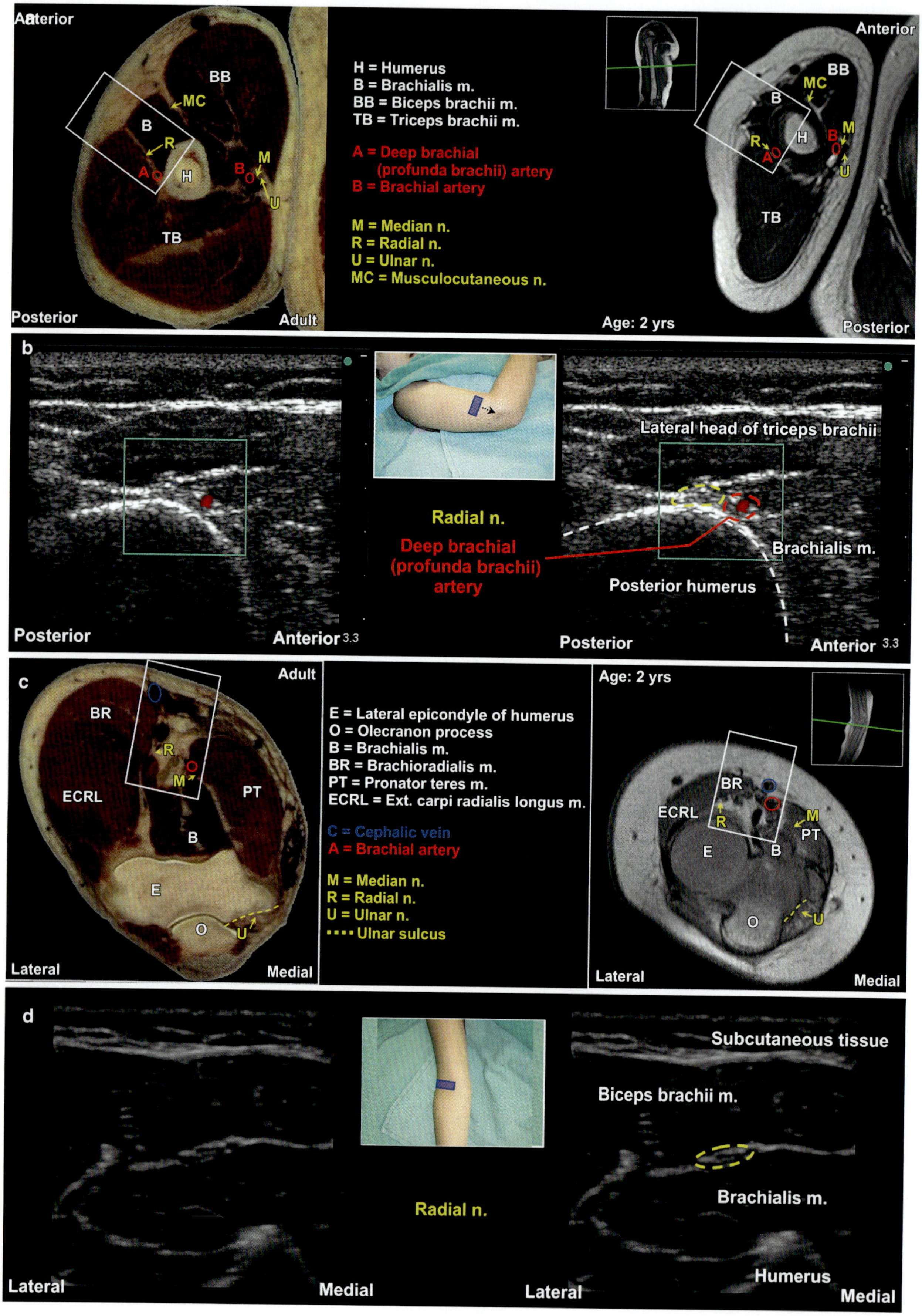

Fig. 23.7 (**a**) VHVS and MRI images of the location of the radial nerve at the level of the humerus. (**b**) Ultrasound image of the location of the radial nerve at the humerus. The dashed arrow indicates that the probe is moved distally from this position to the antecubital fossa. (**c**) VHVS and MRI images of the location of the radial nerve at the level of the antecubital fossa. (**d**) Ultrasound image of the radial nerve at the block location (antecubital fossa)

23.2.3.3 Needle Insertion

- An OOP technique for needle insertion is a good approach due to the short distance to the nerve (Fig. 23.8). Alternatively, an IP technique (see below) using an anterior-to-posterior approach will provide constant visualization of the needle shaft and tip and may help avoid puncture of the deep brachial artery which may be adjacent to the radial nerve. However, an IP technique may cause more discomfort in an awake patient.
- For the OOP approach, position the nerve at the center of the ultrasound screen, and insert the needle in cross section to the transversely placed probe in a cephalad direction. Place the needle initially at a small distance (e.g., 1 cm) from the probe in order to view the needle tip once the needle has reached the nerve.
- For the IP approach, on the posterior aspect of the mid-upper arm, slide the probe caudally looking for the hyperechoic nerve that will eventually run anteriorly along the distal part of the humerus. Move the image of the nerve to the most lateral edge of the screen during IP advancement. The needle is inserted in plane with the ultrasound transducer in a lateral-to-medial or medial-to-lateral direction (Fig. 23.9). The needle shaft and tip should be visualized in real time as it tracks toward the radial nerve. Injecting local anesthetic anteriorly and posteriorly to the nerve may be required to completely surround the nerve.

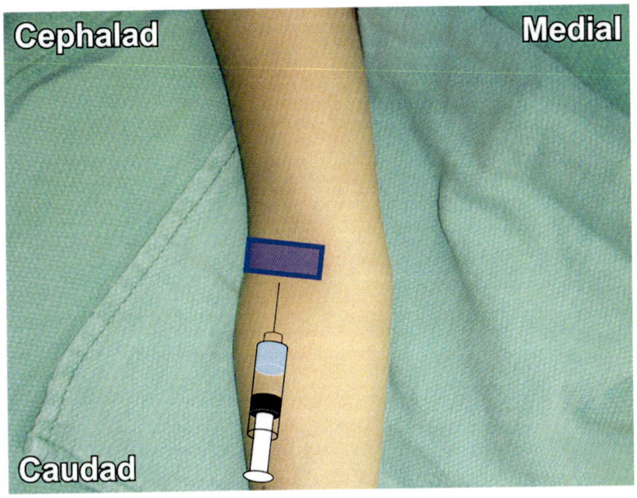

Fig. 23.8 Out-of-plane needling technique for ultrasound-guided radial nerve block. *Blue rectangle* indicates probe footprint

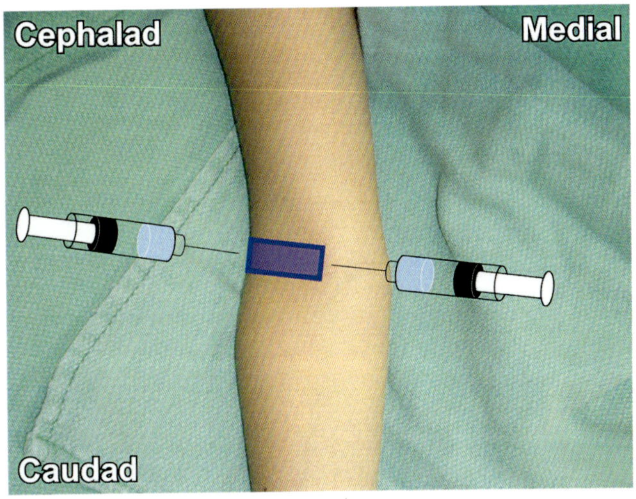

Fig. 23.9 In-plane needling approach for ultrasound-guided radial nerve block. *Blue rectangle* indicates probe footprint

23.2.4 Local Anesthetic Application

- The radial nerve can be blocked using a 30–40 mm needle, insulated if using nerve stimulation, with 2–3 mL of 0.5 % ropivacaine.
- Performing a test dose with D5W is recommended prior to local anesthetic application to visualize the spread and confirm nerve localization. This may not be necessary using the IP technique with good needle tip visualization (see Chap. 4 box on test dose with D5W prior to local anesthetic injection).
- Aim to spread approximately 2–3 mL of local anesthetic (e.g., ropivacaine 0.25–0.5 %) around the nerve in a circular fashion in order to avoid nerve contact but obtain a complete block.
- The local anesthetic injection will appear as an expansion of hypoechogenicity surrounding the nerve.

23.2.5 Case Study

See Sect. 23.1.5 for details on nerve block procedure. Figure 23.10 shows the radial nerve block with a medial-to-lateral approach..

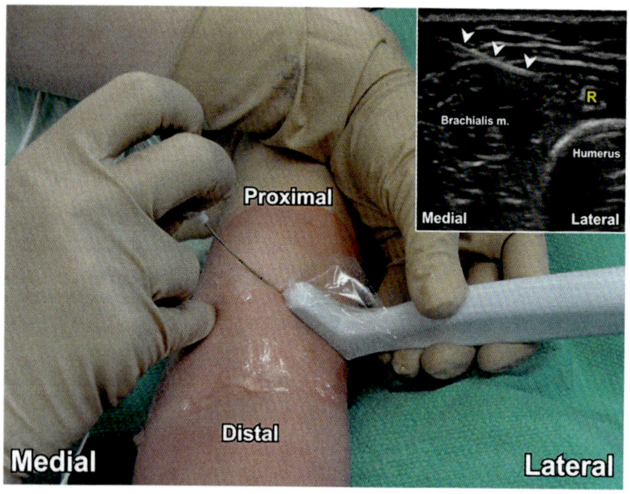

Fig. 23.10 Ultrasound-guided radial nerve block (see median nerve Case Study (Sect. 23.1.5) for details)

23.3 Ulnar Nerve Block

- In the forearm, the ulnar nerve innervates muscles that produce flexion of the ring (fourth) and little (fifth) fingers and ulnar deviation of the wrist. The ulnar nerve is the continuation of the medial cord from the anterior division of the lower trunk of the brachial plexus.
- Initially, the nerve courses between the axillary artery and vein and then along the medial aspect of the brachial artery to the midpoint of the humerus before passing posteriorly and following the anterior surface of the medial head of the triceps brachii muscle (Fig. 10.6).
- It then passes behind the medial epicondyle of the humerus (in the condylar groove), divides between the humeral and ulnar heads of the flexor carpi ulnaris muscle, and lies on the medial aspect of the elbow joint.
- During its descent through the forearm, the nerve courses anteriorly, coming to lie deep to and between the flexor carpi ulnaris and flexor digitorum superficialis muscles, approaching the ulnar artery near the midline of the forearm at its midpoint (Fig. 10.9). The nerve and artery lie directly anterior to the ulna at the junction of the lower third and upper two thirds of the forearm.
- At the wrist, the nerve crosses superficial to the flexor retinaculum immediately lateral to the pisiform bone (medial to the hook of the hamate bone) and divides into superficial and deep branches; the ulnar artery lies anterolateral to the nerve at the wrist.
- The nerve supplies all the intrinsic muscles of the hand except those supplied by the median nerve (i.e., all the interossei, the medial two lumbricals, the hypothenar muscles, the adductor pollicis, and the deep head of flexor pollicis brevis).
- Through its innervation of the interossei and medial two lumbricals, the nerve mediates flexion of the metacarpophalangeal joints and extension of the interphalangeal joints of digits four and five.
- Dorsal and palmar cutaneous branches of the nerve branch 5–10 cm proximal to the wrist and generally supply the medial half of the fourth and the entire fifth digit (there may be some variation in overlap with the cutaneous branches of the median nerve supplying the lateral three and a half digits).

23.3.1 Surface Anatomy (Fig. 23.11)

The patient's arm is flexed at the elbow with the shoulder externally rotated and the forearm supinated and resting on an arm board. Surface landmarks include:

- Ulna: palpate the bone at the junction of the middle and lower thirds of the forearm.
- Ulnar artery pulse: may be difficult to palpate in many individuals.

If using the nerve stimulation technique:

- The needle insertion point is the ulnar groove, which lies between the medial epicondyle of the humerus and the olecranon process.

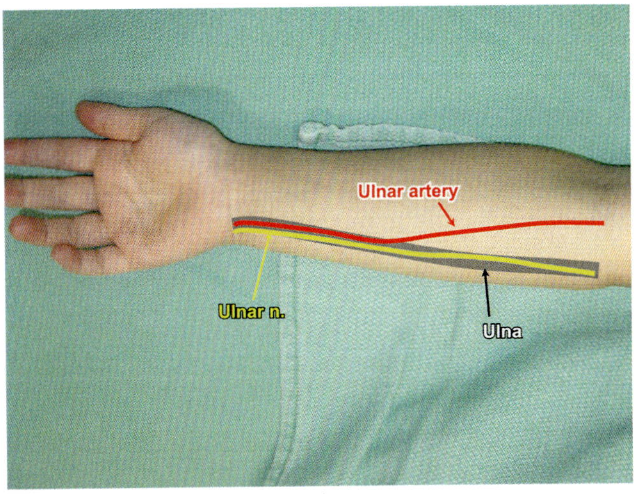

Fig. 23.11 Surface anatomy and landmarks for ulnar nerve block

23.3.2 Nerve Stimulation Technique

- The ulnar nerve is located superficially at the elbow as it passes through the condylar groove.
- With the arm flexed at the elbow, a short-beveled needle (3–5 cm) should be inserted 1–3 cm distal to and in line with the condylar groove. Alternatively, the block may be completed 2–3 cm proximal to the condylar groove.
- Insert the needle in the direction of the ulnar groove using a 45° angle directed proximally and medially.
- Twitches will appear in the ulnar aspect of the hand – motor responses are flexion of the ring and little fingers and ulnar deviation of the wrist.
- Blood withdrawal on aspiration suggests ulnar artery puncture. In this case, the needle should be reinserted after pressure treatment; contact with the ulna indicates that the needle is too deep.

23.3.3 Ultrasound-Guided Technique

Refer to Fig. 23.12 for the VHVS and ultrasound anatomy of this region, respectively.

23.3.3.1 Scanning Technique

The aim is to view the ulnar nerve in short axis as it approaches the ulnar artery:

- Place the probe above the ulna and belly of the flexor carpi ulnaris muscle, on the anterior surface of the forearm, rather than medially to contact the bone. Scan downward slowly until the pulsatile artery and nerve are viewed adjacent to each other (Doppler may be valuable here).
- Confirm the identity of the nerve by dynamically scanning proximally and distally to confirm that it is separate from the artery proximally and that it converges to join the artery at the mid-forearm distally (Fig. 23.12b).
- The block location will be where the nerve and artery are viewed in the same image but remain at sufficient distance apart to avoid arterial puncture during needle insertion.

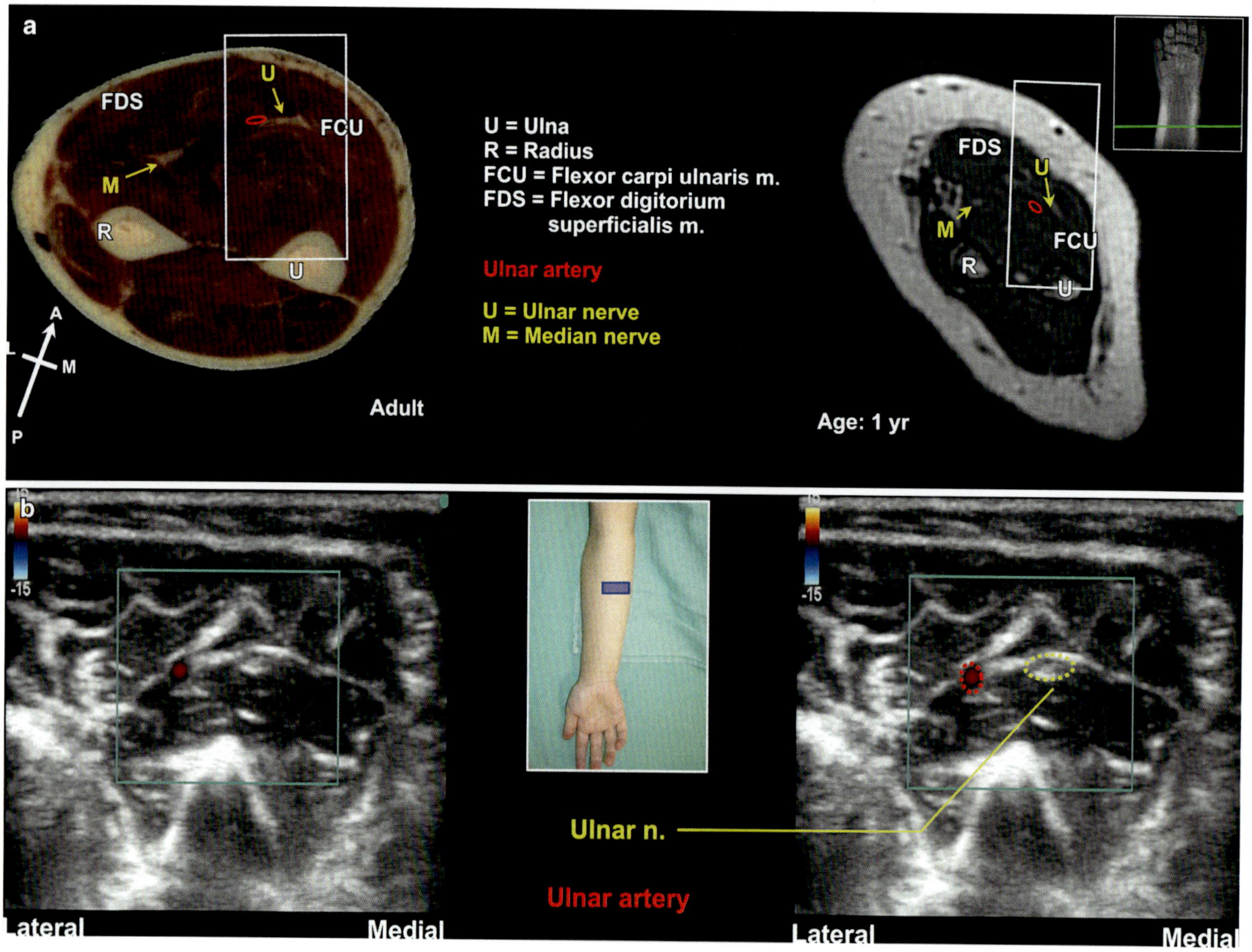

Fig. 23.12 (a) VHVS and MRI images of the ulnar nerve in the forearm. (b) Ultrasound image of the ulnar nerve in the forearm

23.3.3.2 Sonographic Appearance

- The nerve in short axis at a proximal location is viewed as a honeycomb-like, oval-shaped structure, including hypoechoic fascicular structures surrounded significantly by hyperechoic tissue.
- More distally, the nerve appears to take a rounded shape. The adjacent ulnar artery appears anechoic and roughly similar in size to the nerve and lateral to it.
- If able to demarcate the muscles, they are located as follows: the flexor carpi ulnaris is superficial below the skin and subcutaneous layers and has a distinctive linear fascial plane within; the flexor digitorum superficialis is superolateral to the nerve and artery; the flexor digitorum profundus is medial and deep to the nerve and artery (see Fig. 10.9).
- If visible, the deep hyperechoic ulna will have a bony shadow underneath. The median nerve may be seen at the lateral edge of the image and appears similar to the ulnar nerve in size and shape.

23.3.3.3 Needle Insertion

- Our recommended technique is an IP approach to the ulnar nerve at the mid-forearm.
- Position the image of the nerve to the most lateral edge of the screen for good visibility of the needle shaft during IP advancement. Insert the needle above the ulna but below the probe by 0.5–1 cm, in line with the probe's axis (Fig. 23.13).
- An OOP technique can be used, with the needle inserted a small distance from the caudad surface of the probe. For this technique, the nerve should be placed in the center of the image prior to needling (Fig. 23.14).

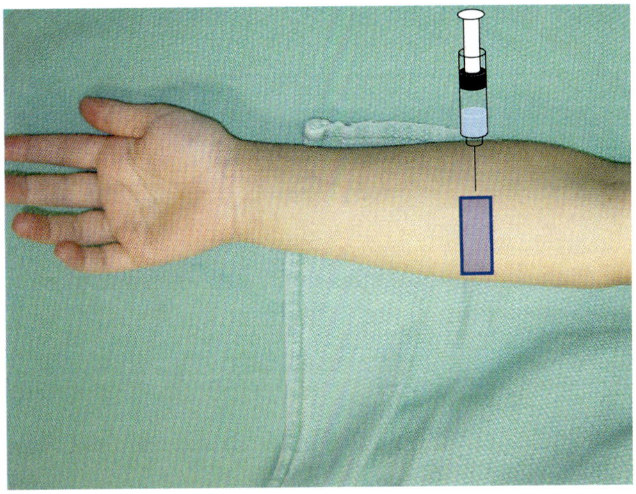

Fig. 23.13 In-plane needling approach for ultrasound-guided ulnar nerve block. *Blue rectangle* indicates probe footprint

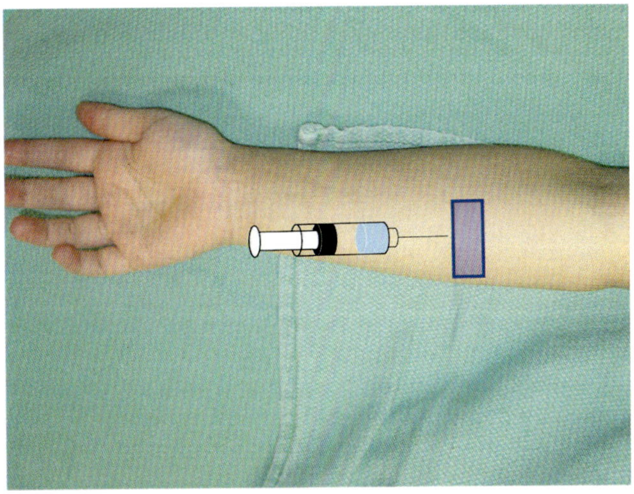

Fig. 23.14 Out-of-plane needling approach for ultrasound-guided ulnar nerve block. *Blue rectangle* indicates probe footprint

23.3.4 Local Anesthetic Application

- The ulnar nerve can be blocked using a 3–5 cm needle, insulated if using nerve stimulation, with 1–3 mL of 0.25–0.5 % ropivacaine or bupivacaine.
- Performing a test dose with D5W to visualize the spread and confirm nerve localization is recommended prior to local anesthetic application.
- Aim to spread approximately 1–3 mL of local anesthetic around the nerve in a circular fashion in order to avoid nerve contact but obtain a complete block.
- The local anesthetic injection will appear as an expansion of hypoechogenicity surrounding the nerve.

23.3.5 Case Study

In the adult population, ulnar nerve block is typically performed as a rescue block in cases of insufficient anesthesia. Blockade of the ulnar nerve is performed rarely as a sole block in the pediatric population.

23.4 Current Literature in Ultrasound-Guided Approaches

A recent letter describes ultrasound-guided blockade of the median and ulnar nerves in children aged 6 and 20 months for syndactyly repair [1]. Pre-procedural scanning allowed visualization of both nerves in one image. Following this, 0.2 mL/kg per nerve of levobupivacaine 0.25 % was injected under ultrasound and nerve stimulation guidance. Postoperative pain control was excellent with no need for opioid analgesics.

Reference

1. Mottard N, James I, Duflo F. Interest of ultrasound guidance for ulnar and median nerve block in the mid forearm in children. Ann Fr Anesth Reanim. 2010;29:406–7.

Suggested Reading

Dalens BJ. Distal conduction blocks. In: Dalens BJ, editor. Pediatric regional anesthesia. Boca Raton: CRC Press; 1990. p. 261–5.

Karmakar MK, Kwok WH. Ultrasound-guided regional anesthesia. In: Cote CJ, Lerman J, Todres ID, editors. A practice of anesthesia for infants and children. 4th ed. Philadelphia: WB Saunders; 2009. p. 926–8.

Mather SJ. Upper limb blocks. In: Peutrell JM, Mather SJ, editors. Regional anaesthesia for babies and children. Oxford: Oxford University Press; 1997. p. 105–8.

Suresh S, Polaner DM, Cote CJ. Regional Anesthesia. In: Cote CJ, Lerman J, Anderson BJ, Eds. 5th ed. Philadelphia: WB Saunders; 2013. p. 835–879.

Tsui BC. Selective terminal nerve blocks of the upper extremity. In: Tsui BC, editor. Atlas of ultrasound and nerve stimulation-guided regional anesthesia. New York: Springer; 2007. p. 109–36.

Part VII

Nerve Blocks of the Lumbar Plexus

Posterior Lumbar Plexus Block

24

Karen R. Boretsky and Ban C.H. Tsui

Contents

K.R. Boretsky, MD
Department of Anesthesia, Perioperative and Pain Medicine,
Harvard Medical School, Boston Children's Hospital,
Boston, MA, USA
e-mail: Karen.boretsky@childrens.harvard.edu

B.C.H. Tsui, Dip Eng, BSc (Math), B Pharm, MSc, MD, FRCPC (✉)
Department of Anesthesiology and Pain Medicine,
Stollery Children's Hospital/University of Alberta Hospital,
2-150 Clinical Sciences Building, Edmonton,
AB T6G 2G3, Canada
e-mail: btsui@ualberta.ca

B.C.H. Tsui, S. Suresh (eds.), *Pediatric Atlas of Ultrasound- and Nerve Stimulation-Guided Regional Anesthesia*,
DOI 10.1007/978-0-387-79964-3_24

24.1 Indications

- Unilateral procedures in the groin area, in the hip, and on the upper and anterior aspect of the lower limb (e.g., femoral osteotomy)
- Combined with a sciatic nerve block for complete surgical anesthesia to the lower extremity
- Situations where neuraxial block is contraindicated for the patient

24.2 Surface Anatomy (Fig. 24.1)

The patient lies in the lateral decubitus position with the operative side up and both hips and knees flexed after general anesthesia has been induced. Surface landmarks include:

- Horizontal line:
  - Intercristal line – a line connecting the upper border of the iliac crests, corresponding to the level of the L4/L5 intervertebral space
- Vertical line:
  - A line perpendicular to the intercristal line and parallel to the spinous processes, crossing through the ipsilateral posterior superior iliac spines (PSIS)

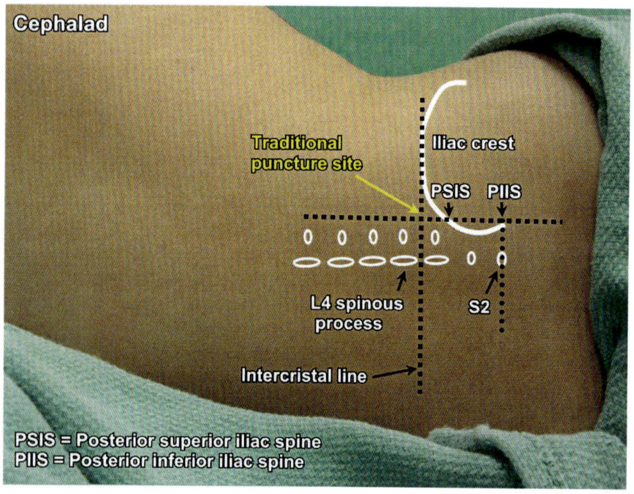

Fig. 24.1 Surface anatomy and landmarks for posterior lumbar plexus block

The site of needle insertion is approximately at the intersection of the two lines described above for Winnie's technique; however, ultrasound imaging may identify a slightly different needle insertion site.

> **Clinical Pearl: Chayen's Technique**
>
> - A more medial and caudal (L5 or below) needle puncture site may be used, following a technique modification described by Chayen and colleagues [1], which places the needle midway between the L5 spinous process and the PSIS.
> - Patients often experience bilateral blockade indicative of epidural spread. This block may be advantageous in cases where epidural anesthesia is contraindicated, such as in patients with scoliosis.
> - Redirections of the needle due to bone contact (iliac bone or vertebral body) may be necessary.
> - The plexus may be reached at a significantly greater depth than when using Winnie's approach.
> - Motor responses to nerve stimulation may be present in both the thigh and lower leg (ankle and foot).
> - The volume of local anesthetic should likely be reduced to that recommended for epidural injections.

24.3 Nerve Stimulation Technique

The authors recommend combining nerve stimulation with ultrasound guidance for lumbar plexus blocks as the nerve roots/plexus can be difficult to visualize, especially for older children.

24.3.1 Needle Insertion

A flowchart illustrating the needle insertion site and procedures is shown in Fig. 24.2.

- Insert an insulated 22–25G, short-bevel needle perpendicular to the skin.
- The needle will pass through the quadratus lumborum muscle before reaching the psoas major muscle and finally the lumbar plexus. The skin-plexus distance correlated strongly with children's weight rather than age and height in a study of children between the ages of 3 and 12 and ranged from 1.24 to 1.74 mm/kg depending on age and the level at which the lumbar plexus was visualized with ultrasound imaging (Table 24.1) [2].
- If the needle contacts the bone (transverse process) at a moderate depth, the needle should be reinserted slightly cranial or caudad. This will occur more frequently if using the needle puncture site described by Chayen et al. [1] (see Clinical Pearl above).

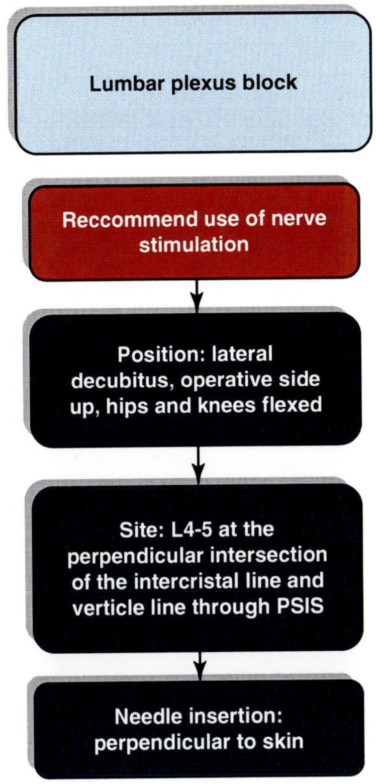

Fig. 24.2 Flowchart of needle insertion and procedures for lumbar plexus blocks

Table 24.1 Distance of skin-plexus at different ages at L3/L4 and L4/L5

Levels where lumbar plexus is delineated	>3–5 years old	>5–8 years old	>8–12 years old
L3/4	1.68 mm/kg	1.55 mm/kg	1.24 mm/kg
L4/5	1.74 mm/kg	1.6 mm/kg	1.31 mm/kg

Based on data from Ref. [2]

24.3.2 Current Application and Appropriate Responses

Figure 24.3 illustrates the procedure for employing nerve stimulation techniques for lumbar plexus block.

- Initially, set the nerve stimulator to apply 1–2 mA current (2 Hz), and aim to elicit motor twitches of the quadriceps muscle at a current intensity threshold of 0.5 mA. See Table 14.3 for expected motor responses during nerve stimulation.

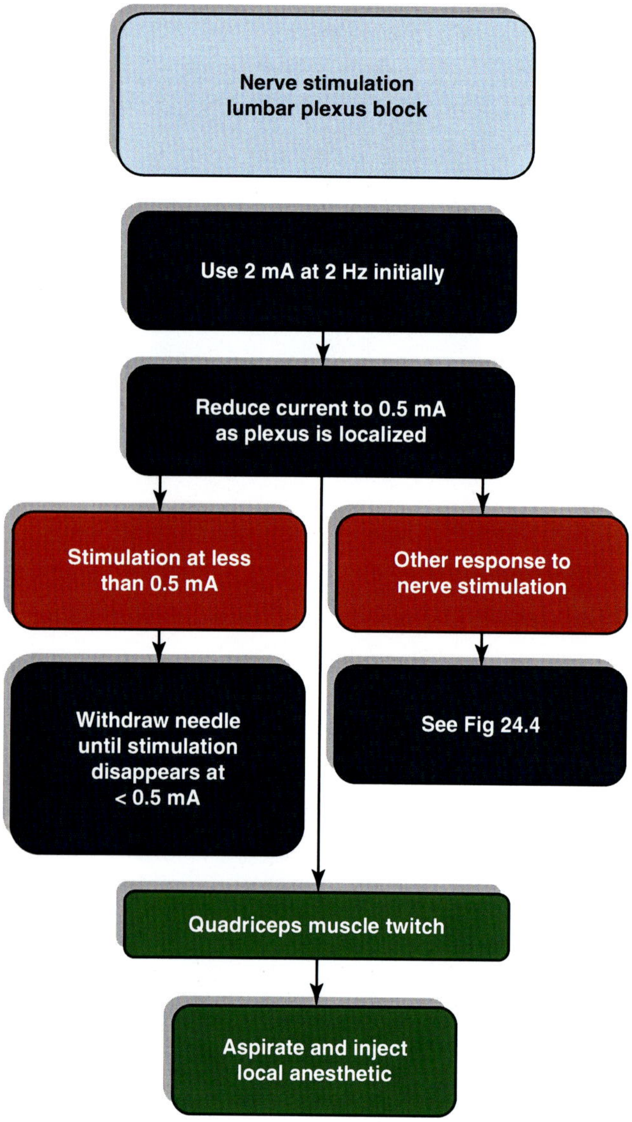

Fig. 24.3 Flowchart of nerve stimulation techniques for lumbar plexus blocks

24.3.3 Modifications to Inappropriate Responses (Table 24.2)

An algorithm of modifications to inappropriate responses to nerve stimulation is shown in Fig. 24.4.

Table 24.2 Responses and recommended needle adjustments for use with nerve stimulation during lumbar plexus blocks

Correct response from nerve stimulation
Quadriceps muscle twitch (palpable or visual) at 0.5–1.0 mA intensity
Other common responses and needle adjustment
Muscle twitches from electrical stimulation
Paraspinal (local twitch from direct stimulation)
Explanation: needle tip too superficial
Needle adjustment: advance needle tip
Hamstring (roots of sciatic nerve)
Explanation: needle inserted too caudally
Needle adjustment: withdraw completely and reinsert 3–5 cm cranially
Thigh flexion (quite deep; psoas major muscle stimulation)
Explanation: needle tip too deep (close to peritoneal cavity)
Needle adjustment: withdraw needle and follow protocol
Bone contact
Transverse process
Explanation: close placement; angle slightly off
Needle adjustment: withdraw to subcutaneous tissue and reinsert with an angle of 5° more cranially or caudally
No response despite deep placement
Past transverse process and lumbar plexus
Explanation: needle tip too deep
Needle adjustment: withdraw completely and reinsert according to protocol

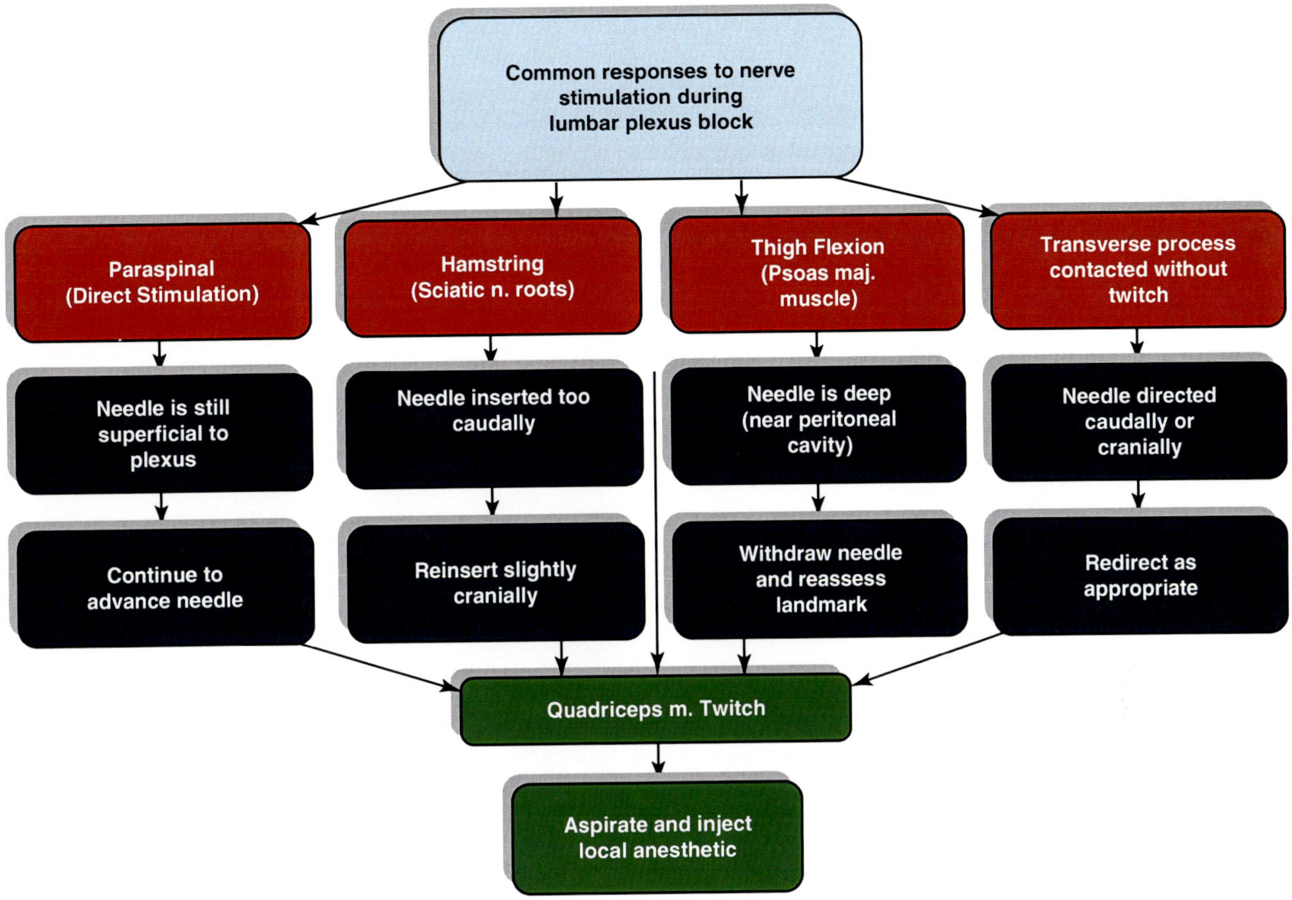

Fig. 24.4 Flowchart of modifications to inappropriate responses to nerve stimulation during lumbar plexus blocks

24.4 Ultrasound-Guided Technique

For a summary of ultrasound guidance techniques in lumbar plexus blocks, see Fig. 24.5.

Major anatomical structures in the lumbar plexus as captured by MRI and VHVS images are shown with the corresponding ultrasound image in Fig. 24.6.

Prepare the needle insertion site and skin surface with an antiseptic solution. Prepare the ultrasound probe surface by applying a sterile adhesive dressing to it prior to needling as discussed in Chap. 4.

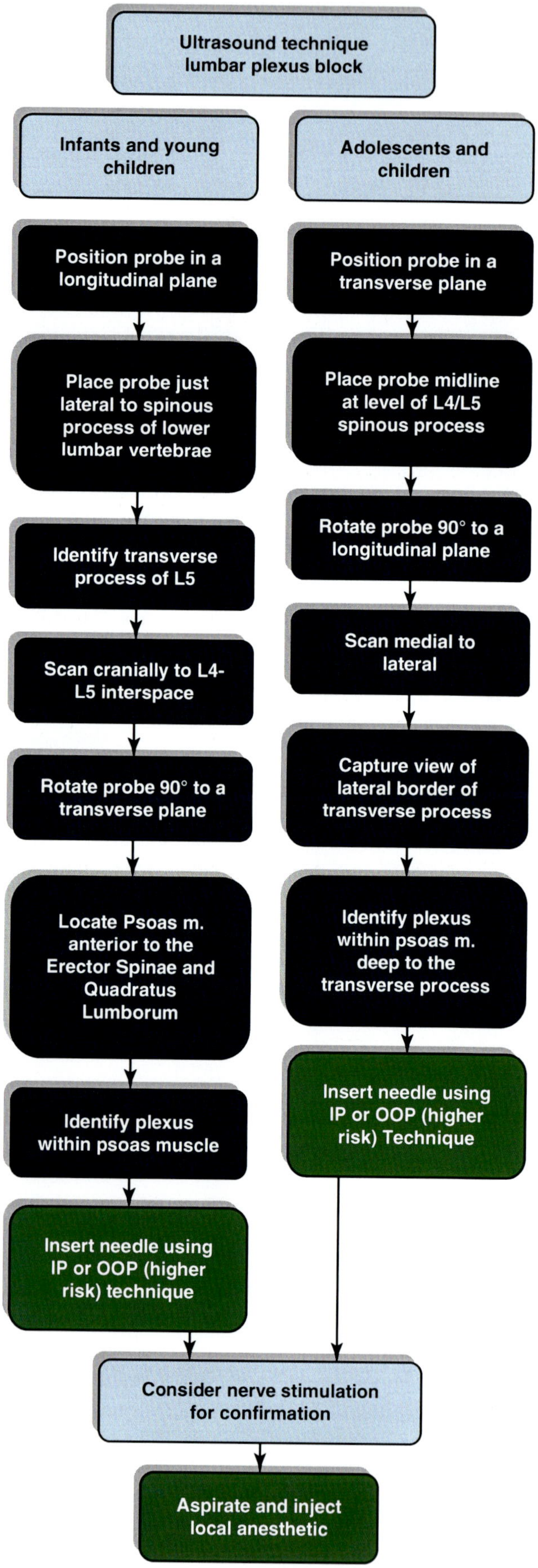

Fig. 24.5 Flowchart of ultrasound-guided techniques in lumbar plexus blocks

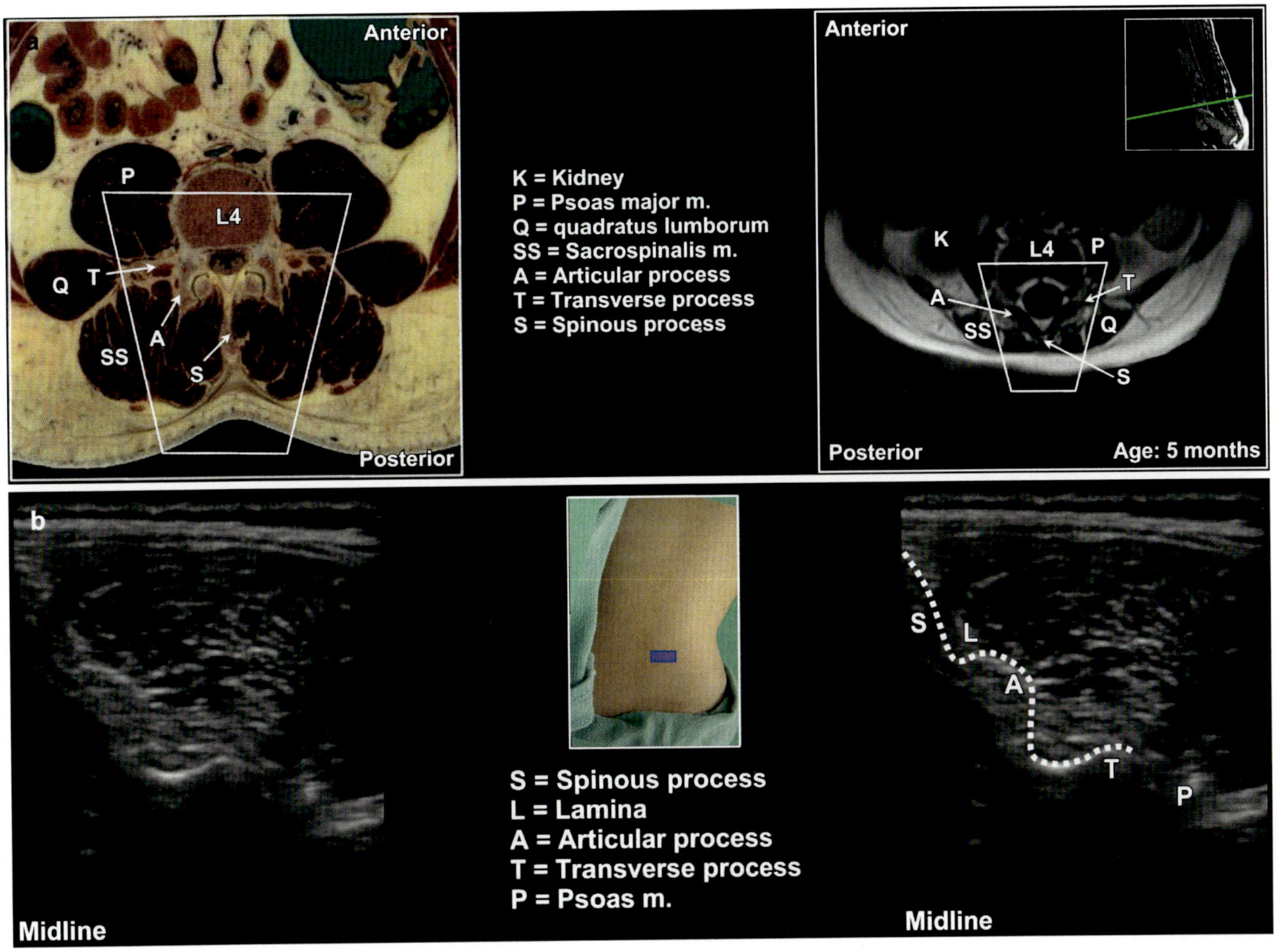

Fig. 24.6 (**a**) VHVS and MRI images of major anatomical structures in the lumbar plexus region. (**b**) Ultrasound image of major anatomical structures in the lumbar plexus region. *Blue rectangle* indicates position of ultrasound probe

24.4.1 Scanning Technique

Traditionally, the approach for the lumbar plexus block has been at the L4–L5 level to avoid renal hematoma or other complications at the level of the kidney (L2–L3). This low approach often results in absence of analgesia in the ilioinguinal/iliohypogastric nerves and occasionally the lateral femoral cutaneous nerve. In the future, ultrasound visualization of the kidneys and vascular structures may allow needle insertion at a more cephalad level (L1–L4) to provide more consistent blockade of these nerves. It must be noted that the lower pole of the kidney can reach down even to the L4–L5 level in young children and infants (Fig. 24.6a).

- In infants and young children:
  - Place a 6–13 MHz "hockey stick" transducer in the posterior longitudinal (parasagittal) plane just lateral to the spinous processes, starting at a caudal level, to view the hyperechoic line and corresponding bony shadowing from the cephalad portion of the sacrum.
  - Identify the first transverse process (L5) and place the probe at the L4/L5 interspace. The L3/L4 interspace may allow higher resolution in some children.
  - Rotate the probe 90° to capture a transverse axis view (Fig. 24.7) in order to visualize (from medial to lateral) the spinous process, the erector spinae muscles, and the quadratus lumborum muscle. Use these landmarks to identify the plexus within the deeper psoas major muscle.
  - Alternate between the transverse and longitudinal views to delineate the plexus.
- In adolescents and children with large amounts of subcutaneous tissue:
  - Place a 5–8 MHz curved array probe (curvilinear) in the transverse plane at the level of the L4 or L5 spinous process (the latter immediately above the intercristal line) to capture an overview of the vertebrae. The more superficial position of the L3/L4 interspace may allow for better resolution of the structures.
  - Rotate the probe to the longitudinal plane and scan laterally from midline, capturing firstly the lamina, articular, and then transverse processes as the probe is moved laterally.
  - The cephalad end of the probe, positioned in the longitudinal plane parallel to the spine, will be over the tip of the transverse processes of L2 or L3 (according to the experience and judgment of the operator), viewing the transverse processes of L2/3/4 or L3/4/5, respectively; the transverse processes and the acoustic shadows cast should be between the psoas muscle seen through the acoustic window between the transverse processes.
- Infants, children, and adolescents: alternate approach:
  - Using a landmark-based technique or pre-scanning with ultrasound, identify and mark the L3 spinous process.
  - Place a 2–6 MHz curved array probe (curvilinear) in the transverse plane in the midaxillary line at the identified L3 level; this is usually immediately cephalad to the iliac crest. A curvilinear probe is preferred even for small infants due to the wide angle of visibility it provides for deep, critical structures.
  - This view positions the probe perpendicular to the spine and allows the transverse process to be viewed on end and exposes the psoas muscle in a position immediately (anatomic) anterior to the transverse process. (The psoas muscle is no longer hidden by/in the acoustic shadow of the transverse process.)
  - Other landmarks that can be verified and identified include the vertebral body, the kidney, the erector spinae, and the quadratus lumborum. See Fig. 24.8.

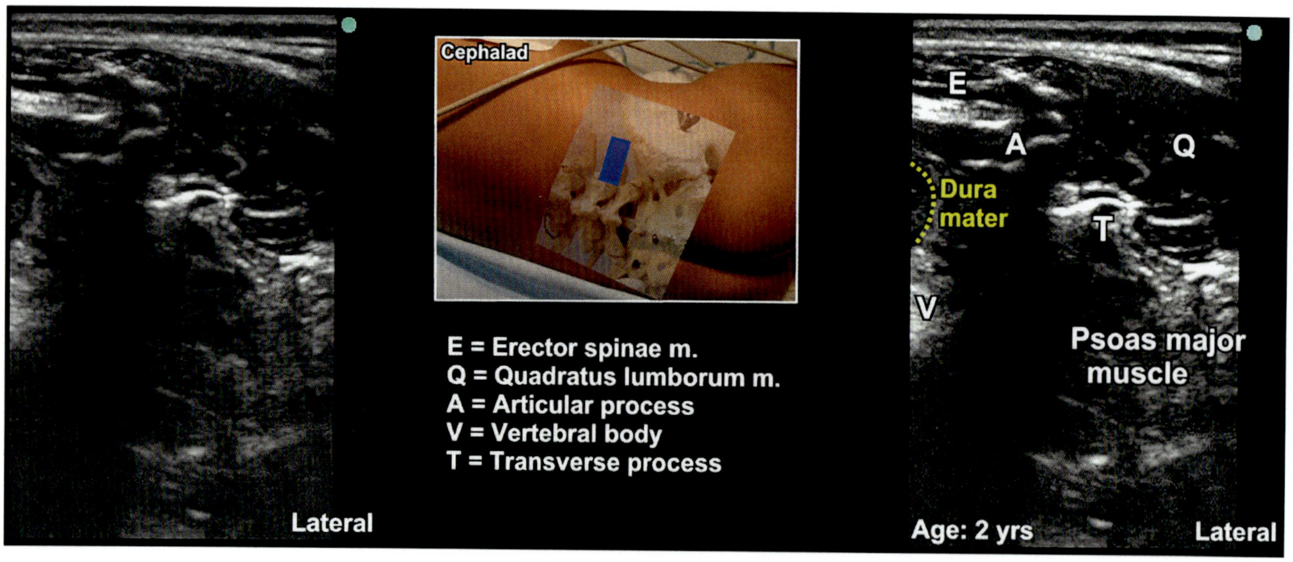

Fig. 24.7 Transverse ultrasound view (from medial to lateral) of the spinous process, the erector spinae muscles, and the quadratus lumborum muscle of infants and young children. *Blue rectangle* indicates position of ultrasound probe

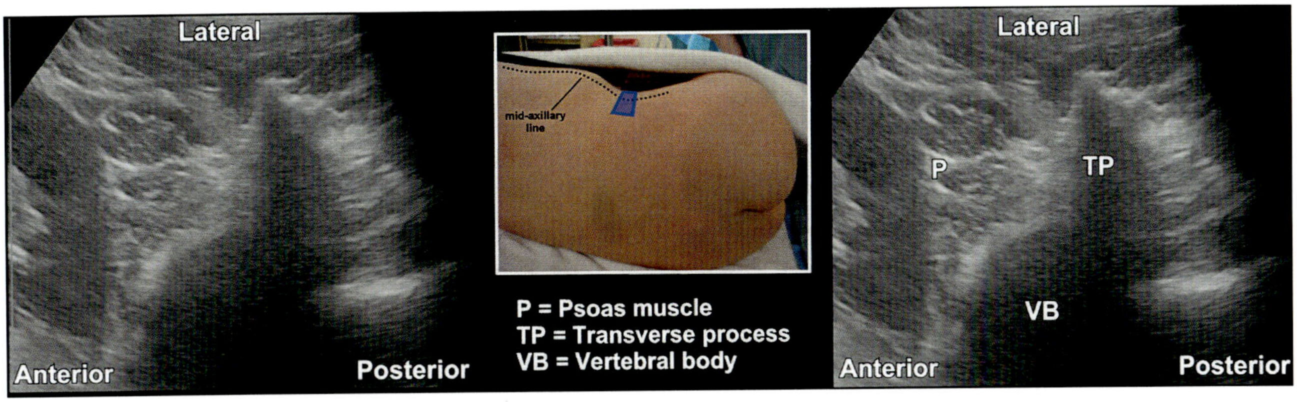

Fig. 24.8 Ultrasound image showing subcutaneous landmarks in a transverse view at L3. *Blue rectangle* indicates position of ultrasound probe

24.4.2 Sonographic Appearance

- In infants and young children (5–10 MHz "hockey stick" probe):
  - Transversely, with the probe lateral to the spinous process (Fig. 24.7), the plexus fascicles or fascicle groups lie within the psoas major muscle and superficial (posterior) to the vertebral body; both the plexus fascicles and the psoas muscle appear hypoechoic.
  - A "starry night" appearance of the muscles is visible, with hyperechoic divisions representing aponeurotic septae; the quadratus lumborum and erector spinae muscles are superficial with the quadratus lumborum muscle deep and lateral to the erector spinae.
  - The nerve fascicles appear as hypoechoic "dots" surrounded by hyperechoic connective tissue.
  - Longitudinally, the plexus appears fascicular with hypoechoic parallel bands bordered by hyperechoic striations and lies embedded within the posterior one third of the hypoechoic-appearing psoas major muscle, deep to the tips of the lumbar transverse processes, and can be visualized in the ultrasound image between hypoechoic acoustic bony shadows cast by the transverse processes of adjacent spinal levels.
  - The superficial erector spinae musculature appears highly hypoechoic and striated.
- In adolescents or children with large amounts of subcutaneous tissue (5–8 MHz curved array probe):
  - The depth of the plexus in older children may limit its visibility. Indeed, the transverse processes (which are the primary landmarks) may be vaguely delineated. Therefore, it is important to switch between transverse and longitudinal scanning within the area of the spinous processes and the tip of the transverse processes.
  - Transverse/short-axis scan:
    - A "starry night" appearance of the muscles is evident, with hyperechoic divisions representing septae, although the individual muscles may not be discernible.
    - The articular and transverse processes are located deep to the erector spinae musculature.
    - The spinous processes appear hypoechoic (likely due to dorsal shadowing effect) and extend superficially.
    - The vertebral body, if visible, is at the deepest aspect of the image and will be dark due to considerable shadowing from the surrounding bony structures.
    - If distinguishable, the psoas major muscle lies superficial and lateral to the vertebral body. The psoas major muscle also lies deep to and at the intersection of the other muscles (quadratus lumborum and erector spinae) and appears largely hypoechoic with few hyperechoic speckles.
    - Plexus fascicles or fascicle groups lie adjacent to both the psoas major muscle and the vertebral body, although it will likely not be seen in this population.
  - Longitudinal/long-axis scan:
    - A striated-appearing erector spinae muscle layer lies most superficial with the "fibrillar-appearing" psoas major muscle between the lumbar transverse processes.
    - The transverse processes are located deep to the erector spinae muscles at roughly equal spacing and appear slightly tubular with bright reflections and adjacent dark (hypoechoic) bony shadowing (Fig. 24.9).
    - Medial to the transverse processes are the "peak-like" hyperechoic edges of the articular processes with bony shadowings (Fig. 24.10). These acoustic shadowings are interspersed between the psoas major musculature. The spinous processes can be captured sonographically and appear broad; like other bony structures, they cast a shadow beneath the bony edge where no other structure is visible (Fig. 24.11).
- Alternate method for all ages: transverse transducer in midaxillary line (Fig. 24.12):
  - A "starry night" appearance of the muscles is evident with hyperechoic divisions representing septae, although the individual muscles may not be discernible.
  - The transverse process appears as a fingerlike projection in the middle of the screen anatomically anterior to the erector spinae (not always visualized) musculature.
  - The rounded vertebral body is at the bottom of the image and has a hyperechoic outline with a dark acoustic shadow underneath.
  - The distinct psoas muscle lies lateral to the vertebral body and anterior to the prominent transverse process and has the "starry night" appearance.
  - The kidney lies anterior to the psoas muscle and appears more homogeneous and hypoechoic.
  - The nerves of the lumbar plexus may sometimes appear as a wafer. If not, the psoas muscle can be mentally divided into quarters; aim the needle for the (anatomic) medial/posterior quarter of the psoas muscle.

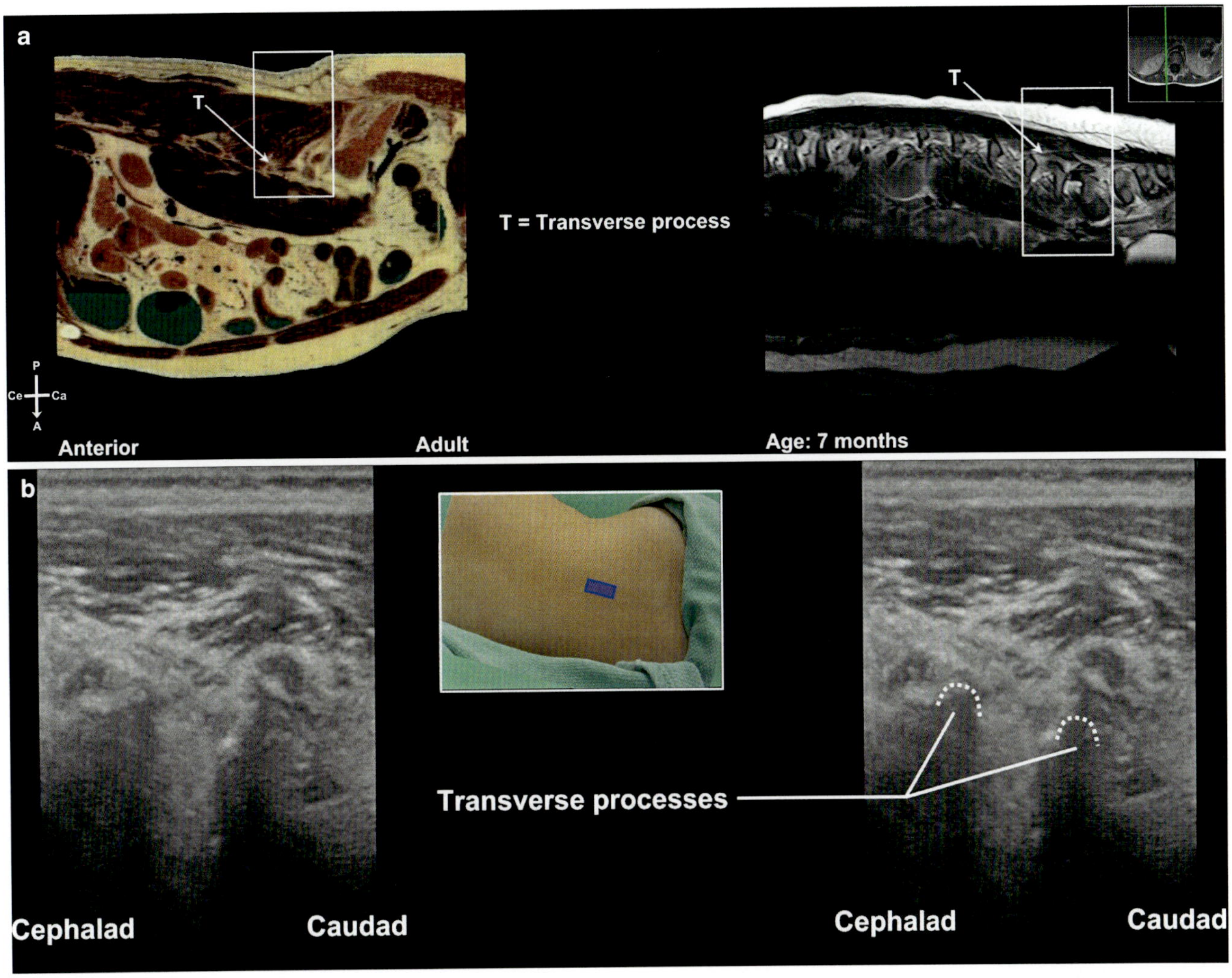

Fig. 24.9 (**a**) VHVS and MRI images of lumbar transverse processes. (**b**) Ultrasound image of lumbar transverse processes. *Blue rectangle* indicates position of ultrasound probe

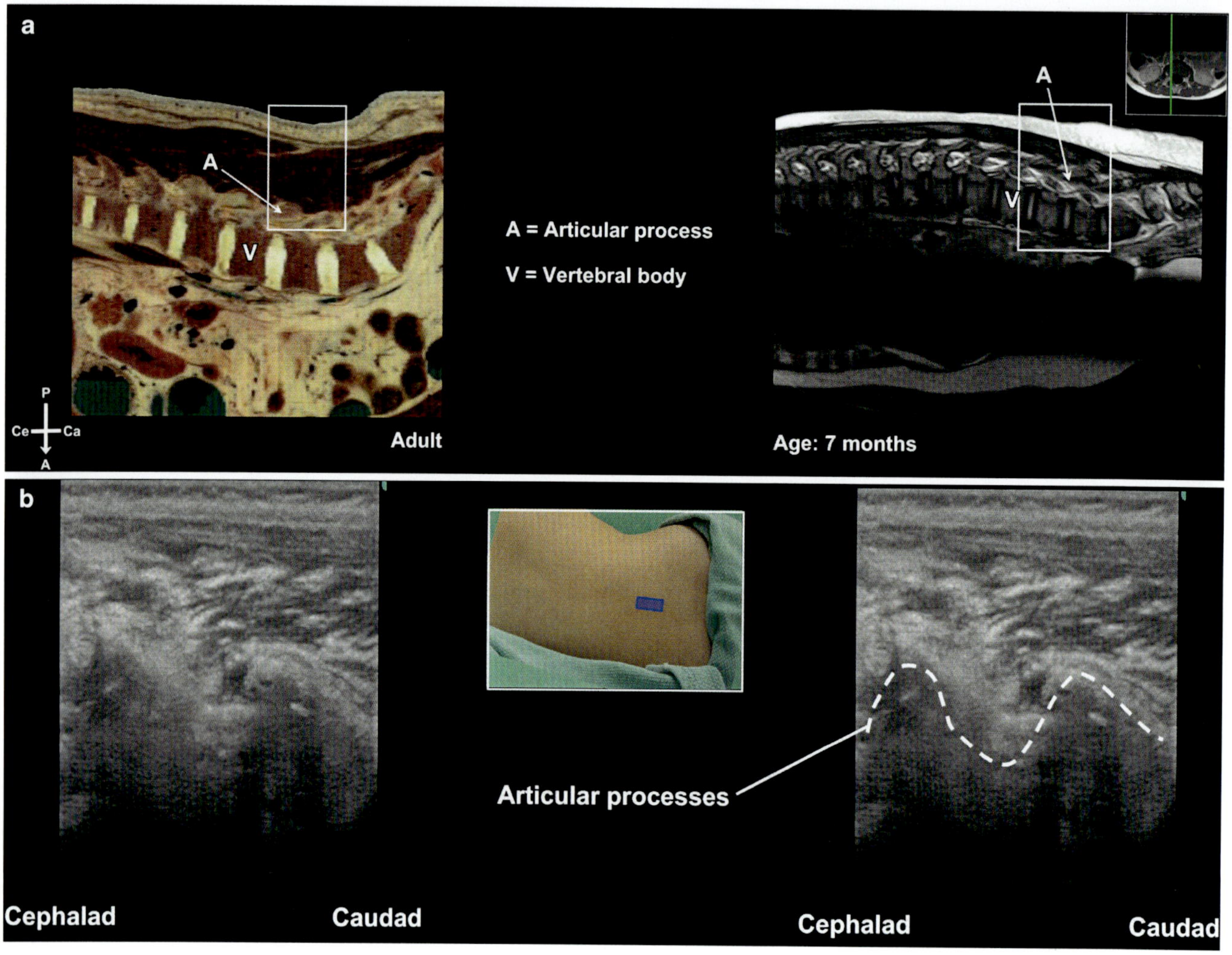

Fig. 24.10 (**a**) VHVS and MRI images of lumbar articular processes. (**b**) Ultrasound image of lumbar articular processes. *Blue rectangle* indicates position of ultrasound probe

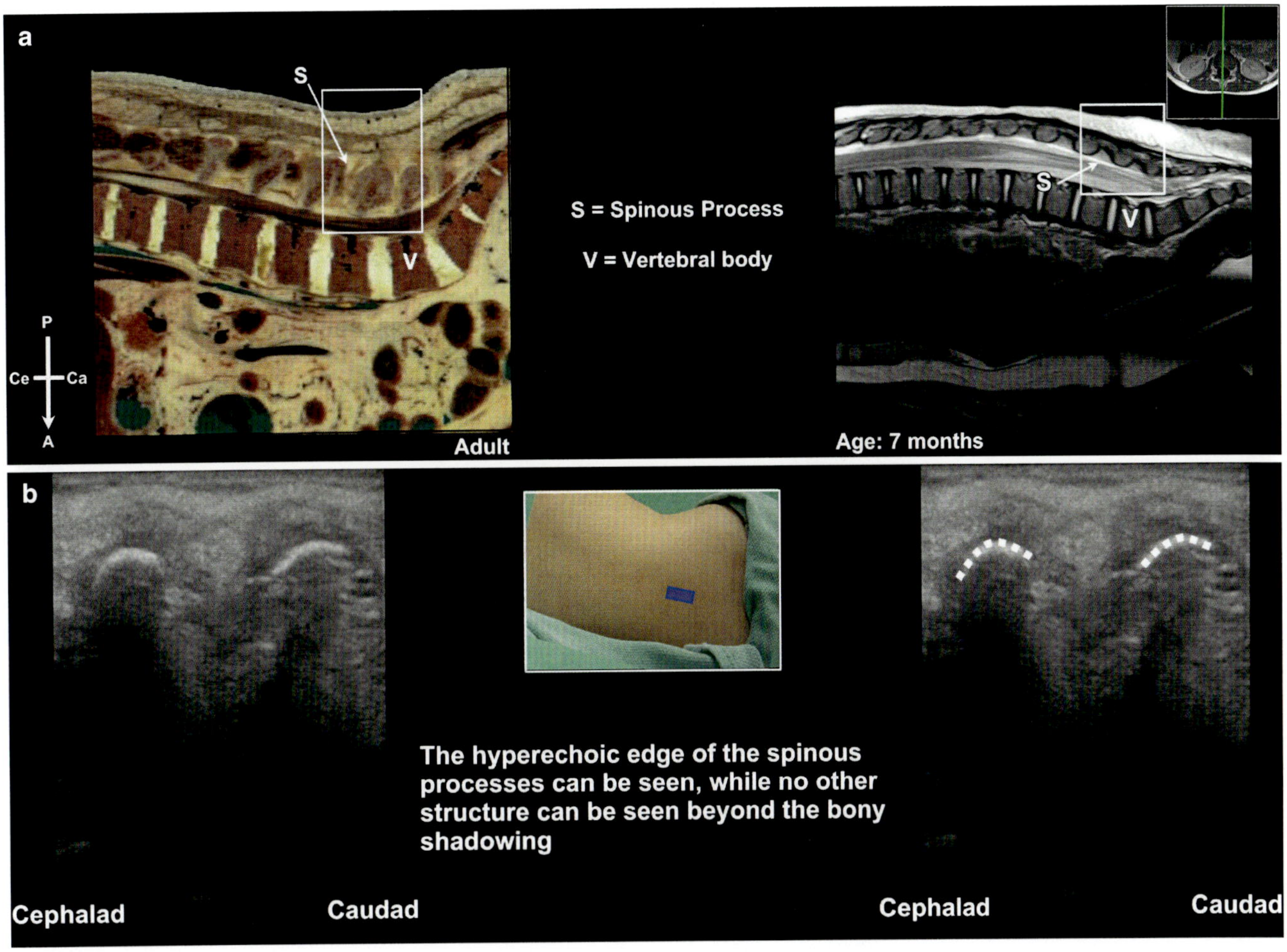

Fig. 24.11 (**a**) VHVS and MRI images of lumbar spinous processes. (**b**) Ultrasound image of lumbar spinous processes. *Blue rectangle* indicates position of ultrasound probe

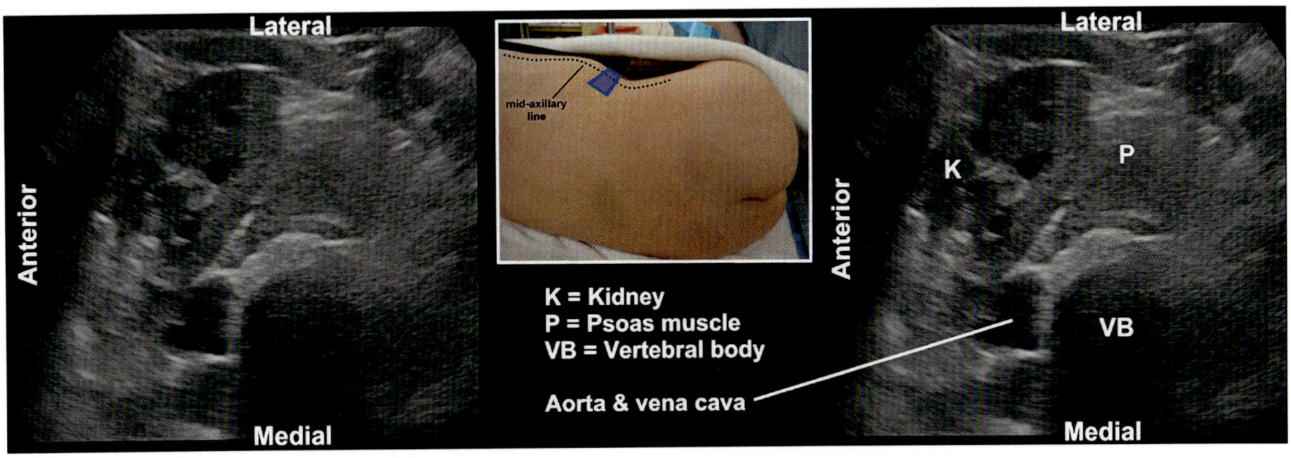

Fig. 24.12 Transverse ultrasound view at the midaxillary line showing landmark structures. *Blue rectangle* indicates position of ultrasound probe

24.4.3 Needle Insertion

Both in-plane (IP) (Fig. 24.13) and out-of-plane (OOP) (Fig. 24.14) techniques using "real-time" ultrasound imaging can be used. In young children, the plexus can be visualized and the needle trajectory controlled to a good degree. In older children, however, we have found that ultrasound imaging is most useful for surveying the region and identifying the location and depth of important bony and muscular anatomical landmarks before performing this block. This is "supported" or "off-line" scanning, often used before performing ultrasound-guided epidurals (see the ultrasound section in Chap. 1).

- "Real-time" technique using ultrasound imaging during the block to control the needle trajectory toward the plexus:
  - An IP alignment to a *longitudinal or transverse* probe and an OOP alignment to a *transverse* probe are the recommended approaches used in real-time needling. A linear, short footprint probe or a curvilinear probe can be used. The primary consideration for choosing an approach is the ability to *view the needle tip in real time as it approaches the plexus*.
  - For IP needling, the needle is inserted from the caudal or anterior end of the probe and advanced to the posterior part of the psoas muscle. Both the needle tip and needle shaft can be seen in real time during this needling approach; thus, it is the preferred method of the authors.
  - For OOP needling (advanced approach), place the probe transversely at the point where a cross section of the plexus is seen at L4/5.
    - Insert the needle (e.g., 25G, 35 mm insulated) approximately 1 cm caudad to the probe at an angle of 45–60° to the skin.
    - The needle tip will be seen as it approaches the plexus through the psoas major muscle; aim to place the needle immediately within the psoas compartment.
    - Verify the needle tip position in both transverse and longitudinal images where possible.
  - An OOP needling approach with a *longitudinally* placed probe, or an IP needling approach with a *transversely* placed probe, may pose a higher risk of injuring neighboring structures. Since it is difficult to track the needle tip on ultrasound, the needle can easily be angled either too medial (i.e., toward the intraforaminal or spinal cord) or lateral (i.e., toward the abdominal cavity or even pleura if too cephalad).
  - Nerve stimulation is recommended to confirm plexus identification.
- "Supported" or "off-line" ultrasound imaging for pre-procedural identification of landmarks:
  - It is critical to use both transverse and longitudinal scanning during off-line scanning to verify the identity and location of the structures:
    - The medial border of the area of interest of the lumbar plexus block is the tips of L4 and L5 transverse processes and lateral border being the ipsilateral iliac crest.
    - Needling at more cephalad levels is possible; however, it is important to visualize the kidney, and the operator should have adequate experience.
  - Mark the lateral edge of the transverse process and record the skin-to-transverse process distance.
  - After assessing the region and identifying landmarks with ultrasound, perform the needling.
  - Insert the needle (e.g., 25G, 35 mm insulated needle) perpendicular to the skin, without any significant medial or lateral angle, to a depth approximately 1 cm beyond the recorded depth of the transverse process with ultrasound during the pre-procedural scan.
  - It is highly recommended to use nerve stimulation to localize the plexus.
  - If the needle contacts the transverse process, redirect the needle caudally, and advance it until a "pop" is felt as the needle enters the psoas major muscle compartment or to the point indicated by nerve stimulation; this caudal direction is used to avoid inadvertent kidney puncture.

Clinical Pearls

- Ultrasound visualization of the plexus is often limited to young patients; thus, the real-time technique may be limited to this population. In older patients, it may be more practical to perform a pre-block scan to mark the location and depth of the bony landmarks (mainly the transverse processes).
- It is important to switch between transverse and longitudinal planes when scanning between the spinous processes and the edge of the transverse processes to survey the area.
- The needle should be inserted in either a cephalad or caudad direction, rather than medially toward the spinal canal.

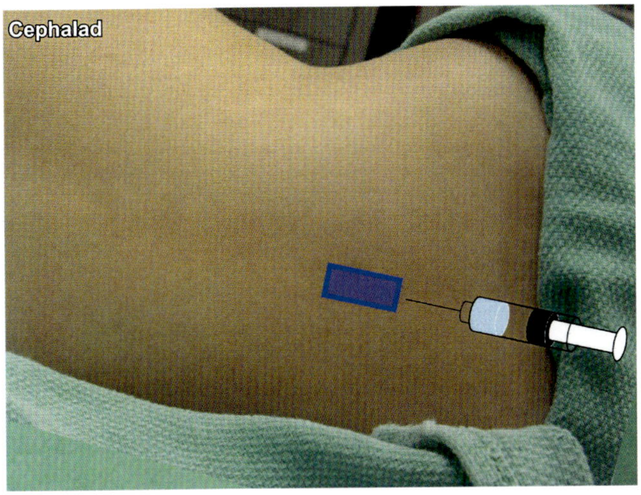

Fig. 24.13 In-plane needling technique for ultrasound-guided lumbar plexus block. *Blue rectangle* indicates probe footprint

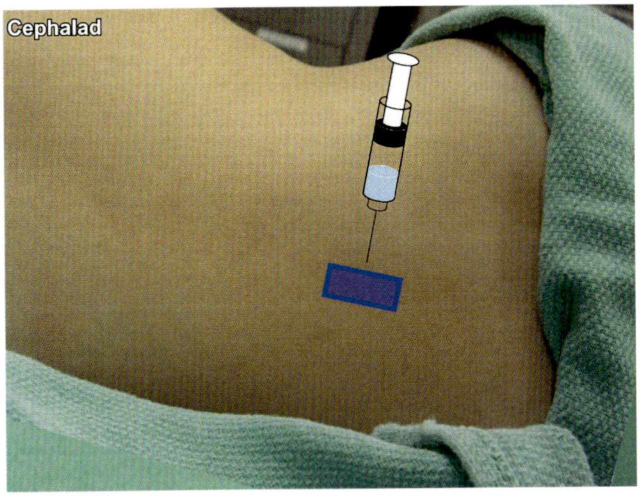

Fig. 24.14 Out-of-plane needling technique for ultrasound-guided lumbar plexus block. *Blue rectangle* indicates probe footprint

24.5 Local Anesthetic Application

- The amount and type of local anesthetic will depend on the duration of the block desired and the age/weight of the patient.
- Kirchmair et al. [2] used 0.3 mL/kg of 0.33 % ropivacaine for blockade in their descriptive study of ultrasound-guided lumbar plexus block in children between the ages of 3 and 12 years and reported successful intra- and post-operative analgesia.
- Generally, 0.2–0.5 mL/kg of 0.25 % bupivacaine or 0.2 % ropivacaine is used. The dose of local anesthetic should not exceed the maximum toxic dose.

Ultrasound Considerations

- The hypoechoic spread of local anesthetic to the posterior portion of the psoas major muscle may be visible. Kirchmair et al. [2] report viewing a "flow-like" pattern within the psoas compartment.
- It will be difficult to view any spread of the local anesthetic in larger patients where the resolution is poor.

Clinical Pearl

- Continuous lumbar plexus catheters provide good analgesia for periacetabular osteotomy, triple Bernese osteotomy, open reduction internal fixation of the hip, femoral osteotomy, and high amputations in children as young as 8 months old.

24.6 Current Literature in Ultrasound-Guided Approaches

The lumbar plexus was primarily detected at the level of L3/L4 and, to a lesser extent, L4/L5 in children older than 8 years old in one study using ultrasound [3]. The lumbar plexus was superficial enough for the use of a high-frequency hockey stick transducer at L4/L5 in patients under the age of 2 years.

Sonographic visualization of the lumbar paravertebral region in children has been described in several studies. Using a HDI 5000 ultrasound system (ATL/Philips, Bothell, WA) with a curved array probe (5–8 MHz, ATL/Philips), Kirchmair et al. [2] placed the probe in longitudinal and transverse planes to view the lumbar plexus and measure the skin-to-plexus distance. The skin-to-plexus distances were significantly correlated with the weight of the child ($r = 0.68$ at L3/4 and 0.64 at L4/5) (Table 24.1). Another study [4] demonstrated a strong correlation between PSIS-intercristal line distance and lumbar plexus depth in 350 individuals aged 1 month to 24 years (mean age 10.4 ± 5.2 years). This is a particularly valuable tool to determine lumbar plexus depth since it varies with age.

Clinical Pearl

- The lumbar plexus is situated deeply within the psoas muscle and is more visible in young children. This is due to the greater contrast between the hypoechoic muscle tissue and the hyperechoic connective tissue of the nerve structures compared with older children and adults [2].
- The needle tip and local anesthetic spread are challenging to visualize adequately for this block, even in young children.
- Nerve stimulation, needle puncture direction (relatively lateral and cranial [5, 6]), and regular aspiration during injection are techniques that will increase the safety of lumbar plexus block.
- There must be a risk-benefit analysis when deciding to use this block; although it will be the most suitable block for achieving anesthesia of the entire lumbar plexus, selective blocks of the separate nerves at more peripheral sites or a caudal block may be more appropriate depending on the procedure.

24.7 Case Study

Lumbar Plexus Block (*Contributed by K. Boretsky*)

A 6-year-old female, 22 kg, presenting with progressive hip pain was diagnosed with developmental dysplasia of the hip. She was scheduled for left femoral derotational osteotomy. After induction of general anesthesia, the patient was placed in the right lateral position for placement of a left lumbar plexus perineural catheter. The L3–L4 spinous processes were palpated at the intercristal line and marked. A curvilinear transducer (2–6 MHz) placed in a transverse orientation in the midaxillary line at the top of the iliac crest was used to identify the L3 transverse process, which appeared as a prominent hyperechoic fingerlike projection (see Fig. 24.8). An 18G, 10 cm insulated block needle was inserted 4 cm lateral to the midline and in plane with the transducer. The needle was advanced until the tip was located in the posterior-medial quadrant of the psoas muscle. Nerve stimulation of the quadriceps femoris confirmed placement near the lumbar plexus. Eleven milliliters (0.5 mL/kg with a maximum of 30 mL) of ropivacaine 0.2 % was bolused through the needle in 5 mL increments, and a 20G single-orifice catheter was inserted 3 cm beyond the needle tip. An infusion of ropivacaine 0.1 % at 5.5 mL/h (0.25 mL/kg) was run throughout the case. At the end of the case, ketorolac 11 mg IV was administered, and acetaminophen 330 mg po was given in PACU. The ropivacaine infusion and the ketorolac and acetaminophen were administered around the clock until postoperative day 2, when the patient was switched to oral oxycodone. Maximum NRS was 3/10, and the patient was comfortable throughout her hospitalization.

References

1. Chayen D, Nathan H, Chayen M. The psoas compartment block. Anesthesiology. 1976;45:95–9.
2. Kirchmair L, Enna B, Mitterschiffthaler G, et al. Lumbar plexus in children. A sonographic study and its relevance to pediatric regional anesthesia. Anesthesiology. 2004;101:445–50.
3. Bosenberg AT. Lower limb nerve blocks in children using unsheathed needles and a nerve stimulator. Anaesthesia. 1995;50:206–10.
4. Walker BJ, Flack SH, Bosenberg AT. Predicting lumbar plexus depth in children and adolescents. Anesth Analg. 2011;112:661–5.
5. Johr M. The right thing in the right place: lumbar plexus block in children. Anesthesiology. 2005;102:865–6.
6. Schuepfer G, Johr M. Psoas compartment block in children: part I–description of the technique. Pediatr Anesth. 2005;15:461–4.

Suggested Reading

Dalens B. Lumbar plexus blocks. In: Dalens B, editor. Regional anesthesia in infants, children, and adolescents. Philadelphia: Lippincott Williams & Wilkins; 1995. p. 313–20.

Karmakar MK, Kwok WH. Ultrasound-Guided Regional Anesthesia. In: Cote CJ, Lerman J, Anderson BJ, Eds. 5th ed. Philadelphia: WB Saunders; 2013. p. 880–908.

Tsui BC. Lumbar plexus/psoas compartment block. In: Tsui BC, editor. Atlas of ultrasound and nerve stimulation-guided regional anesthesia. New York: Springer; 2007. p. 147–60.

Terminal Nerve Blocks of the Lower Extremity

25

Ban C.H. Tsui

Contents

B.C.H. Tsui, Dip Eng, BSc (Math), B Pharm, MSc, MD, FRCPC
Department of Anesthesiology and Pain Medicine,
Stollery Children's Hospital/University of Alberta Hospital,
2-150 Clinical Sciences Building, Edmonton,
AB T6G 2G3, Canada
e-mail: btsui@ualberta.ca

B.C.H. Tsui, S. Suresh (eds.), *Pediatric Atlas of Ultrasound- and Nerve Stimulation-Guided Regional Anesthesia*,
DOI 10.1007/978-0-387-79964-3_25

25.1 Femoral Nerve Block

25.1.1 Indications

Femoral nerve block provides surgical anesthesia and, primarily, postoperative analgesia in the anterior thigh and knee. Combined with a sciatic nerve block, complete anesthesia below the mid-thigh can be achieved.

Indications

- Pain relief and muscle relaxation for femoral fractures, to facilitate transport, physical exams, and clinical and radiological procedures in relation to the fractures.
- For mid-shaft fractures, this block is the best indication for sole femoral nerve anesthesia. Fractures in the upper and lower femoral shaft will benefit from complementary sciatic and obturator nerve blocks, respectively.
- Quadriceps tendon repair.
- Knee surgery (in combination with sciatic nerve block).
- Anesthesia during muscle biopsy and skin grafting procedures. The lateral femoral cutaneous nerve will also need to be blocked for surgical anesthesia if the lateral aspect of the thigh is within the surgical field.

25.1.2 Surface Anatomy (Fig. 25.1)

The patient lies supine with the legs extended and the hip slightly externally rotated after general anesthesia has been induced. Surface landmarks include:

- Inguinal ligament:
  - Attached medially to the pubic tubercle (approximately 0.5–1 cm from midline on upper pubis border, depending on the age and size of the child) and laterally to the anterior superior iliac spine (ASIS).
- Femoral/inguinal crease:
  - Natural oblique skin fold parallel and 0.5–1 cm distal to the inguinal ligament (depending on the age and size of the child); the femoral artery is most superficial here.
- Femoral artery pulse:
  - The femoral artery lies at the "mid-inguinal point," at the junction between the medial third and lateral two thirds of the inguinal ligament, although it is most superficial at the femoral crease.
  - Located medial to the nerve.

The needle is inserted at the inguinal crease: approximately 0.5–1 cm lateral to the femoral artery and approximately 0.5–1 cm below the inguinal ligament, depending on the age and weight of the child. Ultrasound guidance may identify a more optimal needle insertion site.

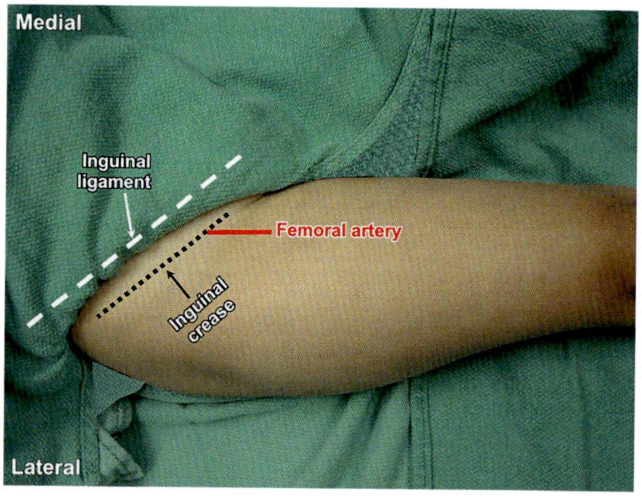

Fig. 25.1 Surface anatomy and landmarks for femoral nerve blocks

25.1.3 Nerve Stimulation Technique

25.1.3.1 Needle Insertion

A flowchart illustrating the needle insertion site and procedures is shown in Fig. 25.2.

- Insert a 35–50 mm, 22G short-beveled, insulated needle using an angle of approximately 30–45° in a cephalad direction.
- Aspirate the needle frequently since the femoral artery is situated close to the nerve.
- As the needle advances, loss-of-resistance "pops" may be felt upon penetration of the fascia lata and iliaca, although penetration of the fascia iliaca may sometimes be difficult to feel. These "pops" may be more pronounced if using a lateral needle puncture point (see "Clinical Pearls" below).
- In the case of femoral arterial puncture, compress the artery for 5–10 min to prevent hematoma formation. Repeat the procedure in a more lateral direction with care.

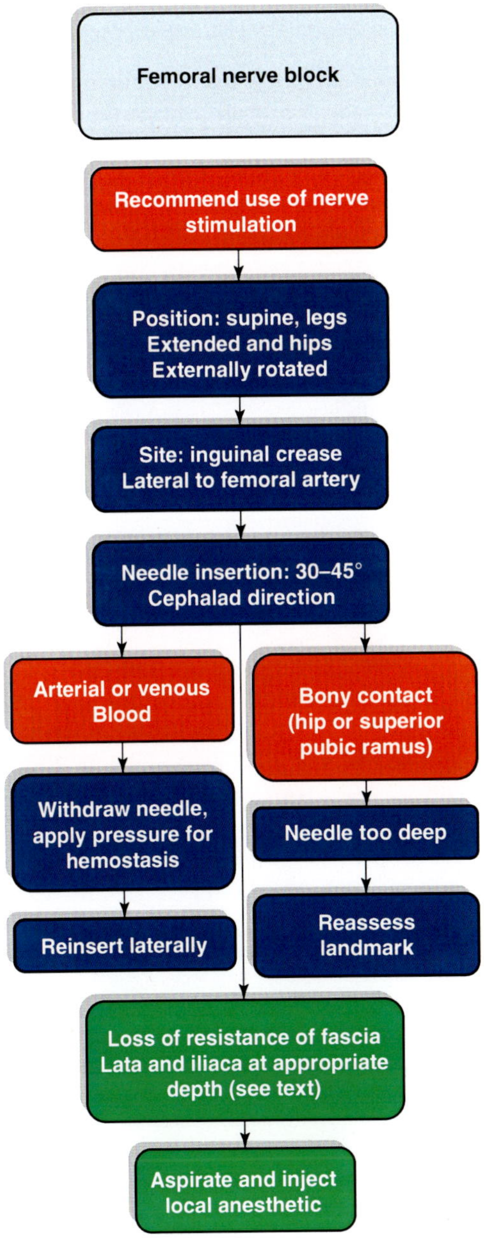

Fig. 25.2 Flowchart of needle insertion and procedures for femoral nerve blocks

25.1.3.2 Current Application and Appropriate Responses

Figure 25.3 illustrates the procedure for employing nerve stimulation techniques for femoral nerve block. See Table 14.3 for expected motor responses during nerve stimulation.

- Using nerve stimulation at an initial current of 0.8–1 mA (1 Hz, 0.1–0.2 ms), a quadriceps femoris muscle response ("patellar kick") is sought. A current threshold of 0.5 mA is used for accurate localization.

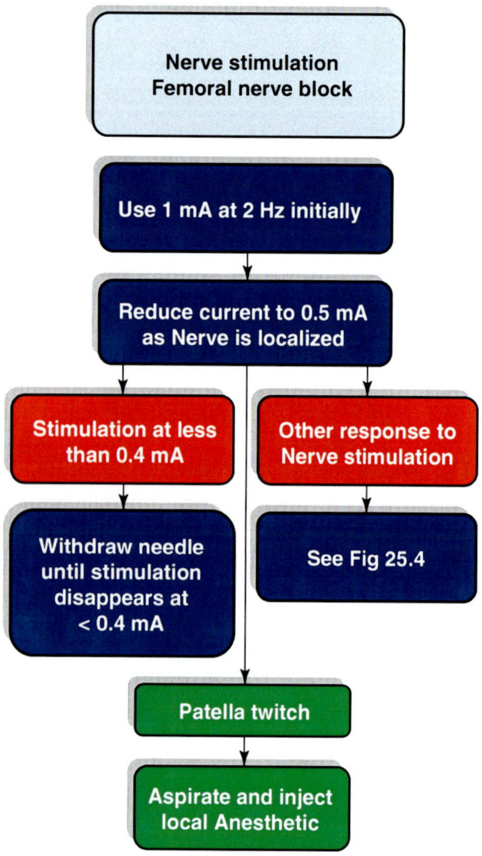

Fig. 25.3 Flowchart of procedure for employing nerve stimulation techniques for femoral nerve blocks

25.1.3.3 Modifications to Inappropriate Responses (Table 25.1)

An algorithm of modifications in the case of inappropriate responses to nerve stimulation is shown in Fig. 25.4.

> **Clinical Pearls**
>
> - For a fascia iliaca block, loss-of-resistance technique is used instead of nerve stimulation since the needle is placed away from the nerve. The puncture point is 0.5–1 cm below the inguinal ligament (depending on the age and size of the child) at the interception of one third lateral and two thirds medial of the inguinal ligament (pubic tubercle-ASIS). The needle is introduced perpendicularly to the skin plane. Two "pops" are felt when the needle traverses the fascia lata and iliacus and enters the iliopsoas muscle.

Table 25.1 Responses and recommended needle adjustments for use with nerve stimulation during femoral nerve block

Correct response from nerve stimulation
The most reliable response is a visible or palpable ipsilateral femoral muscle twitch (patella twitch) at 0.3–0.5 mA current, which indicates that one is stimulating the posterior division of the nerve. If twitches of the sartorius muscle occur, the needle may be outside the nerve sheath, and one may be stimulating the proximal branch which supplies the sartorius muscle
Other common responses and needle adjustments
Muscle twitches from electrical stimulation
Iliopsoas or pectineus (direct stimulation of muscle)
Explanation: too superior or deep needle tip placement
Needle adjustment: withdraw needle completely and reinsert
Sartorius (branches of femoral nerve to sartorius)
Explanation: needle tip too anteromedial to main femoral nerve trunk
Needle adjustment: redirect needle laterally and advance 1–3 mm deeper
Bone contact
Hip or superior ramus of pubic bone
Explanation: needle tip too deep
Needle adjustment: withdraw needle to subcutaneous tissue and reinsert
No response
Explanation: needle tip often too medial or lateral
Needle adjustment: withdraw completely and reinsert after checking landmarks
Vascular puncture
Femoral artery or vein
Explanation: needle tip too medial
Needle adjustment: withdraw needle completely and reinsert laterally

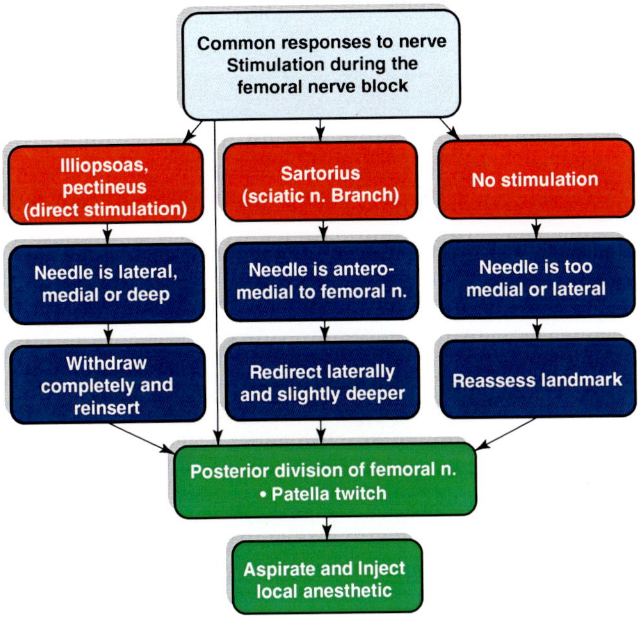

Fig. 25.4 Flowchart of modifications to inappropriate responses to nerve stimulation during femoral nerve blocks

25.1.4 Ultrasound-Guided Technique

For a summary of ultrasound-guided techniques in femoral nerve blocks, see Fig. 25.5. Major anatomical structures surrounding the femoral nerve as captured by MRI and VHVS images are shown with the corresponding ultrasound image in Fig. 25.6.

Prepare the needle insertion site and skin surface with an antiseptic solution. Prepare the ultrasound probe surface by applying a sterile adhesive dressing to it prior to needling as discussed in Chap. 4.

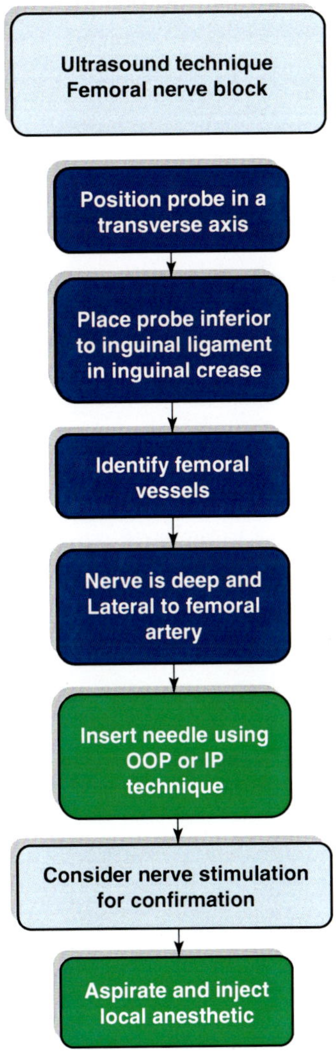

Fig. 25.5 Flowchart of ultrasound-guided techniques in femoral nerve blocks

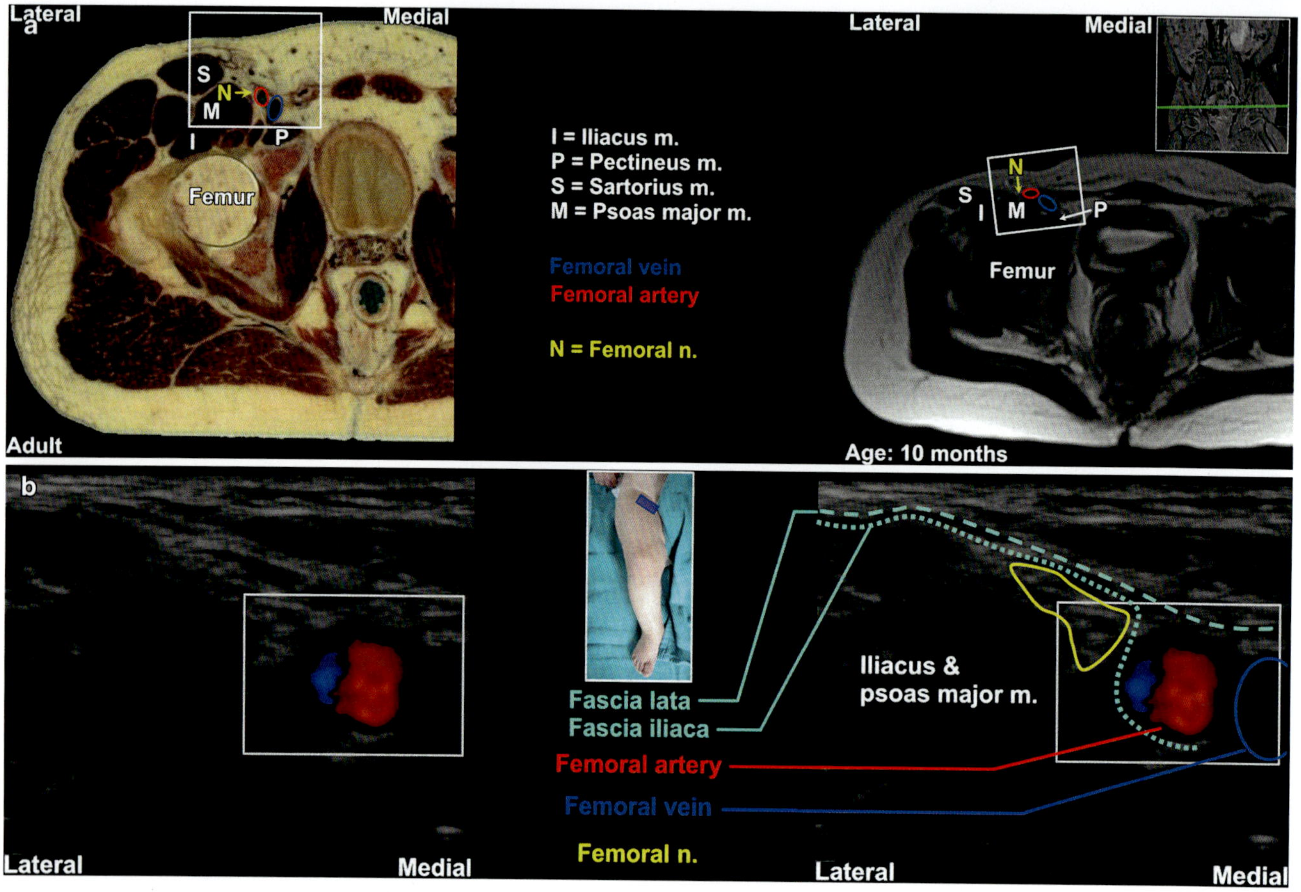

Fig. 25.6 (**a**) VHVS and MRI images of major anatomical structures surrounding the femoral nerve. (**b**) Ultrasound image of major anatomical structures surrounding the femoral nerve

25.1.4.1 Scanning Technique

- A 5–10 MHz hockey stick probe can be used for most children and will allow good axial resolution of the nerve in order to distinguish it from the surrounding structures (vessels and muscles).
- Position the probe transverse to the nerve axis in the proximal thigh, approximately 0.5–1 cm inferior to the inguinal ligament and along the inguinal crease. The nerve should appear approximately 0.5–1 cm deep (depending on the size and age of the child) and just lateral to the femoral artery.
- Color Doppler may be used to localize the femoral artery and vein.
- If the nerve is difficult to characterize, as in obese children, a useful reference landmark is the profunda femoris (deep femoral) artery (Fig. 25.7a). Scan distally to locate the point where profunda femoris artery branches off deep to the femoral artery (Fig. 25.7b). Trace this artery proximally again to its convergence with the femoral artery; the femoral nerve will be located lateral to the artery.
- Tilting the probe from perpendicular usually helps to improve the visualization of the femoral nerve (see "Clinical Pearls" below).
- Color Doppler may be used to localize the profunda femoris artery (Fig. 25.7b).

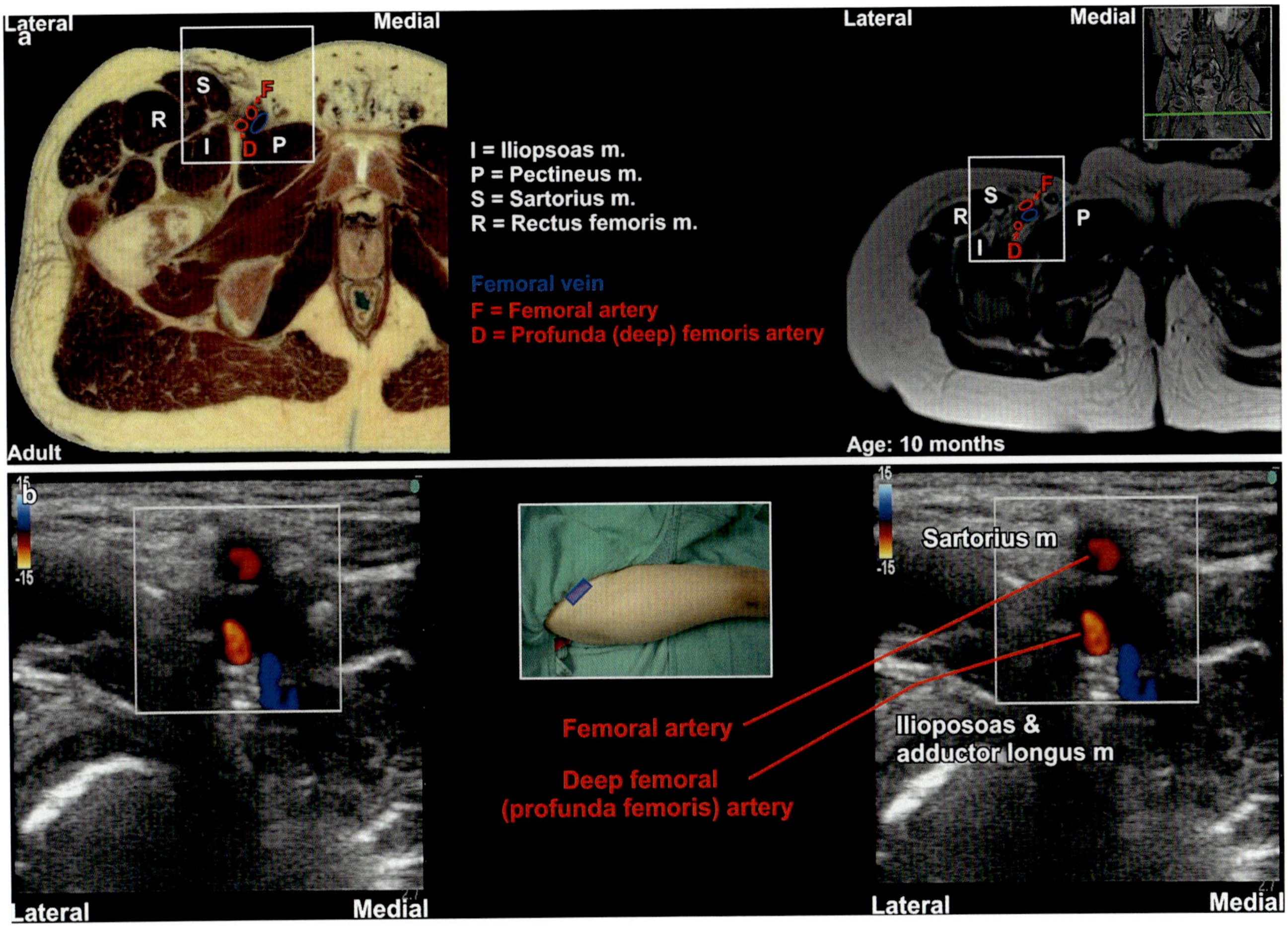

Fig. 25.7 (**a**) VHVS and MRI images of the profunda femoris artery. (**b**) Ultrasound image with color Doppler used to localize the profunda femoris artery

25.1.4.2 Sonographic Appearance

- Short-axis plane below inguinal crease (Fig. 25.6b):
  - The nerve lies lateral and deep to the large, circular, and anechoic femoral artery.
  - The fascia lata (most superficial) and iliaca (immediately adjacent to the nerve, separating the nerve from the artery) are superficial to the femoral nerve and often appear bright and longitudinally angled. The fascia may be better identified in contrast to the hypoechoic injectate after injection.
  - The femoral nerve often appears oval shaped, although it may be triangular and of variable size due to inconsistencies in diameter throughout its course. For example, early division above the inguinal ligament can increase the transverse diameter of the nerve.
  - The iliopsoas muscle may be seen deep to the nerve.

25.1.4.3 Needle Insertion

- Insert a 35–50 mm, 22G–25G needle either in-plane (IP) (Fig. 25.8) or out of plane (OOP) (Fig. 25.9 to the transverse probe at the location identified by ultrasound (approximately at the inguinal crease).
- For an IP approach, insert the needle in a lateral-to-medial direction from the lateral edge of the probe. This will help to ensure that the needle approaches the nerve before the artery or vein.
- For an OOP approach, the needle will be inserted caudad to the probe in one of the following ways:
  - After identifying the nerve, center the screen on the needle target area (just lateral to the nerve). At a distance from the probe that is equal to the depth of the target area, insert the needle caudad to the probe at a 45° angle to the skin, and advance the needle until the tip is visualized at the target location. The hypoechoic spread of a test dose of D5W is helpful to locate the needle tip.
  - An OOP "walk down" approach with incremental, stepwise angulation of the needle will provide immediate localization of the needle tip as a bright dot, allowing the tip to be followed to the required depth.
- Try to localize the needle tip beneath the fascia iliaca.

Clinical Pearls

- It is important to ensure that the ultrasound beam is perpendicular to the nerve's transverse axis to minimize anisotropic effects altering the echogenic properties of the structure. It has been shown that an approximate 10° cephalad or caudad tilt of the transducer can make the nerve isoechoic (similar appearing) to the underlying iliopsoas muscle.

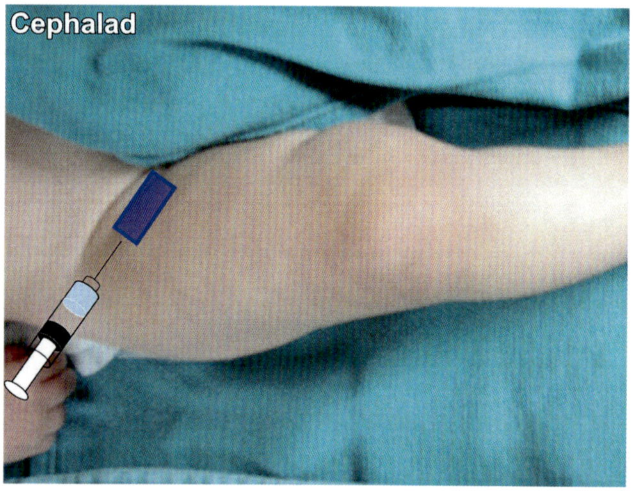

Fig. 25.8 In-plane needling technique for ultrasound-guided femoral nerve block. *Blue rectangle* indicates probe footprint

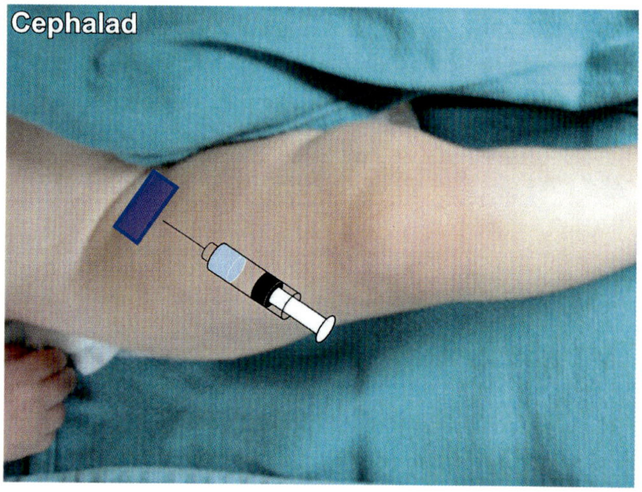

Fig. 25.9 Out-of-plane needling technique for ultrasound-guided femoral nerve block. *Blue rectangle* indicates probe footprint

25.1.5 Local Anesthetic Application

- Inject 0.2–0.5 mL/kg of 0.25 % bupivacaine or 0.2 % ropivacaine without exceeding the recommended toxic dose of local anesthetic (2 mg/kg for bupivacaine and 3–4 mg/kg for ropivacaine without epinephrine).
- Oberndorfer et al. [1] showed that a lower volume of local anesthetic is required when using ultrasound-guided technique as compared to the nerve stimulator approach in children between the ages of 1 and 8 (0.2 mL/kg versus 0.3 mL/kg of 0.5 % levobupivacaine).
- Farid et al. [2] described the use of 0.5 mL/kg of 0.2 % ropivacaine to a maximum volume of 40 mL in patients aged 8–16 years (without US).
- Sethuraman et al. [3] used 0.2 mL/kg 0.5 % bupivacaine with the total dose not exceeding 1–1.5 mg/kg in their cohort of patients <10 years old undergoing muscle biopsy (without ultrasound).
- Perform intermittent injection with interval aspiration.
- If a sciatic nerve block will be administered in addition to the femoral block, use less (e.g., two thirds) of the local anesthetic solution in order to avoid local anesthetic toxicity.

Ultrasound Considerations

- Performing a test dose with D5W is recommended prior to local anesthetic application to visualize the hypoechoic spread and confirm nerve localization.
- Local anesthetic spread can be seen as an expanding hypoechoic area; it should occur beneath the fascia iliaca and should surround the nerve.
- The solution may displace the nerve medially toward or laterally away from the artery, depending on the needle approach.

25.1.6 Current Literature in Ultrasound-Guided Approaches

Oberndorfer et al. [1] compared ultrasound guidance to nerve stimulator technique for sciatic and femoral nerve blocks in a randomized study of 46 children. The primary outcome of the study was the duration of the nerve blockade. The study showed that ultrasound-guided blocks lasted longer (508 vs. 335 min) and that a lower volume of local anesthetic (0.2 mL/kg vs. 0.3 mL/kg of levobupivacaine 0.5 %) was required for an adequate analgesia compared to the nerve stimulator technique.

Gurnaney et al. [4] reported a combined use of ultrasound and nerve stimulation in the placement of a femoral perineural catheter in a pediatric patient with variant anatomy. A 15-year-old presented to the operating room for an arthroscopic chondroplasty of medial and lateral condyles and patella and open lateral release of the knee. After induction of general anesthesia, a linear transducer revealed a nerve-like structure lateral to the femoral artery; stimulation of this structure resulted in a motor response of the sartorius muscle. Stimulation of another hyperechoic structure posterior to the iliacus muscle elicited contraction of quadriceps femoris muscle. Twenty milliliters of 0.2 % ropivacaine was then injected through a stimulating nerve catheter.

A recent case study [5] demonstrated the value of a femoral nerve block for rapid analgesia in an emergency setting: a 3-month-old infant presented with a subtrochanteric femoral neck fracture due to non-accidental trauma. The patient received one dose of morphine and two doses of fentanyl prior to the block. Ultrasound was placed 1 cm distal to the inguinal ligament of the limb in question, allowing visualization of the femoral nerve and surrounding structures. Under ultrasound guidance, a 27G needle was inserted in-plane and used to inject 2 mL 0.25 % bupivacaine (1.25 mg/kg) to surround the nerve. After 15 min, pain control was sufficient to place a Pavlik harness on the patient; only one dose of analgesic was required in the 18 h following the block.

In a recent letter, Miller [6] described combined ultrasound-guided femoral and lateral femoral cutaneous nerve block for pediatric patients undergoing surgical repair of femur fractures. The femoral nerve was blocked first using a 50 mm, 22G needle inserted in-plane in a lateral-to-medial direction, followed by injection of ropivacaine 0.2 % (0.2–0.5 mL/kg; max. volume 20 mL). The needle was withdrawn, and the ultrasound transducer was moved laterally along the inguinal ligament until its lateral aspect is in contact with the ASIS; the lateral femoral cutaneous nerve and local anesthetic from the previous injection was visualized. The same needle was inserted in-plane so that the needle tip was placed between the fascia lata and the fascia iliaca. Ropivacaine 0.2 % (0.05–0.2 mL/kg; max. volume 6 mL) was injected and observed to surround the lateral femoral cutaneous nerve.

Miller also provided the first report of ultrasound-guided fascia iliaca compartment block in pediatric patients [7]. With the ultrasound probe positioned in the long axis and located mid-point over the inguinal ligament, lateral to the border of the middle and lateral third of the ligament, the ilium, iliacus muscle, and fascia can be visualized. A 100 mm, 21G or 50 mm, 22G needle was inserted in-plane approximately 1–2 cm below the inguinal ligament, directed cephalad, and advanced until the tip was just below the fascia iliaca and in the iliacus muscle. An appropriate volume of ropivacaine 0.2 % was injected in this area achieving blockade of the femoral, obturator, and lateral femoral cutaneous nerves. Pain control was excellent in all three cases, with no requirement for narcotics in the recovery unit.

Ponde et al. [8] performed a randomized clinical trial to examine success rates of combined femoral and sciatic block for pediatric patients suffering from arthrogryposis multiplex congenital who were undergoing foot surgery. The results demonstrated significantly higher block success rates using ultrasound guidance compared to guidance by nerve stimulation alone. Interestingly, post-surgery analgesia duration was extended by an hour in the ultrasound group, although the clinical significance of this finding is minimal.

Clinical Pearls

- Although there is no direct evidence to prove that ultrasound can reduce the risk of inadvertent vessel puncture, this has been the case in our experience. Prevention of intraneural local anesthetic injection or direct intravascular puncture may not be possible in all cases (as in situations where the needle tip is not clearly seen and the nerve may not be visible). However, precise placement of local anesthetic, enabled by ultrasound imaging, may lessen the frequency of injecting large volumes of local anesthetic to ensure adequate spread, as is often the case when using blind techniques.
- Our preference is to use an IP technique, which offers the ability to visualize the needle tip and the needle shaft as it advances beneath the fascia iliaca.

25.1.7 Case Study

Case Study: Femoral Nerve Block (Contributed by S. Suresh)

An 8-year-old male, 34.2 kg, with no past medical or relevant family history was presented for physeal-sparing left knee anterior cruciate ligament reconstruction with autogenous iliotibial band and lateral meniscus repair based on MRI of the left knee without contrast. The patient received an in-plane, ultrasound-guided femoral nerve block with a 50 mm 20G needle (10 mL 0.25 % bupivacaine) (see Fig. 25.10), followed by placement of a perineural catheter. Duration of surgery was 2 h, 53 min. Postoperative analgesia reporting was 0/10 (verbal) immediately following surgery and 7/10 (verbal) 30 min after surgery. Postoperatively, the patient received a morphine injection (2 mg) and a continuous infusion of bupivacaine 0.1 % solution.

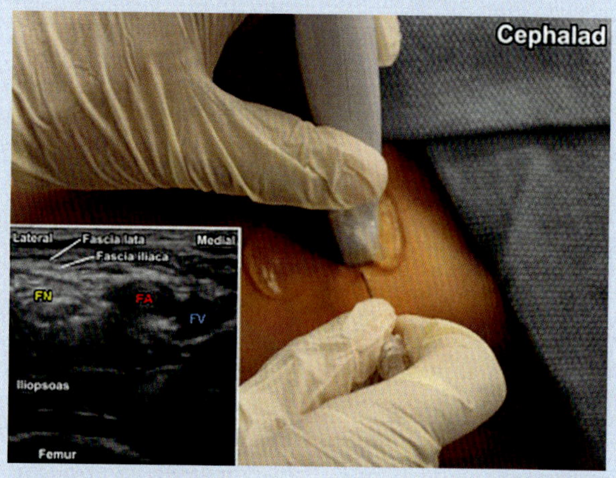

Fig. 25.10 Ultrasound-guided femoral nerve block. *FN* femoral nerve, *FA* femoral artery, *FV* femoral vein. See Case Study for details

25.2 Lateral Femoral Cutaneous Nerve Block

25.2.1 Indications

The lateral cutaneous nerve (L2–L3) of the thigh is a small, subcutaneous sensory nerve that supplies the lateral thigh.

Indications

- Analgesia for:
  - Obtaining a skin graft from the lateral thigh
  - Muscle biopsy
  - Femoral neck pinning
  - Plate placement or removal
- Supplementation of femoral and sciatic nerve blocks when tourniquets are used or when the surgical incision lies within the lateral aspect of the upper thigh.
- Diagnosis of meralgia paresthetica.

25.2.2 Surface Anatomy

The patient is placed supine with slight abduction and external rotation of the leg after general anesthesia has been induced.

The lateral femoral cutaneous nerve is a small nerve; therefore, its relationship with the fascia lata and fascia iliaca plays a key role in identifying the appropriate nerve localization.

- Inguinal ligament: the ligament is attached medially to the pubic tubercle (approximately 0.5–1 cm from midline on upper pubis border depending on the age and size of the child) and laterally to the anterior superior iliac spine.
- ASIS: palpate this landmark by following the iliac crests to their most anterior edge.

The needle puncture site lies approximately 0.5–1 cm caudad to the inguinal ligament and medial to the ASIS. The distance depends on the size and age of the child.

25.2.3 Nerve Stimulation Technique

The lateral femoral cutaneous nerve is purely sensory. Therefore, nerve stimulation is not commonly used for this block, as the elicitation of paresthesia is often difficult and uncomfortable for children.

25.2.3.1 Needle Insertion

- A 35 mm, 22G–25G insulated needle (blunted) is inserted perpendicularly at the puncture site.
- A "pop" is felt as the needle is advanced beyond the fascia lata.

25.2.4 Ultrasound-Guided Technique

Major anatomical structures surrounding the lateral femoral cutaneous nerve as captured by MRI and VHVS images are shown with the corresponding ultrasound image in Fig. 25.11a.

Prepare the needle insertion site and skin surface with an antiseptic solution. Prepare the ultrasound probe surface by applying a sterile adhesive dressing to it prior to needling as discussed in Chap. 4.

25.2.4.1 Scanning Technique

- A 5–10 MHz hockey stick transducer can be used for most children and will allow good axial resolution of the nerve.
- Position the probe on the inguinal crease and scan proximally until the lateral end of transducer lies over the ASIS.
- The nerve should appear approximately 0.5–1 cm medial and inferior to the ASIS, depending on the age and size of the child.
- It can be difficult to identify this small nerve since it is interposed between the fascia lata and iliaca.
- The nerve lies very superficial to the skin surface.

25.2.4.2 Sonographic Appearance (Fig. 25.11b)

- The fascia lata (most superficial) and iliaca (immediately adjacent to the nerve) may be seen superficial to the sartorius muscle and often appear bright and longitudinally angled.
- The lateral femoral cutaneous nerve often appears oval shaped and hyperechoic and can be better identified after injection of D5W or local anesthetic, which will surround the hyperechoic nerve with contrasting hypoechoic injectate.

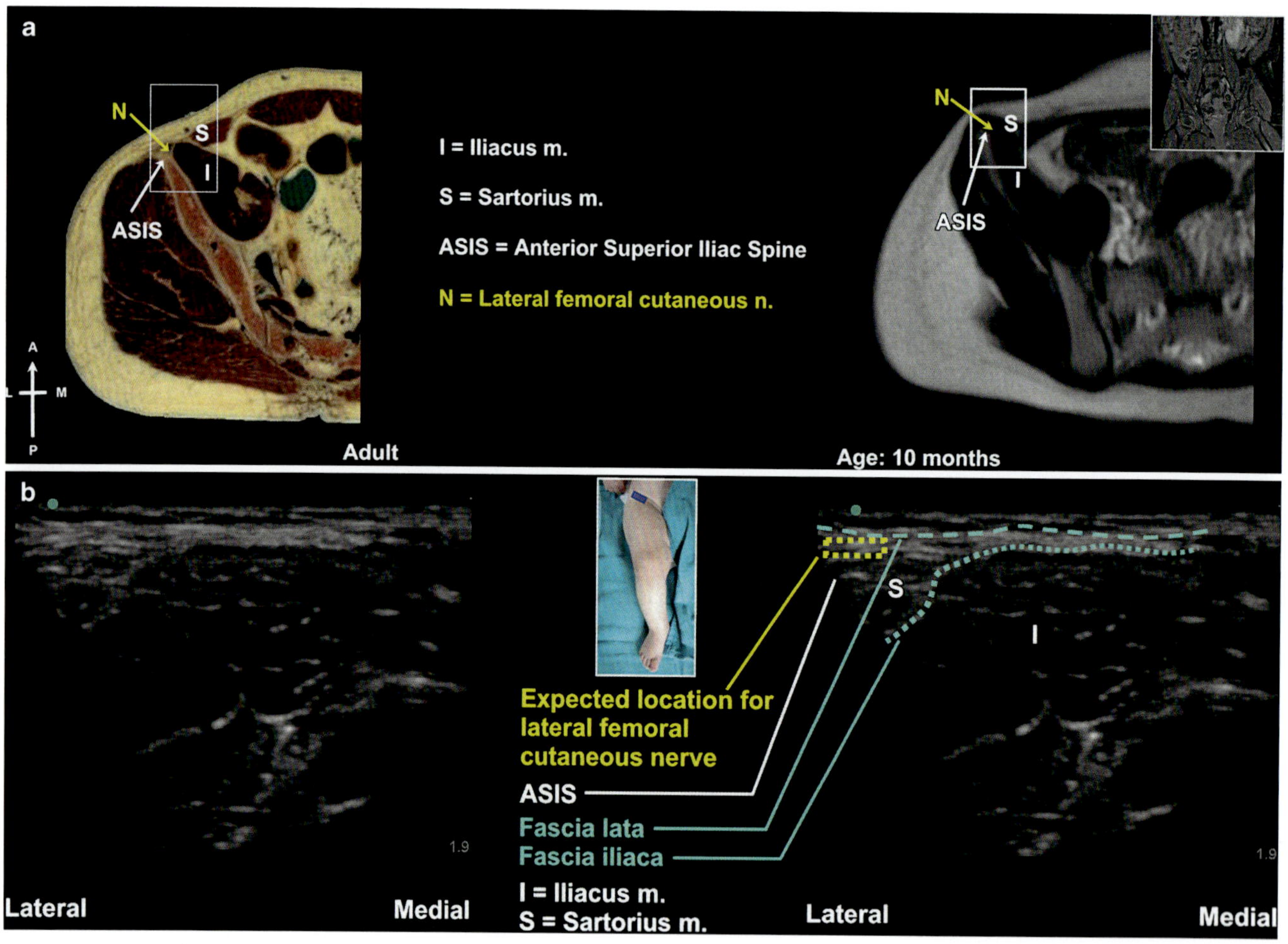

Fig. 25.11 (a) VHVS and MRI images of major anatomical structures surrounding the lateral femoral cutaneous nerve. (b) Ultrasound image of major anatomical structures surrounding the lateral femoral cutaneous nerve

25.2.4.3 Needle Insertion

- Insert a 35 mm, 22G–25G needle IP (Fig. 25.12) or OOP (Fig. 25.13) to the transverse probe at the location identified by ultrasound.
- For an IP approach:
  - Insert the needle in either a lateral-to-medial or medial-to-lateral direction.
  - Localize the needle tip beneath the fascia lata or just medial and inferior to the ASIS.
- For an OOP approach, insert the needle approximately 1 cm caudad to the probe and at a 45° angle to the skin.
  - Where possible, position the nerve in the middle of the screen, or visualize the fascia lata and fascia iliaca medial to the ASIS and inferior to the inguinal ligament. Aim the needle in between the fascial planes, just inferior and medial to the ASIS.
  - An OOP "walk down" approach with incremental, stepwise angulation of the needle will provide immediate localization of the needle tip as a bright dot; the needle tip can be followed to the required depth.

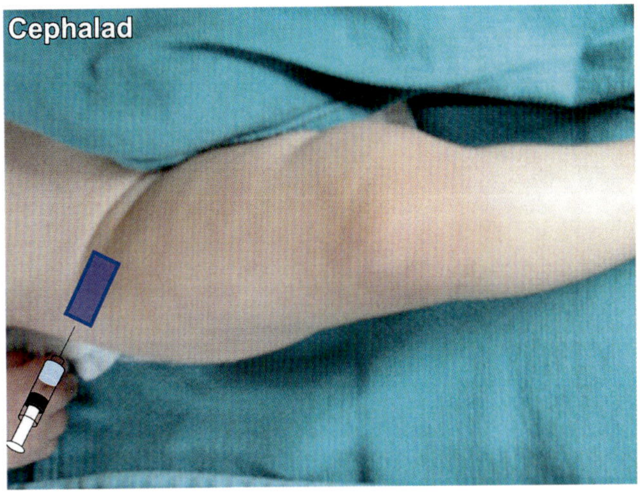

Fig. 25.12 In-plane needling technique for ultrasound-guided lateral femoral cutaneous nerve block. *Blue rectangle* indicates probe footprint

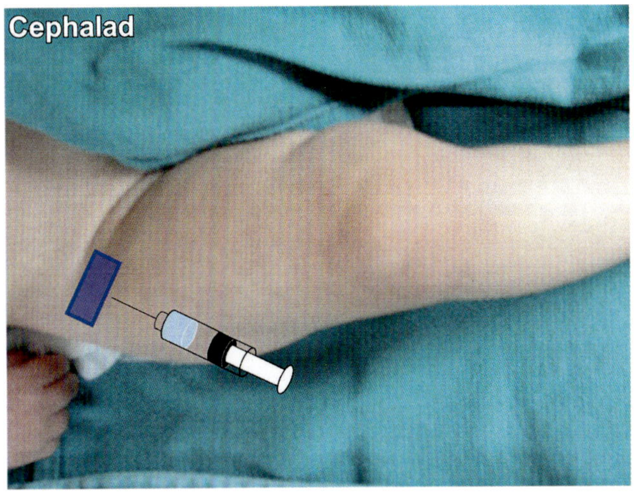

Fig. 25.13 Out-of-plane needling technique for ultrasound-guided lateral femoral cutaneous nerve block. *Blue rectangle* indicates probe footprint

25.2.5 Local Anesthetic Application

- If the lateral femoral cutaneous nerve can easily be identified on ultrasound, inject 1–3 mL of 0.25 % bupivacaine or 0.2 % ropivacaine (depending on the age and size of the child), between the fascia lata and fascia iliaca.
- Prior to the advent of ultrasound-guided lateral femoral cutaneous nerve block, Maccani et al. [9] suggested a "blind" technique of injecting 6.8 mg/kg of lidocaine medial and inferior to the ASIS using a fanlike injection pattern. This method was shown to provide anesthesia (in combination with femoral nerve block and sedation) in children undergoing anterior thigh procedures such as muscle biopsy.

Ultrasound Considerations

- Performing a test dose with D5W is recommended prior to local anesthetic application to visualize the solution spread and confirm nerve localization.
- Local anesthetic spread should occur between the fascial space (fascia lata and fascia iliaca) surrounding the nerve.
- A "donut" shape may appear as the hypoechoic local anesthetic surrounding the nerve and the fascial plane expands.

Clinical Pearls

- It can be difficult to identify the lateral femoral cutaneous nerve in children. Local anesthetic can be deposited between the fascia lata and fascia iliaca, which are easier to identify with their hyperechoic appearance overlying the sartorius muscle.
- When performing this block with conjunction with femoral nerve block, the space between the fascia lata and fascia iliaca can be located easily by slowly withdrawing and simultaneously injecting fluid through the needle following completion of the femoral nerve block.

25.2.6 Current Literature in Ultrasound-Guided Approaches

There is a paucity of literature on the use of ultrasound-guided lateral femoral cutaneous nerve block. Nonetheless, the use of ultrasound guidance in lateral femoral cutaneous and 3-in-1 block allows real-time visualization of the spread of local anesthetic deposited beneath the clearly identifiable fascial layers [10]. This may help predict the success in cases where the nerves may not be seen. There will likely be a reduced reliance on depositing a larger than necessary volume of local anesthetic in hopes of obtaining the block of all related nerves.

A case report by Miller has been published which describes combined femoral and lateral femoral cutaneous nerve block (described in Sect. 25.1) [6].

Clinical Pearls

- Although data on ultrasound-guided techniques for lateral femoral cutaneous block are lacking, ultrasound may improve target nerve localization or identification within the plane of needle entry. Visual confirmation of local anesthetic spread within the correct fascial plane will provide valuable information in cases where the nerve is not visible. The use of ultrasound may, therefore, result in smaller doses of local anesthetic being needed for effective blocks.

25.2.7 Case Study

Lateral Femoral Cutaneous Nerve Block (Contributed by S. Suresh)

A 4-year-old female, 19.7 kg, was scheduled for muscle and skin biopsy and venous port insertion. The patient had previously undergone a bilateral MRI of the lower extremities without contrast and a frontal fluoroscopic spot radiograph. Preadmission medications included folic acid (1 mg tablet), Benadryl 6.25 mg, and Prilosec 10 mg. An ultrasound-guided lateral femoral cutaneous nerve block was indicated, which was performed with a 27G needle and 3 mL 0.25 % bupivacaine (see Fig. 25.14). Surgery lasted 1 h, 38 min; block duration was 12 h.

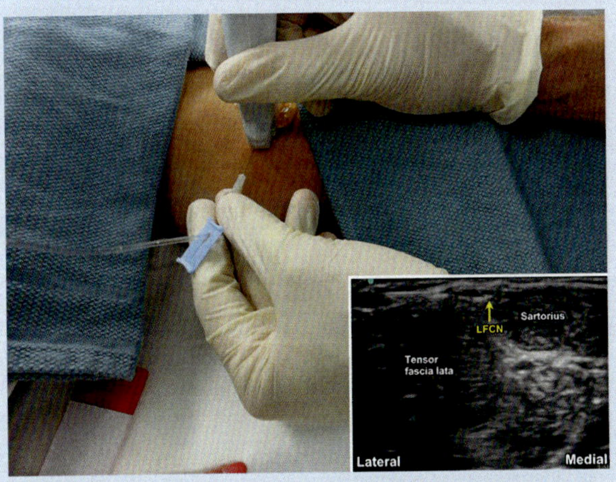

Fig. 25.14 Ultrasound-guided lateral femoral cutaneous nerve (*LFCN*) block. See Case Study for details

25.3 Obturator Nerve Block

25.3.1 Indications

- Prevent obturator reflex during transurethral bladder tumor resections.
- Treatment of pain in the hip area.
- Adductor spasm (as seen in multiple sclerosis patients).
- Diagnostic tool for hip mobility.
- Knee surgery: improved analgesia has been shown when obturator nerve blockade is used in addition to femoral block [11].

25.3.2 Surface Anatomy (Fig. 25.15)

The patient is positioned with the hip externally rotated and the knee slightly flexed to permit maximum exposure of the medial thigh.

The obturator nerve traverses the inguinal ligament medially and lies approximately 0.5–1 cm lateral to the pubic tubercle and 0.5–1 cm below the inguinal ligament (depending on the age and size of the child).

- Pubic tubercle: the tubercle lies approximately 1 cm lateral to the midline.
- ASIS: palpate this landmark by following the iliac crests to their most anterior edge.
- Inguinal ligament: the ligament is attached medially to the pubic tubercle and laterally to the anterior superior iliac spine.
- Landmarks include:
  - Femoral/inguinal crease: a natural oblique skinfold parallel and 0.5–1 cm distal to the inguinal ligament.
  - Adductor longus muscle: the tendon of adductor longus forms the medial border of the upper part of the thigh. The anterior division of the obturator nerve lies immediately deep to the adductor longus muscle.

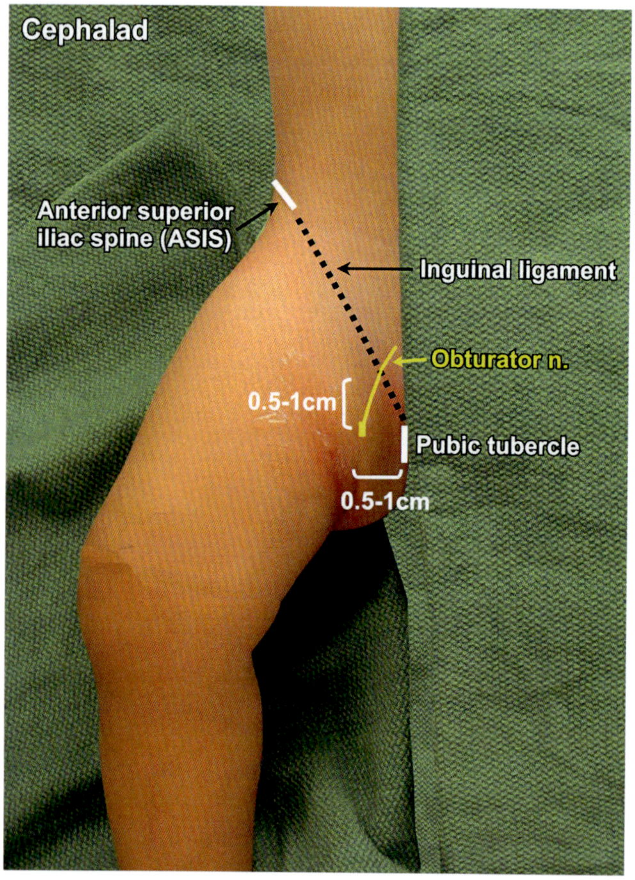

Fig. 25.15 Surface anatomy for obturator nerve block

The needle puncture site is located approximately 0.5–1 cm (depending on the age and size of the child) beneath the inguinal ligament and equidistant laterally to the pubic tubercle.

25.3.3 Nerve Stimulation Technique

Since the obturator nerve branches early after its descent from the obturator canal, blocking this nerve before it branches within the obturator canal near the superior pubic ramus is often indicated for blind techniques. However, in a small proportion of children, the obturator nerve divides either before or far from the obturator canal.

25.3.3.1 Needle Insertion

- Insert a 35–50 mm, 22G–25G insulated needle 0.5–1 cm caudad to the inguinal ligament and 0.5–1 cm lateral to the pubic tubercle, almost perpendicular to the skin, using a slight (15°) lateral direction.
- If contact with the pubic ramus occurs, "walk" the needle caudally off the pubic ramus and then advance the needle.

25.3.3.2 Current Application and Appropriate Responses

- Apply an initial current of 0.8–1 mA (1 Hz, 0.1–0.2 ms) and aim to elicit muscle twitches in the adductor muscles using a current of 0.5 mA. See Table 14.3 for expected motor responses during nerve stimulation.

25.3.3.3 Modifications to Inappropriate Responses

- If no motor response occurs with a needle depth of one third of the anteroposterior diameter of the thigh, the direction of the needle is incorrect, and the procedure should be repeated after reassessing the landmark.
- Adduction of the adductor muscles can be obtained by direct muscle stimulation at 1 mA. Decreasing the current intensity to 0.5 mA will help with nerve localization.

> **Clinical Pearls**
>
> - Aspiration is essential when injecting near the unbranched obturator nerve, as the obturator artery lies adjacent to the nerve. Hemorrhage involving this artery can be life-threatening [12].

25.3.4 Ultrasound-Guided Technique

Major anatomical structures surrounding the obturator nerve as captured by MRI and VHVS images are shown with the corresponding ultrasound image in Fig. 25.16.

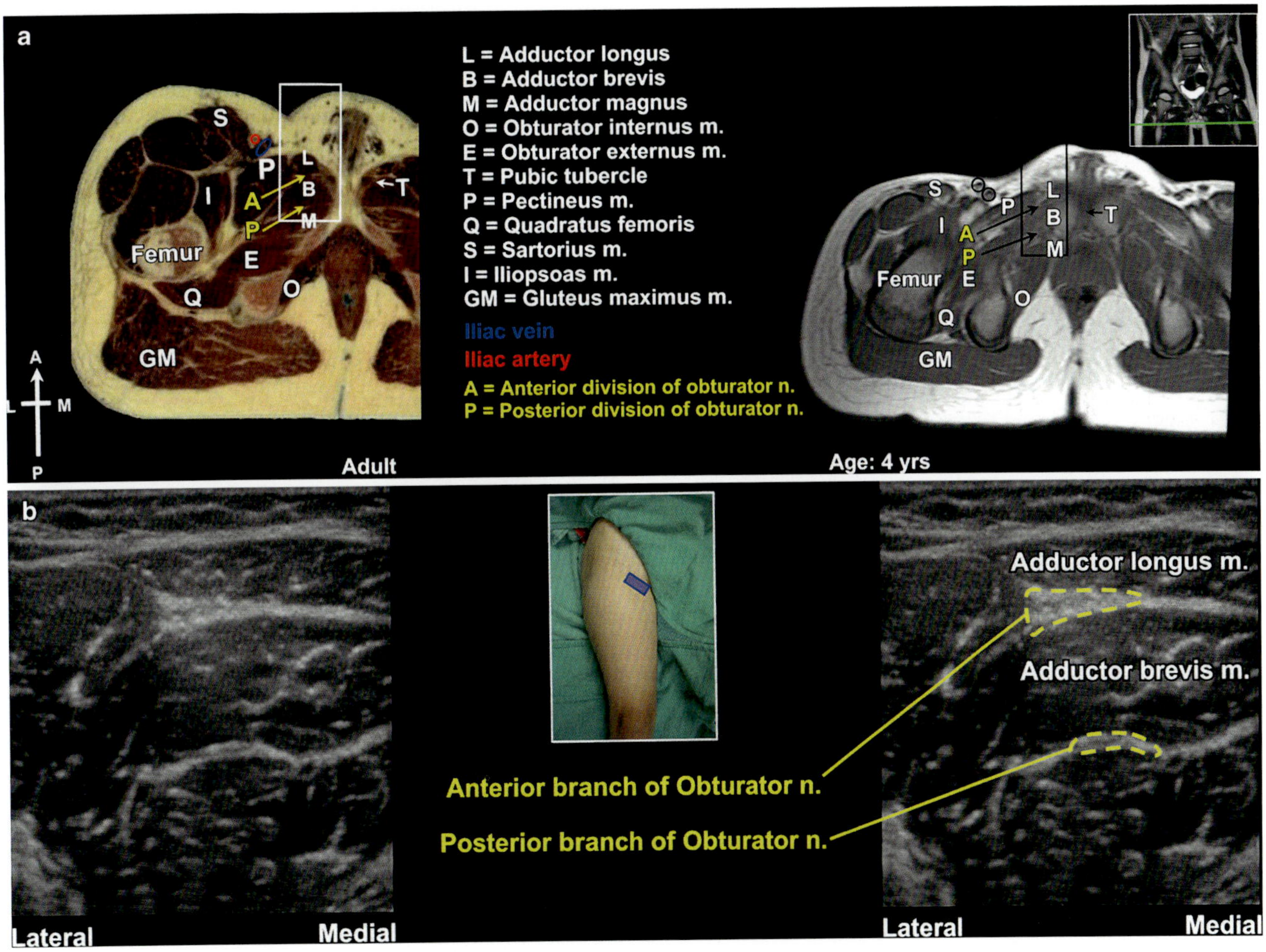

Fig. 25.16 (**a**) VHVS and MRI images of major anatomical structures surrounding the anterior and posterior obturator nerves. (**b**) Ultrasound image of major anatomical structures surrounding the anterior and posterior obturator nerves

25.3.4.1 Scanning Technique

- A linear (6–15 MHz) transducer is placed in a transverse location over the anterior surface of the proximal thigh approximately 0.5–2 cm inferior to the inguinal ligament along the inguinal crease.
- Depth of penetration is 1–4 cm from the skin surface.
- The femoral vessels are identified using the Doppler function if necessary. The femoral vein is medial to the artery.
- The pectineus muscle can be found medial to the femoral vein. Further medial movement of the probe along the inguinal crease reveals the adductor longus, brevis, and magnus muscles. At this location, the anterior division of the obturator nerve lies in the fascial plane between adductor longus and brevis, while the posterior division lies between adductor brevis and magnus.
- If the transducer is moved cranially toward the inguinal ligament until the superior pubic ramus is identified, the fascia separating pectineus from obturator externus may be visualized. At this location, the anterior division of the nerve runs between the obturator externus and pectineus, while the posterior division pierces the obturator externus.

25.3.4.2 Sonographic Appearance

- The nerves may not be visible. In this case, the target for injection is the intermuscular fascial plane in which the nerves traverse.
- The adductor muscles – adductor longus, brevis, and magnus – are arranged vertically from superficial to deep. The pectineus muscle is located lateral to the adductor muscles (Fig. 25.16b).
- A hyperechoic fascial plane separates the adductor muscles from each other.
- The anterior division may be seen as a hyperechoic, elongated oval structure between the adductor longus and brevis muscles. The posterior division has a similar appearance and lies between the adductor brevis and magnus muscles.

25.3.4.3 Needle Insertion

- Use a 35–50 cm, 22–25G insulated needle.
- An in-plane (IP) approach is used for ultrasound-guided obturator nerve block (Fig. 25.17).
- The block needle is advanced from lateral to medial. It is important not to puncture the femoral vessels using this approach. In addition, the medial circumflex artery and vein (arising from the profunda femoris vessels) may traverse between the obturator externus, adductor magnus, and adductor brevis muscles [3]. The needle is first directed into the fascial plane between the adductor longus and adductor brevis. After injection of local anesthetic at this location, the needle is redirected to the deeper plane between the adductor brevis and adductor magnus.

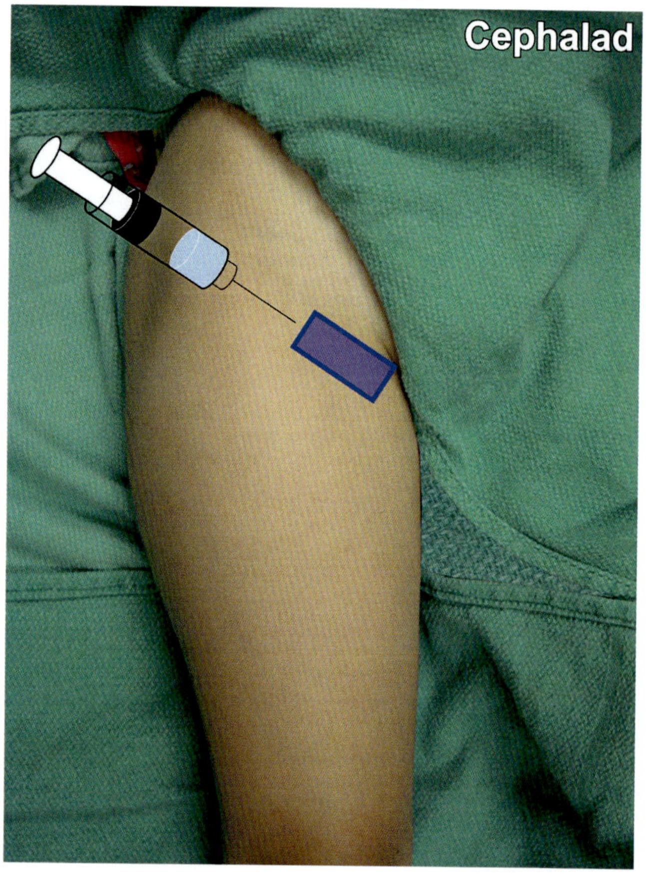

Fig. 25.17 In-plane needling technique for ultrasound-guided obturator nerve block. *Blue rectangle* indicates probe footprint

25.3.4.4 Local Anesthetic Application

- Performing a test dose with D5W is recommended prior to local anesthetic application to visualize the spread and confirm needle tip localization.
- 0.25 mL/kg (maximum 10 mL) of 0.25 % bupivacaine or 0.2 % ropivacaine is injected at each interfascial plane.
- Upon injection, one should visualize longitudinal spread of the hypoechoic-appearing local anesthetic within the interfascial plane.

Clinical Pearls

- Performing a test dose with D5W is recommended prior to local anesthetic application to visualize the spread and confirm nerve localization.
- Local anesthetic spread should appear as a hypoechoic expansion around the nerve between the fascial planes of the muscles.
- Locate the femoral artery as a single vessel first, then scan medially to locate the femoral vein. The pectineus muscle can be found medial to the femoral vein; finally, locate the adductor muscles medial to pectineus muscle.

25.3.5 Current Literature in Ultrasound-Guided Approaches

To date, there have been no clinical reports in the pediatric literature describing ultrasound guidance for obturator nerve block.

25.3.6 Case Study

Obturator Nerve Block (Contributed by A. Spencer)

An 8-year-old male, 25 kg, presented for obturator nerve block and multiple orthopedic procedures including percutaneous hip adductor tenotomy and botox injections, bilateral medial release, and tibialis anterior tendon lengthening. The patient had a complex history, including mixed cerebral palsy with spastic and dyskinetic components. The patient was ex-premature and suffering from intellectual disability and was also wheelchair bound. Clinically, the patient also suffered from adductor muscle spasm and contractures and required repeated obturator nerve phenol blocks. Other history included central sleep-disordered breathing and mild obstructive sleep apnea. The patient's preadmission medications included baclofen, Sinemet, and Prevacid.

The patient underwent a general anesthetic with endotracheal intubation and lower lumbar epidural for perioperative pain control. Phenol blocks were completed prior to the scheduled orthopedic procedures; the upper thighs and groin areas were prepped with chlorhexidine solution, and the leg was externally rotated and slightly flexed to provide good exposure for ultrasound scanning. An 80 mm, 22G echogenic needle and an in-plane approach was used for the blocks (see Fig. 25.18). Phenol 6 % solution ×1.5 mL was deposited bilaterally in the fascia containing the anterior division of the obturator nerve. Duration of surgery was 4 h. The patient was comfortable in the recovery area under epidural analgesia; postoperative analgesia consisted of a continuous epidural infusion of bupivacaine 0.08 % at 5 mL per hour for 48 h. Acetaminophen 375 mg po q6h regular and ketorolac 8 mg IV q8h regular for 48 h were also used.

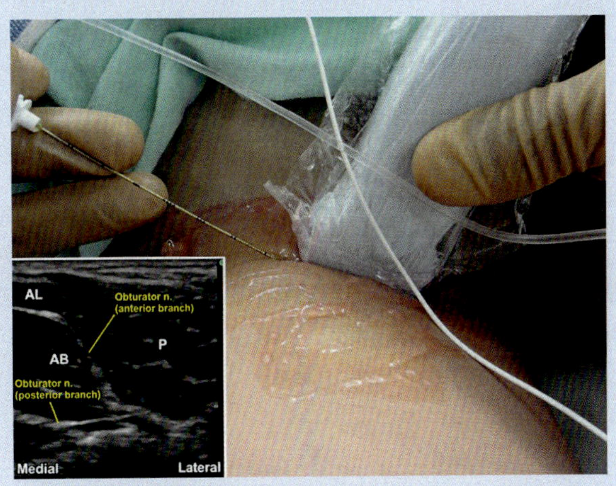

Fig. 25.18 Ultrasound-guided obturator nerve block. *AL* adductor longus, *AB* adductor brevis, *P* pectineus. See Case Study for details

25.4 Saphenous Nerve Block

25.4.1 Indications

The saphenous nerve is a sensory nerve providing cutaneous innervation to the medial side of the thigh and foot. A saphenous nerve block is a useful adjunct to a sciatic nerve block when complete sensory blockade of the lower leg and foot is desired (e.g., following major foot and ankle surgery).

Indications

- Surgical procedures of the medial aspect of the lower leg and ankle (in combination with sciatic nerve block).

25.4.2 Surface Anatomy (Fig. 25.19)

After general anesthesia has been induced, the patient is placed supine with the hip slightly externally rotated and the knee slightly flexed. Surface landmarks include:

- Femoral triangle
  - Formed by the inguinal ligament superiorly, sartorius laterally, and adductor longus medially.
- Vastus medialis
  - Part of the quadriceps muscle group. It is a prominent muscle on the medial side of the lower half of the thigh.
- Tibial tuberosity
  - Bony prominence on the anteromedial aspect of the tibia and inferior to the patella. Useful when performing subcutaneous landmark-based block

The needle puncture site is located approximately distal one third of the thigh above the medial aspect of the knee.

Clinical Pearls: Landmark-Based Technique (Transsartorial Approach)

- After raising a skin wheal of local anesthetic over the sartorius muscle at the level of one finger width above the patella, advance a 20G Tuohy pediatric epidural needle in a caudad (45°) and slightly posterior direction into the sartorius muscle in the medial aspect of the lower thigh.
- A loss of resistance should be felt as the needle penetrates the fat pad underneath the sartorius muscle (approximately 1–2 cm, depending on the age and size of the child).
- This "blind" transsartorial block approach described first by van der Wal et al. [13] has shown to be more effective than those performed at other block locations for producing anesthesia to the medial aspect of the foot. The approaches using needle insertion below the knee may limit the efficacy of the block (i.e., failure to provide complete anesthesia of the medial ankle), due to the oftentimes significant branching of the nerve once it passes the knee [14].

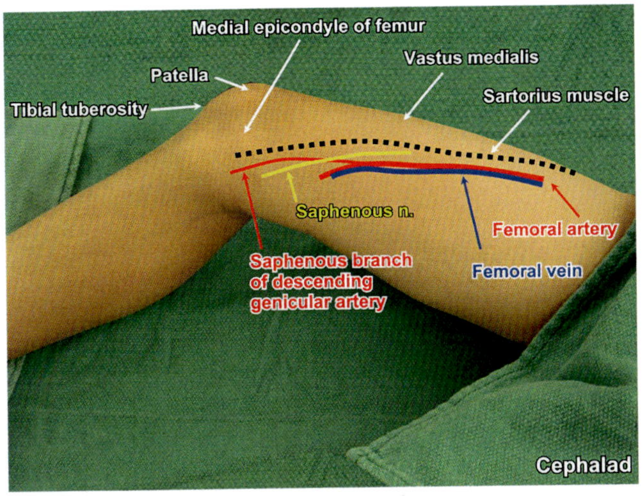

Fig. 25.19 Surface anatomy for saphenous nerve block

25.4.3 Nerve Stimulation Technique

The saphenous nerve is purely sensory, and elicitation of paresthesia, which is often difficult and uncomfortable for children, remains the only means to confirm the appropriate needle placement. Therefore, nerve stimulators are not commonly used in children to localize this nerve.

25.4.4 Ultrasound-Guided Technique

Major anatomical structures in the thigh as captured by MRI and VHVS images are shown with the corresponding ultrasound image in Fig. 25.20a.

Ultrasound guidance has been used successfully at different locations, depending on the visibility of landmarks in the vicinity of the nerve. Two techniques (transsartorius and perifemoral approach) place the needle near the adductor canal, and one uses a paravenous (saphenous vein) approach. While each approach may be effective, disadvantages to the paravenous approach include the limited visibility of the nerve at this distal location and the fact that the nerve may have already branched significantly at this point [15]. The transsartorius perifemoral approach, which occurs at the mid-lower thigh (adductor canal) level and uses the large femoral artery instead of the more distal saphenous branch of the descending genicular artery [16] as a primary visible landmark (via color Doppler), may be a superior option and is described below.

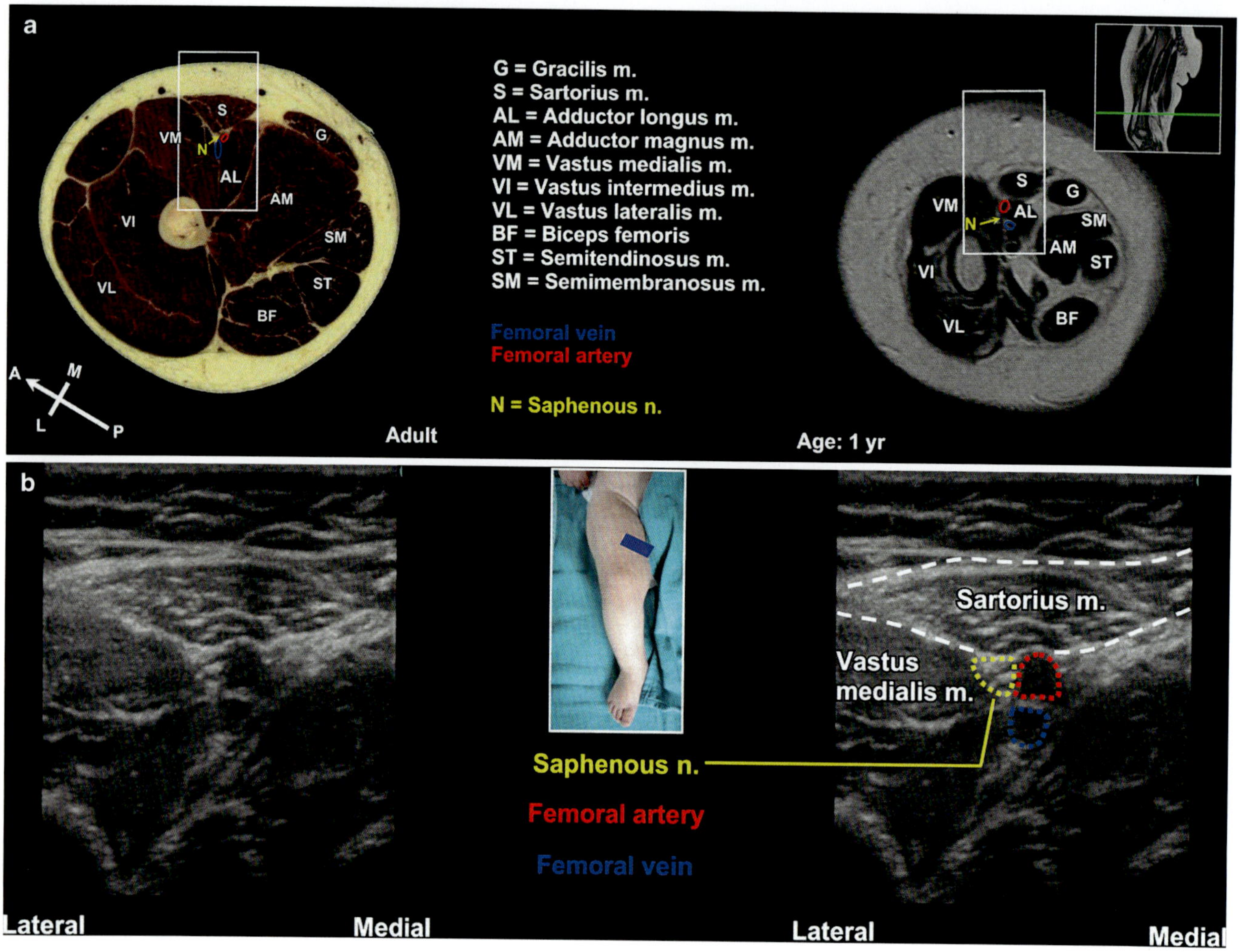

Fig. 25.20 (**a**) VHVS and MRI images showing the saphenous nerve just above the medial aspect of the patella. (**b**) Ultrasound image showing the saphenous nerve just above the medial aspect of the patella

25.4.4.1 Scanning Technique (Fig. 25.20b)

- A linear (6–15 MHz) transducer is placed in a transverse location over the anteromedial surface of the mid-thigh.
- The femoral artery is identified here along with the overlying sartorius muscle. The vastus medialis is anterolateral to the sartorius muscle at this location.
- The probe is scanned distally to the point where the femoral artery begins to move posteriorly. (The artery exits the adductor canal through the adductor hiatus to become the popliteal artery.)
- At this point, the saphenous nerve begins to cross from anterolateral to anteromedial along with the artery within the adductor canal.

25.4.4.2 Sonographic Appearance

- The saphenous nerve is occasionally too small to be visible (Fig. 25.20b).
- The sartorius, vastus medialis, and adductor magnus muscles are viewed in transverse with overlying subcutaneous fat.
- The femoral artery lies deep to the sartorius and is anechoic in appearance.
- The femoral vein is deep to the artery and is compressible.

25.4.4.3 Needle Insertion

- Use a 5 cm, 22G needle. Nerve stimulation is unnecessary since the saphenous nerve is purely sensory.
- The needle is advanced using an in-plane (IP) technique until it is medial to the artery and between the artery and the sartorius muscle (Fig. 25.21).
- A distinct "pop" may be felt as the needle passes through the adductor membrane (between adductor magnus and vastus medialis).

Clinical Pearls

- Only a small volume of local anesthetic is required for an effective saphenous nerve block. Too much local anesthetic could result in nerve injury secondary to increased pressure within the compartment.
- The saphenous nerve is small and can be difficult to locate even with ultrasound. However, the nerve usually lies in the fascial plane between the sartorius and the vastus medialis muscles. Local anesthetic can be deposited in this plane.
- Locate and follow the sartorius muscle with the femoral artery underneath.

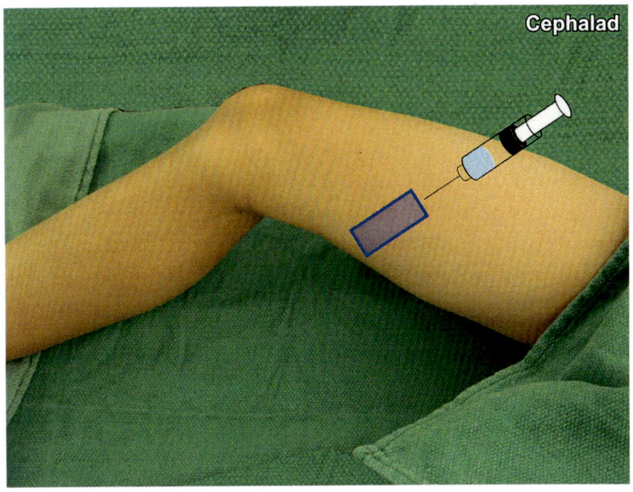

Fig. 25.21 In-plane needling technique for ultrasound-guided saphenous nerve block at the lower thigh

25.4.4.4 Local Anesthetic Application

- Performing a test dose with D5W is recommended prior to local anesthetic application to visualize the spread and confirm needle tip localization.
- 0.15–0.25 mL/kg (maximum 10 mL) of 0.25 % bupivacaine or 0.2 % ropivacaine is injected.

Clinical Pearls

- During injection, expansion of the hypoechoic solution in the fascial plane between the sartorius muscle and the vastus medialis muscle can be observed.

25.4.5 Current Literature in Ultrasound-Guided Approaches

There has been a limited amount of literature describing or evaluating the efficacy of the saphenous nerve block and its various approaches. A paravenous approach of the saphenous nerve block under ultrasound guidance in children has recently been described [17]. At the level of the proximal tibia, the saphenous nerve usually lies posteromedial to the saphenous vein (although this position can vary). The saphenous nerve can also be identified at the level of the ankle where the nerve is in close proximity to the saphenous vein (paravenous approach). A tourniquet can be tied around the lower leg to distend the saphenous vein just proximal to the ankle. Color Doppler can be used to aid identification of the saphenous vein. The nerve is adjacent to the vein in the subcutaneous tissue.

An ultrasound-guided transsartorial perifemoral approach has also been described in adults [18] and can also be adopted in children. This is a more proximal approach in the mid-thigh position using the easily identifiable femoral artery. When the high frequency 5–10 MHz hockey stick probe is placed transversely in the mid-thigh position, the femoral artery can be identified lying deep to the sartorius muscle. By scanning distally, the point where the femoral artery courses deep to become the popliteal artery can be determined. Just proximal to this location – deep to the sartorius muscle and medial to the femoral artery – is where local anesthetic can be deposited.

25.4.6 Case Study

Saphenous Nerve Block (Contributed by S. Suresh)

An 8-year-old male, 23 kg, was scheduled for a left calcaneal osteotomy following an X-ray of the left foot. A left calcaneal osteotomy and lengthening and cuboid closing wedge osteotomy were performed following a sciatic nerve block. The block was performed under ultrasound guidance using a 22G needle and 5 mL 0.25 % bupivacaine with 1:200,000 epinephrine (see Fig. 25.22). Surgery lasted 2 h, 18 min; block duration was 6–12 h. Pain reporting was 8/10 half an hour following surgery and 0/10 1 h after surgery. Postoperative analgesia consisted of a morphine (Duramorph) injection, 1.2 mg 30 min after surgery.

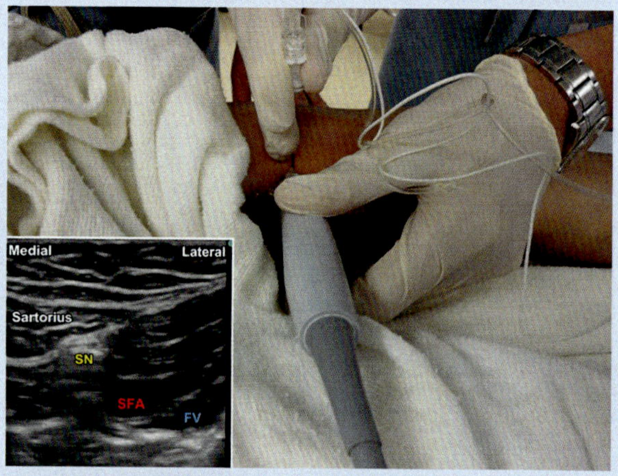

Fig. 25.22 Ultrasound-guided saphenous nerve block. *SN* saphenous nerve, *SFA* superficial femoral artery, *FV* femoral vein. See Case Study for details

References

1. Oberndorfer U, Marhofer P, Bosenberg A, et al. Ultrasonographic guidance for sciatic and femoral nerve blocks in children. Br J Anaesth. 2007;98:797–801.
2. Farid IS, Heiner EJ, Fleissner PR. Comparison of femoral nerve block and fascia iliaca block for analgesia following reconstructive knee surgery in adolescents. J Clin Anesth. 2010;22:256–9.
3. Sethuraman M, Neema PK, Rathod RC. Combined monitored anesthesia care and femoral nerve block for muscle biopsy in children with myopathies. Paediatr Anaesth. 2008;18:691.
4. Gurnaney H, Kraemer F, Ganesh A. Ultrasound and nerve stimulation to identify an abnormal location of the femoral nerve. Reg Anesth Pain Med. 2009;34:615.
5. Frenkel O, Mansour K, Fischer JW. Ultrasound-guided femoral nerve block for pain control in an infant with a femur fracture due to nonaccidental trauma. Pediatr Emerg Care. 2012;28:183–4.
6. Miller BR. Combined ultrasound-guided femoral and lateral femoral cutaneous nerve blocks in pediatric patients requiring surgical repair of femur fractures. Paediatr Anaesth. 2011;21:1163–4.
7. Miller BR. Ultrasound-guided fascia iliaca compartment block in pediatric patients using a long-axis, in-plane needle technique: a report of three cases. Paediatr Anaesth. 2011;21:1261–4.
8. Ponde V, Desai AP, Shah D. Comparison of success rate of ultrasound-guided sciatic and femoral nerve block and neurostimulation in children with arthrogryposis multiplex congenita: a randomized clinical trial. Paediatr Anaesth. 2013;23:74–8.
9. Maccani RM, Wedel DJ, Melton A, Gronert GA. Femoral and lateral femoral cutaneous nerve block for muscle biopsies in children. Paediatr Anaesth. 1995;5:223–7.
10. Simion C, Suresh S. Lower extremity peripheral nerve blocks in children. Tech Reg Anesth Pain Manag. 2007;11:222–8.
11. Macalou D, Trueck S, Meuret P, et al. Postoperative analgesia after total knee replacement: the effect of an obturator nerve block added to the femoral 3-in-1 nerve block. Anesth Analg. 2004;99:251–4.
12. Akata T, Murakami J, Yoshinaga A. Life-threatening haemorrhage following obturator artery injury during transurethral bladder surgery: a sequel of an unsuccessful obturator nerve block. Acta Anaesthesiol Scand. 1999;43:784–8.
13. van der Wal M, Lang SA, Yip RW. Transsartorial approach for saphenous nerve block. Can J Anaesth. 1993;40:542–6.
14. Benzon HT, Sharma S, Calimaran A. Comparison of the different approaches to saphenous nerve block. Anesthesiology. 2005;102:633–8.
15. Krombach J, Gray AT. Sonography for saphenous nerve block near the adductor canal. Reg Anesth Pain Med. 2007;32:369–70.
16. Gray AT, Collins AB. Ultrasound-guided saphenous nerve block. Reg Anesth Pain Med. 2003;28:148.
17. Miller BR. Ultrasound-guided proximal tibial paravenous saphenous nerve block in pediatric patients. Paediatr Anaesth. 2010;20:1059–60.
18. Tsui BC, Ozelsel T. Ultrasound-guided transsartorial perifemoral artery approach for saphenous nerve block. Reg Anesth Pain Med. 2009;34:177–8.

Suggested Reading

Dalens BJ. Blocks of nerves of the lumbar plexus supplying the lower extremities. In: Dalens BJ, editor. Pediatric regional anesthesia. Boca Raton: CRC Press; 1990. p. 287–97.

Dalens B. Lumbar plexus blocks. In: Dalens B, editor. Regional anesthesia in infants, children, and adolescents. Philadelphia: Lippincott Williams & Wilkins; 1995. p. 321–33.

Karmakar MK, Kwok WH. Ultrasound-Guided Regional Anesthesia. In: Cote CJ, Lerman J, Anderson BJ, Eds. 5th ed. Philadelphia: WB Saunders; 2013. p. 880–908.

Suresh S, Polaner DM, Cote CJ. Regional Anesthesia. In: Cote CJ, Lerman J, Anderson BJ, Eds. 5th ed. Philadelphia: WB Saunders; 2013. p. 835–879.

Tsui BC. Femoral block. In: Tsui BC, editor. Atlas of ultrasound and nerve stimulation-guided regional anesthesia. New York: Springer; 2007. p. 161–70.

Part VIII

Nerve Blocks of the Sacral Plexus

Sciatic and Popliteal Nerve Blocks

26

Heather Y.Z. Ting and Ban C.H. Tsui

Contents

H.Y.Z. Ting, MD, FRCPC
Department of Anesthesiology and Pain Medicine,
University of Alberta Hospital, 8440-112 St NW, 2-150 Clinical Sciences Building, Edmonton, AB T6G 2G3, Canada
e-mail: yizhenhe@ualberta.ca

B.C.H. Tsui, Dip Eng, BSc (Math), B Pharm, MSc, MD, FRCPC (✉)
Department of Anesthesiology and Pain Medicine,
Stollery Children's Hospital/University of Alberta Hospital,
2-150 Clinical Sciences Building, Edmonton, AB T6G 2G3, Canada
e-mail: btsui@ualberta.ca

B.C.H. Tsui, S. Suresh (eds.), *Pediatric Atlas of Ultrasound- and Nerve Stimulation-Guided Regional Anesthesia*,
DOI 10.1007/978-0-387-79964-3_26

26.1 Indications

Indications

- Sciatic nerve before bifurcation:
  - Knee surgery (with supplemental blockade of the femoral nerve)
  - Removal of leg implants
- Sciatic nerve after bifurcation (may require supplemental blockade of the saphenous nerve):
  - Surgery on the lower limb
  - Foot and ankle surgery

26.2 Posterior Gluteal (Labat) Sciatic Nerve Block

The sciatic nerve at this location is deep compared to other approaches described in the subsequent sections of this chapter and can therefore be more challenging technically.

26.2.1 Surface Anatomy (Figs. 26.1 and 26.2)

The patient is placed in the lateral decubitus position with the legs flexed at the hip and knee. Surface landmarks include:

- Greater trochanter of the femur
- Sacral hiatus
- Posterior superior iliac spine

The point of needle entry when using the landmark technique is where a perpendicular line drawn at the midpoint between the greater trochanter and posterior superior iliac spine intercepts a line drawn between the greater trochanter and the sacral hiatus.

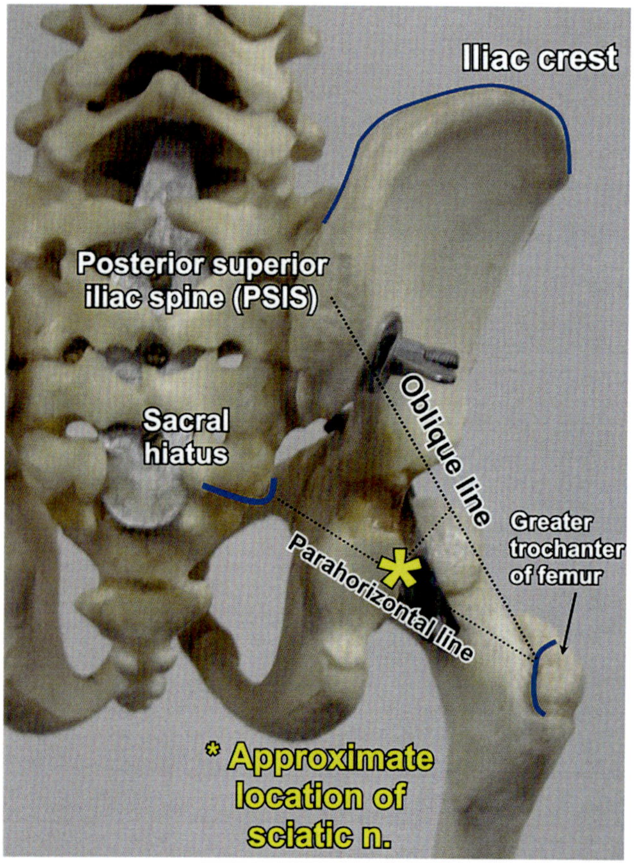

Fig. 26.1 Skeletal model showing anatomical landmarks for posterior gluteal sciatic nerve blockade

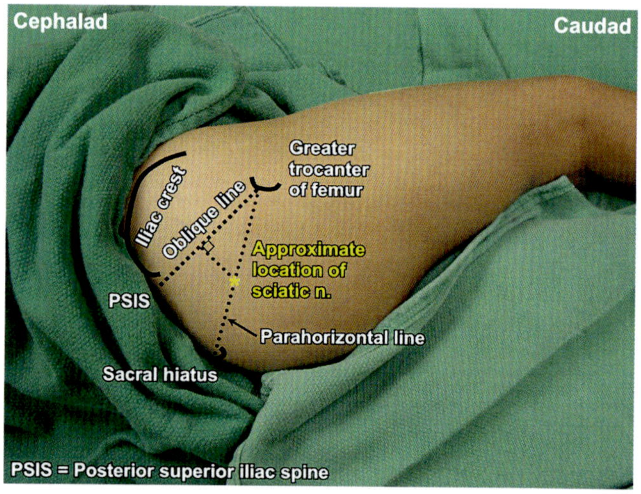

Fig. 26.2 Surface landmarks for posterior gluteal sciatic nerve block

26.2.2 Nerve Stimulation Technique

The approach described here is a modification of the landmark-based approach described by Winnie [1] with simplified landmarks and is typically easier to perform than the lateral or anterior approach [2].

Nerve stimulation in conjunction with ultrasound guidance is recommended for enhanced nerve localization using a posterior approach due to the depth of the sciatic nerve in the gluteal region.

26.2.2.1 Needle Insertion

A flowchart illustrating the needle insertion site and procedures is shown in Fig. 26.3.

- With the operator facing the patient's back, a 50–80 mm, 22G–25G needle (depending on the age and size of the child) is inserted perpendicular to the skin at the landmark described above and advanced in the direction of the ischium.
- The sciatic nerve may be reached at a variable depth, depending on the child's size and adiposity, but the depth may be approximated as about 1 mm per kg of weight (especially between 20 and 40 kg) with relatively less depth for younger children and greater depth for older children [2].
- If there is bony contact, the needle may either be touching the iliac bone or the ischial spine. In these cases, the needle tip has been placed too cephalad or too medial, respectively, or the needle is too deep.
- The inferior gluteal and internal pudendal vessels are at risk for puncture if the needle is directed too medially.

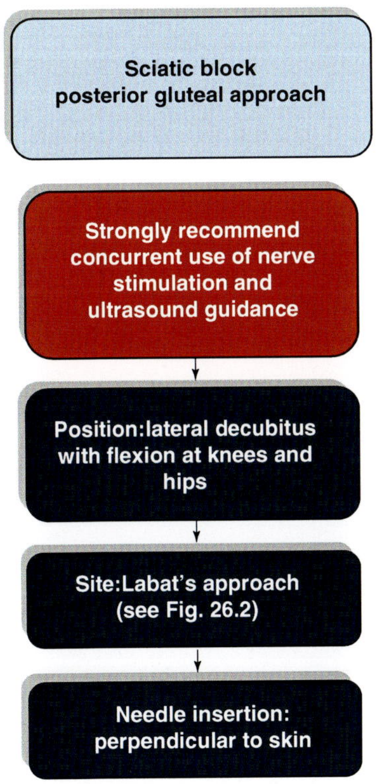

Fig. 26.3 Flowchart of needle insertion and procedures for posterior gluteal sciatic nerve block

26.2.2.2 Current Application and Appropriate Responses

Figure 26.4 illustrates the procedure for employing nerve stimulation techniques for lumbar plexus block.

- Initially, set the nerve stimulator to apply a current of 1–1.5 mA (2 Hz, 0.1–0.2 ms), and aim to elicit motor twitches at a current intensity threshold of 0.4 mA (0.1–0.2 ms) once the nerve is localized. Motor response cessation at currents less than 0.2 mA indicates that the needle is probably at an intraneural location.
- Visible or palpable twitches of the hamstring, calf muscles, foot, or toes verify stimulation of the sciatic nerve.
- Inversion of the foot or plantar flexion is sought, with inversion producing a more rapid onset and increased success of complete block than plantar flexion. Foot eversion indicates stimulation of the superficial peroneal nerves only and is associated with incomplete block [3].
- See Table 14.4 for expected motor responses during nerve stimulation.

Clinical Pearl

A double-injection technique has been used for proximal and popliteal sciatic nerve blocks in order to accurately localize the two components of the sciatic nerve and thus provide greater block success (with shorter latency) and allow lower total doses of local anesthetic. However, this may increase the potential risk of needling trauma.

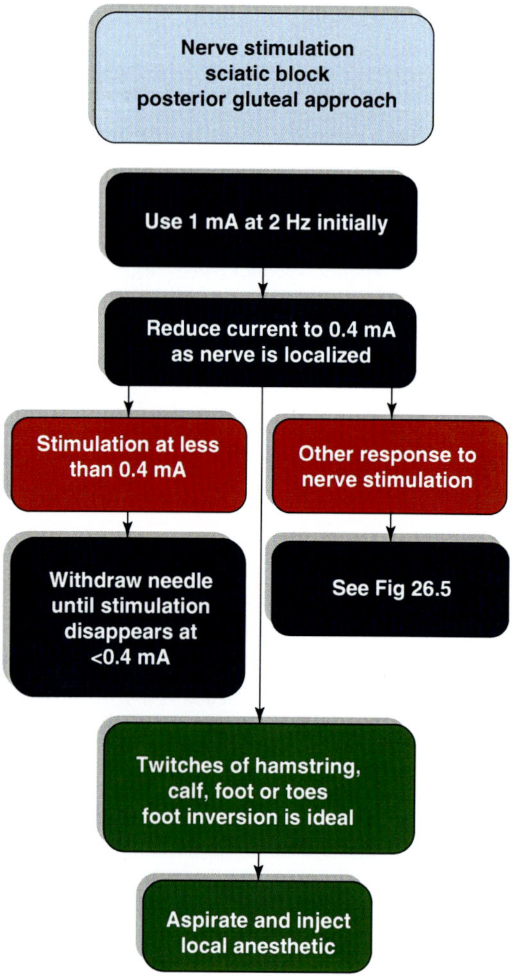

Fig. 26.4 Flowchart for employing nerve stimulation technique for posterior gluteal sciatic nerve block

26.2.2.3 Modifications to Inappropriate Responses (Table 26.1)

An algorithm of modifications in case of inappropriate responses to nerve stimulation is shown in Fig. 26.5.

Table 26.1 Responses and recommended needle adjustments for use with nerve stimulation during sciatic nerve block (posterior gluteal approach)

Correct response from nerve stimulation
Visible or palpable twitches in any of the hamstring or calf muscles, foot, or toes, at 0.2–0.5 mA. Up to 1.0 mA may be required in some patients (diabetic, peripheral vascular disease, sepsis)
Other common responses and needle adjustment
Muscle twitches from electrical stimulation
Gluteus maximus (local twitch from direct stimulation)
Explanation: needle tip too superficial
Needle adjustment: advance needle tip
Deep muscle layer (local twitch of inferior or superior gemellus, obturator internus, or quadratus femoris muscles)
Explanation: needle advanced too deep and beyond the nerve
Needle adjustment: withdraw needle to the skin and redirect slightly medially or laterally
Vascular puncture
Inferior gluteal or internal pudendal vessels puncture
Explanation: needle tip placed too medially
Needle adjustment: withdraw needle to skin and reinsert more laterally
Bone contact
Iliac bone (close to gluteus insertion)
Explanation: needle tip too superior
Needle adjustment: withdraw completely and reinsert according to protocol (check landmarks)
Ischial spine
Explanation: needle inserted at too medial position or angled in a medial direction
Needle adjustment: withdraw completely and reinsert in a more lateral direction

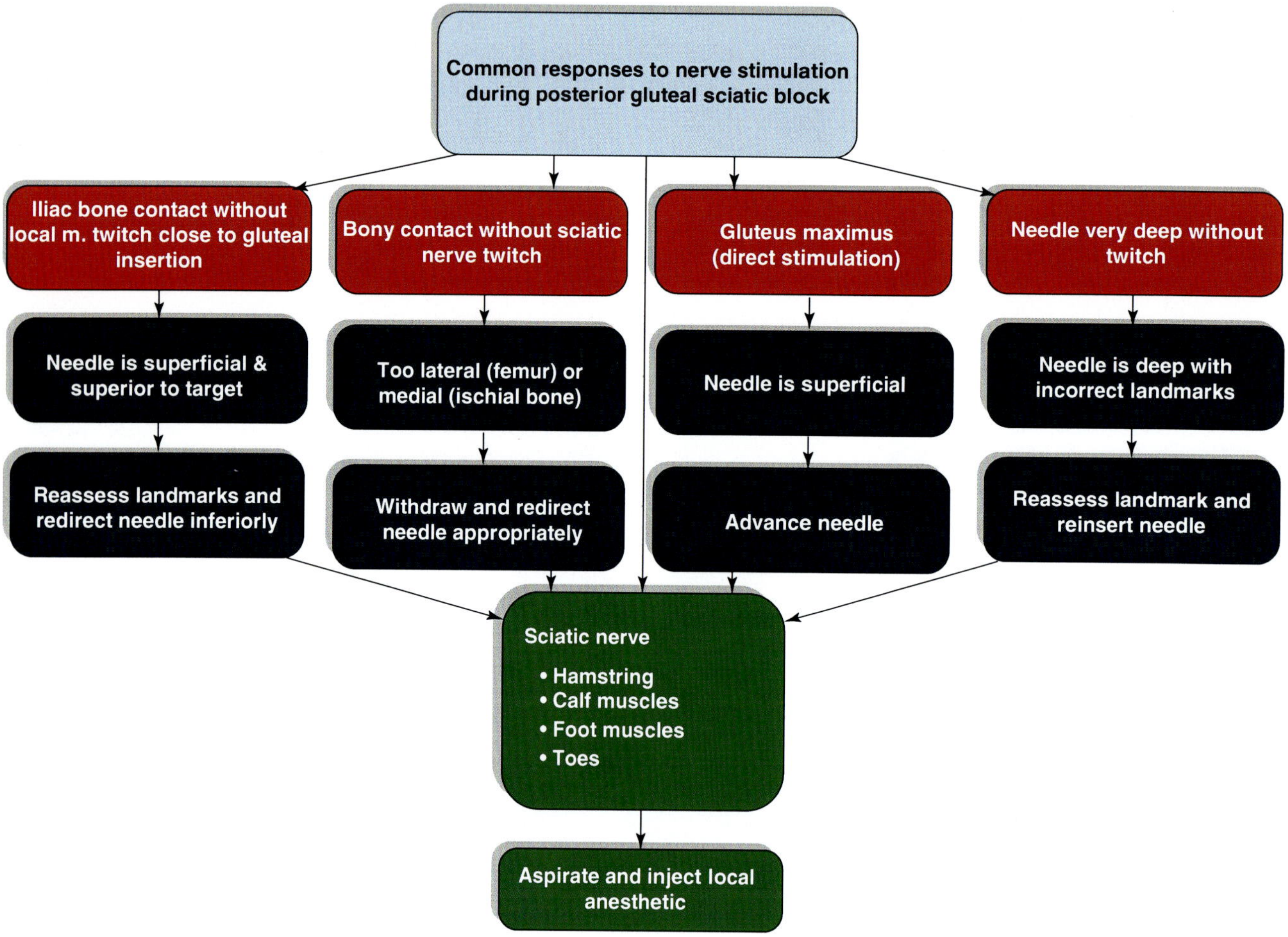

Fig. 26.5 Flowchart of modifications to inappropriate responses to nerve stimulation during posterior gluteal sciatic nerve block

26.2.3 Ultrasound-Guided Technique

For a summary of ultrasound guidance techniques for posterior gluteal sciatic nerve blocks, see Fig. 26.6.

Major anatomical structures of the sciatic nerve in the gluteal region as captured by MRI and VHVS images are shown with the corresponding ultrasound image in Fig. 26.7a.

Prepare the needle insertion site and skin surface with an antiseptic solution. Prepare the ultrasound probe surface by applying a sterile adhesive dressing to it prior to needling as discussed in Chap. 4.

There are some differences between adults and children in terms of their anatomical landmarks and sonoanatomy. The ischial tuberosity is very thin in children under 1 year of age and may be more difficult to palpate or view sonographically [4]. Laterally, the medial aspect of the greater trochanter will appear largely hypoechoic, although its size will depend on the age of the child, and it will only become highly recognizable at 6–8 years of age [5]. The femoral condyles are cartilaginous between the first and third years of life and do not ossify and develop their distinctive shape with visible sonographic appearance until 7–9 years of age; therefore, the borders of the femur may not be as hyperechoic in young children.

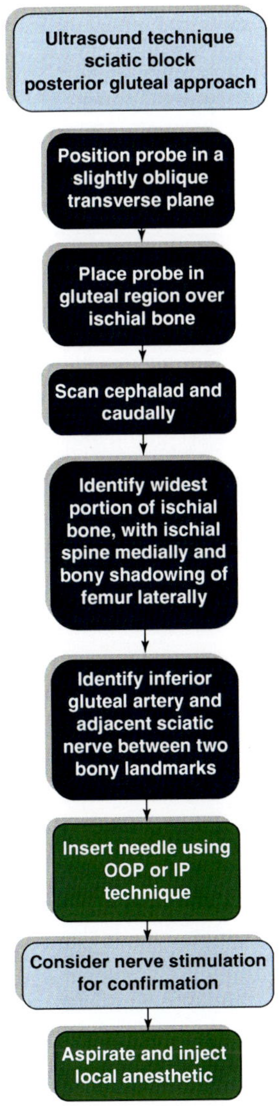

Fig. 26.6 Flowchart of ultrasound guidance technique for posterior gluteal sciatic nerve block

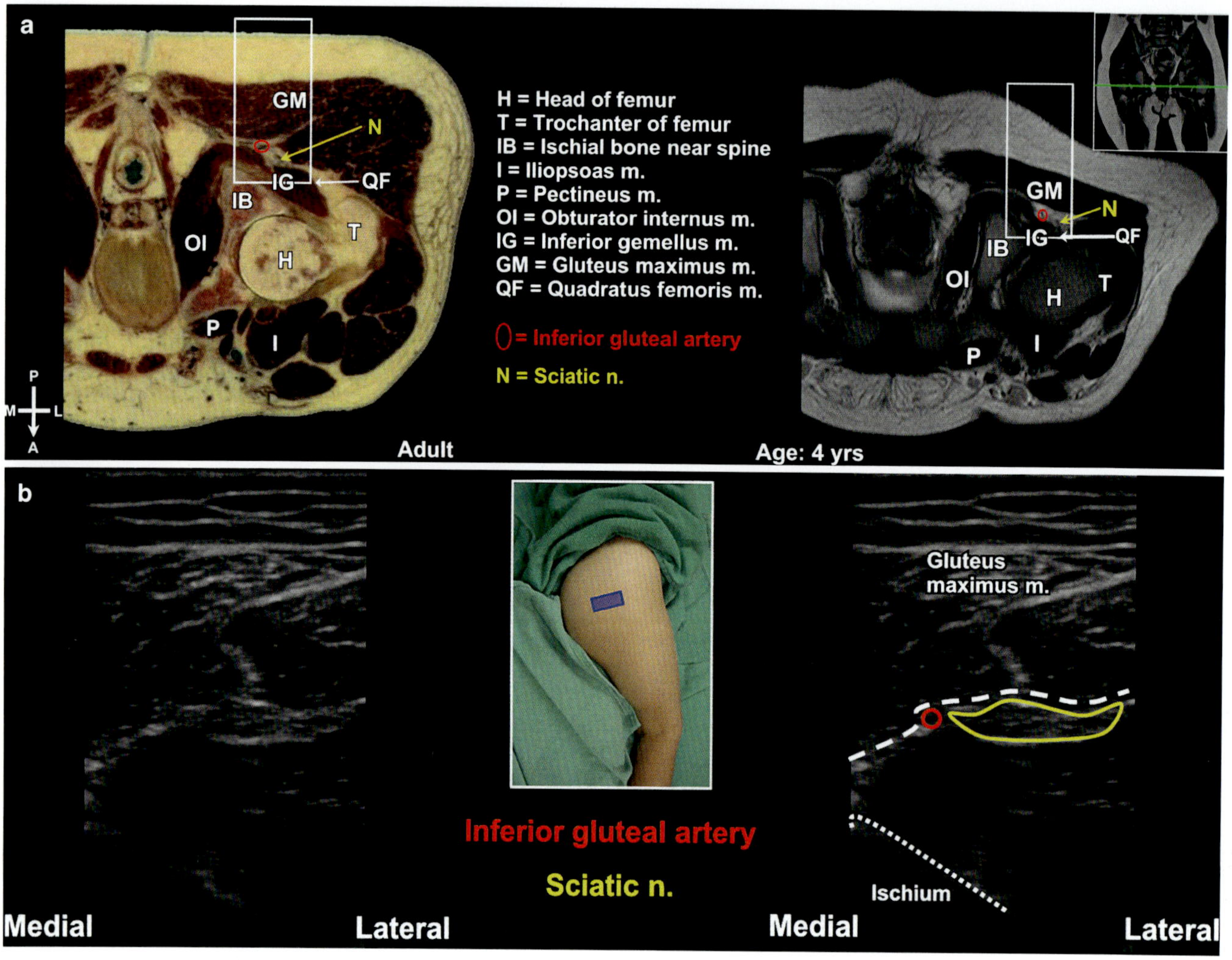

Fig. 26.7 (**a**) VHVS and MRI images of anatomical structures surrounding the sciatic nerve in the posterior gluteal region. (**b**) Ultrasound image of the posterior gluteal sciatic nerve block location

26.2.3.1 Scanning Technique

- The choice of ultrasound probe for this block will depend on the size of the patient. For young children, a high-frequency linear probe (10–5 MHz) can be used, although in older or larger patients, a curved, lower-frequency (5–2 MHz) probe may be required for increased depth of penetration.
- The probe is moved cephalad and caudad in the gluteal region to examine the ischial bone (a hyperechoic line with bony shadowing). Locate the widest portion of this bone that includes the ischial spine in the medial aspect.
- The gluteus maximus muscle will be visible superficial and posterior to the sciatic nerve.
- Alternatively, the sciatic nerve can be first located in the subgluteal region at approximately the midpoint between the greater trochanter and ischial tuberosity and traced proximally.
- Identification of the internal pudendal artery and vein adjacent to the ischial spine, as well as the inferior gluteal artery immediately adjacent to the sciatic nerve, may be facilitated with color Doppler.

26.2.3.2 Sonographic Appearance

- The sciatic nerve is hyperechoic and often appears wide and flat in short axis (Fig. 26.7b).
- Overlying the sciatic nerve is the distinctive gluteus maximus, which has a "starry night" pattern, and the inner muscle layers (superior and inferior gemellus muscles and quadratus femoris muscle) are often indistinct.

26.2.3.3 Needle Insertion

- Both in-plane (IP) and out-of-plane (OOP) approaches are appropriate for ultrasound-guided sciatic nerve block using the posterior gluteal approach.
- OOP approach (Fig. 26.8): the needle is inserted inferior to the probe in a cephalo-anterior direction. Since the nerve is deep at the gluteal region, needle insertion at a steep angle immediately next the transducer may increase the visibility of the needle tip.
- IP approach (Fig. 26.9): the needle may be advanced in a lateral-to-medial direction, penetrating the gluteus maximus muscle prior to reaching the sciatic nerve above the ischial bone.

26.2.4 Local Anesthetic Application

- Ensure negative aspiration of blood prior to injection of local anesthetic.
- Dalens et al. [2] described the use of four anesthetic solutions, each with 1:200,000 epinephrine (15 patients in each group): (1) 1 % lidocaine, (2) 0.5 % bupivacaine, (3) a mixture of equal volumes of 0.5 % bupivacaine and 1 % lidocaine, and (4) a mixture of equal volumes of 0.5 % bupivacaine and 1 % etidocaine. The local anesthetic solution was administered on a weight basis: 0.5 mL/kg in patients weighing less than 20 kg and 10 mL plus 0.25 mL/kg of patient's weight exceeding 20 kg, up to 25 mL maximum injected volumes.
- Small amounts of local anesthetic (0.3–0.5 mL/kg of 0.5 % bupivacaine for single limb blocks and 0.3 mL/kg 0.25 % bupivacaine per side for bilateral blocks) have also proven effective [6–8].
- Ivani et al. [9] suggested a bolus dose of 0.4–0.6 mL/kg of 0.2 % ropivacaine for postoperative analgesia and a higher concentration of 0.5 % ropivacaine if intraoperative pain control is required. They also described the use of clonidine 2 μg/kg in their local anesthetic mixture.
- The same group also suggested that ropivacaine and levobupivacaine are probably the best choice for longer operations when pain is more intense and long-lasting [10].
- Due to the anatomy of the nerves in children (smaller diameter and shorter distance between the nodes of Ranvier), larger volumes with lower concentrations are key to obtaining effective analgesia [11].
- We recommend the use of ropivacaine 0.2 %, bupivacaine 0.25 %, or levobupivacaine 0.25 %, with a volume of 0.25–0.5 mL/kg.
- As a guideline, lower concentrations should be used in children below the age of 6 years. Based on clinical experience, 6–12 h of analgesia can be expected [12].
- The dose of local anesthetic should not exceed the maximum toxic dose.

Ultrasound Considerations

- Performing a test dose with D5W is recommended prior to local anesthetic application to visualize the spread and confirm nerve localization. Deposit the local anesthetic solution over and around the sciatic nerve.

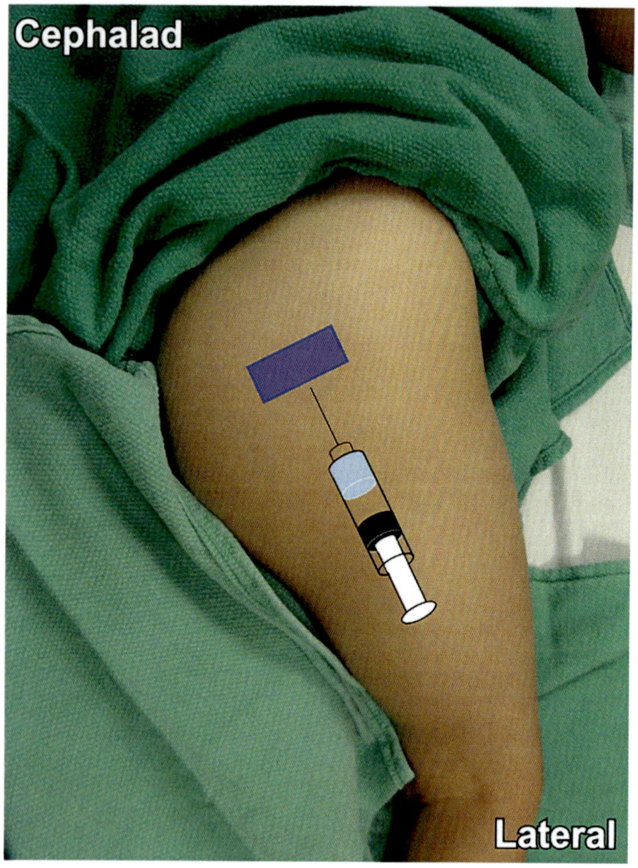

Fig. 26.8 Out-of-plane needling technique for ultrasound-guided posterior gluteal sciatic nerve block. *Blue rectangle* indicates probe footprint

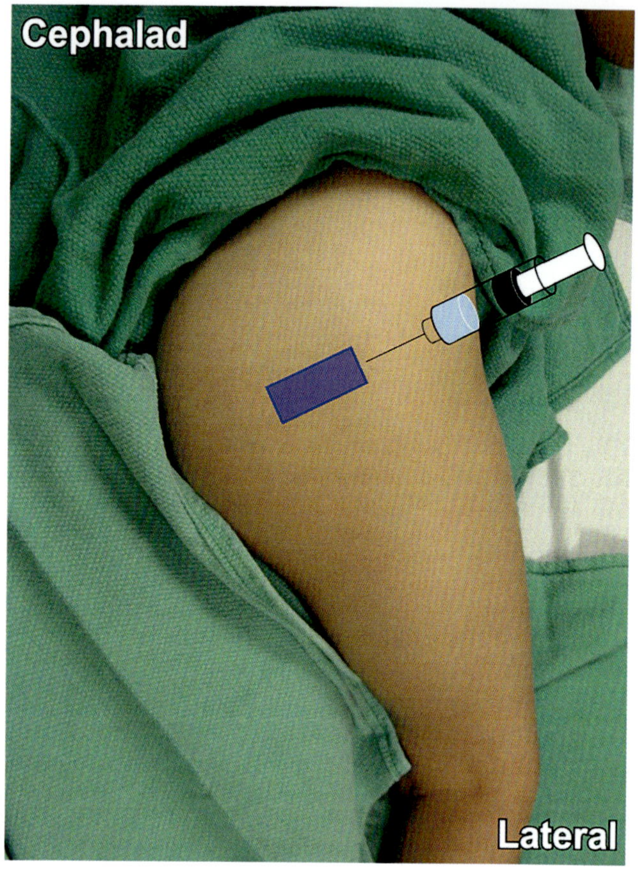

Fig. 26.9 In-plane needling technique for ultrasound-guided posterior gluteal sciatic nerve block. *Blue rectangle* indicates probe footprint

26.3 Infragluteal/Subgluteal Sciatic Nerve Block Approach

In contrast to the Labat/gluteal sciatic nerve block, the infragluteal/subgluteal approach targets the sciatic nerve at a more superficial location.

26.3.1 Surface Anatomy (Fig. 26.10)

The patient can be placed in the lateral decubitus position with the hip flexed and knee slightly extended, or they may be positioned prone. Surface landmarks include:

- Ischial tuberosity
- Greater trochanter

The needle is inserted at the midpoint of a line drawn between the greater trochanter and the ischial tuberosity at the level of the gluteal crease (Figs. 26.10 and 26.11).

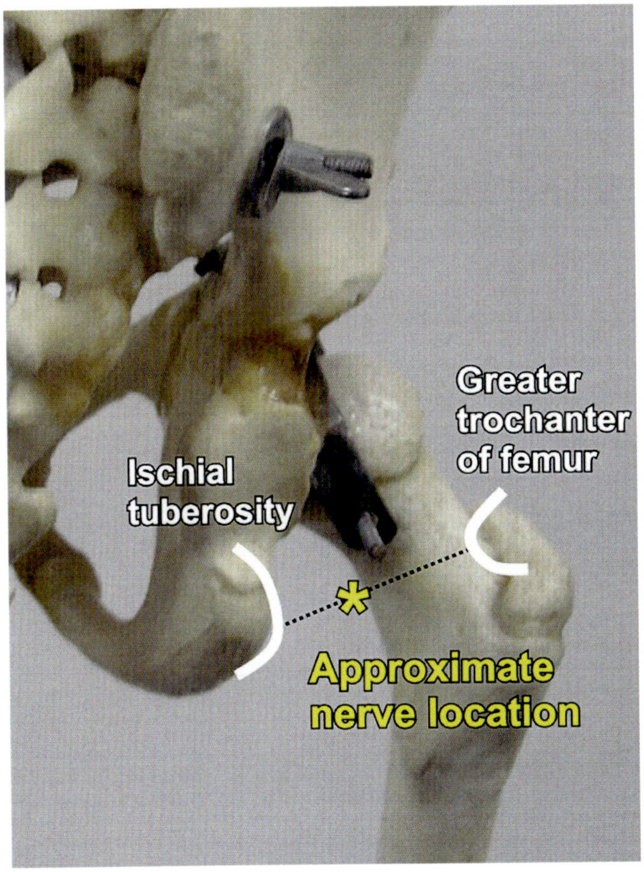

Fig. 26.10 Skeletal model showing anatomical landmarks for subgluteal sciatic nerve blockade

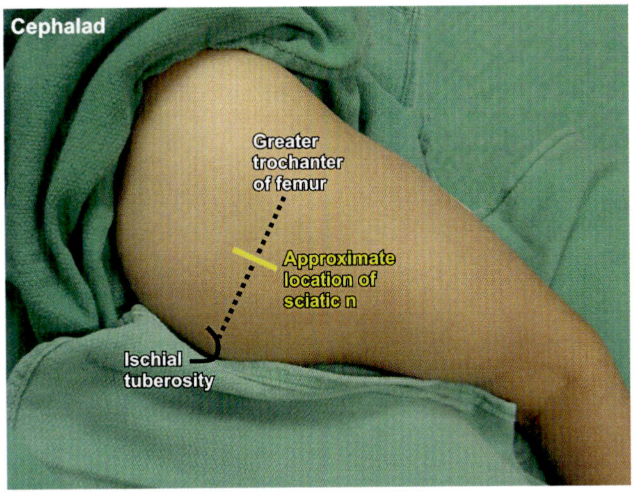

Fig. 26.11 Surface landmarks for subgluteal approach to sciatic nerve block

26.3.2 Nerve Stimulation Technique

The authors recommend combining nerve stimulation with ultrasound guidance for infragluteal/subgluteal sciatic blocks.

26.3.2.1 Needle Insertion

A flowchart illustrating the needle insertion site and procedures is shown in Fig. 26.12.

- A 50–80 mm, 22G–25G needle (depending on the child's age and size) is inserted perpendicularly to the skin until a loss of resistance is felt upon entrance to the common sheath.
- The depth of the sciatic nerve will be variable and age dependent.
- In situations of needle contact with bone:
  - Touching the iliac bone: needle tip is placed too cephalad.
  - Touching the hip joint: needle is located too deep and lateral.
  - Touching the ischium: needle is deep and medial.

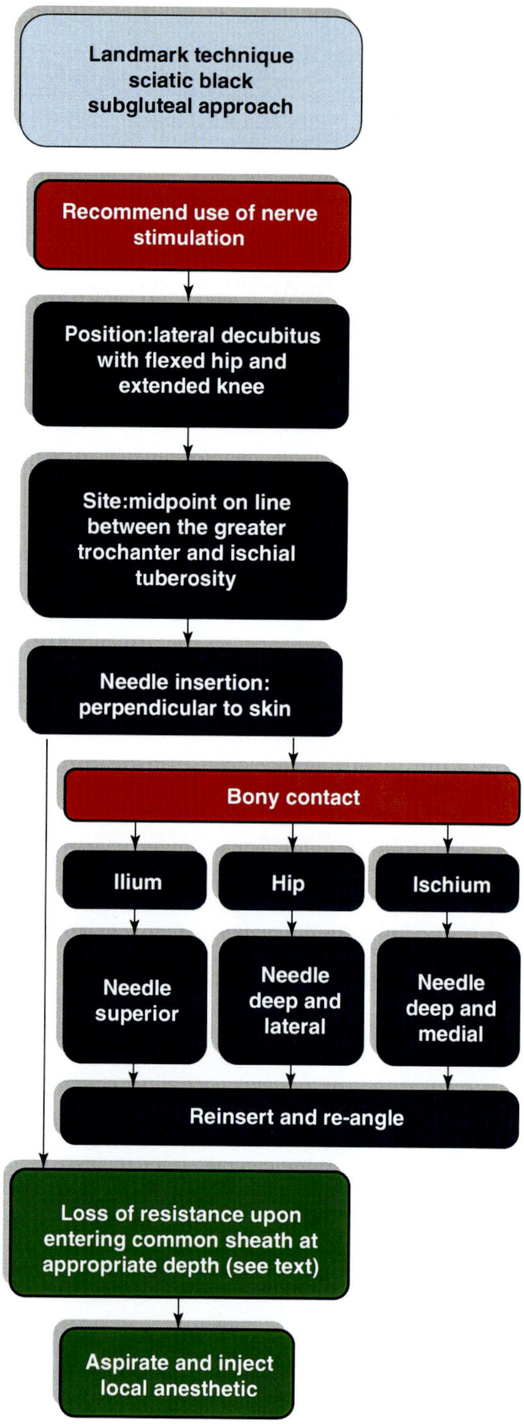

Fig. 26.12 Flowchart of needle insertion and procedures for subgluteal sciatic nerve block

26.3.2.2 Current Application and Appropriate Responses

Figure 26.13 illustrates the procedure for employing nerve stimulation techniques for subgluteal sciatic nerve block.

- Applying an initial current of 1–1.5 mA (2 Hz, 0.1–0.2 ms) is sufficient for stimulation of the sciatic nerve. After obtaining the appropriate motor response, the current is reduced to aim for a threshold current of 0.4 mA (0.1–0.2 ms). Motor response cessation at currents less than 0.2 mA indicates that the needle is probably in an intraneural location.

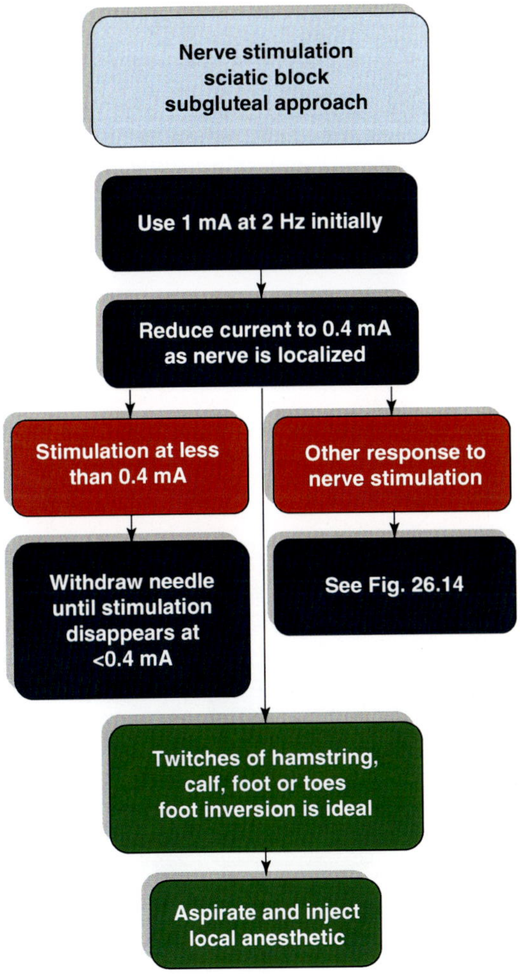

Fig. 26.13 Procedure for employing nerve stimulation technique during subgluteal sciatic nerve block

- Visible or palpable twitches of the hamstring or calf muscles, foot, or toes verify stimulation of the sciatic nerve.
- Twitches in the foot indicate stimulation of the tibial and common peroneal nerves rather than the proximal branches of the sciatic nerve and suggest optimal needle placement. Ideally, inversion of the foot, which is indicative of tibial nerve stimulation, is sought [3].
- See Table 14.4 for expected motor responses during nerve stimulation.

26.3.2.3 Modifications to Inappropriate Responses (Table 26.2)

An algorithm of modifications in case of inappropriate responses to nerve stimulation is shown in Fig. 26.14.

Table 26.2 Responses and recommended needle adjustments for use with nerve stimulation during sciatic nerve block (subgluteal approach)

Correct response from nerve stimulation
Twitches (visible or palpable) in any of the hamstring or calf muscles, foot, or toes, at 0.2–0.5 mA. Up to 1.0 mA may be required in some patients (diabetic, peripheral vascular disease, sepsis)
Other common responses and needle adjustments
Muscle twitches from electrical stimulation
Gluteus maximus (local twitch from direct stimulation)
Explanation: needle tip too superficial
Needle adjustment: advance needle tip
Bone contact
Iliac bone (close to gluteus insertion)
Explanation: needle tip too superior
Needle adjustment: withdraw completely and reinsert according to protocol (check landmarks)
Ischial or hip joint
Explanation: needle missed the plane of the sciatic nerve and the tip is placed too far medially (ischial) or laterally (hip)
Needle adjustment: withdraw completely and reinsert with a 5–10° angle adjustment
No response despite deep placement
Deep (10 cm) but no response; it is likely that the needle has been placed in the greater sciatic notch
Explanation: needle tip too inferior and medial
Needle adjustment: withdraw completely and reinsert slightly superiorly

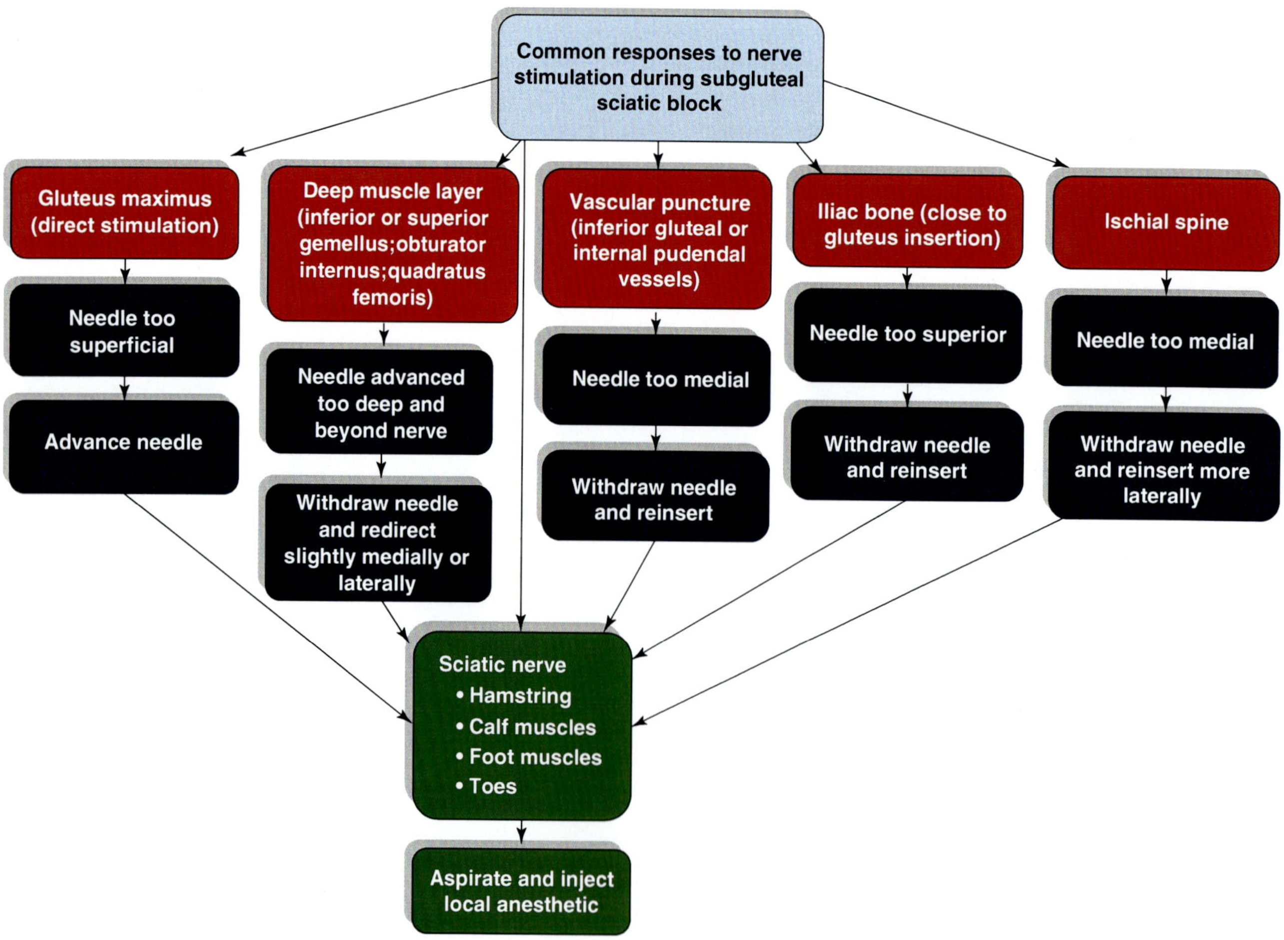

Fig. 26.14 Flowchart of modifications to inappropriate responses to nerve stimulation during subgluteal sciatic nerve block

26.3.3 Ultrasound-Guided Technique

For a summary of ultrasound guidance techniques in subgluteal sciatic nerve blocks, see Fig. 26.15.

Major anatomical structures surrounding the sciatic nerve using a subgluteal approach as captured by MRI and VHVS images are shown with the corresponding ultrasound image in Fig. 26.16.

Prepare the needle insertion site and skin surface with an antiseptic solution. Prepare the ultrasound probe surface by applying a sterile adhesive dressing to it prior to needling as discussed in Chap. 4.

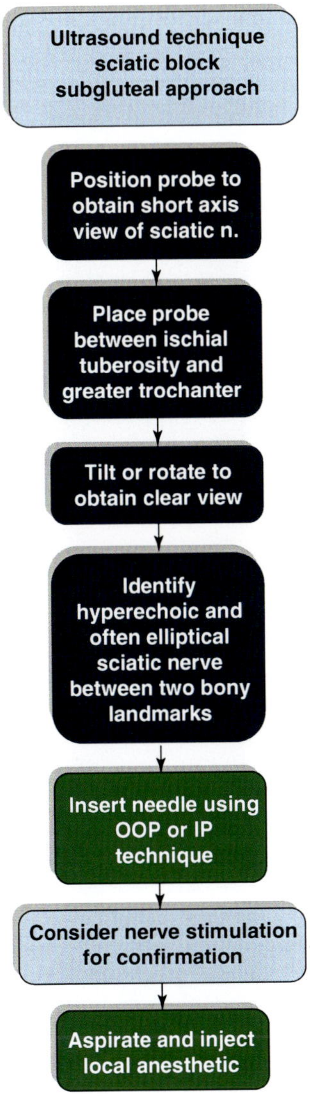

Fig. 26.15 Flowchart of ultrasound guidance technique for subgluteal sciatic nerve block

26.3.3.1 Scanning Technique

- A high-frequency (10–5 MHz) linear probe is appropriate for most children. Larger children and adolescents may require the use of a curved, low-frequency (5–2 MHz) probe.
- Position the probe to obtain a short-axis view of the sciatic nerve, usually between the ischial tuberosity and the greater trochanter of the femur.
- Tilt and/or rotate the probe to optimize the ultrasound image of the sciatic nerve.
- If the sciatic nerve is hard to localize at the subgluteal region, it can be traced proximally from the bifurcation point at or near the apex of the popliteal fossa

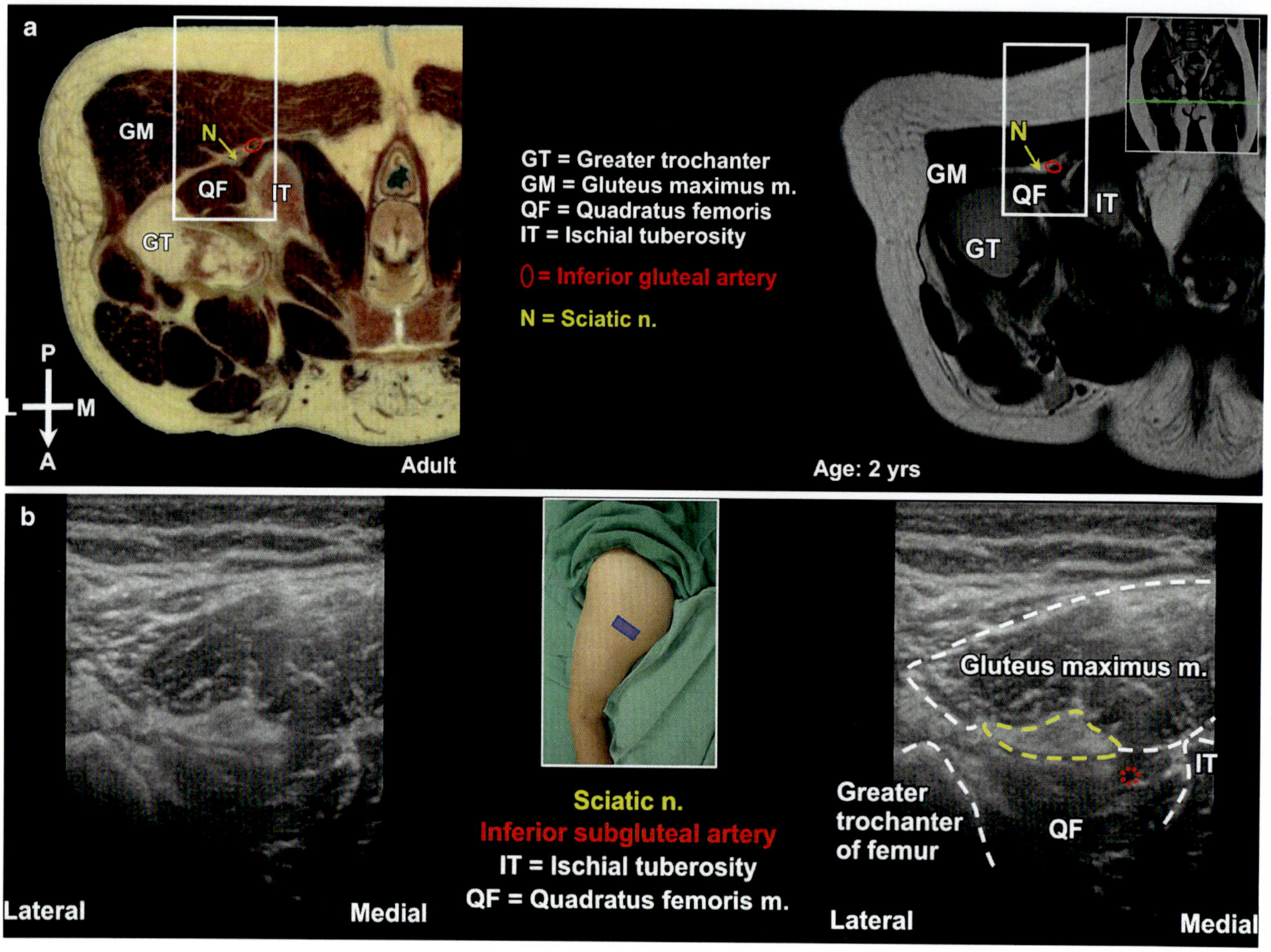

Fig. 26.16 (**a**) VHVS and MRI images of anatomical structures surrounding the sciatic nerve in the subgluteal region. (**b**) Ultrasound image of the subgluteal sciatic nerve block location

26.3.3.2 Sonographic Appearance

- On the lateral side, the greater trochanter appears round with a hyperechoic edge and associated hypoechoic bony shadowing.
- The sciatic nerve in the subgluteal region appears predominantly hyperechoic and is often elliptical in a short-axis view (Fig. 26.16b).

26.3.3.3 Needle Insertion

- An OOP technique will result in the shortest possible needle path (Fig. 26.17). Since the nerve is deep, inserting the needle at a steep angle immediately next the transducer may increase the visibility of the needle tip.
- An IP alignment (Fig. 26.18) may allow for greater ease of needle shaft and tip recognition than OOP alignment. Use color Doppler to identify any blood vessels, such that the needle trajectory can be modified to avoid vascular puncture.

26.3.3.4 Local Anesthetic Application

See Sect. 26.2.4.

Ultrasound Considerations

- Ultrasound guidance may allow for lower volumes of local anesthetic compared to the nerve stimulation technique.
- Local anesthetic is injected following careful aspiration and injection of a test dose of D5W to visualize the spread and confirm nerve localization.
- Deposit local anesthetic next to, but not directly within, the sciatic nerve structure in the subgluteal region. A hypoechoic local anesthetic fluid collection is often seen around the hyperechoic nerve during injection.

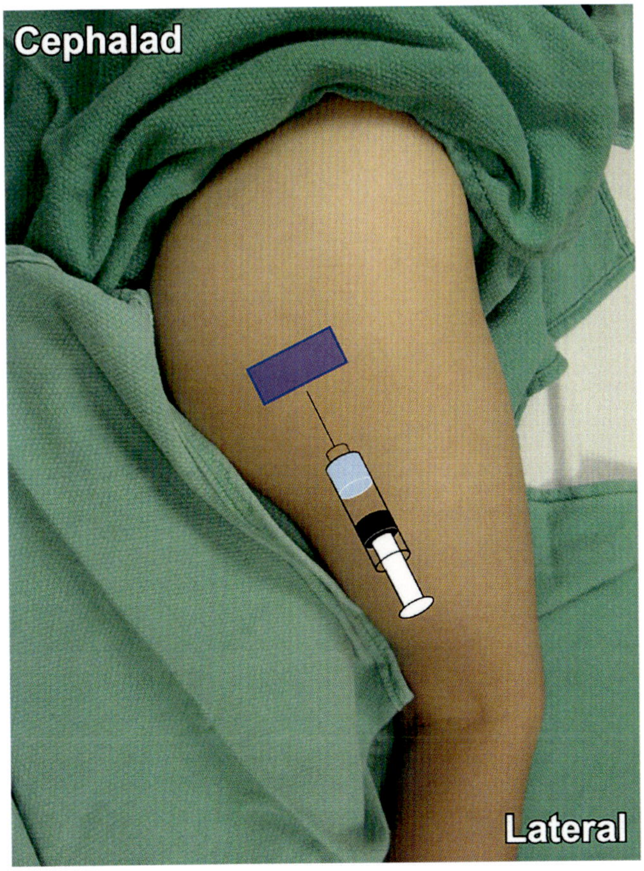

Fig. 26.17 Out-of-plane needling technique for ultrasound-guided subgluteal sciatic nerve block. *Blue rectangle* indicates probe footprint

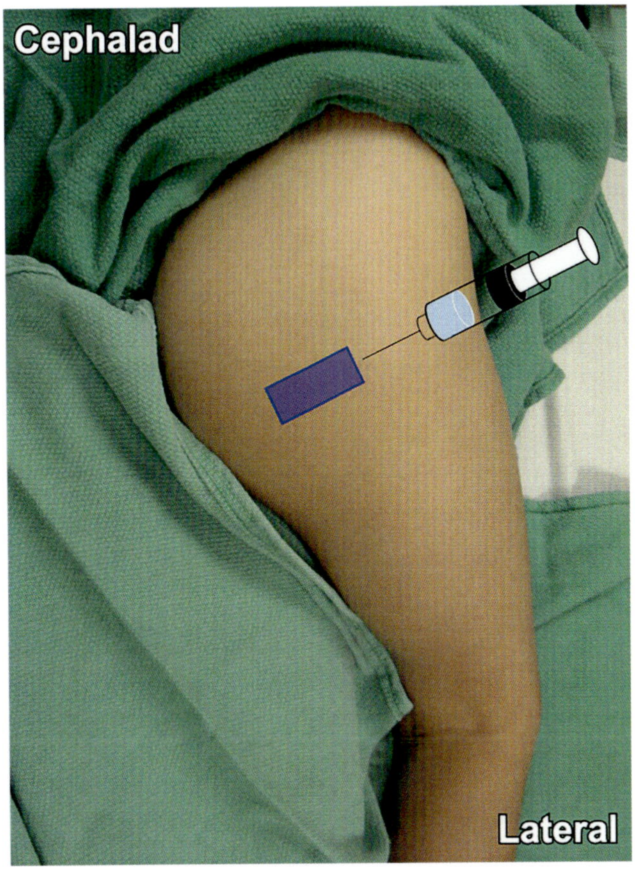

Fig. 26.18 In-plane needling technique for ultrasound-guided subgluteal sciatic nerve block. *Blue rectangle* indicates probe footprint

26.3.4 Case Study

Sciatic Nerve Block (Subgluteal Approach)
(Contributed by A. Sawardekar)

A 10-year-old girl, 40 kg, with no previous medical history, presented with a left ankle fracture after falling while playing basketball. The fracture was confirmed by X-ray. Open reduction and internal fixation of the ankle was scheduled, and a left sciatic nerve block was chosen for pain control. An ultrasound-guided sciatic nerve block with a subgluteal approach was administered. A 22G, 80 mm needle and a 13–6 MHz linear high-frequency probe were used; the sciatic nerve was visualized at the subgluteal-parabiceps area, medial to the femur (Fig. 26.19). Ten mL 0.25 % bupivacaine was injected, and the block lasted for 8 h. Duration of surgery was 120 min. No additional analgesics were needed in the recovery room. The patient was discharged home after 2 h in the recovery room and was given instructions to take oral hydrocodone once sensation had returned to the operative extremity.

Note: As seen in the figure, the nerve appears to expand following suspected injection into the epineurium and encompasses the needle tip. Although no neurologic sequelae were noted in this case, this practice is debatable, as some practitioners prefer to inject outside the epineurium.

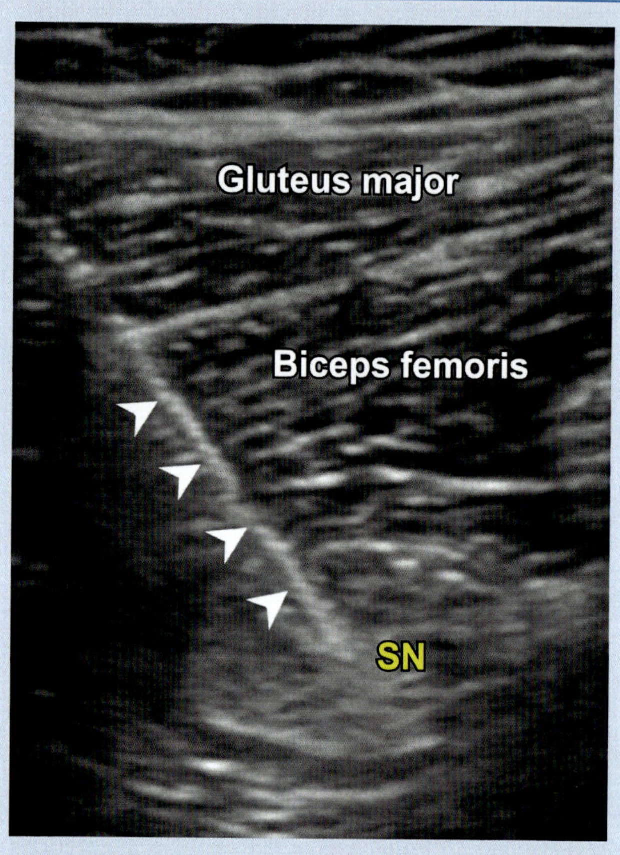

Fig. 26.19 Ultrasound-guided sciatic nerve block using a subgluteal approach. *SN* sciatic nerve, *arrowheads* indicate needle position (see Case Study for details)

26.4 Anterior Sciatic Nerve Block Approach

Compared to the posterior approach, the anterior approach is more difficult to perform due to the requirement of deeper needle insertion. In adults, it is a viable and important alternative when the patient must be kept in a supine position.

26.4.1 Surface Anatomy

The patient is placed in the supine position with the hip and knee slightly flexed and the hip externally rotated. Alternatively, the leg can be kept straight with slight internal rotation. These approaches move the lesser trochanter away from the sciatic nerve to facilitate easy nerve access (Fig. 26.20). Surface landmarks include:

- Anterior superior iliac spine (ASIS)
- Pubic tubercle
- Greater trochanter
- Lesser trochanter
- Femoral crease

Three lines are drawn: (1) between the ASIS and the pubic tubercle (inguinal ligament); (2) from the greater trochanter towards the inner thigh, parallel to the inguinal ligament; and (3) perpendicular to the first line, beginning at the junction of its medial one-third and lateral two-thirds. The needle insertion site is approximately at the intersection of the latter two lines (Fig. 26.21).

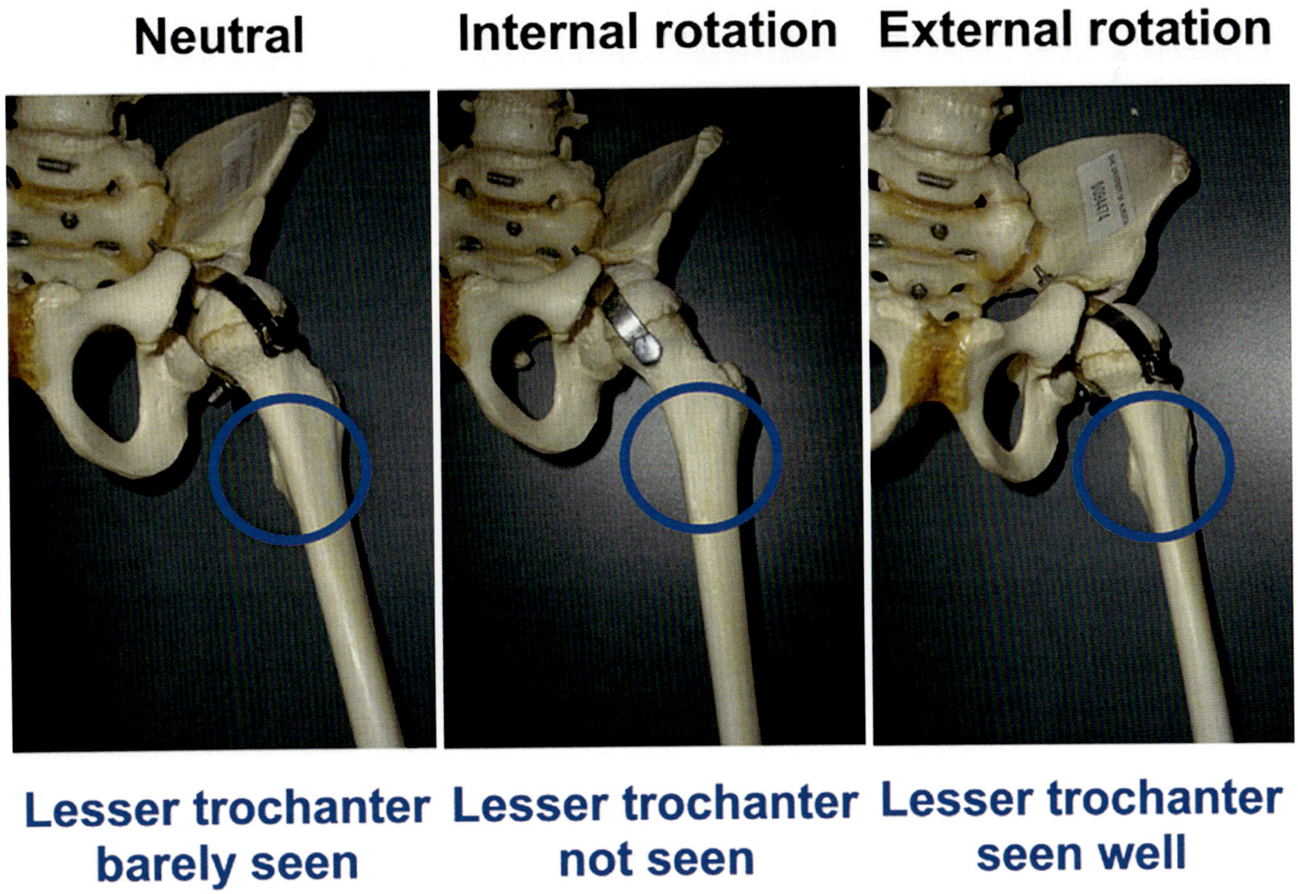

Fig. 26.20 Skeletal model illustrating the appearance of the lesser trochanter with neutral, internal, and external rotation of the hip

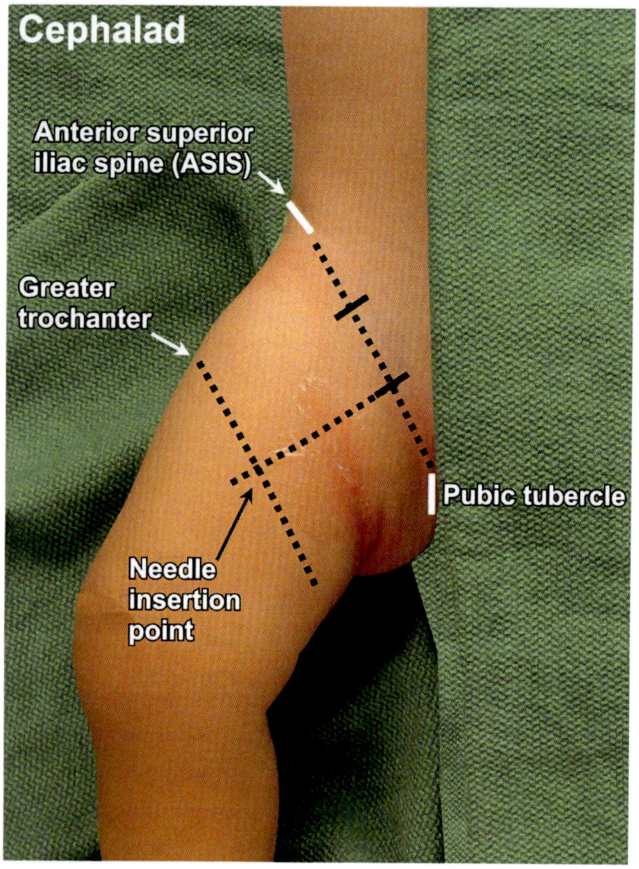

Fig. 26.21 Surface landmarks for anterior sciatic nerve block

26.4.2 Nerve Stimulation Technique

26.4.2.1 Needle Insertion

A flowchart illustrating the needle insertion site and procedures is shown in Fig. 26.22.

- A 50–100 mm, 22G–25G insulated block needle (depends on the age and size of the child) is inserted at the location described above and advanced perpendicularly to the operating table until the bone (lesser trochanter) is encountered. The needle is "walked off" the bone medially and cephalad to enter the adductor magnus muscle.
- When the needle has penetrated the adductor magnus muscle and entered the sciatic neurovascular compartment, loss of resistance may be felt.
- The depth of needle insertion will be at least twice that of the posterior approach [2].

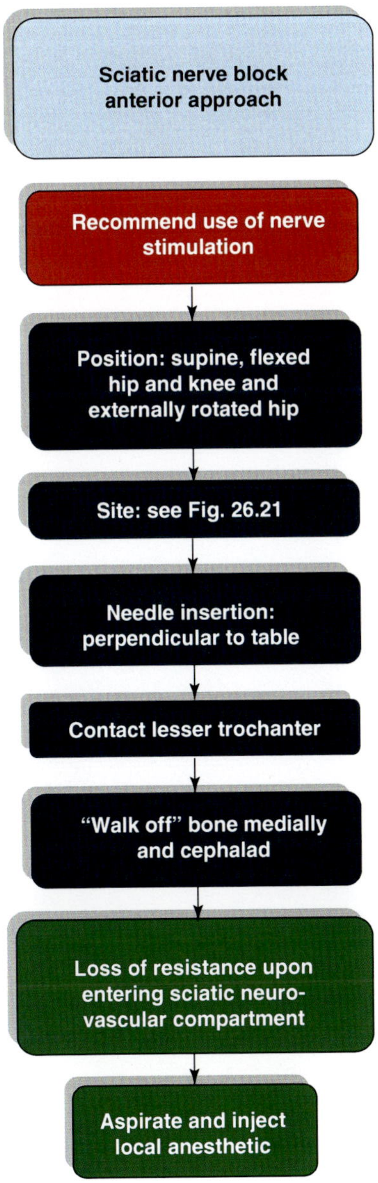

Fig. 26.22 Flowchart of needle insertion and procedures for anterior sciatic nerve block

26.4.2.2 Current Application and Appropriate Responses

Figure 26.23 illustrates the procedure for employing nerve stimulation techniques for anterior sciatic nerve block.

- An initial current of 1–2 mA (2 Hz, 0.1–0.2 ms) is sufficient for stimulation of the sciatic nerve. After obtaining the appropriate motor response, the current is reduced to aim for a threshold current of 0.4 mA (0.1–0.2 ms). Motor response cessation less than 0.2 mA indicates that the needle is probably in an intraneural location.
- Visible or palpable twitches in the leg, foot, or toes verify stimulation of the sciatic nerve.
- See Table 14.4 for expected motor responses during nerve stimulation.

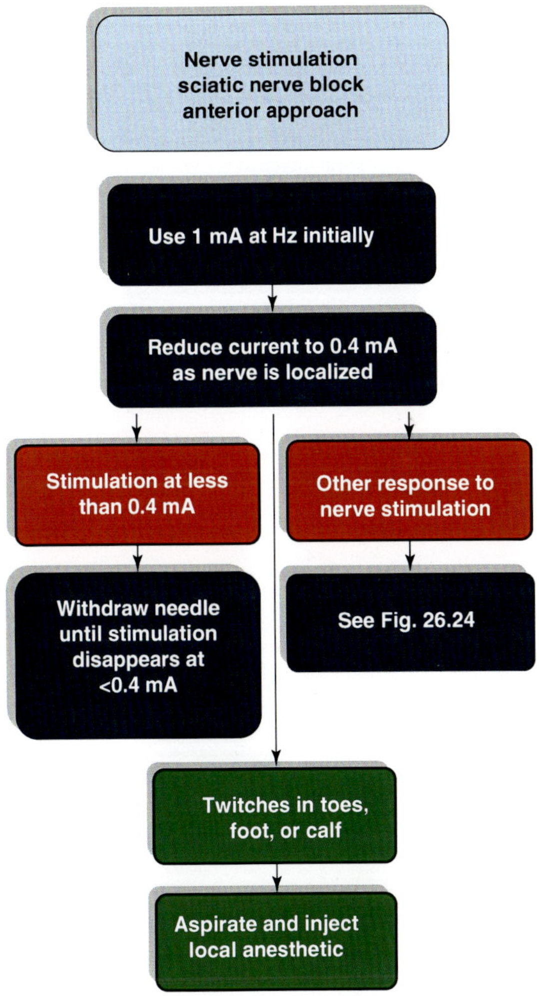

Fig. 26.23 Procedure for employing nerve stimulation technique for anterior sciatic nerve block

26.4.2.3 Modifications to Inappropriate Responses (Table 26.3)

An algorithm of modifications in case of inappropriate responses to nerve stimulation is shown in Fig. 26.24.

Table 26.3 Responses and recommended needle adjustments for use with nerve stimulation during sciatic nerve block (anterior approach)

Correct response from nerve stimulation
Twitches obtained (visible or palpable) from the calf, foot, or toe muscles at 0.2–0.5 mA current. Twitches of the quadriceps muscles will likely occur during advancement
Other common responses and needle adjustments
Muscle twitches from electrical stimulation
Quadriceps (patella twitch):
Explanation: needle placement too superficial
Needle adjustment: continue to advance the needle
Iliopsoas or pectineus (local twitch at femoral crease area):
Explanation: needle tip placement is too superior
Needle adjustment: withdraw needle completely and reinsert more inferiorly
Hamstrings (branches of the sciatic nerve or direct stimulation of muscles)
Explanation: needle possibly too inferior and caudally directed, although often this is not specific
Needle adjustment: withdraw needle completely and reinsert in a slightly more medial or lateral direction (5–10° in transverse plane)
Bone contact
Femur (usually lesser trochanter)
Explanation: needle tip directed too laterally or excessive lateral rotation of the femur
Needle adjustment: withdraw needle 2–3 cm and internally rotate the leg, then continue; if this fails withdraw the needle to the subcutaneous tissue and reinsert it in a more medial direction
No response despite deep placement
Deep needle advancement but no response
Explanation: needle tip is often too medial
Needle adjustment: withdraw completely and reinsert at a slightly more lateral position

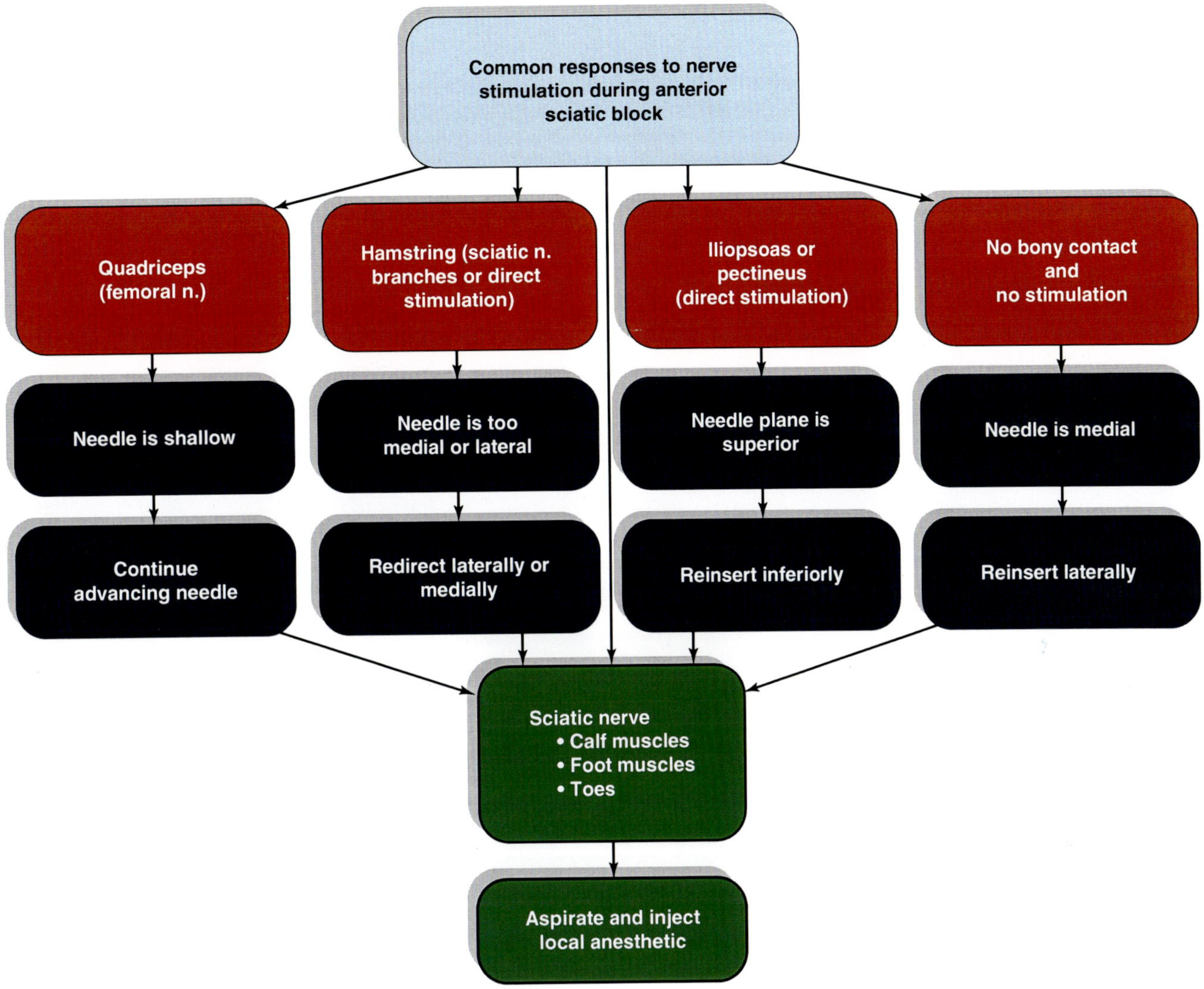

Fig. 26.24 Flowchart of modifications to inappropriate responses to nerve stimulation during anterior sciatic nerve block

26.4.3 Ultrasound-Guided Technique

For a summary of ultrasound guidance techniques in anterior sciatic nerve blocks, see Fig. 26.25.

Anatomical details of the sciatic nerve in the anterior aspect of the upper thigh as captured by MRI and VHVS images are shown with the corresponding ultrasound image in Fig. 26.26.

Prepare the needle insertion site and skin surface with an antiseptic solution. Prepare the ultrasound probe surface by applying a sterile adhesive dressing to it prior to needling as discussed in Chap. 4.

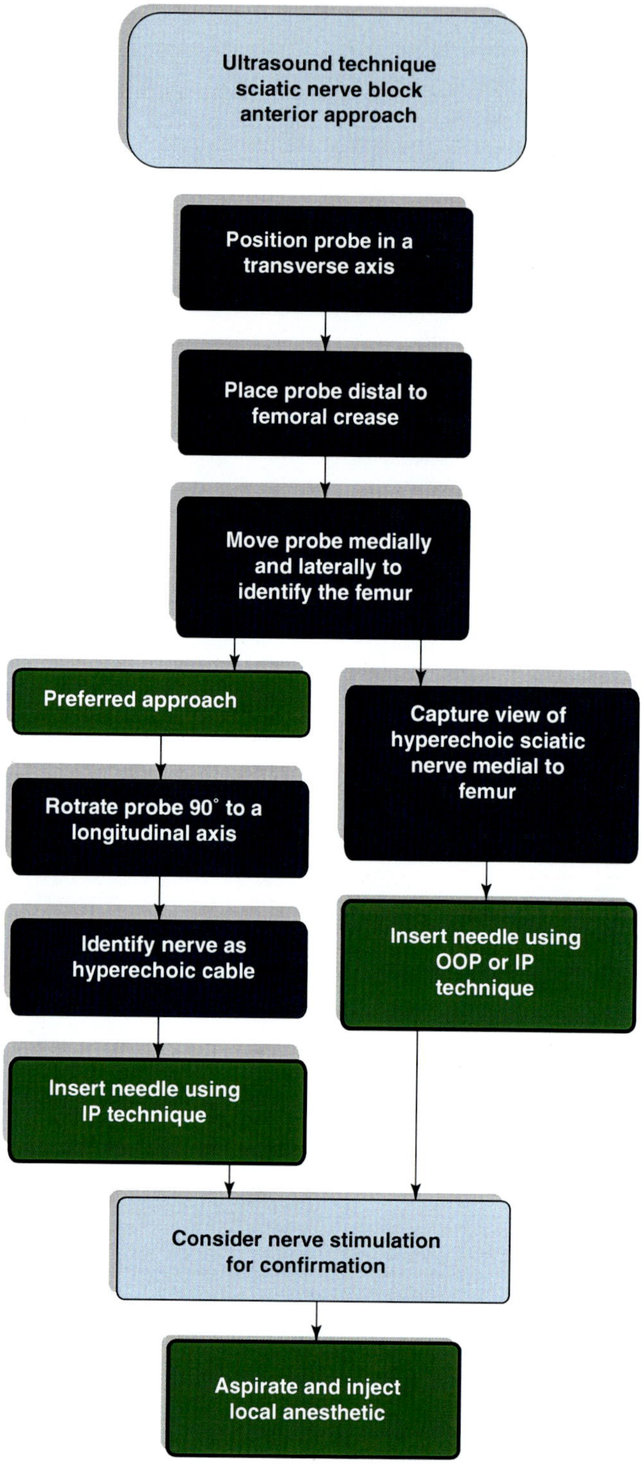

Fig. 26.25 Flowchart of ultrasound guidance technique during anterior sciatic nerve block

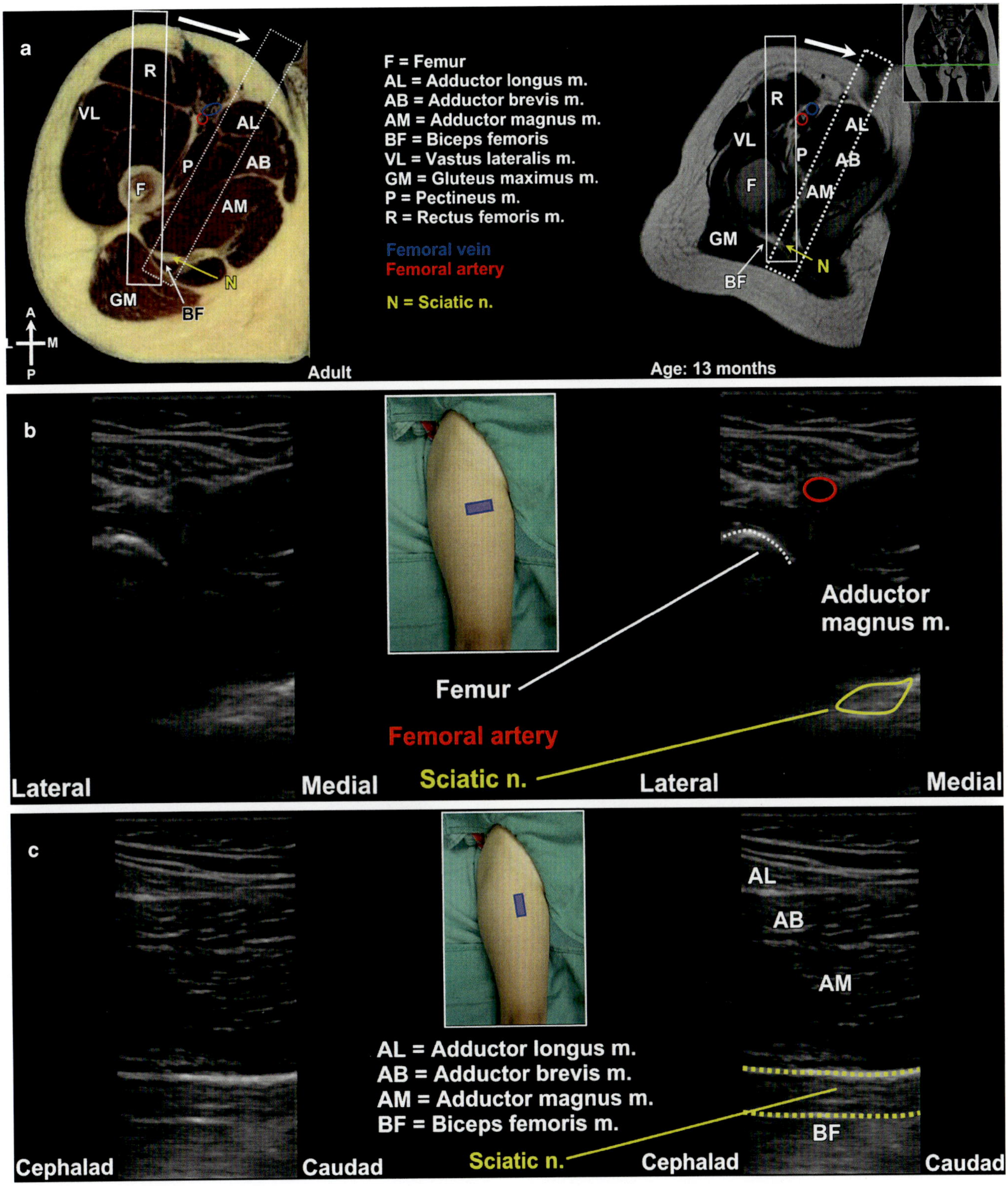

Fig. 26.26 (**a**) VHVS and MRI images of anatomical structures surrounding the sciatic nerve in the anterior aspect of the upper thigh. The *white box* depicts ultrasound scanning from a lateral-to-medial direction to improve visualization. (**b**) Ultrasound image of anterior sciatic nerve block location. (**c**) Ultrasound image showing a longitudinal view of the sciatic nerve during the anterior approach. The nerve appears as a hyperechoic "cable" when turning the transducer 90° relative to the transverse view

26.4.3.1 Scanning Technique

- A curved, low-frequency (5–2 MHz) probe is suitable for scanning the sciatic nerve in the proximal thigh.
- Place the probe over the proximal one-third of the thigh.
- A transversely placed probe tends to be commonly used to view the sciatic nerve in the short axis, although the nerve may be best visualized by rotating the probe 90° to view the nerve longitudinally. The nerve appears as a "cable," which may aid in its identification and needle placement [13].
- Moving in a lateral-to-medial direction may also aid in nerve imaging with a longitudinally placed transducer. At first, the femur, which casts a hypoechoic bony shadow, is seen. As the probe is moved medially, a long, hyperechoic cable-like structure can be seen.

26.4.3.2 Sonographic Appearance

As the sciatic nerve courses along the upper thigh, it is mostly obscured by the femur when viewed from the anterior aspect. The nerve is located deep to the adductor magnus muscle within the posterior medial thigh compartment.

- In transverse axis, the sciatic nerve often appears oval or round, predominantly hyperechoic, and is medial and posterior to the lesser trochanter and deep to the adductor magus muscle (Fig. 26.26b).
- The femoral neurovascular structures can be identified using the Doppler and are visible superficial to the hyperechoic fascial tissue and lateral to the sciatic nerve. The neurovascular structures are better visualized when the leg is externally rotated. A longitudinal view captures a broad, linear, and hyperechoic cable of fibers and may allow for easier identification of the nerve [13] (Fig. 26.26c).
- Color Doppler should be employed to identify any branches of the femoral artery or inferior gluteal artery in close proximity to the sciatic nerve or in the needle trajectory.

26.4.3.3 Needle Insertion

- When using a probe positioned in transverse axis to the nerve, an IP approach (Fig. 26.27) involves advancing the needle in an anteromedial to posterolateral direction. An OOP approach (Fig. 26.28) involves inserting the needle at a steep angle, almost perpendicular, along the midline of the probe. A steep angle is used since the nerve is deep, and it may be easier to visualize the needle with this approach.
- If the probe is placed longitudinally (Fig. 26.29), the sciatic nerve appears as a long, linear "cable," expanding the visible surface area of the nerve. Therefore, an IP approach will be useful and will maximize the chance of success since a "wider" target is presented.

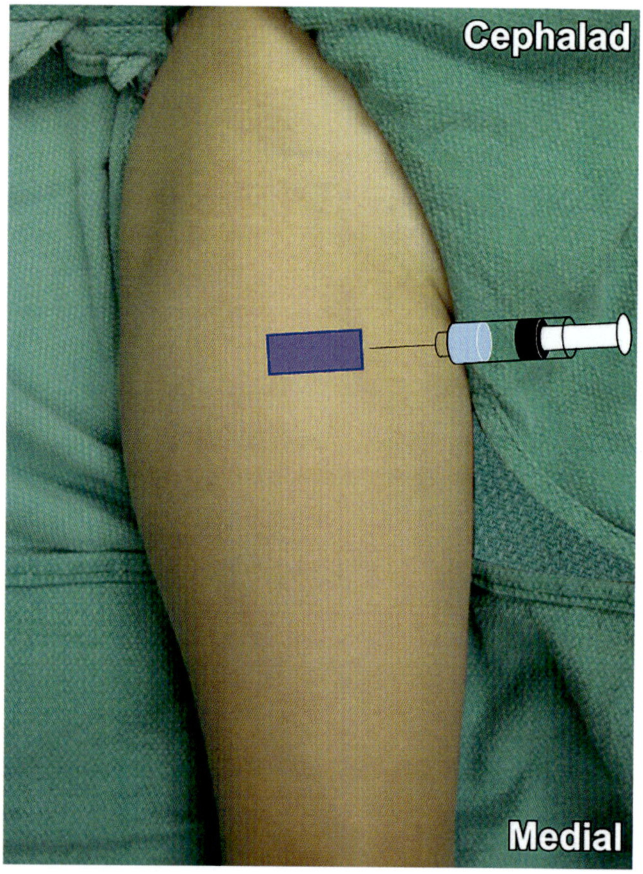

Fig. 26.27 Needling technique for anterior sciatic nerve block using an in-plane needle approach with a transverse view. *Blue rectangle* indicates probe footprint

26.4.4 Local Anesthetic Application

See Sect. 26.2.4.

Ultrasound Considerations

- After careful aspiration and injection of a test dose of D5W to visualize the anesthetic spread and confirm nerve localization, inject the local anesthetic so that it spreads over and around the sciatic nerve.

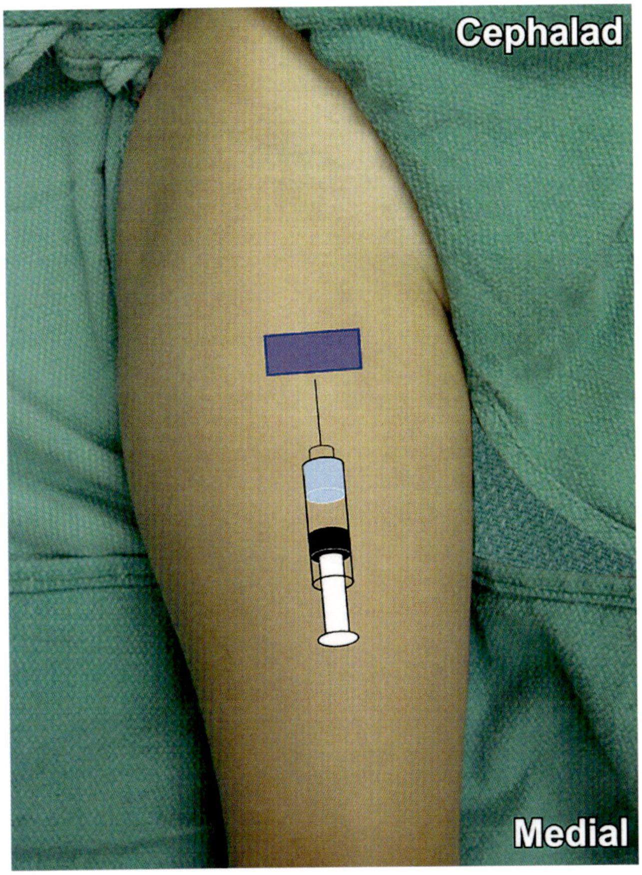

Fig. 26.28 Needling technique for anterior sciatic nerve block using an out-of-plane approach with a transverse view. *Blue rectangle* indicates probe footprint

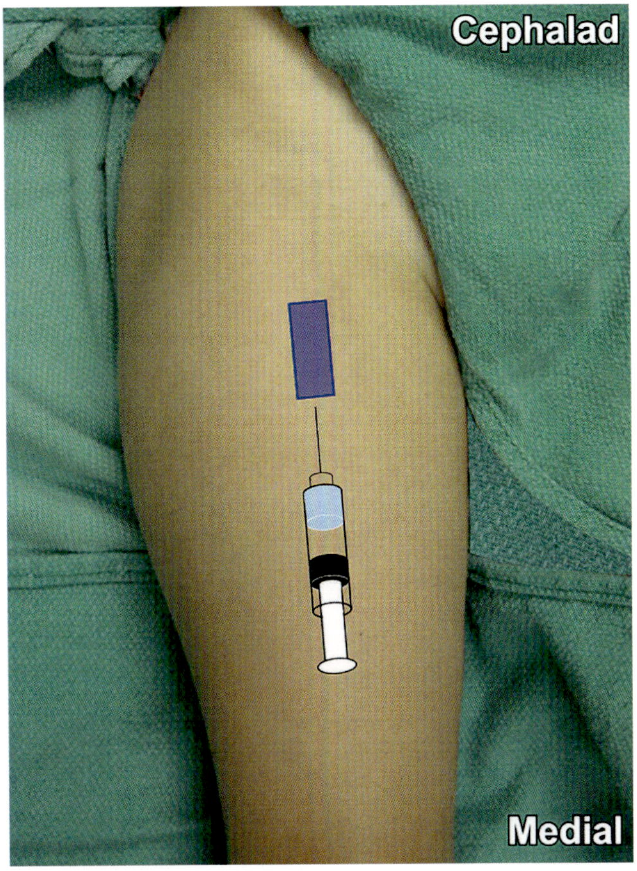

Fig. 26.29 Needling technique for anterior sciatic nerve block using an in-plane approach with a longitudinal view. *Blue rectangle* indicates probe footprint

26.5 Popliteal or Mid-Thigh Sciatic Nerve Block

Blocking the sciatic nerve in the popliteal fossa is a relatively easy procedure, making it desirable for blocks at or below the knee. Due to the variable and oftentimes proximal division of the sciatic nerve, a landmark-based approach to the popliteal block may result in blockade of the distinct (posterior) tibial or common peroneal nerves, rather than the common sciatic nerve. It is useful to place the needle proximal in the popliteal fossa in attempt to locate the sciatic nerve [14]. Table 26.1 describes methods for locating the common sciatic nerve when performing this block using the landmark/blind technique. With the use of ultrasound, it is possible to locate the bifurcation of the sciatic nerve, thus enabling blockade of both branches at the popliteal fossa.

Indications

- Foot and ankle surgery
- Other procedures involving the tibia and fibula, for example, amputation below the knee

26.5.1 Surface Anatomy

The patient may be placed in the lateral position with the knee extended as much as possible or in the prone position. A supine position can be modified by elevating the child's leg with the hip and knee flexed. If nerve stimulation will be used, the ankle should be extended off the end of the table. Surface landmarks include:

- Superior triangle of the popliteal fossa: formed by the popliteal crease (base), biceps femoris tendon (lateral), and semimembranosus and semitendinosus tendons (medial) (Fig. 26.30).

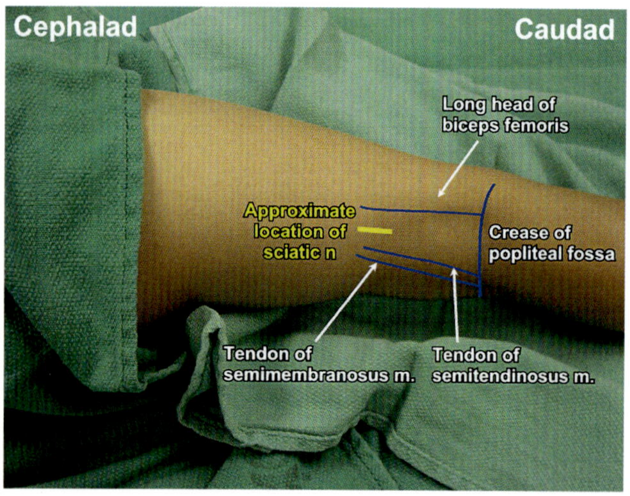

Fig. 26.30 Surface anatomy of the superior triangle of the popliteal fossa

- Inferior triangle of the popliteal fossa: located below the popliteal crease and bordered by the gastrocnemius; this triangle is an inversion of the superior triangle.

Typically, the point of needle insertion is within the superior triangle of the popliteal fossa at the lower third of the triangle, immediately medial to the biceps femoris tendon. This point will be lateral to the popliteal artery. The knee can be flexed for palpation of the tendons, allowing the boundaries of the popliteal fossa to be marked. If the tendons are indistinguishable, it may be possible to palpate the apex of the triangle, where the muscle bellies of the semitendinosus (medial) and biceps femoris (lateral) muscles join. Otherwise, tightening the posterior thigh musculature by applying slight passive extension of the knee with the hip flexed may also be helpful for landmark identification [15].

The distance from the popliteal fold to the point of needle insertion can also be defined relative to patient weight. If the weight of the patient <10 kg, the distance from the popliteal fold to the point of insertion is 1 cm. If the patient's weight is 10–20 kg, the point of insertion is 2 cm, 20–30 kg is 3 cm, etc. [7].

Clinical Pearl

A lateral approach to the sciatic nerve at the popliteal fossa may also be used. With this approach, the patient is positioned supine, and the leg and hip do not need to be flexed. The needle is inserted at a posterior angle (30° from the horizontal) at the junction of the tendon of the biceps femoris and the vastus lateralis muscles. One drawback may be the need for double injection to block both divisions of the sciatic nerve [16].

26.5.2 Nerve Stimulation Technique

A landmark-based technique, which relies on loss of resistance as the needle enters the popliteal membrane, has shown to be successful [15, 17]. However, with such a wide variability of the location of the sciatic nerve bifurcation, nerve stimulation is useful to verify nerve localization, especially when blockade of either the tibial or common peroneal nerves is desired. Furthermore, the use of nerve stimulation together with ultrasound guidance (a method the authors recommend) enables more precise needle positioning and thus greater block success using lower local anesthetic volumes. The nerve stimulation technique will rely upon the same landmarks, needle insertion considerations, and local anesthetic application as the landmark-based techniques.

26.5.2.1 Needle Insertion

A flowchart illustrating the needle insertion site and procedures is shown in Fig. 26.31.

- A short-beveled or insulated block needle 30–40 mm, 22G–25G (depending on the age and size of the child) is inserted in a cephalad direction at an angle of 45° to the skin.
- High in the popliteal fossa, the nerve is located at a mean distance of 4.1 ± 0.8 cm in children under 8 years and at 5.8 ± 1.3 cm in those older than 8 years [18].
- A distinct "pop" may be felt as the needle enters the popliteal fossa membrane.
- If blood is aspirated, the needle may have punctured one of the popliteal vessels. This likely indicates that the needle is positioned too medial and should be withdrawn; pressure should be applied for 3 min on the puncture site before needle reinsertion.

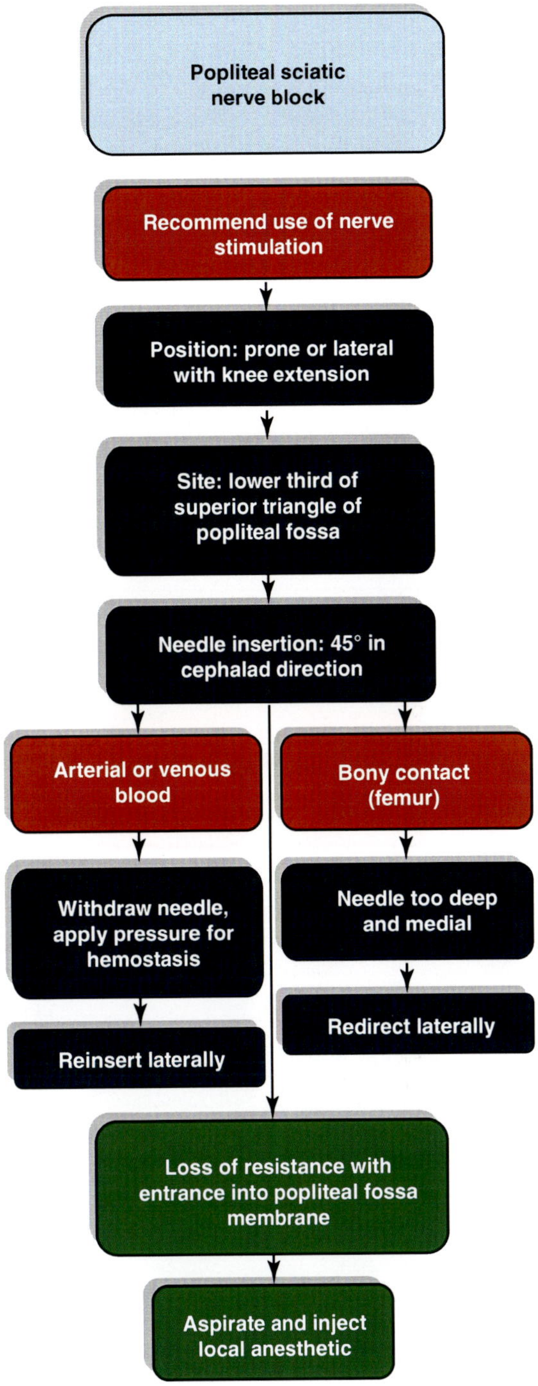

Fig. 26.31 Flowchart of needle insertion and procedures for popliteal sciatic nerve block

26.5.2.2 Current Application and Appropriate Responses

Figure 26.32 illustrates the procedure for employing nerve stimulation techniques for the sciatic nerve block.

- Using an initial current of 1 mA, advance the needle until a motor response is elicited in the foot and/or toes. Adjust the needle depth to obtain a minimal motor response at a current of approximately 0.4 mA. Motor response cessation at currents less than 0.2 mA indicates that the needle is probably in an intraneural location.
- There is no clear influence of age and depth of needle insertion on the elicitation of motor responses [17]. Obtaining a tibial nerve response (plantar flexion or foot inversion) may be preferable to a common peroneal nerve response (dorsiflexion or foot eversion), since local anesthetic injected around the common peroneal nerve may not reach the tibial nerve.
- One study found that foot inversion was the best predictor of complete sensory blockade of the foot [19].
- See Table 14.4 for expected motor responses during nerve stimulation.

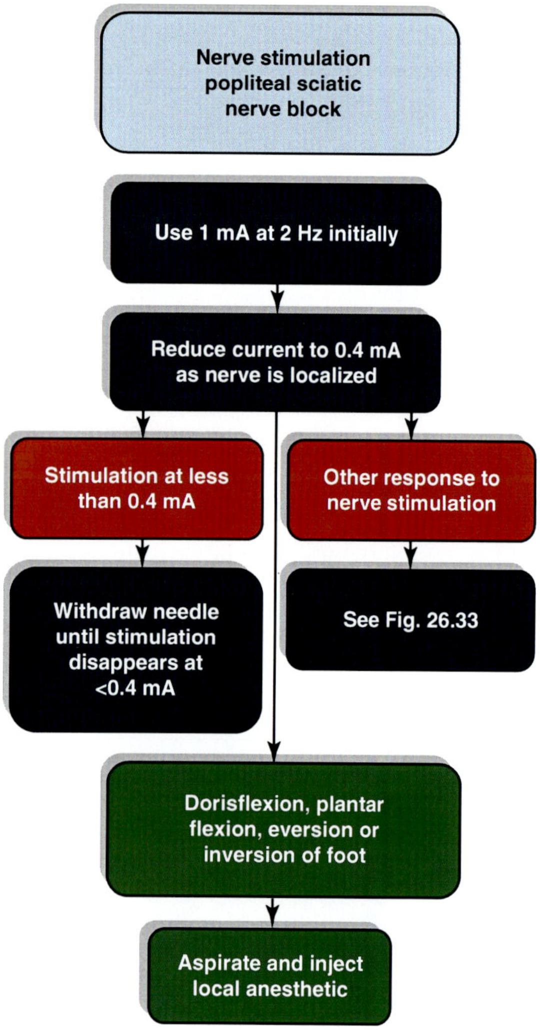

Fig. 26.32 Procedure for employing nerve stimulation technique for popliteal sciatic nerve block

26.5.2.3 Modifications to Inappropriate Responses (Tables 26.4 and 26.5)

An algorithm of modifications in case of inappropriate responses to nerve stimulation is shown in Fig. 26.33.

Table 26.4 Responses and recommended needle adjustments for use with nerve stimulation during sciatic nerve block (posterior popliteal approach)

Correct response from nerve stimulation
Twitches (visible or palpable) in the foot or toes with 0.3–0.5 mA current. Either a common peroneal (fibular) or tibial nerve response may result and both indicate correct needle positioning even slightly below the sciatic nerve bifurcation as the large volume of local anesthetic will spread within the sheath. The common peroneal (fibular) response is ankle dorsiflexion and eversion; the tibia is ankle plantar flexion and inversion. If eliciting a response is difficult in this current range, 0.7 mA may be used reliably with a tibial nerve response
Other common responses and needle adjustments
Muscle twitches from electrical stimulation
Biceps femoris (local twitch)
Explanation: needle placement too lateral
Needle adjustment: withdraw needle completely and reinsert slightly more medial
Semimembranosus or semitendinosus (local twitch)
Explanation: needle placement too medial
Needle adjustment: withdraw needle completely and reinsert slightly more laterally
Calf muscles without foot or toe movement (muscular branches of sciatic nerve)
Explanation: needle probably too superficial
Needle adjustment: continue advancement
Bone contact
Femur
Explanation: needle tip advanced too deeply
Needle adjustment: withdraw needle to look for response at more superficial location; withdraw if not seen
Vascular puncture
Popliteal artery or vein
Explanation: needle tip too medial
Needle adjustment: withdraw completely and reinsert at slightly more lateral position

Table 26.5 Responses and recommended needle adjustments for use with nerve stimulation during sciatic nerve block (lateral popliteal approach)

Correct response from nerve stimulation
Twitches (visible or palpable) in the foot or toes at 0.3–0.5 mA current
It is common to encounter a biceps femoris twitch at a location superficial to the sciatic nerve. Once this ceases, proceed slowly and the sciatic response should be detected at about 2 cm beyond this location
With this approach, it is common to stimulate the common peroneal portion (i.e., dorsiflexion) of the sciatic nerve first
Other common responses and needle adjustments
Muscle twitches from electrical stimulation
Biceps femoris (local twitch)
Explanation: needle placement too superficial
Needle adjustment: advance needle slowly, approximately 2 cm
Vastus lateralis (local twitch)
Explanation: needle placement too anterior
Needle adjustment: withdraw needle completely and reinsert slightly more posterior
Calf muscles without foot or toe movement (muscular branches of sciatic nerve)
Explanation: needle probably too superficial
Needle adjustment: continue advancement
Vascular puncture
Popliteal artery or vein
Explanation: needle tip too deep and anterior
Needle adjustment: withdraw completely and reinsert posteriorly with less depth
Bone contact
Femur
Explanation: needle tip too anterior and deep
Needle adjustment: withdraw completely and reinsert at slightly more posterior location

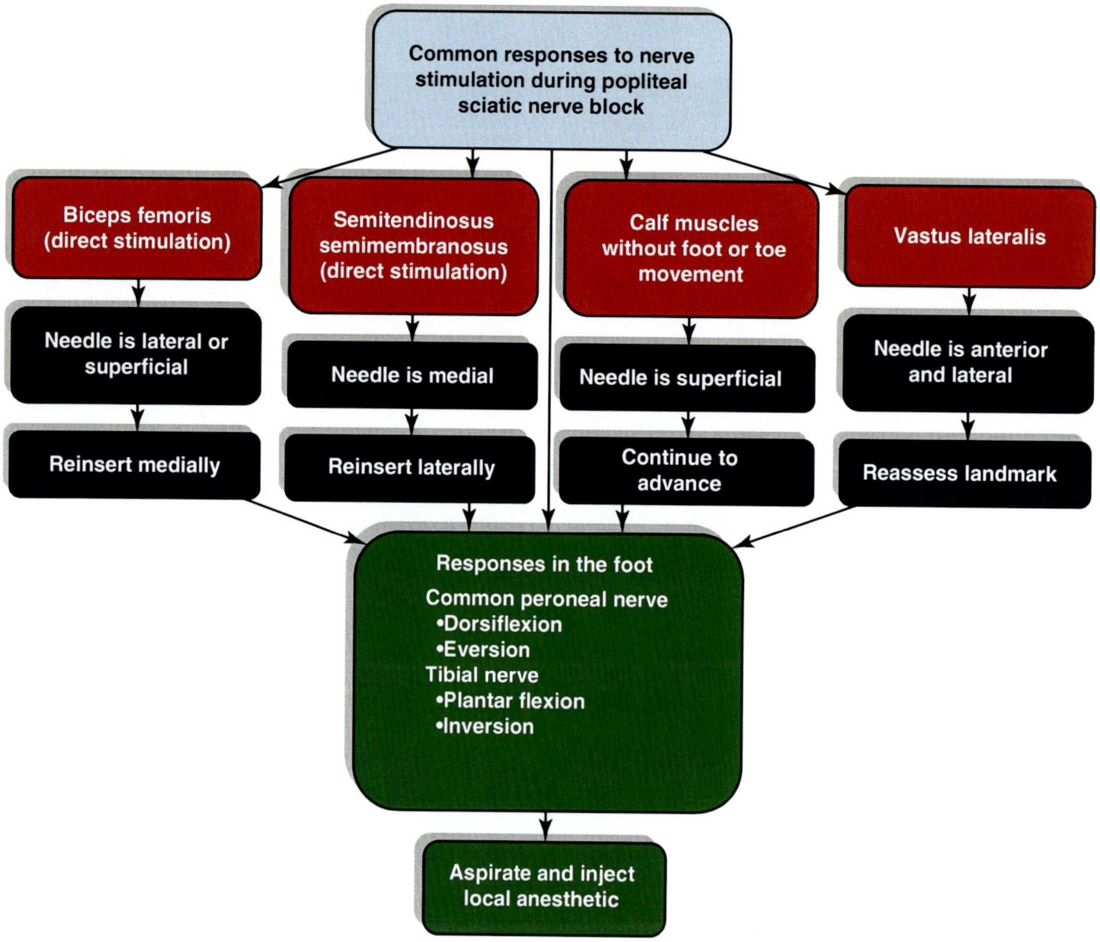

Fig. 26.33 Flowchart of modifications to inappropriate responses to nerve stimulation during popliteal sciatic nerve block

26.5.3 Ultrasound-Guided Technique

For a summary of ultrasound guidance techniques in popliteal sciatic nerve blocks, see Fig. 26.34.

Major anatomical structures surrounding the branches of the sciatic nerve at the popliteal fossa as captured by MRI and VHVS images are shown with the corresponding ultrasound image in Fig. 26.35. The schematic drawing in Fig. 26.36 depicts a posterior view showing the position of the sciatic nerve in the mid-thigh (prior to bifurcation) and associated landmarks.

Prepare the needle insertion site and skin surface with an antiseptic solution. Prepare the ultrasound probe surface by applying a sterile adhesive dressing to it prior to needling as discussed in Chap. 4.

The bifurcation point of the sciatic nerve varies widely between individuals (Table 26.6); thus, ultrasound imaging is highly valuable for accurate nerve localization. Placing the needle in close proximity to the nerve will maximize block success with the need for minimal dosages of local anesthetic.

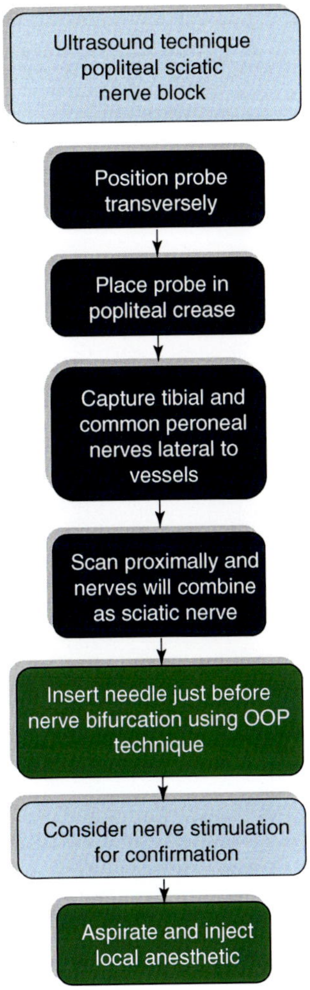

Fig. 26.34 Flowchart of ultrasound guidance technique during popliteal sciatic nerve block

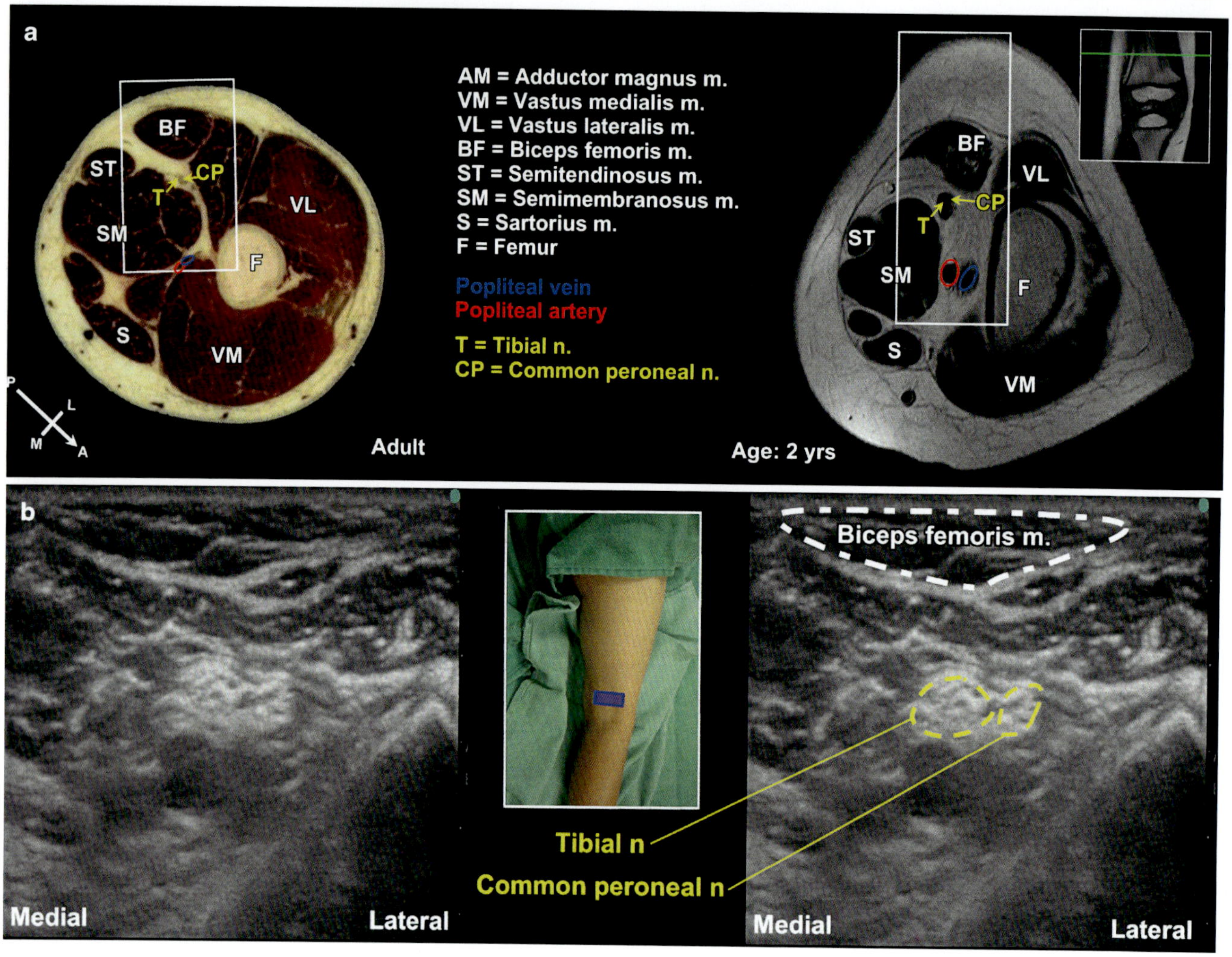

Fig. 26.35 (**a**) VHVS and MRI images of anatomical structures surrounding the branches of the sciatic nerve at the popliteal fossa. (**b**) Ultrasound image of the popliteal sciatic nerve block location

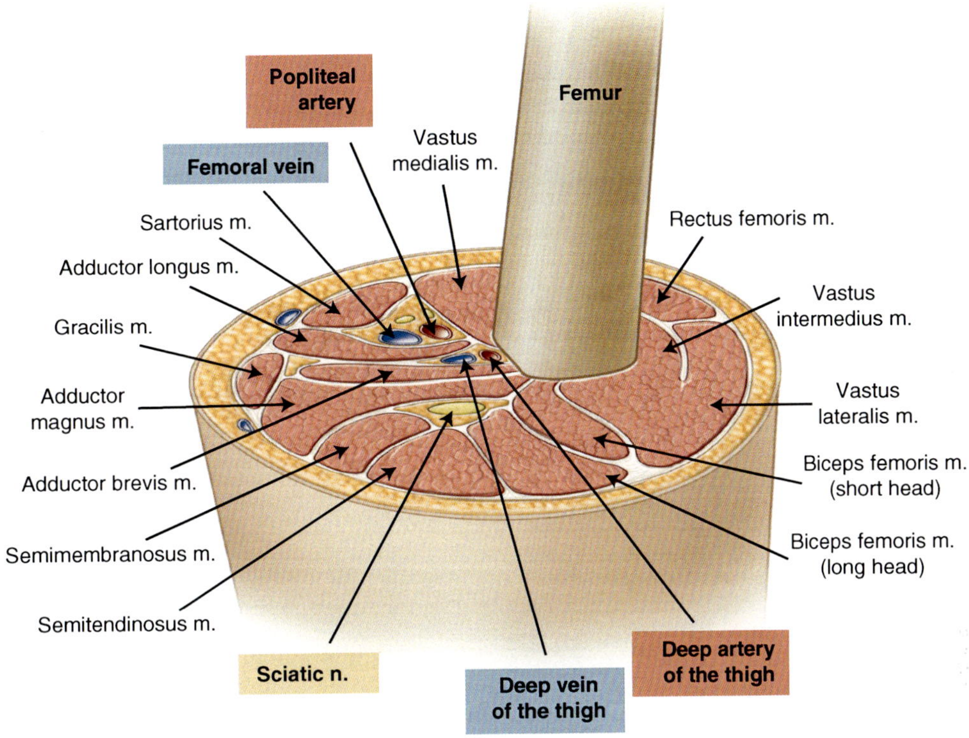

Fig. 26.36 Posterior view of the thigh showing position of the sciatic nerve and major muscles and vessels

Table 26.6 Location of needle insertion for popliteal sciatic nerve block and position of sciatic nerve bifurcation

- A general guideline for determining the needle insertion distance is 1 cm from the popliteal crease for every 10 kg of the patient [7]
- Another method to determine a needle insertion point prior to sciatic nerve bifurcation is to use a ratio of femoral shaft lengths between children (according to their age) and adults. This method assumes that the bifurcation is approximately 10 cm above the popliteal crease in adults; the ratio is factored to this length of 10 cm to determine the needle location in the child [20]. Although Berniere et al. demonstrated successful blocks using this method, block success and motor responses associated with either the tibial or common peroneal nerves were used as endpoints. There was no verification using imaging
- Using MRI, Suresh et al. [21] found that the position of the sciatic nerve bifurcation correlated to age ($R^2=0.73$) and created a formula [27 + 4 × age (years) mm] to determine the point of bifurcation in children
- Ultrasound imaging has shown that, in the posterior thigh, the bifurcation point is highly variable (32–76 cm) [22]. This finding suggests that ultrasound may be a superior method for performing the block when it is desirable to locate the sciatic nerve

26.5.3.1 Scanning Technique

- A linear or hockey stick, high-frequency (10–5 MHz) probe is commonly used for scanning the sciatic nerve transversely in the popliteal fossa. A distal-to-proximal traceback approach (Fig. 26.37a) can effectively locate the sciatic nerve in the posterior popliteal fossa at the bifurcation point.
- At the popliteal crease, a transversely positioned probe captures the tibial and common peroneal nerves, with both nerves located posterior and superficial to the popliteal vessels. Doppler can be valuable to visualize the popliteal vessels (see Fig. 26.37b).
- As the probe is moved proximally from the crease, the tibial and common peroneal nerves approach each other and finally join to form the sciatic nerve (Fig. 26.37b).

26.5.3.2 Sonographic Appearance

- At the level of the popliteal crease, the tibial and common peroneal nerves lie superficial and lateral to the popliteal vessels. Both nerves appear round to oval and hyperechoic (Fig. 26.37a).
- The hyperechoic border of the femur (condyles) may be visible.
- As the probe is moved more proximally, the common peroneal nerve appears to move towards the tibial nerve, merging to form the sciatic nerve.
- More proximal in the thigh, the lip-shaped, hypoechoic biceps femoris muscle lies superficial to the round hyperechoic sciatic nerve (Fig. 26.37b).

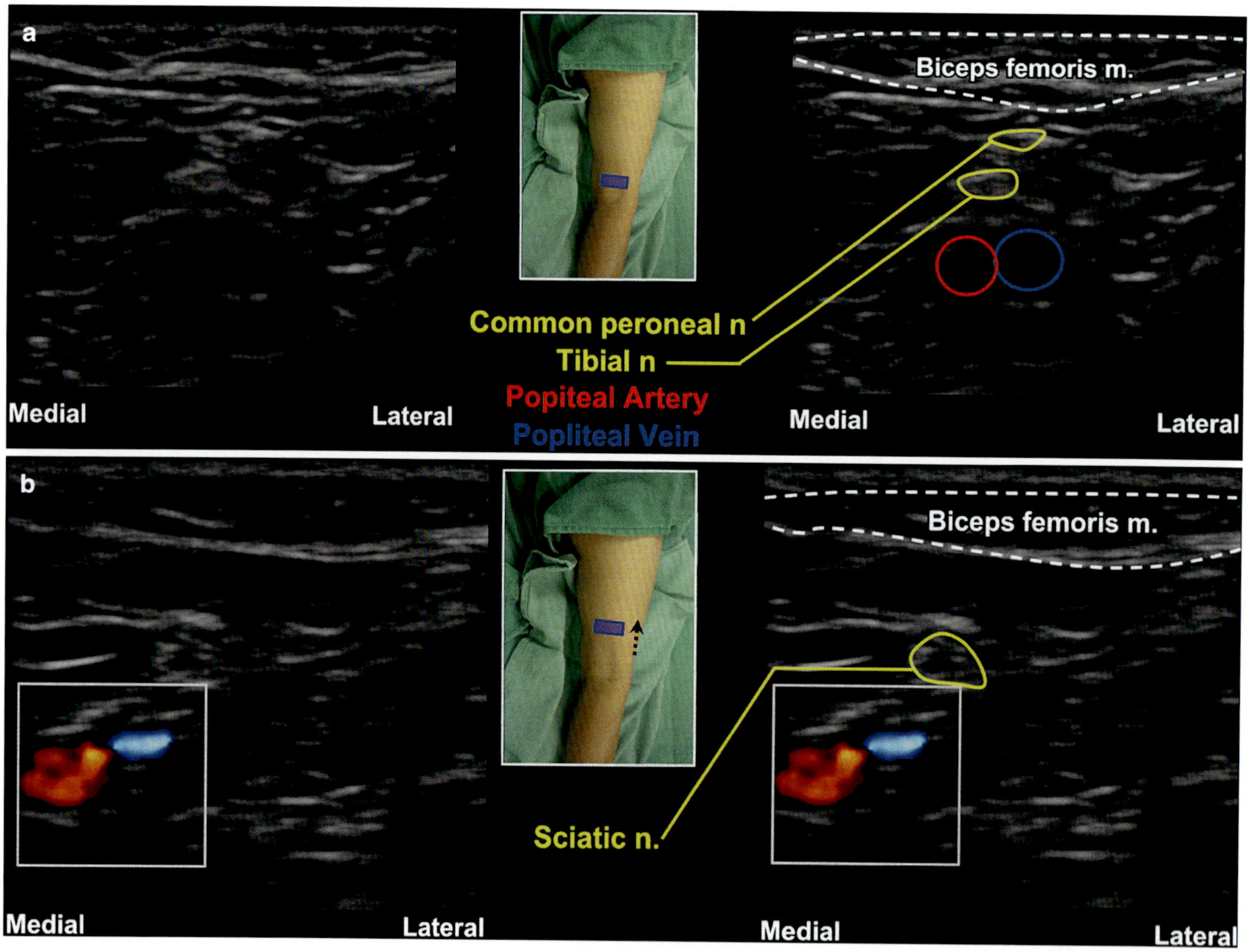

Fig. 26.37 Ultrasound image showing the distal-to-proximal scanning technique to locate the bifurcation of the sciatic nerve at the popliteal fossa. (**a**) Ultrasound probe is placed distally to visualize the separate common peroneal and tibial nerves. (**b**) Ultrasound probe is moved proximal to view the sciatic nerve. Doppler ultrasound highlights the popliteal vessels

26.5.3.3 Needle Insertion

- An OOP approach at the bifurcation of the sciatic nerve (Fig. 26.38) is preferable, although the IP approach shown in Fig. 26.39 can also be used.
- The OOP approach is a useful technique since the needle can be seen piercing through the epineural sheath at the bifurcation between the two branches of the sciatic nerve. This approach also enables a catheter to be threaded cephalad along the sciatic nerve.
- For the OOP approach, the probe is positioned directly above the sciatic nerve at its bifurcation point so that the nerve is placed in the center of the image. The needle should be inserted equidistant caudad or cephalad (caudad when inserting a catheter) to the probe at a 45° angle, such that the tip of the needle can be visualized as it approaches the nerve.

26.5.4 Local Anesthetic Application

- Ensure negative aspiration of the blood prior to injection of local anesthetic.
- There is a limited amount of literature on ultrasound-guided popliteal blocks in the pediatric population. Ivani et al. [10] suggested that ropivacaine and levobupivacaine are probably the best choice for longer operations when pain is more intense and long-lasting.
- Due to the anatomy of the nerves in children (smaller diameter and shorter distance between the nodes of Ranvier), larger volumes with lower concentrations are key to obtaining effective analgesia [11].
- We recommend the use of ropivacaine 0.2 %, bupivacaine 0.25 %, or levobupivacaine 0.25 %, with a volume of 0.25–0.5 mL/kg.
- The dose of local anesthetic should not exceed the maximum toxic dose, especially if a saphenous nerve block or femoral nerve block is required to provide anesthesia/analgesia to the medial aspect of the leg and foot.

Ultrasound Consideration

- The onset of anesthesia is more rapid if there is circumferential spread around both branches of the sciatic nerve. Injection at the bifurcation or multiple injections may be required for complete circumferential spread.

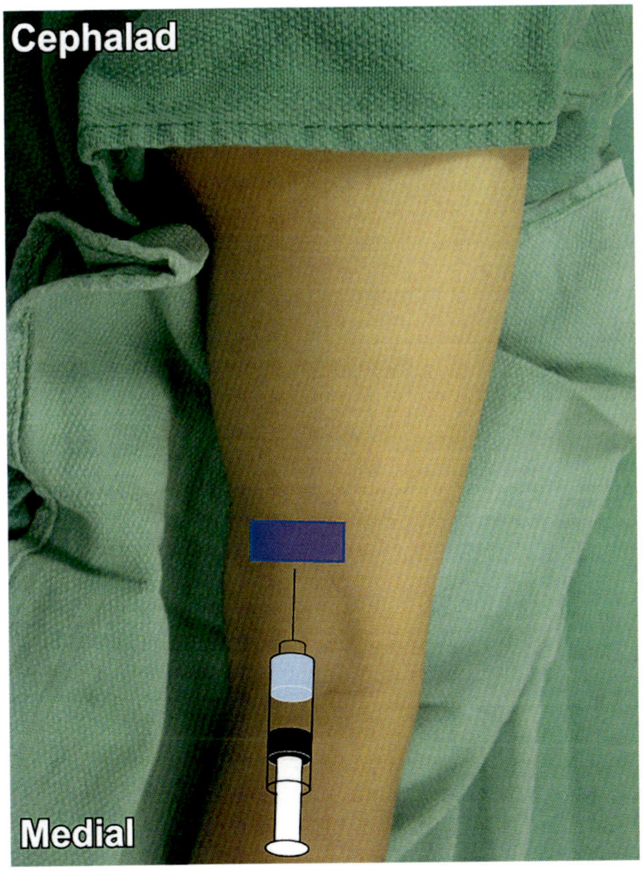

Fig. 26.38 Out-of-plane needling technique for ultrasound-guided popliteal sciatic nerve block. *Blue rectangle* indicates probe footprint

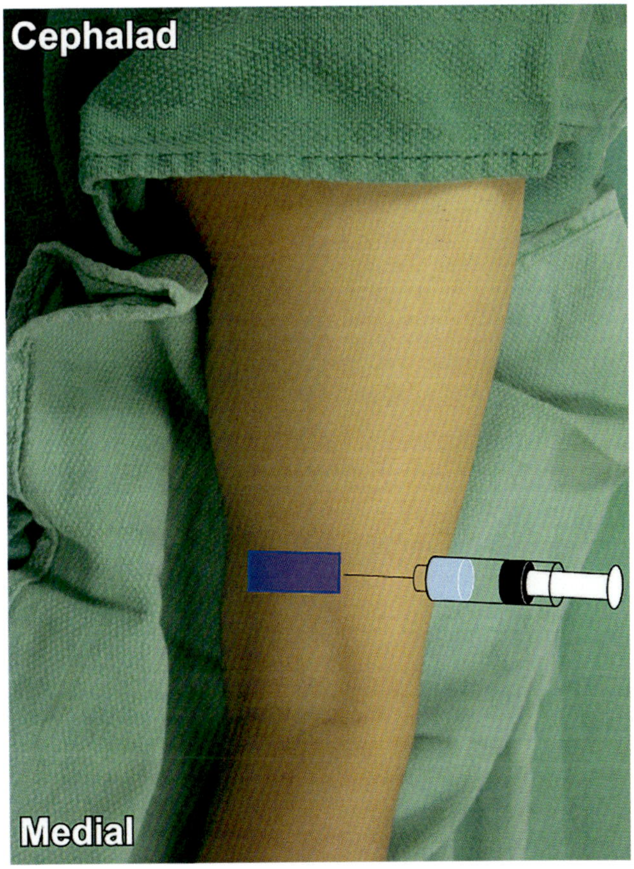

Fig. 26.39 In-plane needling technique for ultrasound-guided popliteal sciatic nerve block. *Blue rectangle* indicates probe footprint

26.5.5 Case Study

Sciatic Nerve Block (Lateral Popliteal Approach) (Contributed by S. Suresh)

A 16-year-old male, 81.8 kg in weight, was diagnosed with a left knee ACL tear and left knee lateral meniscus tear based on knee X-rays and MR with contrast. Preadmission medications included docusate (Colace) 100 mg and hydrocodone-acetaminophen (Norco) 5–325 mg. Surgery lasted 3 h and 28 min and involved a left knee ACL reconstruction with patellar tendon autograft and partial meniscectomy. An ultrasound-guided tibial nerve block with 20 mL 0.25 % bupivacaine in the popliteal fossa was used (Fig. 26.40). Pain control in recovery was reported as 0/10 at PACU admission and 2/10 at PACU discharge. Postoperative analgesia included morphine 2 mg injection, acetaminophen tablet 650 mg, hydrocodone-acetaminophen (Norco) 10 mg, and 400 mL/h 0.1 % bupivacaine (continuous nerve block).

Note: This patient also received a femoral nerve block and femoral nerve catheter.

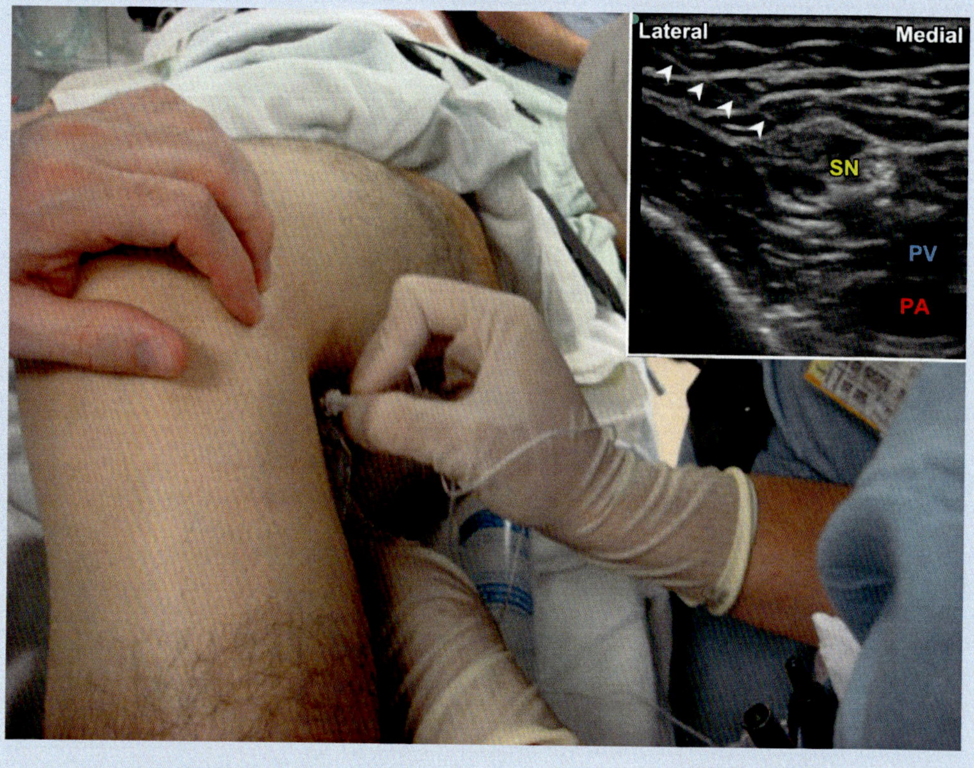

Fig. 26.40 Ultrasound-guided lateral popliteal sciatic nerve block. *SN* sciatic nerve, *PV* popliteal vein, *PA* popliteal artery, *arrowheads* indicate needle position (see Case Study for details)

26.6 Current Literature in Ultrasound-Guided Approaches

The first published case of sciatic nerve blockade under ultrasound in a child was in 2003 by Gray and colleagues [23]. Several case reports have described ultrasound guidance during continuous sciatic/popliteal blocks in children [18, 24–26], and Ponde et al. [27] showed that successful continuous sciatic blocks can be achieved when placing catheters under ultrasound guidance alone. For sciatic (subgluteal and popliteal) and femoral nerve blocks in children, Oberndorfer et al. [7] found that ultrasound guidance prolongs the duration of sensory block (mean of 508 min vs. 335 min) compared to the nerve stimulation technique, while allowing for reduced volumes of local anesthetic. A recent randomized controlled study compared ultrasound- and nerve stimulation-guided approaches to femoro-sciatic block in patients with arthrogryposis multiplex congenita. The results showed that block success and duration of analgesia were increased significantly in the ultrasound group. van Geffen et al. compared proximal, subgluteal, and distal approaches to sciatic nerve block and demonstrated that good pain control and good visualization of the sciatic nerve can be achieved using each technique.

A parasacral approach to sciatic nerve block has been used in adults and has been reported to block the entirety of the sacral plexus at the exit of the greater sciatic notch [28–31]. A recent case series by Dillow et al. [32] studied the parasacral approach in pediatric patients undergoing lower limb surgery; both ultrasound and nerve stimulation were used, and 0.5 mL/kg ropivacaine 0.2 % was injected. In all cases using the parasacral approach, block success was 100 %. Pain control was excellent, and mean block duration was 17.3 ± 5.4 h. These results demonstrate that the parasacral approach is effective for children as well as adults.

Ultrasound imaging may increase the use of the anterior approach to the sciatic nerve, which would be favorable because the patient can remain in the supine position. Ultrasound guidance may also aid in the precise placement of local anesthetic around the sciatic (or other) nerve. This concept has been promoted by two recent studies on the use of ultrasound techniques alone in sciatic nerve block in infants and toddlers [8, 27].

There is a paucity of literature on ultrasound-guided popliteal nerve blocks in children. Nonetheless, popliteal approaches to the sciatic nerve have been used successfully in infants and children undergoing surgery of the ankle and foot [7, 15, 20, 33, 34]. Blind techniques using either loss of resistance or nerve stimulation (including surface nerve mapping [35]) have typically been used for sciatic nerve localization in the posterior thigh. In an imaging study, Schwemmer et al. [22] found that there was high variability (32–76 mm) in the point of sciatic nerve division in the popliteal fossa in children. These authors' results indicate, in contrast to age-dependent formulas, that there was no consistent age-related distance in their sample of patients, which is not surprising given the range of body habitus in children today. Direct visualization may be the key to accurate localization on a case-by-case basis. Miller [36] described an alternative approach to ultrasound-guided popliteal sciatic block using the biceps femoris muscle, rather than the popliteal artery, as a landmark. The ultrasound transducer is placed distal to the bifurcation with the lateral aspect of the transducer medial to the biceps femoris muscle. The common peroneal nerve may or may not be visible; however, moving the transducer cephalad along the medial aspect of the biceps femoris reveals the tibial nerve, whose path can be traced back to the bifurcation point. This approach allows the block to be performed with the patient in a prone or "near-prone" position.

Using nerve stimulation, elicitation of foot inversion has been shown to be the best predictor of complete sciatic nerve blockade [19]; however, Ponde et al. [8] demonstrated, in a case series of infants and toddlers scheduled for congenital talipes equinovarus or vertical talus repair, that the success rate of ultrasound-guided sciatic nerve block was unaffected by the ability to elicit a motor response with nerve stimulation. Nevertheless, it is our opinion that nerve stimulation, when combined with ultrasound imaging, can both confirm the location of the nerve and act as an adjunct to monitoring, thus preventing intraneural injury. Therefore, we strongly recommend the concurrent use of ultrasound and nerve stimulation wherever possible.

References

1. Winnie AP. Regional anesthesia. Surg Clin North Am. 1975;55: 861–92.
2. Dalens B, Tanguy A, Vanneuville G. Sciatic nerve blocks in children: comparison of the posterior, anterior, and lateral approaches in 180 pediatric patients. Anesth Analg. 1990;70:131–7.
3. Sukhani R, Candido KD, Doty Jr R, et al. Infragluteal-parabiceps sciatic nerve block: an evaluation of a novel approach using a single-injection technique. Anesth Analg. 2003;96:868–73.
4. Scheuer L, Black S, Christie A. The pelvic girdle. In: Scheuer L, editor. Developmental juvenile osteology. London: Academic; 2000. p. 341–73.
5. Scheuer L. The lower extremity. In: Scheuer L, editor. Developmental juvenile osteology. London: Academic; 2000. p. 374–467.
6. Bosenberg AT. Lower limb nerve blocks in children using unsheathed needles and a nerve stimulator. Anaesthesia. 1995;50: 206–10.
7. Oberndorfer U, Marhofer P, Bosenberg A, et al. Ultrasonographic guidance for sciatic and femoral nerve blocks in children. Br J Anaesth. 2007;98:797–801.
8. Ponde VC, Desai AP, Dhir S. Ultrasound-guided sciatic nerve block in infants and toddlers produces successful anesthesia regardless of the motor response. Pediatr Anesth. 2010;20:633–7.
9. Ivani G, Tonetti F. Postoperative analgesia in infants and children: new developments. Minerva Anestesiol. 2004;70:399–403.
10. Ivani G, DeNegri P, Conio A, et al. Comparison of racemic bupivacaine, ropivacaine, and levo-bupivacaine for pediatric caudal anesthesia: effects on postoperative analgesia and motor block. Reg Anesth Pain Med. 2002;27:157–61.
11. Bosenberg AT, Ivani G. Regional anaesthesia – children are different. Pediatr Anesth. 1998;8:447–50.
12. Eck JB, Ross AK. Paediatric regional anaesthesia – what makes a difference? Best Pract Res Clin Anaesthesiol. 2002;16:159–74.
13. Tsui BC, Ozelsel TJ. Ultrasound-guided anterior sciatic nerve block using a longitudinal approach: "expanding the view". Reg Anesth Pain Med. 2008;33:275–6.
14. Singelyn FJ, Gouverneur JM, Gribomont BF. Popliteal sciatic nerve block aided by a nerve stimulator: a reliable technique for foot and ankle surgery. Reg Anesth. 1991;16:278–81.
15. Tobias JD, Mencio GA. Popliteal fossa block for postoperative analgesia after foot surgery in infants and children. J Pediatr Orthop. 1999;19:511–4.
16. Zetlaoui PJ, Bouaziz H. Lateral approach to the sciatic nerve in the popliteal fossa. Anesth Analg. 1998;87:79–82.
17. Kempthorne PM, Brown TC. Nerve blocks around the knee in children. Anaesth Intensive Care. 1984;12:14–7.
18. van Geffen GJ, Bruhn J, Gielen M. Ultrasound-guided continuous sciatic nerve blocks in two children with venous malformations in the lower limb. Can J Anesth. 2007;54:952–3.
19. Benzon HT, Kim C, Benzon HP, et al. Correlation between evoked motor response of the sciatic nerve and sensory blockade. Anesthesiology. 1997;87:547–52.
20. Berniere J, Schrayer S, Piana F, et al. A new formula of age-related anatomical landmarks for blockade of the sciatic nerve in the popliteal fossa in children using the posterior approach. Pediatr Anesth. 2008;18:602–5.
21. Suresh S, Simion C, Wyers M, et al. Anatomical location of the bifurcation of the sciatic nerve in the posterior thigh in infants and children: a formula derived from MRI imaging for nerve localization. Reg Anesth Pain Med. 2007;32:351–3.
22. Schwemmer U, Markus CK, Greim CA, et al. Sonographic imaging of the sciatic nerve and its division in the popliteal fossa in children. Pediatr Anesth. 2004;14:1005–8.
23. Gray AT, Collins AB, Schafhalter-Zoppoth I. Sciatic nerve block in a child: a sonographic approach. Anesth Analg. 2003;97:1300–2.
24. van Geffen GJ, Gielen M. Ultrasound-guided subgluteal sciatic nerve blocks with stimulating catheters in children: a descriptive study. Anesth Analg. 2006;103:328–33.
25. van Geffen GJ, Scheuer M, Muller A, et al. Ultrasound-guided bilateral continuous sciatic nerve blocks with stimulating catheters for postoperative pain relief after bilateral lower limb amputations. Anaesthesia. 2006;61:1204–7.
26. van Geffen GJ, McCartney CJ, Gielen M, Chan VW. Ultrasound as the only nerve localization technique for peripheral nerve block. J Clin Anesth. 2007;19:381–5.
27. Ponde VC, Desai AP, Shah DM, Johari AN. Feasibility and efficacy of placement of continuous sciatic perineural catheters solely under ultrasound guidance in children: a descriptive study. Pediatr Anesth. 2011;21:406–10.
28. Ben-Ari AY, Joshi R, Uskova A, Chelly JE. Ultrasound localization of the sacral plexus using a parasacral approach. Anesth Analg. 2009;108:1977–80.
29. Bendtsen TF, Lonnqvist PA, Jepsen KV, et al. Preliminary results of a new ultrasound-guided approach to block the sacral plexus: the parasacral parallel shift. Br J Anaesth. 2011;107:278–80.
30. Ripart J, Cuvillon P, Nouvellon E, et al. Parasacral approach to block the sciatic nerve: a 400-case survey. Reg Anesth Pain Med. 2005;30:193–7.
31. Taha AM. A simple and successful sonographic technique to identify the sciatic nerve in the parasacral area. Can J Anesth. 2012;59: 263–7.
32. Dillow JM, Rosett RL, Petersen TR, et al. Ultrasound-guided parasacral approach to the sciatic nerve block in children. Pediatr Anesth. 2013;23:1042–7.
33. Dadure C, Bringuier S, Nicolas F, et al. Continuous epidural block versus continuous popliteal nerve block for postoperative pain relief after major podiatric surgery in children: a prospective, comparative randomized study. Anesth Analg. 2006;102:744–9.
34. Konrad C, Johr M. Blockade of the sciatic nerve in the popliteal fossa: a system for standardization in children. Anesth Analg. 1998;87:1256–8.
35. Bosenberg AT, Raw R, Boezaart AP. Surface mapping of peripheral nerves in children with a nerve stimulator. Pediatr Anesth. 2002;12: 398–403.
36. Miller BR. The biceps femoris muscle as a landmark for performing the popliteal sciatic nerve block using ultrasound guidance in pediatric patients. Pediatr Anesth. 2010;20:960–1.

Suggested Reading

Karmakar MK, Kwok WH. Ultrasound-Guided Regional Anesthesia. In: Cote CJ, Lerman J, Anderson BJ, Eds. 5th ed. Philadelphia: WB Saunders; 2013. p. 880–908.

Suresh S, Polaner DM, Cote CJ. Regional Anesthesia. In: Cote CJ, Lerman J, Anderson BJ, Eds. 5th ed. Philadelphia: WB Saunders; 2013. p. 835–79.

Tsui BC. Sciatic and popliteal blocks. In: Tsui BC, editor. Atlas of ultrasound and nerve stimulation-guided regional anesthesia. New York: Springer; 2007. p. 171–203.

Part IX

Nerve Blocks at the Ankle

Ankle Blocks

27

Ban C.H. Tsui

Contents

B.C.H. Tsui, Dip Eng, BSc (Math), B Pharm, MSc, MD, FRCPC
Department of Anesthesiology and Pain Medicine,
Stollery Children's Hospital/University of Alberta Hospital,
2-150 Clinical Sciences Building, Edmonton, AB T6G 2G3, Canada
e-mail: btsui@ualberta.ca

B.C.H. Tsui, S. Suresh (eds.), *Pediatric Atlas of Ultrasound- and Nerve Stimulation-Guided Regional Anesthesia*,
DOI 10.1007/978-0-387-79964-3_27

27.1 Indications

- Club foot repair.
- Reconstructive surgeries (e.g., polydactyly).
- Removal of a foreign body.
- Ankle blocks can also be used as a diagnostic tool to determine surgical procedures to correct foot deformities in children with cerebral palsy [1].

27.2 Surface Anatomy

The patient is positioned supine with the foot placed on the table or extended (for deep peroneal nerve block). If using nerve stimulation, it will be necessary to either support the foot above the table or extend the leg beyond the table. Surface landmarks include:

- Medial malleolus.
- Lateral malleolus.
- Extensor hallucis tendon: This tendon can be located in an awake child by asking them to extend their big toe.
- Achilles tendon.
- Anterior tibial artery: Pulsation of the artery is sought at the level of the skin crease on the anterior midline surface of the ankle.

To block all five nerves at the ankle, more than one point of needle insertion is necessary. For the superficial nerves (superficial peroneal and saphenous), a line is drawn on the anterior surface of the ankle, uniting the medial and lateral malleoli. The point of needle entry for the posterior tibial nerve is midway between the medial malleolus and the medial border of the Achilles tendon; the nerve is located just posterior to the tibial artery (Fig. 27.1). The deep peroneal nerve is located between the extensor hallucis longus tendon and the extensor digitorum longus tendon (Fig. 27.2). To block the deep peroneal nerve, insert the needle either lateral to the extensor hallucis tendon or to the anterior tibial artery.

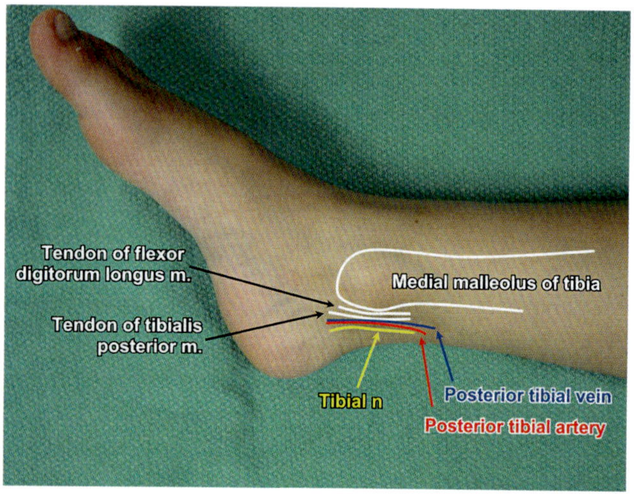

Fig. 27.1 Surface anatomy and landmarks for posterior tibial nerve block

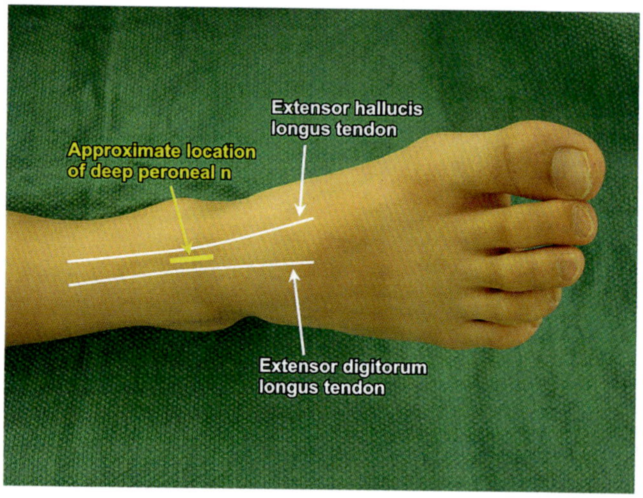

Fig. 27.2 Surface anatomy and landmarks for deep peroneal nerve block

27.3 Nerve Stimulation Technique

The posterior tibial nerve and the peroneal nerve are the only motor nerves at the ankle. Table 14.5 summarizes motor responses associated with nerve stimulation.

27.3.1 Needle Insertion

- The nerves are all superficially located, and a short (20–30 mm) 25G–27G needle with a short bevel (or a hypodermic needle) should be used for the blocks.
- Superficial nerves: Insert the needle to deposit local anesthetic subcutaneously in a ringlike fashion along the line drawn between the malleoli.
- Isolated saphenous nerve block: Infiltrate the area overlying and anterior to the medial malleolus.
- Posterior tibial nerve: Insert the needle perpendicular to the skin between the medial malleolus and the medial border of the Achilles tendon, directed toward the pulsation of the posterior tibial artery. The nerve is located behind the posterior tibial artery.
  - Aspiration will be important to rule out intravascular placement.
- Deep peroneal nerve: Insert the needle perpendicular to the skin and with a slight anterior tilt either lateral to the extensor hallucis longus tendon or the anterior tibial artery (whichever is used) and inject into the deep planes below the fascia.
- Sural nerve: Insert the needle perpendicular to the skin between the lateral malleolus and the calcaneus.

27.3.2 Current Application and Appropriate Responses

- Applying an initial current of 0.8 mA (2 Hz, 0.1–0.3 ms) is sufficient for nerve stimulation. After obtaining the appropriate motor response, the current is reduced to aim for a threshold current of 0.4 mA (0.1–0.2 ms) before injection.
- Twitches of the first (medial plantar branch) and fifth (lateral plantar branch) toes are typical responses to nerve stimulation.
- For the deep peroneal nerve, toe extension is seen.

27.3.3 Modifications to Inappropriate Responses

- In general, alternate motor responses from direct muscle stimulation will not be elicited since this region is mainly composed of tendons rather than muscle fibers.

27.4 Ultrasound-Guided Technique

Ultrasound imaging may be suitable for visualizing the deep nerves (posterior tibial and deep peroneal). Imaging at the medial aspect of the ankle will enable the block to be localized to the posterior tibial nerve prior to its division into the medial and lateral plantar nerves. Imaging for the deep peroneal block may be helpful in children since the voluntary extension of the toe, to localize the extensor hallucis tendon, will not be possible in anesthetized patients.

27.4.1 Scanning Technique

- High-frequency, short footprint probes (e.g., SLA 6–13 MHz, 25 mm footprint hockey stick probe, MicroMaxx, SonoSite, Bothell, WA) are used for these blocks.
- Posterior tibial nerve: The probe is positioned in transverse (short) axis to the nerve just posterior and inferior to the medial malleolus. Alternatively, the nerve can be identified in the distal quarter of the lower leg above the medial malleolus (Fig. 27.3).
  - Color Doppler is helpful to localize the nerve at the above locations since in each one the nerve lies posterior and deep to the posterior tibial artery (Fig. 27.4). The nerve should be localized before it branches into the medial and lateral plantar nerves.
- Deep peroneal nerve: The probe is placed in transverse (short) axis to the nerve at the anterior surface of the ankle joint. Alternatively, the nerve can also be found in the distal quarter of the lower leg above the ankle joint (Fig. 27.5). However, the nerve itself can be difficult to see, and only the artery can be consistently located.
  - Color Doppler can be used at both locations to illuminate the anterior tibial artery lying medial to the nerve (Fig. 27.4).

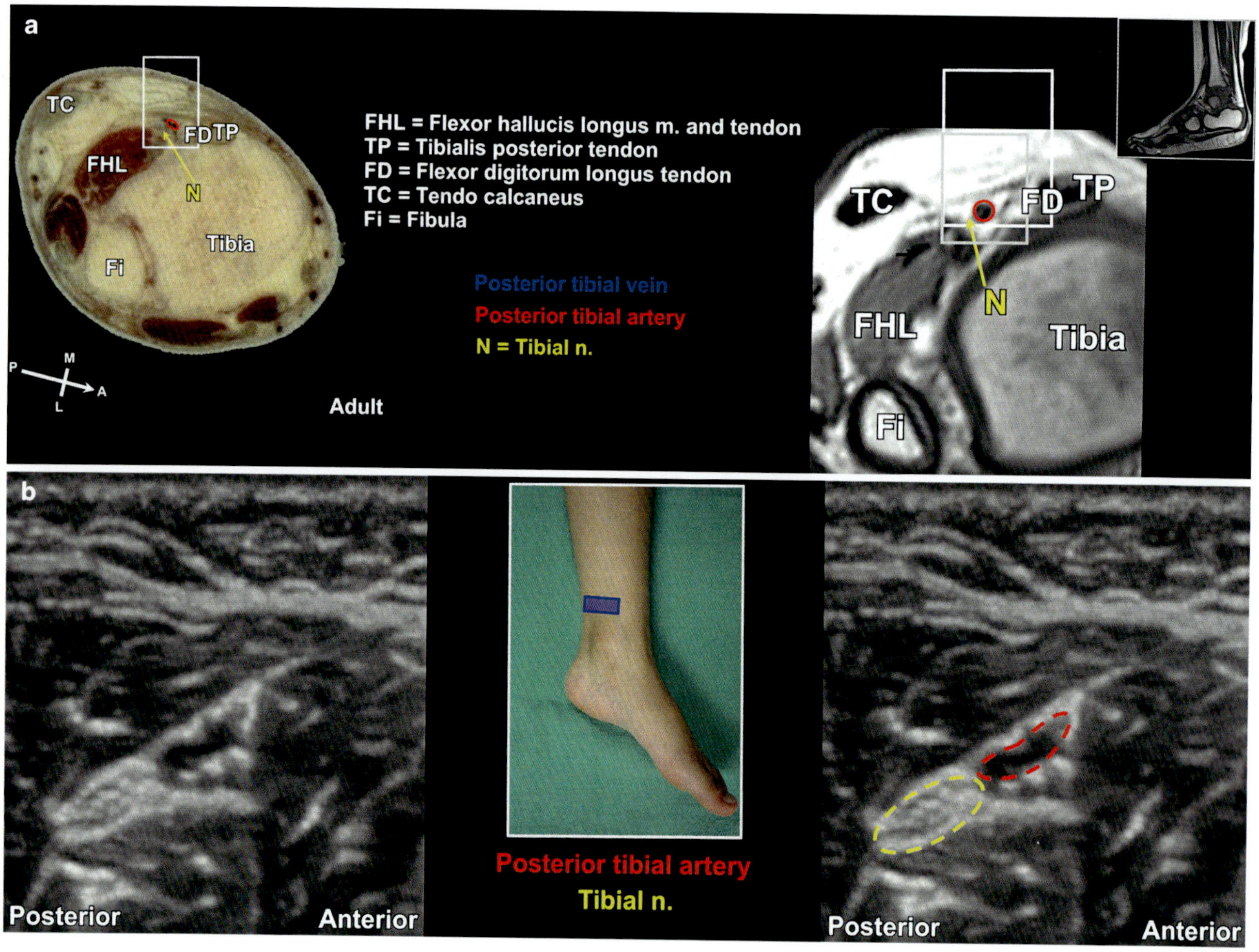

Fig. 27.3 (a) VHVS and MRI images of major anatomical structures surrounding the tibial nerve. (b) Ultrasound image of major anatomical structures surrounding the tibial nerve

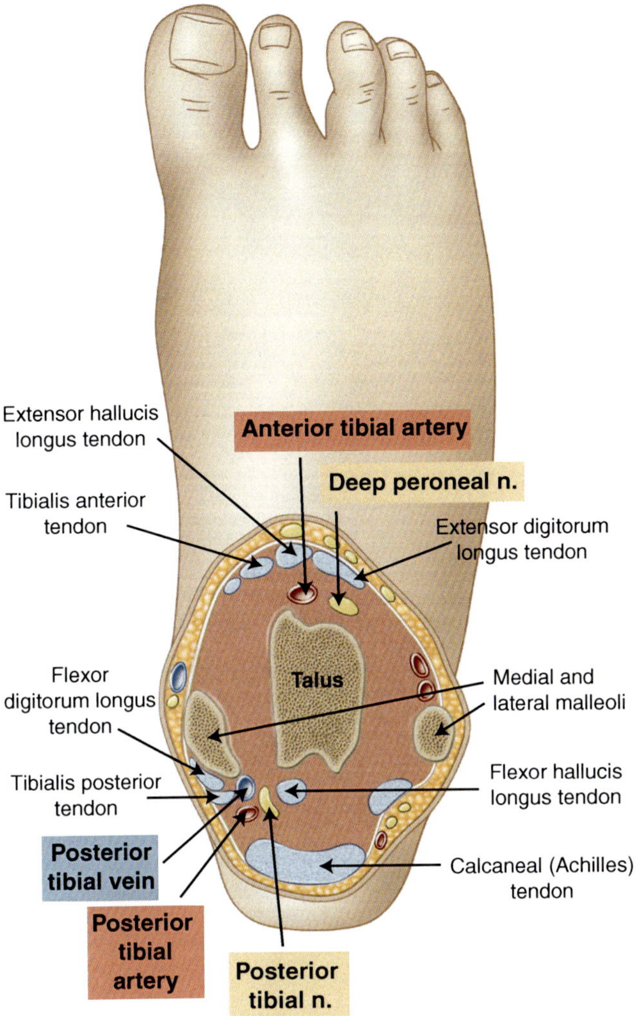

Fig. 27.4 Transverse section at the ankle showing spatial relationship of subcutaneous structures

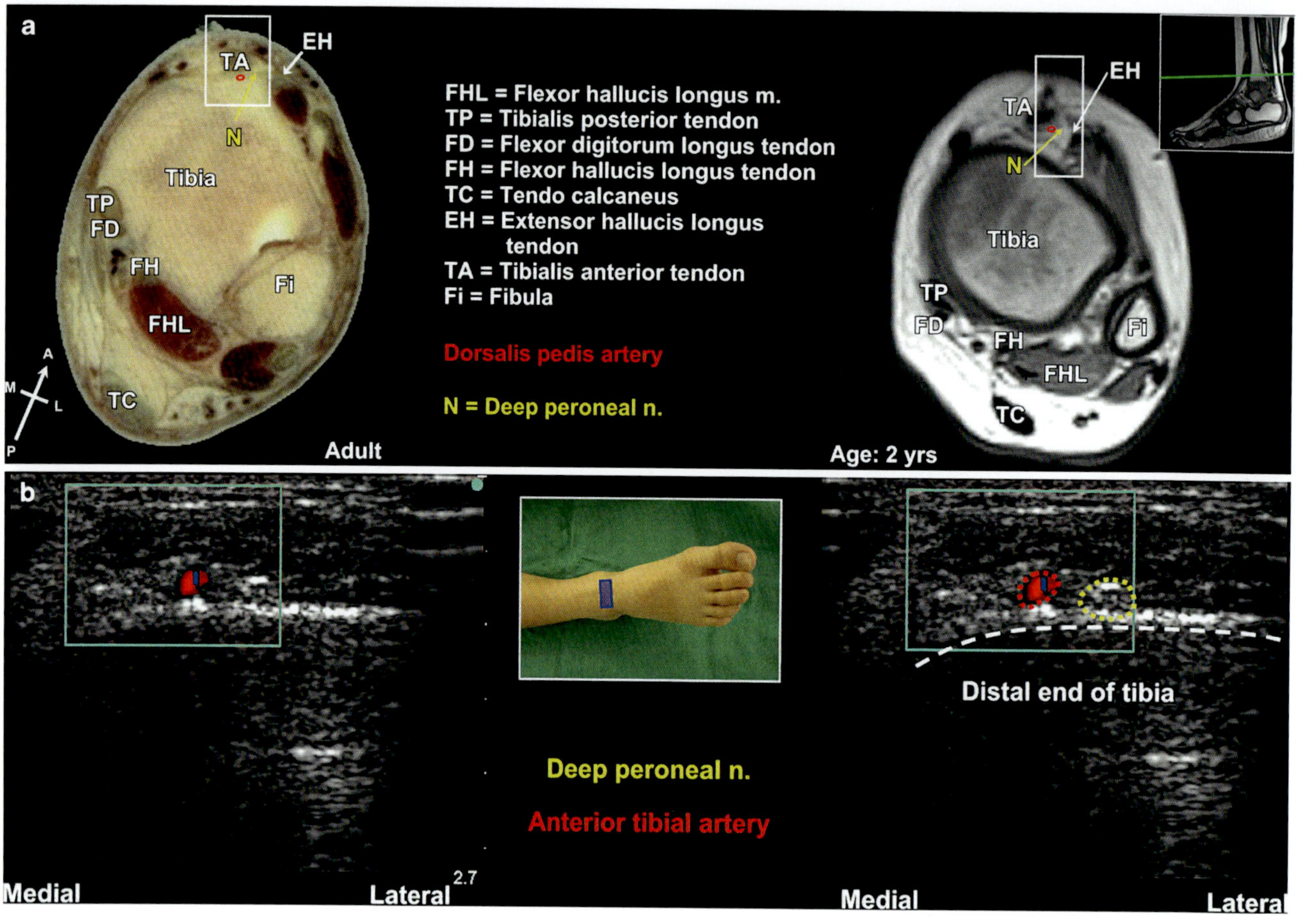

Fig. 27.5 (**a**) VHVS and MRI images of major anatomical structures surrounding the deep peroneal nerve. (**b**) Ultrasound image of major anatomical structures surrounding the deep peroneal nerve

27.4.2 Sonographic Appearance

- Posterior tibial nerve: The hypoechoic circular posterior tibial vein lies immediately posterior to the artery; the vein may be compressed and not apparent on the screen. Posterior to the artery, the nerve appears slightly more hyperechoic than the surrounding tissues and looks like a condensed "honeycomb-appearing" structure [2] (Fig. 27.3b).
- Deep peroneal nerve: If seen, the nerve appears as a small cluster of hyperechoic fascicular-appearing fibers immediately lateral to the artery, with both the nerve and artery adjacent to the well-demarcated distal end of the tibia (Fig. 27.5b).

27.4.3 Needle Insertion

- Posterior tibial nerve: A 3.5–5 cm needle is inserted using either an OOP approach (Fig. 27.6) with the needle caudal or an IP approach (Fig. 27.7) with the needle posterior to the transversely positioned probe.
- Deep peroneal nerve: An OOP approach (Fig. 27.8) will be most suitable here since the tendons lie on either side of the nerve, although an IP approach can also be employed (Fig. 27.9). A 3.5–5 cm needle is inserted OOP and caudal to the transversely positioned small footprint probe.

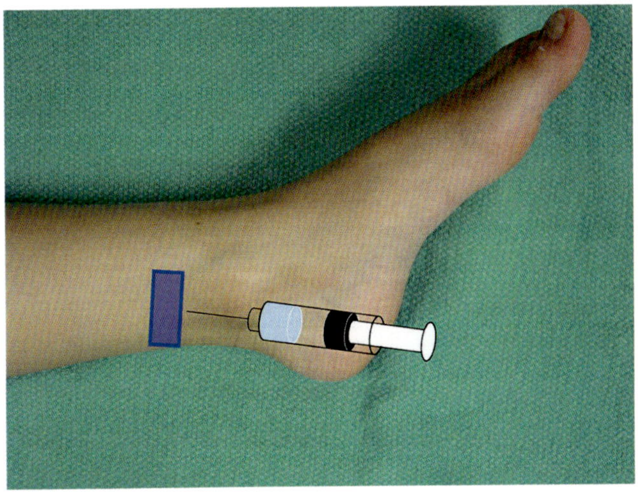

Fig. 27.6 Out-of-plane needling technique for ultrasound-guided posterior tibial nerve block. *Blue rectangle* indicates probe footprint

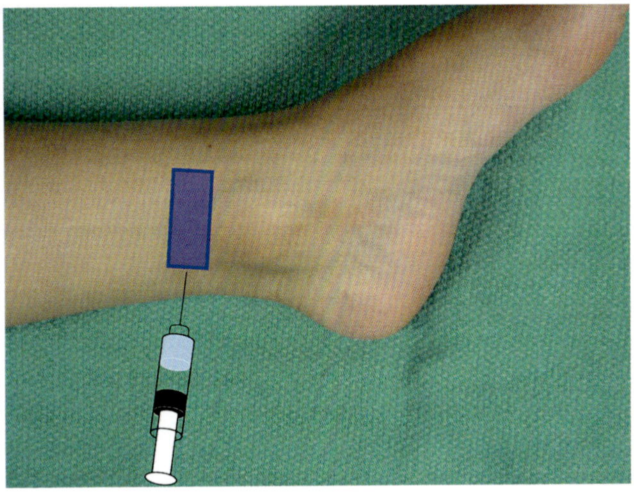

Fig. 27.7 In-plane needling technique for ultrasound-guided posterior tibial nerve block. *Blue rectangle* indicates probe footprint

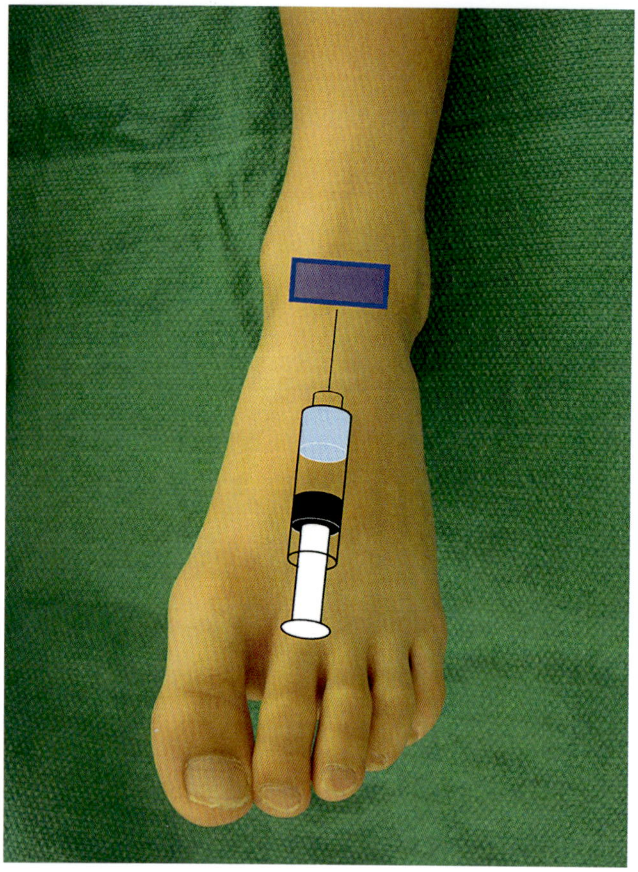

Fig. 27.8 Out-of-plane needling technique for ultrasound-guided deep peroneal nerve block. *Blue rectangle* indicates probe footprint

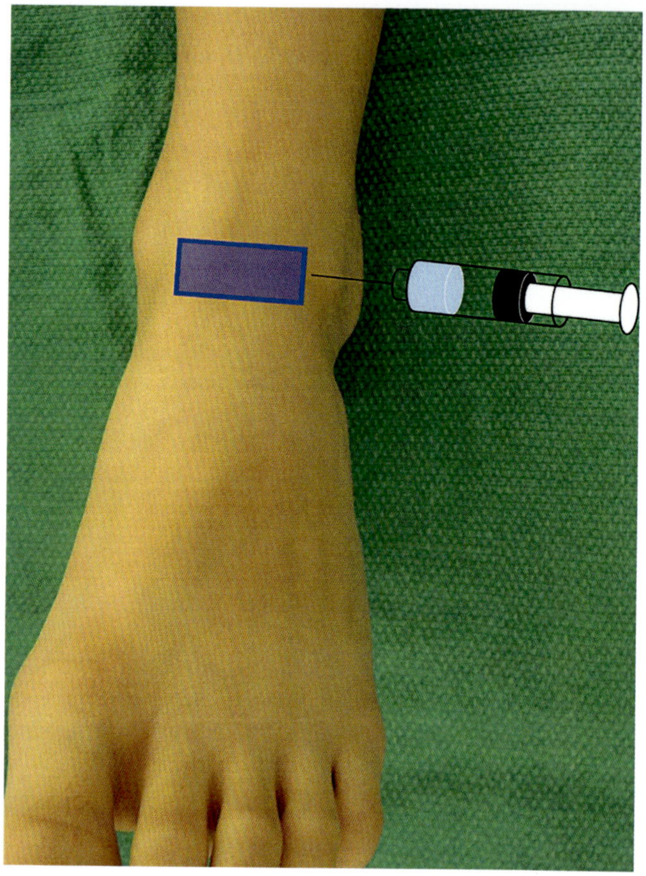

Fig. 27.9 In-plane needling technique for ultrasound-guided deep peroneal nerve block. *Blue rectangle* indicates probe footprint

27.5 Local Anesthetic Application

- The total amount of local anesthetic should be monitored and will depend on the size of the child. 0.1 mL/kg of 0.25 % bupivacaine or 0.2 % ropivacaine may be given, but generally, a small volume, such as 1–3 mL, is sufficient without overexerting pressure in the perineural space.
- A volume of 1–3 mL is adequate for an isolated block of the saphenous nerve.
- For the posterior tibial nerve, a fan-shaped injection of 1–3 mL can be performed in the triangle formed by the artery, the Achilles tendon, and the tibia.
- Epinephrine should **not** be added to the anesthetic solution.

Clinical Pearls

- For both nerves, injection of 1–3 mL (depending on the age and size of the child) of local anesthetic solution near the nerve will anesthetize the nerve. Care should be taken to avoid the nearby vessels; it is important to perform aspiration prior to injection.
- Due to the limited and compact space at the ankle, OOP needling approaches are easier to perform than IP approaches, although IP or OOP needling may be possible if the probe is moved proximally 3–4 cm cephalad to the ankle.
- Ankle blocks can be very stimulating; therefore, adequate depth of anesthesia is required.
- Placing a bolster under the foot improves access for ankle block.

27.6 Current Literature in Ultrasound-Guided Approaches

There is limited evidence documenting the use of ultrasound in ankle blocks in children. Nonetheless, ultrasound has been shown to improve success in posterior tibial and sural nerve blocks in adults [3, 4]. For deep peroneal nerve block at the ankle, ultrasound improved the onset of the block without improving the overall block quality [5].

27.7 Case Study

Ankle blocks can be useful if popliteal sciatic nerve block is contraindicated. Since popliteal sciatic blocks can be performed easily and reliably under ultrasound with a single injection, ankle blocks – which usually require multiple injections – are now often administered by the surgeon for supplementary analgesia following surgery.

References

1. Carpenter EB. Role of nerve blocks in the foot and ankle in cerebral palsy: therapeutic and diagnostic. Foot Ankle. 1983;4:164–6.
2. Silvestri E, Martinoli C, Derchi LE, Bertolotto M, Chiaramondia M, Rosenberg I. Echotexture of peripheral nerves: correlation between US and histologic findings and criteria to differentiate tendons. Radiology. 1995;197:291–6.
3. Redborg KE, Antonakakis, Beach M, Chinn C, Sites B. Ultrasound improves the success rate of a tibial nerve block at the ankle. Reg Anesth Pain Med. 2009;34:256–60.
4. Redborg KE, Sites BD, Chinn CD, Gallagher JD, Ball PA, Antonakakis JG, Beach ML. Ultrasound improves the success rate of a sural nerve block at the ankle. Reg Anesth Pain Med. 2009;34: 24–8.
5. Antonakakis JG, Scalzo DC, Jorgenson AS, Figg KK, Ting P, Zuo Z, Sites BD. Ultrasound does not improve the success rate of a deep peroneal nerve block at the ankle. Reg Anesth Pain Med. 2010;35: 217–21.

Suggested Reading

Dalens B. Complementary and distal blocks of the extremities. In: Dalens B, editor. Regional anesthesia in infants, children, and adolescents. Philadelphia: Lippincott Williams & Wilkins; 1995. p. 384–8.

Dalens BJ. Distal conduction blocks. In: Dalens BJ, editor. Pediatric regional anesthesia. Boca Raton: CRC Press, Inc; 1990. p. 340–4.

Peutrell JM, Mather SJ. Regional anaesthesia for babies and children. Oxford: Oxford University Press; 1997. p. 174–84.

Tsui BC. Ankle blocks. In: Tsui BC, editor. Atlas of ultrasound and nerve stimulation-guided regional anesthesia. New York: Springer; 2007. p. 205–13.

Part X

Nerve Blocks at the Trunk

Paravertebral Blocks

28

Heather Yizhen Z. Ting, Karen R. Boretsky, and Ban C.H. Tsui

Contents

H.Y.Z. Ting, MD, FRCPC
Department of Anesthesiology and Pain Medicine, University of Alberta Hospital, 8440-112 St NW, 2-150 Clinical Sciences Building, Edmonton, AB T6G 2G3, Canada
e-mail: yizhenhe@ualberta.ca

K.R. Boretsky, MD
Department of Anesthesia, Perioperative and Pain Medicine, Harvard Medical School, Boston Children's Hospital, 300 Longwood Avenue, Boston, MA 02115, USA
e-mail: Karen.boretsky@childrens.harvard.edu

B.C.H. Tsui, Dip Eng, BSc (Math), B Pharm, MSc, MD, FRCPC (✉)
Department of Anesthesiology and Pain Medicine, Stollery Children's Hospital/University of Alberta Hospital, 2-150 Clinical Sciences Building, Edmonton, AB T6G 2G3, Canada
e-mail: btsui@ualberta.ca

B.C.H. Tsui, S. Suresh (eds.), *Pediatric Atlas of Ultrasound- and Nerve Stimulation-Guided Regional Anesthesia*, DOI 10.1007/978-0-387-79964-3_28

28.1 Indications

Paravertebral blocks are indicated for unilateral surgical procedures, such as renal surgery and thoracotomy (thoracic paravertebral blocks) and lower limb (hip and thigh) surgeries (lumbar paravertebral blocks). Paravertebral blocks can provide postoperative analgesia lasting 12–48 h, often longer than what is expected of the local anesthetic used. There is generally less motor blockade of the extremities than with epidurals, unless lumbar spinal levels are incorporated (L2 and below). Visceral pain may not be blocked, and there may be a need to increase the depth of anesthesia compared to caudal or epidural blockade. Although placement of a catheter under direct vision during thoracic surgery can be performed in children and provides effective postoperative analgesia for cholecystectomy and renal surgery [1], only percutaneous techniques (mainly single-shot blocks) will be described in this chapter.

28.2 Clinical Anatomy

On either side of the vertebral column, there is a wedge-shaped paravertebral space through which the spinal nerves depart after exiting from the intervertebral foramina. In the thoracic region, the boundaries of the paravertebral space are as follows: medially lies the vertebral body, intervertebral disc and foramen, and spinous processes; anterolaterally is the parietal pleura; and posteriorly lies the anterior surface of the transverse process and superior costotransverse ligament positioned between the adjacent ribs (Fig. 13.1). The space often has a slightly caudal orientation. The paravertebral space communicates medially with the intervertebral foramen and laterally with the intercostal space. In the thoracic region, adjacent levels of the paravertebral space communicate with each other, and some spread of the local anesthetic solution will occur.

The lumbar paravertebral space is surrounded by the psoas major muscle anteriorly, which makes up most of the lumbar paravertebral space; the vertebral bodies, the intervertebral disks, and the intervertebral foramen medially; and the lumbar transverse process along with its ligaments between adjacent transverse processes posteriorly. The psoas major muscle consists of a fleshy anterior part and a thin posterior (accessory) part. The anterior part originates from the anterolateral surface of the vertebral bodies, while the posterior part originates from the anterior surface of transverse process. The ventral rami of the spinal nerve roots extend laterally within the psoas muscle, and the paravertebral space at the lumbar level is divided segmentally by the origins of the psoas muscle.

Since there is large interindividual variation in respect to patient size, knowledge of the depth of the paravertebral space is important to accurately position the needle at the correct location. The depth of the paravertebral space has been found to correlate well with patient parameters (i.e., weight, height, and body surface area), and a formula using patient weight has been reported for calculating the depth of needle penetration when using a medially orientated puncture site [2] (see below). Alternatively, ultrasound imaging can be used to view anatomical structures relevant to the paravertebral block (e.g., transverse processes) and to help determine the accurate depth for needle placement. With some patients, ultrasound imaging may also allow the operator to view the local anesthetic spread and to dynamically control the needle trajectory in order to avoid penetration of the epidural space and the pleura. The ability to use dynamic, "real-time" ultrasound guidance will usually depend on the patient's age and visibility of the anatomical structures (including nerves). Young patients will have little ossification of many bony elements in the vertebral column, and the ultrasound beam will therefore more effectively penetrate to the paravertebral space.

28.3 Block Techniques

Prepare the needle insertion site and skin surface with an antiseptic solution. If using ultrasound, prepare the probe surface by applying a sterile adhesive dressing prior to needling (see Chap. 4).

28.3.1 Landmark-Based Technique

28.3.1.1 Patient Positioning

- The patient is often placed in the prone position, although the lateral decubitus position may be used. Conscious patients may adopt a seated position, but this is rare.
- In the prone position, the arms should be abducted when performing thoracic blocks. A pillow can be placed under the abdomen to minimize the lumbar lordosis.
- Rounding out the back (increasing the thoracic kyphotic curve) in the lateral or sitting position will increase the distance between the transverse processes and may ease injection.

28.3.1.2 Landmarks and Surface Anatomy

Thoracic Paravertebral Block

- *Spinous processes*: Locate T7 at the tips of the scapulae (Fig. 28.1a). Look for scoliosis, which may require further study of the anatomy of the spinal column with ultrasound.
- *Transverse processes*: At T1, the transverse process is located directly lateral to its corresponding spinous process. Subsequent transverse processes are extended to increasingly cephalad locations (i.e., the T7 transverse process is lateral to T6 spinous process) due to the increasingly inferior angulation of the spinous processes. The inferior borders of the relevant transverse processes are marked on the skin, and a line is drawn through these marks.

Lumbar Paravertebral Block

- *Spinous processes*: Typically, the spinous process of L4 is at the level of the iliac crests (neonates and infants have a proportionally smaller pelvis, and the sacrum is located more cephalad relative to the iliac crests; in neonates and infants, the intercristal line crosses the midline of the vertebral column at the L4–L5 or L5–S1 interspace [3, 4]). A vertical line intersecting the posterior superior iliac spine (S2 level) is drawn (Fig. 28.1b).
- *Transverse processes*: The transverse processes of the lumbar spine are long and slender and are located directly lateral to their corresponding spinous process. The inferior borders of the relevant transverse processes are marked on the skin, and a line is drawn through these marks.

The distance between the spinous process and the corresponding transverse process is variable, depending on the patient's age. At the thoracic level, the needle puncture site is lateral to the spinous process but may be 1 cm or larger (2.5 cm) (Fig. 28.1a). For the lumbar levels, the puncture site is also 1–2.5 cm lateral to the corresponding spinous process (Fig. 28.2).

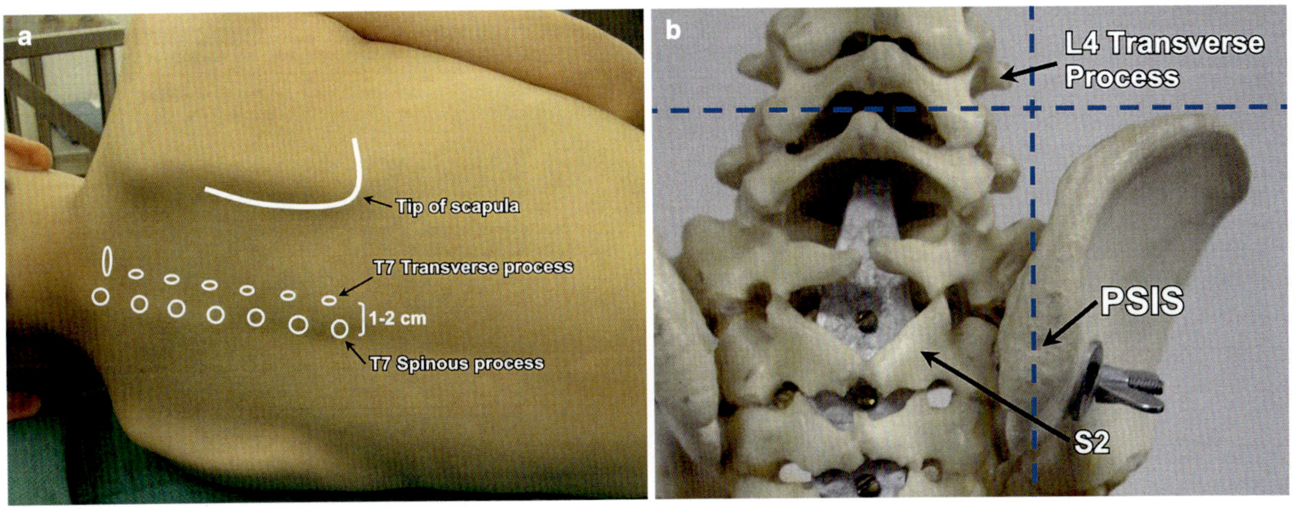

Fig. 28.1 (**a**) Surface anatomy for thoracic paravertebral block. (**b**) Skeletal model showing the L4 transverse process and posterior superior iliac spine (*PSIS*) landmarks

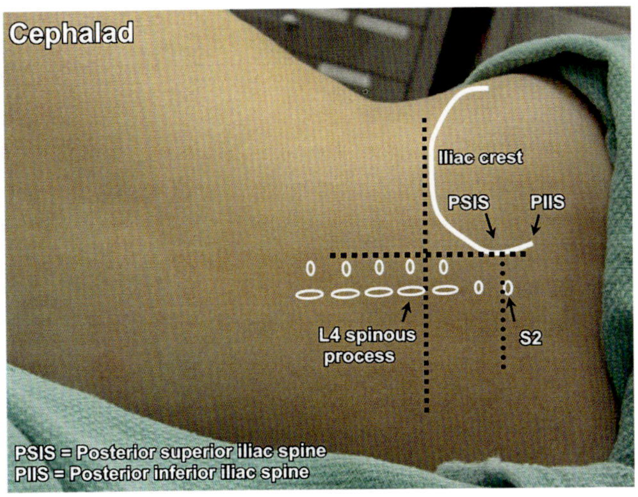

Fig. 28.2 Surface anatomy for lumbar paravertebral block

28.3.1.3 Needle Insertion

Thoracic Paravertebral Block

- After aseptic skin preparation and patient sedation, local anesthetic skin wheals are raised at the marked transverse processes.
- If using nerve stimulation, an insulated needle (5–8 cm, 22G needles are used, depending on the size of the child) is introduced through the skin wheal in the sagittal plane and directed slightly cephalad to contact the transverse process or, sometimes, likely the costotransverse ligament.
- Gentle cephalad or caudad exploration may be required to identify the bone.
- The depth of the transverse process should be carefully noted on the needle shaft.
- The needle is now withdrawn from the transverse process to the skin level and reinserted 10° superiorly (to target the spinal nerve corresponding to the spinous process) or inferiorly (corresponding to the vertebral level below the spinous process) and slightly deeper (usually up to a maximum of 1 cm) than the previously marked point of bone contact.
- The needle should be angled slightly medially to avoid causing pneumothorax. There will be a subtle "give" at the midpoint between these landmarks (spinous and transverse processes), indicating entrance into the paravertebral space.
- For the loss-of-resistance technique, an epidural set containing an 18G–22G (the latter for children under 6 months of age) Tuohy needle with a syringe is used. After walking off the transverse processes, a "pop" or loss of resistance to air or D5W may be felt when entering the paravertebral space through the costotransverse ligament.
- Lonnqvist et al. [1] reported calculations using computed tomography for determining both the depth of the paravertebral space from the skin (S-PVS depth) and the lateral distance of the paravertebral space from the spinous process (SP-PVS distance) since they correlate with the patient's body weight:

1. $\text{S}-\text{PVS depth}\ (\text{mm}) = 0.48 \times \text{body weight}\ (\text{kg}) + 18.7$
2. $\text{SP}-\text{PVS distance}\ (\text{mm}) = 0.12 \times \text{body weight}\ (\text{kg}) + 10.2$

Lumbar Paravertebral Block

- After aseptic skin preparation and patient sedation, local anesthetic skin wheals are raised at the marked transverse processes.
- If using nerve stimulation, an insulated needle (5–8 cm, 22G needles are used, depending on the size of the child) is introduced through the skin wheal in the sagittal plane, penetrating the fascia surrounding the quadratus lumborum muscle to contact the transverse process.
- Gentle cephalad or caudad exploration may be required to identify the bone.
- The depth of the transverse process should be noted on the needle shaft.
- The needle is now withdrawn from the transverse process to the skin level and reinserted 10° superiorly (to target the spinal nerve corresponding to the spinous process) or inferiorly (corresponding to the vertebral level below the spinous process) and slightly deeper (up to a maximum of 1 cm) than the previously marked point of bone contact, sliding off the superior or inferior edge of the transverse process.
- There will be a subtle "give" at the midpoint between these landmarks (spinous and transverse processes), indicating entrance into the paravertebral space.
- For the loss-of-resistance technique, an epidural set containing an 18G–22G (the latter for children under 6 months of age) Tuohy needle with a syringe is used. After walking off the transverse processes, a "pop" or loss of resistance to air or D5W may be felt when entering the paravertebral space through the ligament.

Clinical Pearl

For intermittent or continuous blocks, an epidural catheter set is used, and the catheter is advanced 2–3 cm into the paravertebral space. After aspiration of the catheter, a test dose using lidocaine 1 % (0.1 mL/kg) with 1:200,000 epinephrine (0.5 μg/kg), followed by a bolus dose (0.5 mL/kg) of local anesthetic (0.125–0.25 % bupivacaine, depending on age and weight of the child), can be injected over 5–10 min. Note that the heart rate increase can be unreliable, especially under anesthesia [5]. The continuous block may be maintained with hourly injections of 0.1–0.25 mL/kg/h of the same solution.

28.3.1.4 Local Anesthetic Application

- Since the paravertebral space is well-vascularized, inadvertent vascular puncture will often occur, highlighting the need for frequent aspiration and injection in small aliquots.
- If depending on multi-segmental block at the thoracic level, inject 0.5 mL/kg of local anesthetic solution (e.g., 0.25 % bupivacaine) with or without epinephrine. This volume should cover at least four to five segments of spinal nerves. If using individual blocks for each segment, the volume of local anesthetic will be reduced to 0.1 mL/kg. Vertical spread of local anesthetic is limited at the lumbar level, so reduced volumes injected at each level will be required. The dose of bupivacaine should not exceed 2 mg/kg. Dilution with normal saline can help increase the volume (to more effectively produce the block) while maintaining safe doses of local anesthetic.

28.3.2 Nerve Stimulation Technique

28.3.2.1 Current Application and Appropriate Responses

- An initial current of 1.5–3 mA is used, and the needle is advanced until contractions of the appropriate muscles (e.g., abdominal muscles with thoracic paravertebral block and quadriceps muscle twitch with lumbar paravertebral block) are observed. The current intensity is then reduced to localize the nerves at 0.4–0.6 mA.
- Until the paravertebral space is entered, the motor response will be from the paraspinal muscles.
- A test dose of local anesthetic (0.1 mL/kg of 1 % lidocaine) will confirm nerve localization, and current dissipation at the needle tip by the conducting solution will eliminate the nerve response.

28.3.2.2 Modifications to Inappropriate Responses

- Bilateral muscle twitches of the lower extremity may indicate epidural needle placement. Bilateral twitches at low current (<1 mA) may indicate subdural needle placement.

28.3.3 Ultrasound-Guided Technique

Traditionally, ultrasound imaging has been used prior to (i.e., "pre-procedural," "supported," or "off-line" imaging) rather than during (i.e., "real-time" or "on-line" imaging) block performance to identify the deep bony landmarks, including the articular and transverse processes. Real-time imaging for paravertebral blocks is now used widely for both single-shot blocks and catheter insertion [6, 7]. Ultrasound guidance can be used to help identify the paravertebral space and needle placement and to monitor the spread of the local anesthetic. The MRI images in Figs. 28.3, 28.4, 28.5, 28.6, 28.7, and 28.8 correlate to the ultrasound images in these figures, allowing the reader to better understand the anatomy of the region.

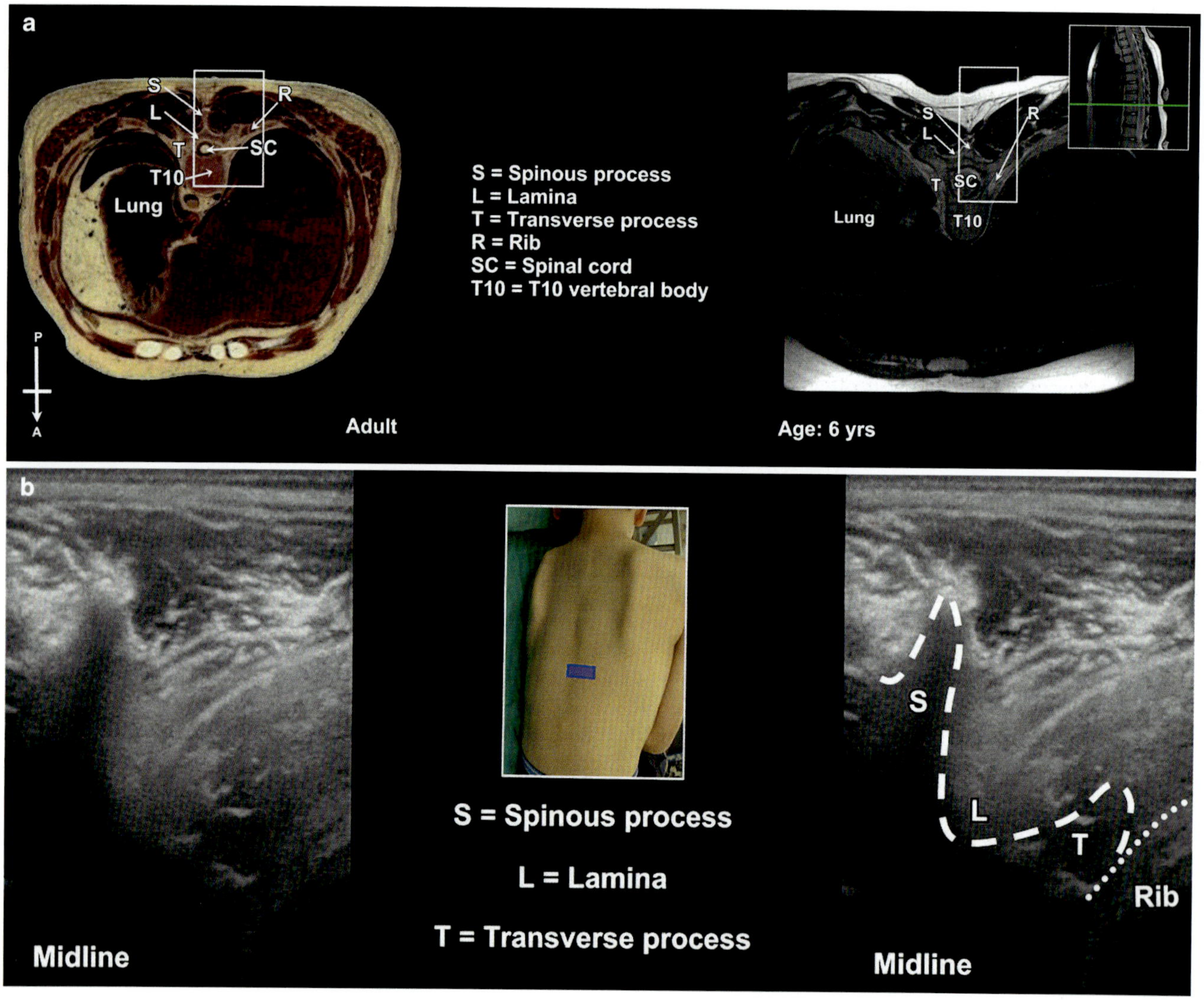

Fig. 28.3 (a) VHVS and MRI images of transverse section at T9–10. (b) Ultrasound images of transverse section at T9–10

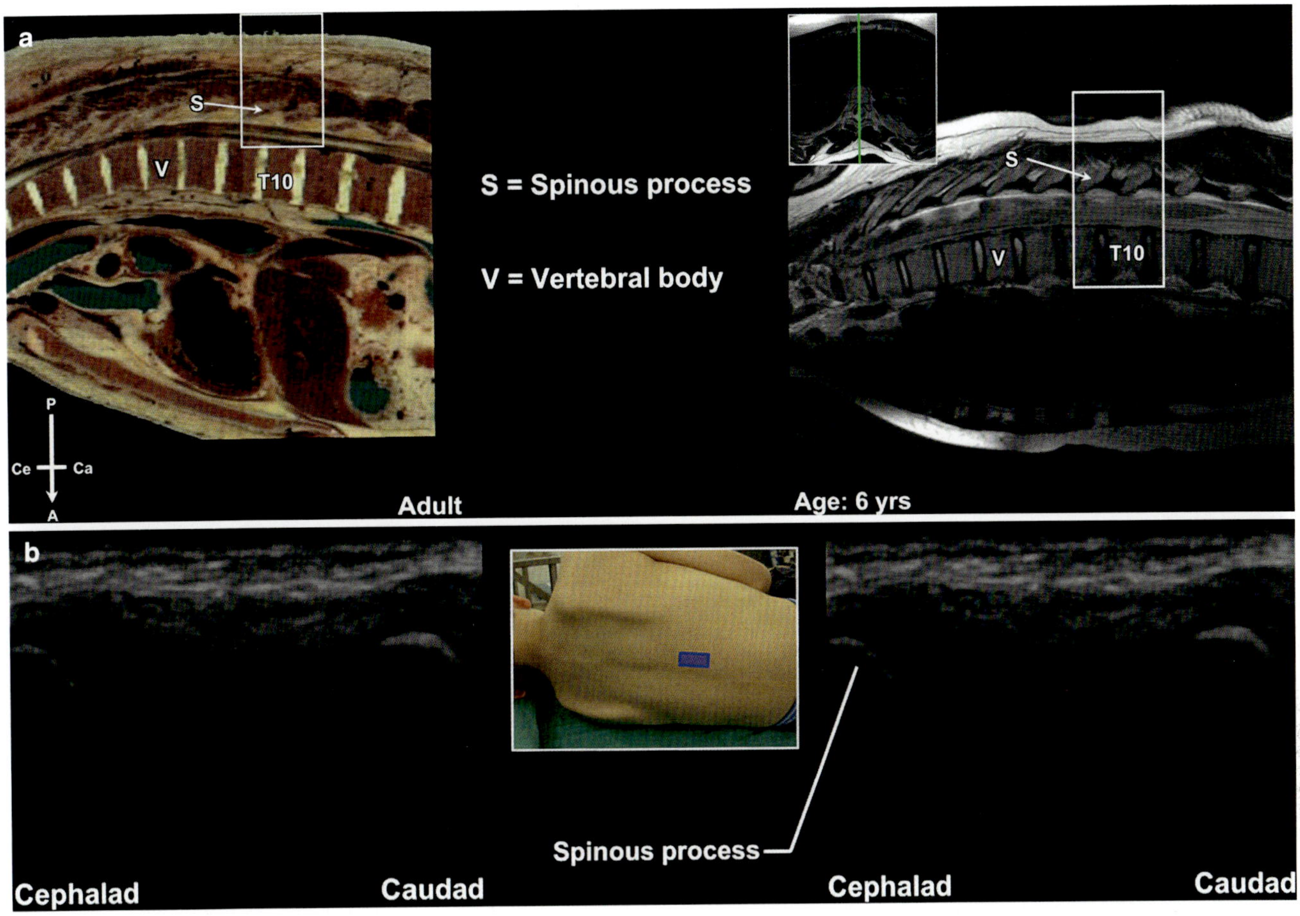

Fig. 28.4 (**a**) VHVS and MRI images of longitudinal section at the midline showing the spinous process of T9 and T10. (**b**) Ultrasound images of longitudinal section at the midline showing the spinous process of T9 and T10

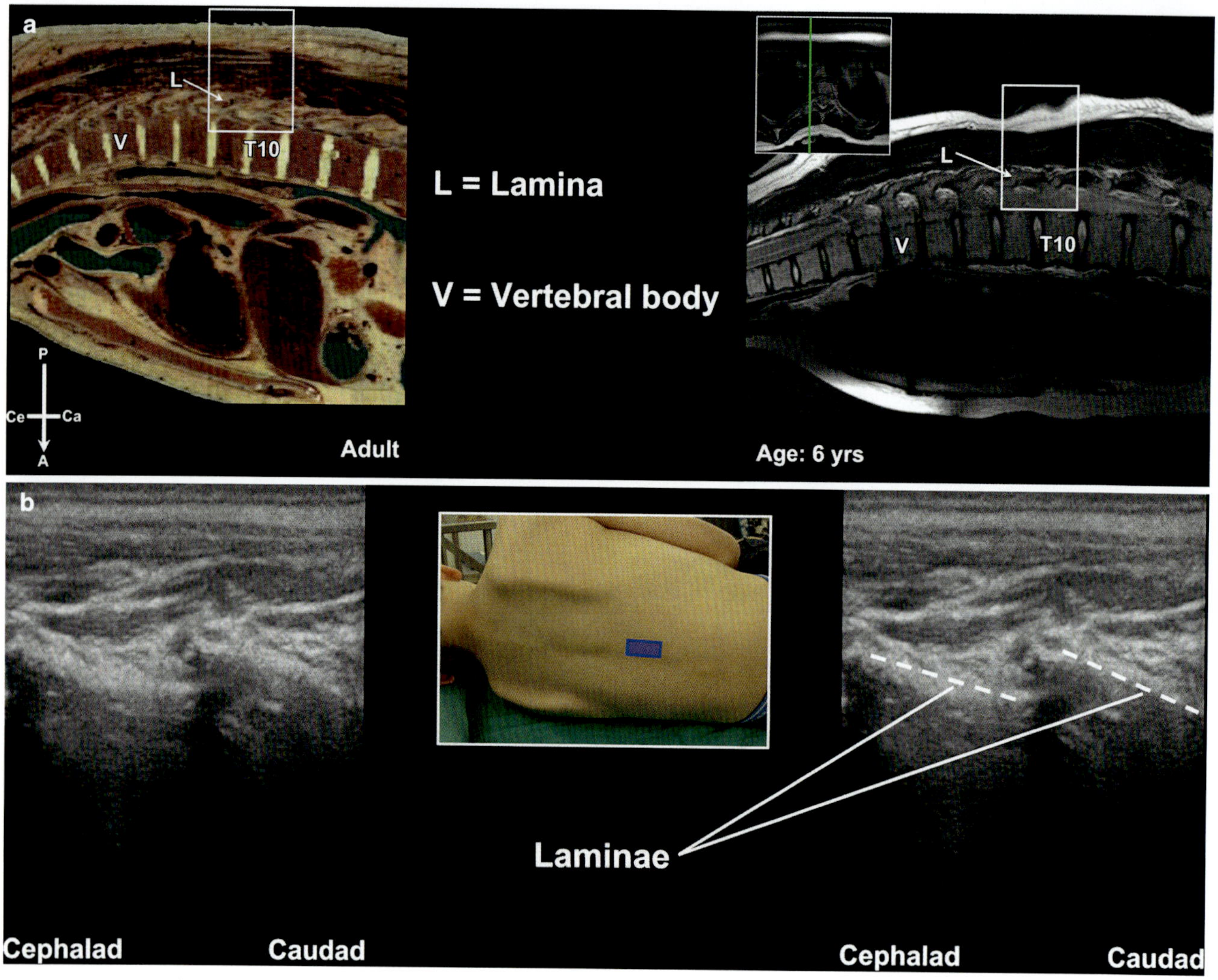

Fig. 28.5 (**a**) VHVS and MRI images of longitudinal section at the midline showing the laminae of T9 and T10. (**b**) Ultrasound images of longitudinal section at the midline showing the laminae of T9 and T10

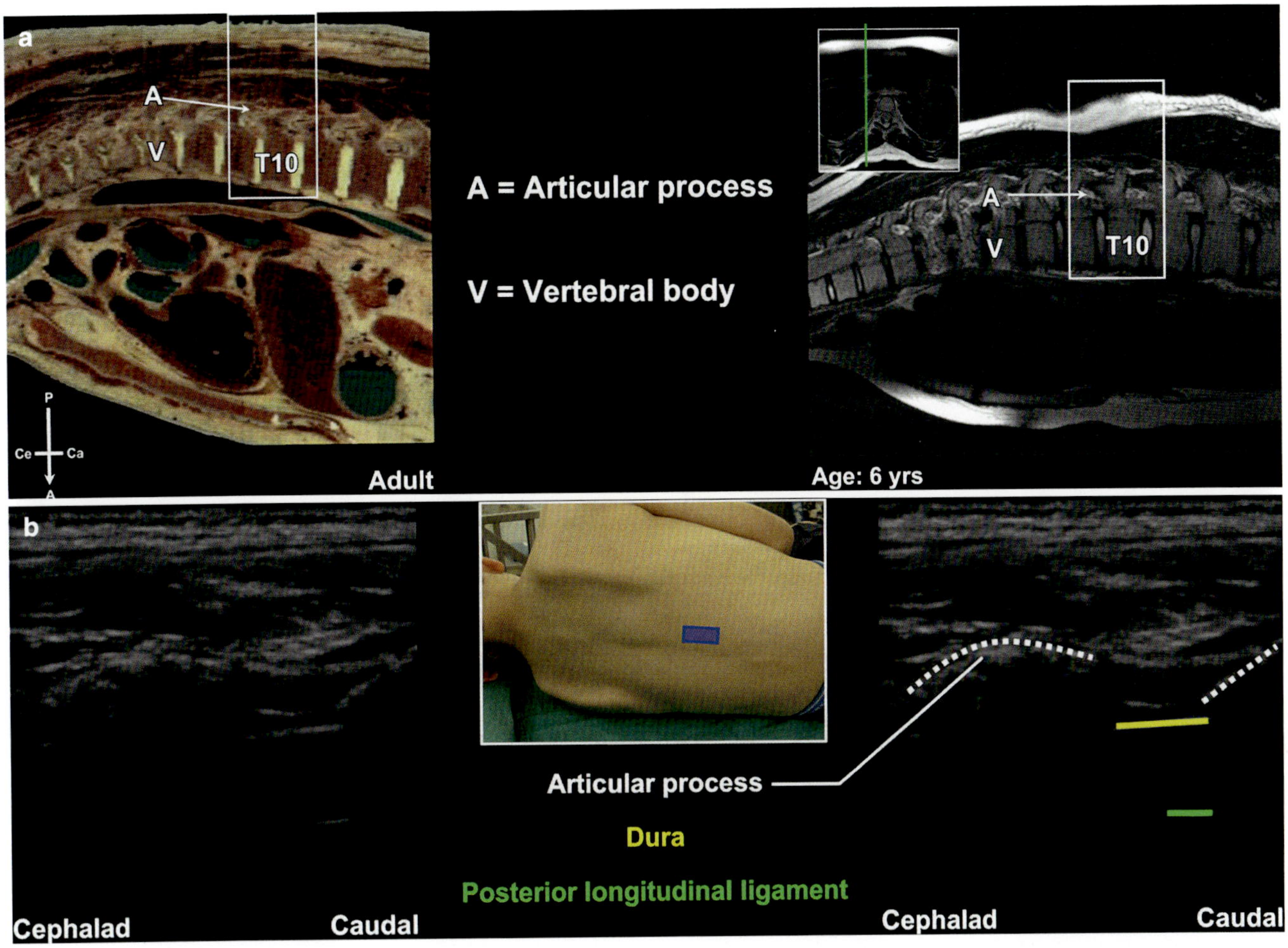

Fig. 28.6 (**a**) VHVS and MRI images of longitudinal section at the midline showing the articular processes of T9 and T10. (**b**) Ultrasound images of longitudinal section at the midline showing the articular processes of T9 and T10

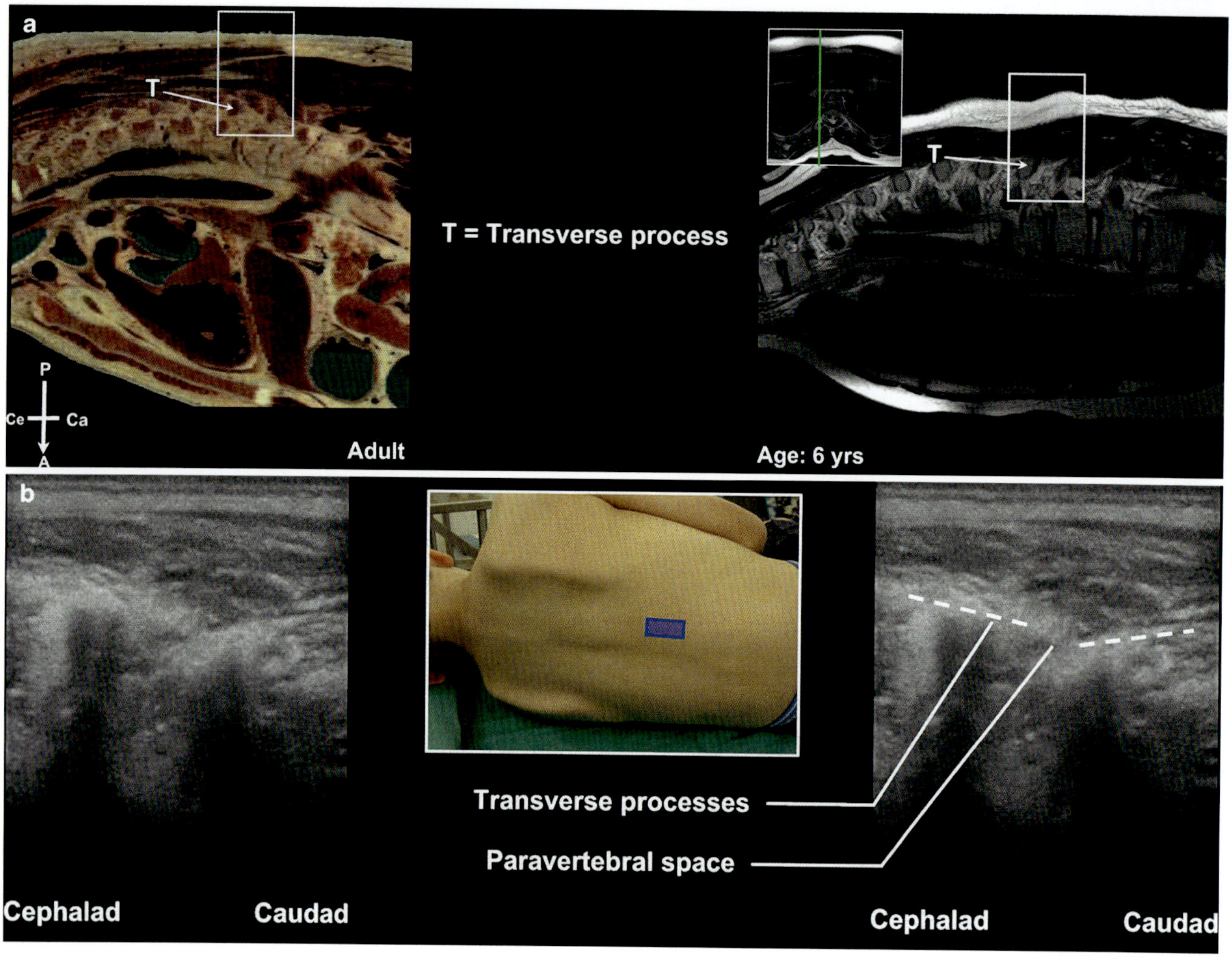

Fig. 28.7 (**a**) VHVS and MRI images of longitudinal section at the midline showing the transverse processes of T9 and T10. (**b**) Ultrasound images of longitudinal section at the midline showing the transverse processes of T9 and T10

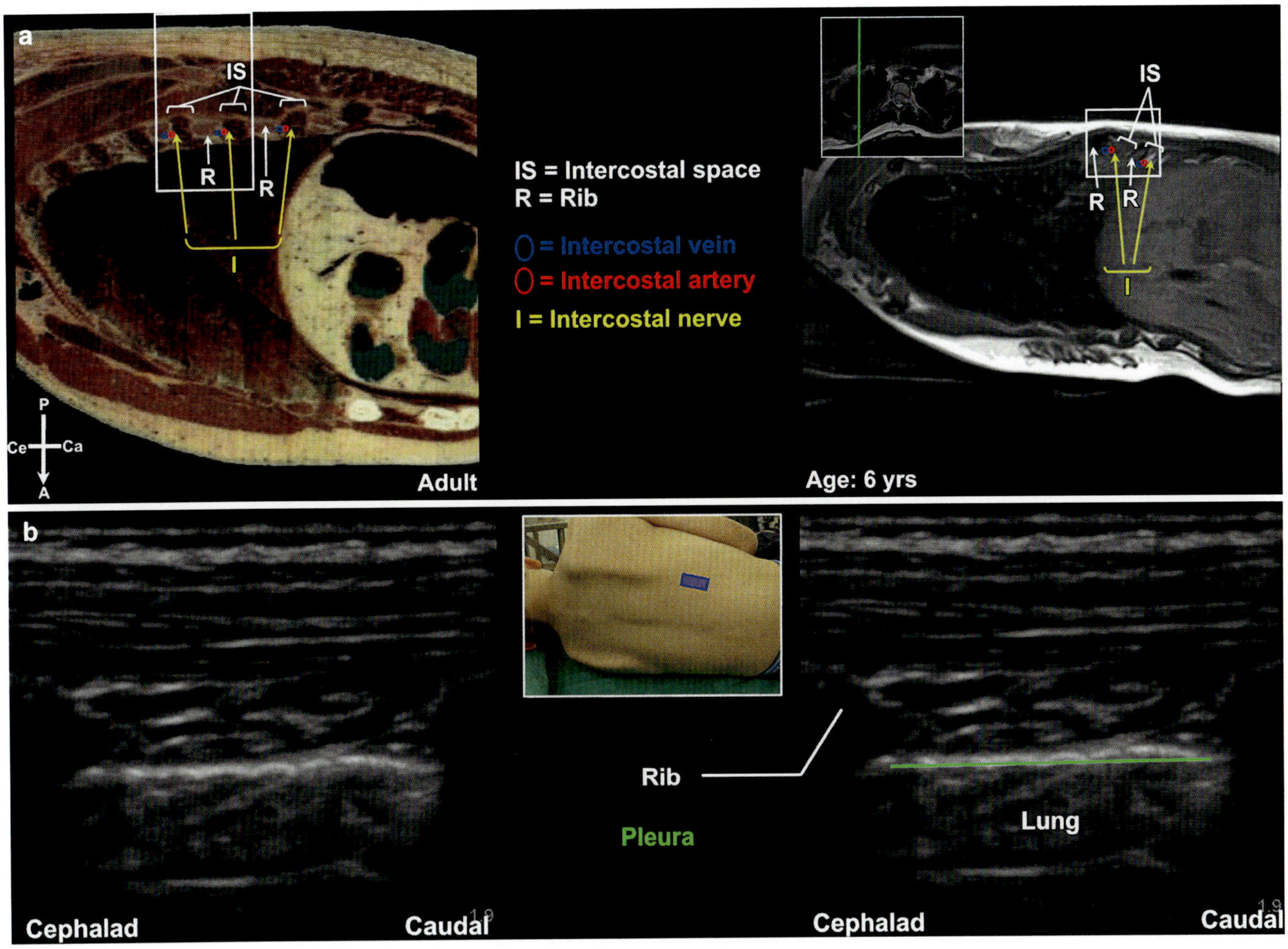

Fig. 28.8 (**a**) VHVS and MRI images of longitudinal section lateral to the midline showing the ninth and tenth ribs and the underlying pleural space. (**b**) Ultrasound images of longitudinal section lateral to the midline showing the ninth and tenth ribs and the underlying pleural space

28.3.3.1 Scanning Technique

- Position a linear high-frequency (10–12 MHz) probe in the transverse plane in the midline to capture an overview of the vertebrae (Fig. 28.3). The vertebral laminae and processes will be viewed, allowing the lateral distance to the transverse processes to be marked.
- To obtain a more accurate localization (lateral distance and depth) of the transverse processes, rotate the probe to the longitudinal plane, and scan in a medial-to-lateral direction. Starting at the spinous processes (Fig. 28.4), the scan will capture (in sequence) the lamina (Fig. 28.5), articular (Fig. 28.6) and transverse processes (Fig. 28.7), and, in the thoracic spine, the ribs (Fig. 28.8).
- To locate the desired segment at the lumbar spine, place the probe in the longitudinal plane at the lateral distance of the transverse processes and shift the probe caudally to capture the cephalad aspect of the sacrum. The transverse processes can then be counted during a cephalad scan.

28.3.3.2 Sonographic Appearance

- The initial transverse scan will show a hyperechoic outline of the vertebral spinous and transverse processes, the lamina, and, in the thoracic spine, associated rib (Fig. 28.3).
- The midline image in the longitudinal plane will capture the spinous processes (Fig. 28.4).
- During the lateral scan with the probe placed longitudinally to the spine, the laminae will appear first as largely overlapping linear structures (Fig. 28.5).
- The articular processes in long-axis appear as multiple "lumps" just lateral to the spinous processes and laminae and are short, rectangular structures with hyperechoic lines with underlying hypoechoic bony shadowing (Fig. 28.6).
- Moving laterally, the transverse processes appear (Fig. 28.7) and look similar to the articular processes. The transverse processes will disappear from view when the probe is moved beyond their tips, which can help distinguish them from the articular processes and mark the lateral block location.
- Beyond the transverse processes in the thoracic region, the rib heads appear as long shadows within hyperechoic borders deep to the linear hyperechoic muscle fibers of the paravertebral muscles (Fig. 28.8).
- The paravertebral space lies deep to the transverse processes between the intercostal muscle and parietal pleura (Fig. 28.7), and the pleura can often be identified as a bright hyperechoic line under the ribs (Fig. 28.8).
- At the lumbar spine, the relatively bulky erector spinae muscles appear highly linear and overlay the vertebrae and spinal nerves during the scan.
- Deep to the medial aspect of the transverse processes, the lumbar nerve roots may be seen between the hypoechoic shadows of the bones, as hypoechoic parallel bands interspersed with the hyperechoic striations of the related connective tissue.
- In the lumbar paravertebral space, the lumbar plexus lies in the "psoas compartment" bordered by the psoas major anteriorly and quadratus lumborum posteriorly (Figs. 11.4 and 24.6a).

Clinical Pearl

Lumbar plexus vs. lumbar paravertebral block:

Lumbar plexus block, also known as the psoas sheath block, is performed by injecting local anesthetic within the psoas sheath and into the psoas muscle. The lumbar paravertebral block, which is also known as psoas compartment block, involves injection of local anesthetic posterior to the psoas sheath, between the psoas muscle and quadratus lumborum.

28.3.3.3 Needle Insertion

- When using ultrasound guidance for paravertebral block, it is important to carefully observe the angulation of the needle. Using an IP needle alignment to a longitudinal probe may be most prudent (Fig. 28.9).
- The needle should not be inserted in a significantly medial direction due to a risk of spinal cord injury from intraforaminal insertion and injection. Likewise, a lateral direction bears the risk of pneumothorax.
- Under real-time ultrasound guidance, please note:
  1. With the probe placed in the sagittal/longitudinal plane, OOP needling (Fig. 28.10) may be more risky, as it often requires medial or lateral angulations (described above).
  2. An IP needling approach can be more risky when the probe is placed in the coronal/transverse plane if the needle is advanced blindly.

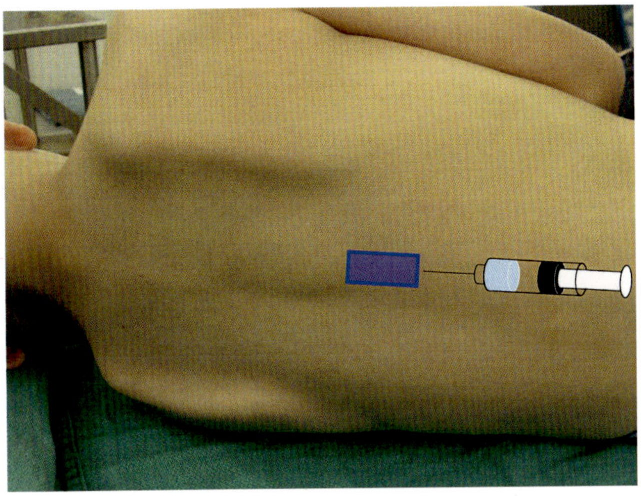

Fig. 28.9 In-plane needling technique for ultrasound-guided paravertebral block at T9–10. *Blue rectangle* indicates probe footprint

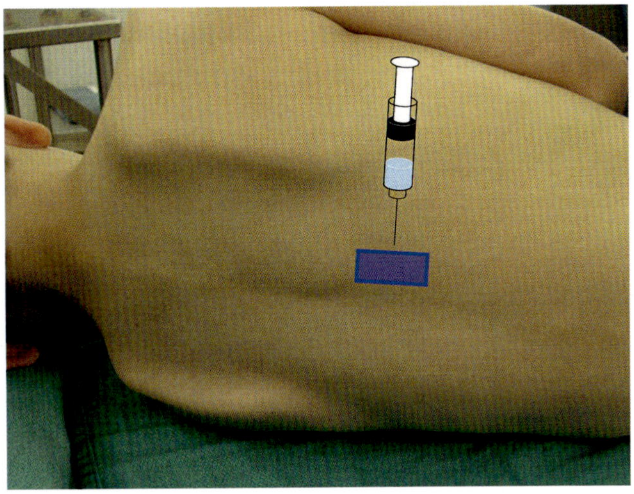

Fig. 28.10 Out-of-plane needling technique for ultrasound-guided paravertebral block at T9–10. *Blue rectangle* indicates probe footprint

28.3.3.4 Alternate Scanning Technique: Transverse Approach

The miniscule distance between transverse processes and the resultant steep angle of the needle required to access the paravertebral space makes a parasagittal approach difficult in very small patients. A transverse (lateral-to-medial) approach allows continuous visualization of the advancing needle and, providing that the needle is never advanced blindly, is a safe alternate technique.

- The appropriate thoracic level is identified using surface landmarks or ultrasound pre-scanning and marked (see parasagittal approach).
- Place a high-frequency linear transducer in a transverse orientation over the spinous process corresponding to the dermatomal level to be blocked. The spinous process is identified as a hyperechoic inverted V-shape with an acoustic shadow beneath.
- Slide the probe lateral and rotate to a slightly oblique orientation following the direction of the rib (lateral probe edge slightly caudal) until the tip of the transverse process is visualized as a characteristic thumb shape (Fig. 28.11). Locate the transverse process in the center of the screen. The pleura is seen just lateral and deep to the transverse process.
- If the rib is seen articulating with the transverse process and the pleura is not visualized, slide the probe caudal or cephalad a few millimeters until the pleura and transverse process are visualized with no overshadowing rib.
- When visible, the internal intercostal membrane (IICM) (the lateral continuation of the costotransverse ligament) is identified as a linear hyperechoic structure connecting the edge of the internal intercostal muscle to the lower edge of the transverse process.
- The paravertebral space is located in the triangle formed by the anatomic anterior surface of the transverse process and IICM, the anatomic posterior surface of the parietal pleura, and the lateral surface of the vertebral body.
- The needle is introduced with the bevel toward and in-plane with the probe, several centimeters from the lateral edge of the probe. The needle is advanced at an angle from lateral to medial until the needle tip penetrates the IICM and passes into the paravertebral space immediately underneath the transverse process.
- Correct positioning within the paravertebral space can be confirmed by real-time ultrasound visualization of anterior displacement of the pleura following injection of a small amount of sterile saline or D5W.

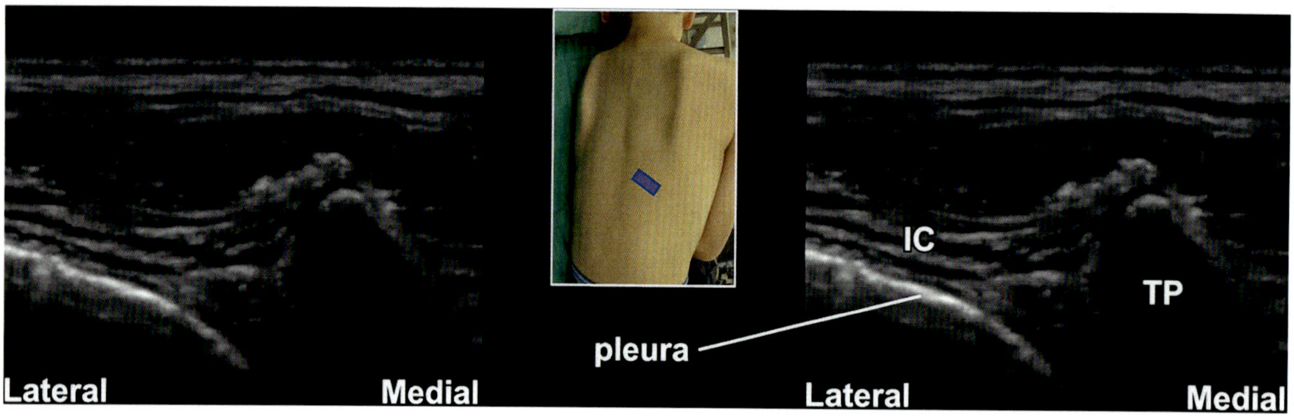

Fig. 28.11 Transverse view of transverse process and surrounding anatomy for medial-to-lateral approach for paravertebral block, *IC* intercostal muscles; *TP* transverse process

28.3.3.5 Local Anesthetic Application

- Local anesthetic spread will be difficult to view in most patients if using real-time ultrasound guidance during this block. The overlying bones largely reflect the US beam and obstruct visibility of the paravertebral space. The spread may be captured in young patients (generally <2–3 years), since their neural arches have yet to fuse with the vertebral bodies (centrums), allowing the ultrasound beam to better penetrate to the paravertebral space.
- In young patients, the hypoechoic spread of local anesthetic can be seen as it displaces the parietal pleura anteriorly during thoracic paravertebral block. During lumbar paravertebral block, local anesthetic spread can be seen posterior to the psoas major muscle.
- Chest X-ray following injection of omnipaque contrast dye (0.25 mL/kg) in a 6-month-old infant shows the anterior-posterior spread of injectate across eight dermatomes following ultrasound-guided injection into the paravertebral space (Fig. 28.12).

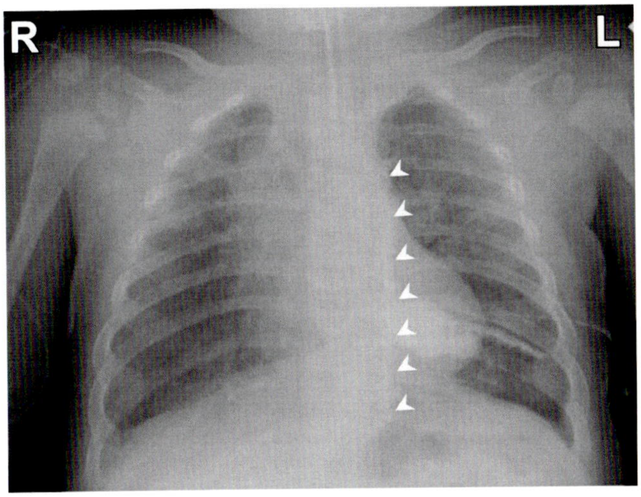

Fig. 28.12 Chest X-ray showing anterior-posterior dermatomal spread of contrast agent (*arrowheads*) following injection into paravertebral space

28.4 Current Literature in Ultrasound-Guided Approaches

Recently, Ponde et al. [8] attempted to create formulae that would allow determination of the distances from the spine to the needle insertion point and from the insertion point to the paravertebral space at the thoracic (T1–T12), lumbar (L1), and cervical (C6) levels in children up to 5 years old. The formulae use ultrasound measurements and account for age and weight, allowing easy calculation of the two distances.

A case report by Visoiu and Yang described the use of continuous bilateral paravertebral blocks in a 16-year-old patient with Denys-Drash syndrome and history of end-stage renal failure who underwent exploratory laparotomy and small bowel resection [9]. Despite the presence of mild coagulopathy at the time of admission, bilateral paravertebral catheters were installed at the T8 level; under ultrasound guidance, a 90 mm, 18G Tuohy needle was inserted in-plane, lateral to medial, followed by injection of 10 mL ropivacaine 0.5 % into the paravertebral space. A catheter was threaded 3 cm into the paravertebral space, and placement was confirmed with 2 mL of local anesthetic. Pain management following surgery was satisfactory, and the catheters were removed without any problems on postoperative day 5.

28.5 Case Study

Thoracic Paravertebral Block (*Provided by A. Sawardekar*)

A 16-year-old male, 76 kg, with a history of pectus excavatum presented with ongoing pain in the right chest wall. The patient had received a Nuss procedure to repair the defect 18 months prior, and upon chest X-ray, it was determined that the Nuss bar should be removed. An ultrasound-guided paravertebral block was administered with a 22G needle (see Fig. 28.13). The right T6 paravertebral space was identified using a 13–6 MHz linear high-frequency probe. A longitudinal, out-of-plane approach was used to advance the needle with saline hydrodissection below the costotransverse ligament. Ten mL of 0.25 % bupivacaine was injected at this site. Duration of surgery was 60 min, and block duration was 12 h. No additional analgesics were needed in the recovery room or on the ward.

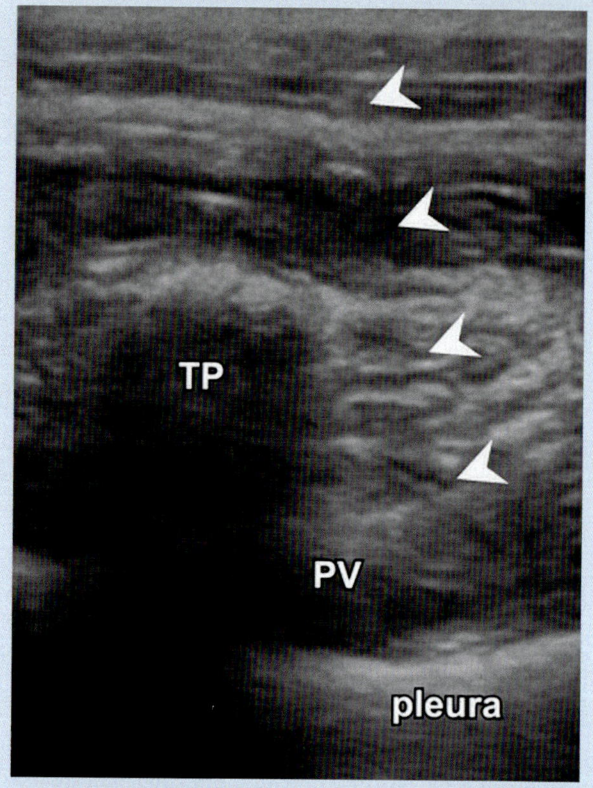

Fig. 28.13 Ultrasound image of thoracic paravertebral block. *TP* transverse process, *PV* paravertebral space; *arrowheads* indicate shadow of needle. See Case Study for details

References

1. Lonnqvist PA. Continuous paravertebral block in children. Initial experience. Anaesthesia. 1992;47:607–9.
2. Lonnqvist PA, Hildingsson U. The caudal boundary of the thoracic paravertebral space. A study in human cadavers. Anaesthesia. 1992;47:1051–2.
3. Busoni P, Messeri A. Spinal anesthesia in children: surface anatomy. Anesth Analg. 1989;68:418–9.
4. Busoni P, Messeri A. Spinal anesthesia in infants: could a L5–S1 approach be safer? Anesthesiology. 1991;75:168–9.
5. Tanaka M, Nishikawa T. Simulation of an epidural test dose with intravenous epinephrine in sevoflurane-anesthetized children. Anesth Analg. 1998;86:952–7.
6. Bhalla T, Sawardekar A, Dewhirst E, Jagannathan N, Tobias JD. Ultrasound-guided trunk and core blocks in infants and children. J Anesth. 2013;27:109–23.

7. Boretsky K, Visoiu M, Bigeleisen P. Ultrasound-guided approach to the paravertebral space for catheter insertion in infants and children. Pediatr Anesth. 2013;23:1193–8.
8. Ponde VC, Desai AP. Echo-guided estimation of formula for paravertebral block in neonates, infants and children till 5 years. Indian J Anaesth. 2012;56:382–6.
9. Visoiu M, Yang C. Ultrasound-guided bilateral paravertebral continuous nerve blocks for a mildly coagulopathic patient undergoing exploratory laparotomy for bowel resection. Pediatr Anesth. 2011;21:459–62.

Suggested Reading

Dalens BJ. Blocks of nerves of the trunk. In: Dalens BJ, editor. Pediatric regional anesthesia. Boca Raton: CRC Press, Inc.; 1990. p. 459–3.

Suresh S, Polaner DM, Cote CJ. Regional Anesthesia. In: Cote CJ, Lerman J, Anderson BJ, Eds. 5th ed. Philadelphia: WB Saunders; 2013. p. 835–879.

Tsui BC. Paravertebral and intercostal blockade. In: Tsui BC, editor. Atlas of ultrasound and nerve stimulation-guided regional anesthesia. New York: Springer; 2007. p. 257–70.

Intercostal Nerve Blocks

29

Ban C.H. Tsui

Contents

B.C.H. Tsui, Dip Eng, BSc (Math), B Pharm, MSc, MD, FRCPC
Department of Anesthesiology and Pain Medicine,
Stollery Children's Hospital/University of Alberta Hospital,
2-150 Clinical Sciences Building, Edmonton,
AB T6G 2G3, Canada
e-mail: btsui@ualberta.ca

B.C.H. Tsui, S. Suresh (eds.), *Pediatric Atlas of Ultrasound- and Nerve Stimulation-Guided Regional Anesthesia*,
DOI 10.1007/978-0-387-79964-3_29

29.1 Clinical Anatomy

29.1.1 Intercostal Nerves

Figure 13.10 illustrates a transverse section of the hemithorax. Thoracic spinal nerves emerge from the intervertebral (spinal) foramina, between the superior and inferior articulations of the vertebral bodies and ribs. The spinal nerves divide to supply paraspinal muscles and skin of the back (*dorsal ramus*) and the intercostal spaces (*ventral ramus*). The ventral rami of the thoracic spinal nerves form 11 pairs of *intercostal nerves* (T1–T11) for the 11 intercostal spaces (the ventral rami of T1 split into two and the larger branch serves as the brachial plexus) and the *subcostal nerve* (T12), which courses below the 12th rib. The nerves relay and receive information with the ganglia of the paravertebral sympathetic chain through gray and white rami communicantes. The intercostal nerves give off cutaneous branches at the anterior and lateral aspects of the thoracic wall.

Initially, the intercostal nerves run along the dorsal aspect of the intercostal space, between the intercostal membrane and the parietal pleura. From here, they course laterally past the angle of the rib, pierce the internal intercostal membrane, and run between the internal and middle intercostal muscles (also referred to as the innermost and internal intercostal muscles, respectively). Laterally, the nerves give off both collateral (running adjacent to the nerve within the intercostal space) and lateral cutaneous branches, the latter dividing into ventral and dorsal branches. Rather than branching, the second intercostal nerve supplies the intercostobrachial nerve, which innervates the axillary region. As they travel anteriorly, the nerves again contact the parietal pleura before dividing into the anterior cutaneous nerves of the thorax. The tenth intercostal nerve, supplying the umbilical area, travels laterally between the transversus abdominis and the internal oblique muscles and then courses between the rectus sheath and the posterior wall of the rectus abdominis muscle (see Chap. 30). Within each intercostal groove, the nerve runs inferior to the intercostal artery, with the vein located uppermost.

29.1.2 Costovertebral Articulations

The ribs articulate with the vertebral column through two synovial joints (Fig. 13.6). The costovertebral joint is formed by the head of the rib articulating with the demifacets on the adjacent thoracic vertebral bodies and the corresponding intervertebral disk of the upper vertebral joint. The costotransverse joint is formed by the articular facets on the tubercles of the ribs articulating with the transverse processes of the thoracic vertebrae. Ultrasound imaging may help determine the needle puncture point for intercostal nerve block by marking the location of the costotransverse joint.

29.2 Landmark-Based Technique

29.2.1 Patient Positioning

- For unilateral intercostal nerve block, the patient is usually placed in the lateral decubitus position with the upper arm resting on a support.
- For bilateral blockade, the patient may be placed in the prone position or (if conscious) asked to sit. Their arms are draped over the edge of the stretcher or operating table so that the scapula falls away laterally from the midline.
- For anterior blocks, the patient may be supine or sitting.

29.2.2 Landmarks and Surface Anatomy (Fig. 29.1)

- Midaxillary line: This line is drawn longitudinally from the midpoint of the axilla and is used in younger children (younger than 10 years). At this more lateral location, the nerves are separated from the parietal pleura by the internal intercostal muscle.
- Scapular line: This line is drawn downward at the inferior angle of the scapula. The insertion site is immediately medial to the scapula or along the scapular line. This line is more suitable for older children (older than 10 years) and adolescents.
- Ribs: The lower border of each rib marks the needle puncture site for the nerve of the same level.
- Nipples and sternum (anterior block).

Needle insertion typically occurs at the intersection of the midaxillary line (for children <10 years old) or scapular line (for children >10 years old) or immediately medial to the scapula (Fig. 29.1). For the 11th intercostal nerve and the subcostal nerve (T12), the puncture point will be medial to the scapular line, with the length of the corresponding rib determining the point. Although an anterior approach has been described [1], it is rarely indicated and will not be discussed here.

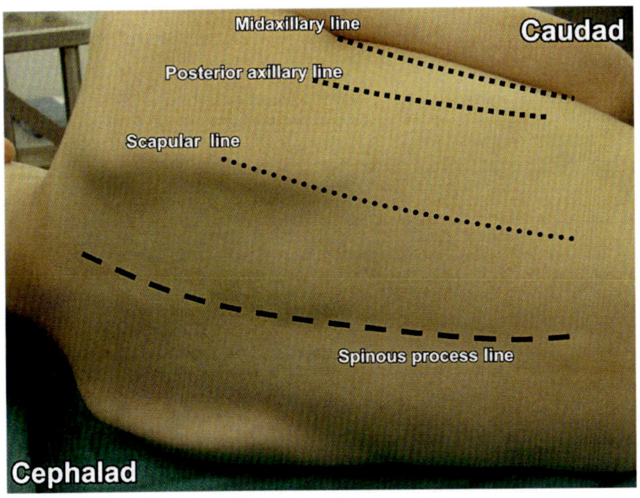

Fig. 29.1 Surface anatomy and needle insertion points for intercostal nerve block

29.2.3 Needle Insertion

- The same procedure will be repeated at all levels to be blocked. Posterior blocks are described here.
- Most anesthesiologists prefer to stand on the side that allows their dominant hand to hold the syringe at the caudal end of the patient.
- A short-beveled needle with a length of no longer than 3 cm should be used to allow maximum appreciation, or "feel," of the tissue resistances and to avoid trauma.
- Generally, 22G–24G needles will be used. A Tuohy needle will allow a catheter to be placed for continuous blocks.
- Plastic tubing should be placed between the needle and syringe containing the local anesthetic solution in order to avoid needle disturbances from chest movements during respiration.
- Starting with the lowest rib, the index finger of the cephalad hand retracts the skin overlying the rib in a cephalad direction.
- With the bevel of the needle directed cephalad, insert the needle, maintaining a constant 20° cephalad angulation.
- After contact is made with the inferior border of the rib, withdraw the needle slightly, and release the cephalad traction slowly.
- The cephalad hand takes over the needle and syringe, and the needle is allowed to "walk down" to below the rib at the same angle.
- Advance the needle slightly (2–3 mm) while maintaining the cephalad angle.
- Maintaining pressure on the syringe will allow a loss of resistance to be felt upon penetration of the intercostal space.

29.2.4 Local Anesthetic Application

- The needle is placed within the intercostal space, inferior to the overlying rib, and after obtaining a negative aspiration test, 0.5–1 mL (depending on the patient) of local anesthetic solution is injected. The lower volume is typically used in patients under the age of three. Since larger volumes may produce a more effective block, the solution should be diluted with normal saline to avoid overdose.
- Since absorption of local anesthetic by the blood is high at the intercostal space, peak plasma levels of local anesthetic are reached after injection, and high toxicity potential exists. To reduce the solution's absorption, the use of epinephrine is advised, although a maximum dose of 4 μg/kg, with typical concentrations of 1:400,000, is used. Incremental injection with frequent aspiration is an additional measure to avoid toxicity.
- A shorter duration block will be achieved when using lidocaine (0.25–1 %), while longer duration (up to 16–18 h) will be attainable with bupivacaine (0.125–0.25 %).

Clinical Pearl

- Despite frequent concern about the incidence of pneumothorax with intercostal blocks, this complication is rare in experienced hands. This depends primarily on maintaining strict safety features of the described technique. Emphasis should be placed on absolute control of the syringe and needle at all times, particularly during injection.

29.3 Nerve Stimulation Technique

Generally, nerve stimulation is not used to confirm nerve localization.

29.4 Ultrasound-Guided Technique

The intercostal space is depicted in the MRI and corresponding ultrasound images in Fig. 29.2.

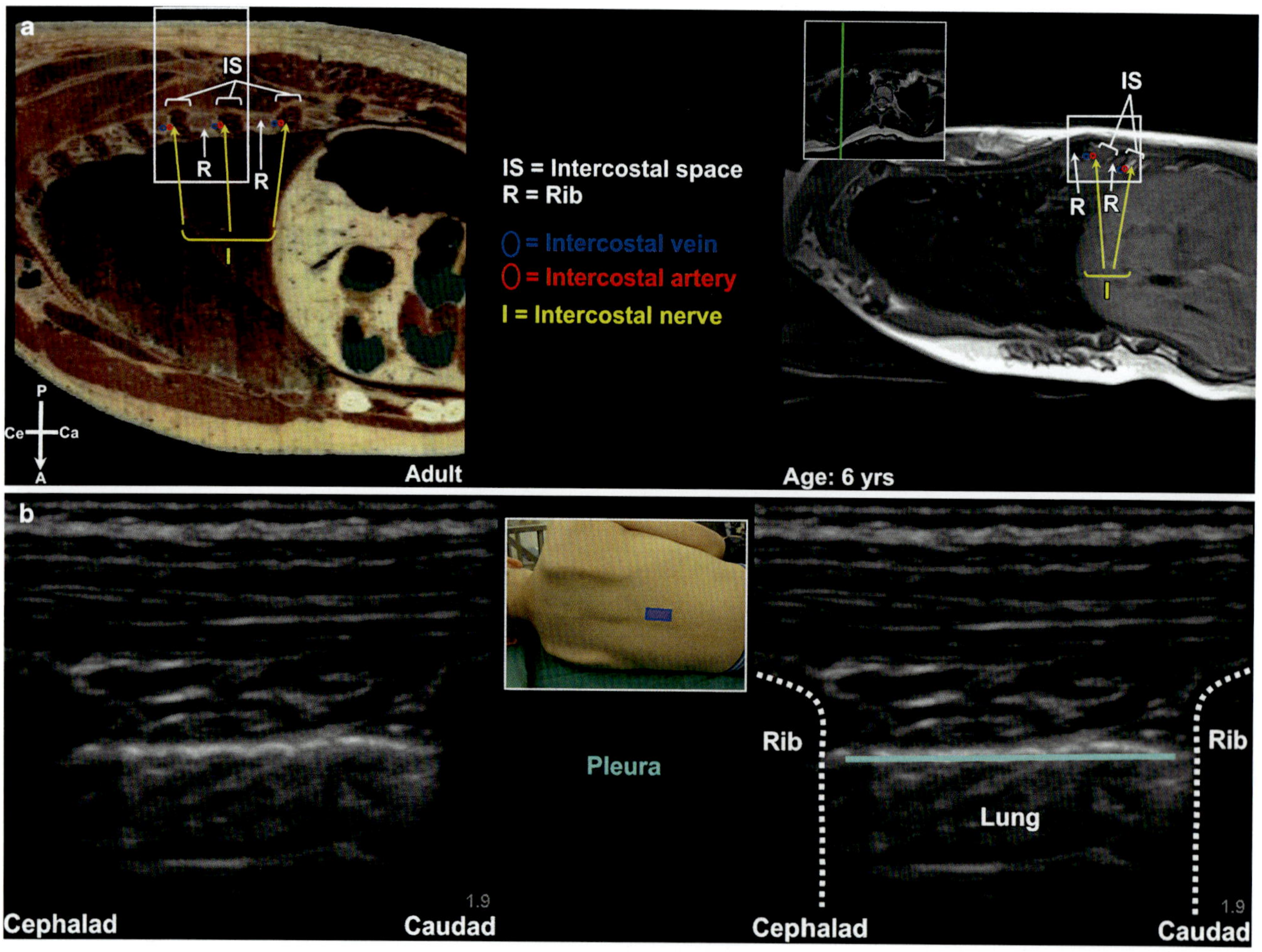

Fig. 29.2 (a) VHVS and MRI images of sagittal section showing the intercostal space. (b) Ultrasound images of sagittal section showing the intercostal space

29.4.1 Scanning Technique

- At each level, place a high-frequency probe perpendicular to the ribs at the appropriate position (mid-axillary line or scapular line or immediately medial to the scapular line) to capture an image of the cephalad and caudal rib and the underlying pleura.

29.4.2 Sonographic Appearance

- The ribs will appear hyperechoic with dorsal shadowing, and the hypoechoic pleural cavity will appear interspersed between and deep to the ribs (Fig. 29.2b).
- When using the M-mode to visualize the intercostal space, the typical "seashore sign" illustrating the position of the pleura and lung tissue can be better appreciated (Fig. 29.3).
- The muscles appear hypoechoic with a pennate pattern.
- The neurovascular space can be difficult to visualize, but the vascular bundle can be made more obvious with color Doppler.

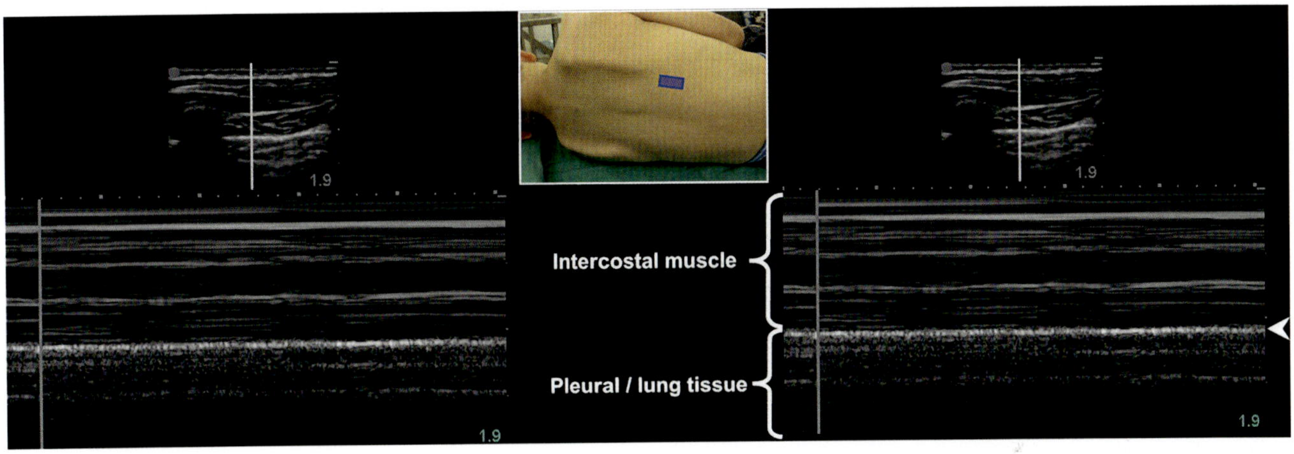

Fig. 29.3 Ultrasound image showing the intercostal space in M-mode. The linear pattern is tissue superficial to the pleura (*arrowhead*). The granular or "sandy" appearance below the pleura is lung tissue; this "seashore sign" indicates normal lung sliding. *Blue rectangle* indicates ultrasound probe footprint

29.4.3 Needle Insertion

- Insert a short-beveled, 22G–24G needle using an OOP alignment to the probe (Fig. 29.4).
- Apply color Doppler to help confirm the location of the intercostal blood vessels.
- Position the needle immediately inferior to the cephalad rib and inferior to the artery.
- For the IP technique, the needle is inserted caudad to the ultrasound probe which is placed in a parasagittal plane. The needle is aimed at the inferior part of the rib, where the neurovascular bundle is situated: between the innermost intercostal membrane and internal intercostal muscle (Fig. 29.5).

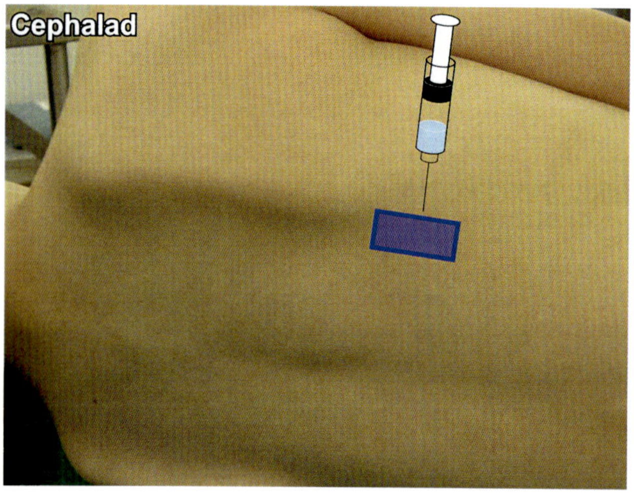

Fig. 29.4 Out-of-plane needling technique for ultrasound-guided intercostal nerve block. *Blue rectangle* indicates probe footprint

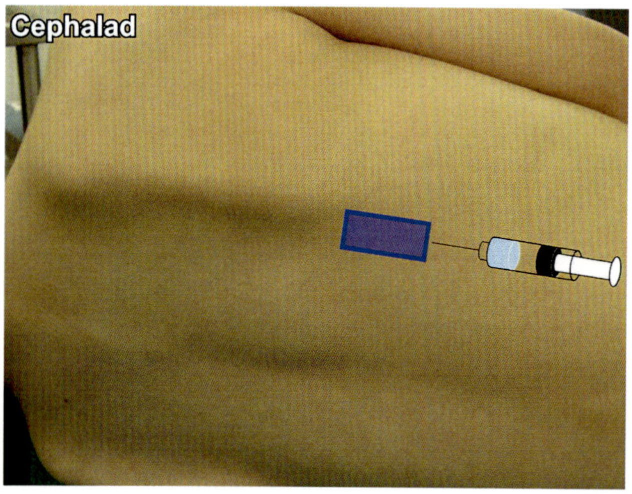

Fig. 29.5 In-plane needling technique for ultrasound-guided intercostal nerve block. *Blue rectangle* indicates probe footprint

29.4.4 Local Anesthetic Application

- Inject 0.5–1 mL of local anesthetic solution into each level, and view the spread between the middle and internal intercostal muscles in the vicinity of the neurovascular space.
- The spread will appear as a small expansion of hypoechogenicity.

29.5 Current Literature in Ultrasound-Guided Approaches

Local anesthetic absorption for intercostal block is the highest of all peripheral blocks due to the area's abundant vascularity. Peak plasma concentration of bupivacaine 0.5 % occurs between 5 and 15 min in children; [2] thus, addition of epinephrine can help slow the systemic absorption.

A retrospective review was performed by Shelly and Park on liver transplant patients who received intercostal blocks [3]. This study showed that children who received intercostal block had much lower opioid requirements than those not receiving intercostal blocks. A prospective study of 20 children (5–12 years) who received intercostal block for thoracotomy also showed improved pain control compared to those maintained on opioids alone [4].

29.6 Case Study

Intercostal Nerve Block (*Contributed by S. Suresh*)

A 6-year-old female, 25.7 kg, presented with arhinia due to congenital anomalies of the skull and face bones. A nasal reconstruction was scheduled using a cartilage graft from the left sixth rib to the nose. A one-view chest X-ray was taken prior to surgery. An in-plane, ultrasound-guided intercostal block was performed using a 22G needle and 3 mL 0.25 % bupivacaine with epinephrine 1:200,000 (see Fig. 29.6). Duration of the surgery was 5 h, 25 min; block duration was 6–8 h.

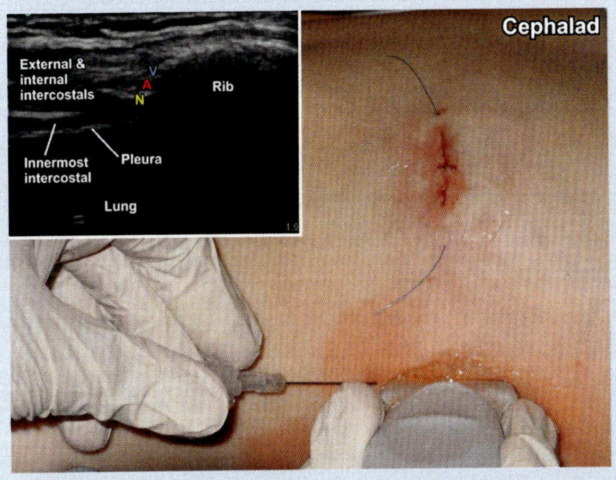

Fig. 29.6 Ultrasound-guided intercostal nerve block. *N* intercostal nerve, *A* intercostal artery, *V* intercostal vein (See "Case Study" for details)

References

1. Dalens B. Regional anesthesia in infants, children, and adolescents. Baltimore: Williams & Wilkins; 1995. p. 464–5.
2. Rothstein P, Arthur GR, Feldman HS, Kopf GS, Covino BG. Bupivacaine for intercostal nerve blocks in children: blood concentrations and pharmacokinetics. Anesth Analg. 1986;65:625–32.
3. Shelly MP, Park GR. Intercostal nerve blockade for children. Anaesthesia. 1987;42:541–4.
4. Matsota P, Livanios S, Marinopoulou E. Intercostal nerve block with bupivacaine for post-thoracotomy pain relief in children. Eur J Pediatr Surg. 2001;11:219–22.

Suggested Reading

Dalens BJ. Blocks of nerves of the trunk. In: Dalens BJ, editor. Pediatric regional anesthesia. Boca Raton: CRC Press; 1990. p. 441–50.

Peutrell JM, Mather SJ. Regional anaesthesia for babies and children. Oxford: Oxford University Press; 1997. p. 117–24.

Suresh S, Polaner DM, Cote CJ. Regional Anesthesia. In: Cote CJ, Lerman J, Anderson BJ, Eds. 5th ed. Philadelphia: WB Saunders; 2013. p. 835–79.

Tsui BC. Paravertebral and intercostal blockade. In: Tsui BC, editor. Atlas of ultrasound and nerve stimulation-guided regional anesthesia. New York: Springer; 2007. p. 257–70.

Rectus Sheath and Transversus Abdominis Plane (TAP) Blocks

30

Bryan J. Dicken and Ban C.H. Tsui

Contents

B.J. Dicken, MSc, MD, FRCSC
Division of Pediatric Surgery, Department of Surgery,
University of Alberta Hospital, Edmonton, AB, Canada
e-mail: bdicken@ualberta.ca

B.C.H. Tsui, Dip Eng, BSc (Math), B Pharm, MSc, MD, FRCPC (✉)
Department of Anesthesiology and Pain Medicine,
Stollery Children's Hospital/University of Alberta Hospital,
2-150 Clinical Sciences Building, Edmonton,
AB T6G 2G3, Canada
e-mail: btsui@ualberta.ca

B.C.H. Tsui, S. Suresh (eds.), *Pediatric Atlas of Ultrasound- and Nerve Stimulation-Guided Regional Anesthesia*,
DOI 10.1007/978-0-387-79964-3_30

30.1 Rectus Sheath Block

30.1.1 Clinical Anatomy

- The anterior abdominal wall is innervated by the inferior seven thoracic nerves (T6–T12) and one lumbar nerve (L1). These nerves travel laterally between the transversus abdominis and the internal oblique muscles and then, at the level of the linea semilunaris (or lateral edge of the rectus abdominis muscle), penetrates the rectus sheath to travel between the posterior wall of the rectus sheath and the rectus abdominis muscle. From there, the nerves penetrate anteriorly through the rectus muscle to innervate the skin.
- The rectus sheath is formed by the aponeuroses of the lateral three abdominal muscles and encloses the rectus abdominis muscle (Fig. 13.9). Bilateral sheaths are joined at the linea alba above the arcuate line. The arcuate line is the horizontal line separating the lower limit of the posterior layer of the rectus sheath, which is derived from the posterior layer of the internal oblique aponeurosis and the transversus abdominal aponeurosis.
- The arcuate line also marks the point where the inferior epigastric vessels are separated by the posterior fascia of the rectus abdominis.
- The posterior wall of the sheath is not attached to muscle, and the area between the rectus abdominis muscle and sheath can be separated for the block.
- The nerve's anterior cutaneous branch, formed as it crosses the rectus muscle, supplies the skin of the umbilical area.
- The rectus sheath block aims to place local anesthetic between the posterior aspect of the rectus sheath and the rectus abdominis muscle. The posterior wall of the sheath is not attached to the muscle and thus can be separated during the block injection (i.e., represents a potential space).

30.1.2 Landmark-Based Technique

30.1.2.1 Patient Positioning

- A supine position is most appropriate for this block.

30.1.2.2 Landmarks and Surface Anatomy (Fig. 30.1)

- Umbilicus
- Linea semilunaris: the lateral edge of the rectus abdominal muscle

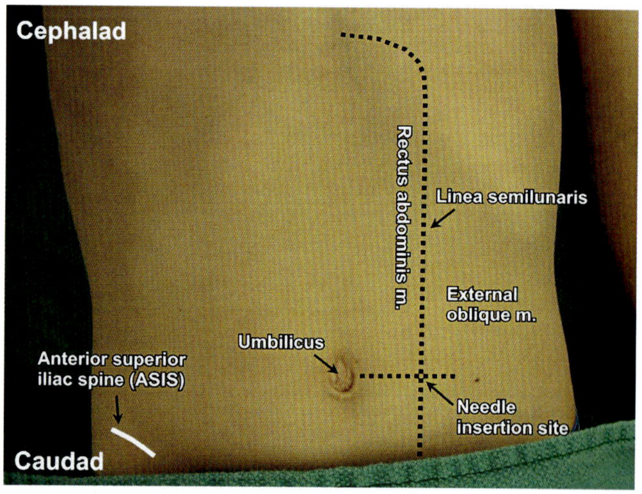

Fig. 30.1 Surface anatomy for rectus sheath block

30.1.2.3 Needle Insertion

- After marking the external layer of the rectus sheath on both sides of the abdomen, insert a short-bevel needle at the point where the outer border of the rectus sheath intersects a horizontal line at the level of the umbilicus.
- Advance the needle 60° to the skin toward the umbilicus until a loss of resistance and a "pop" is felt, indicating puncture of the anterior rectus sheath.
- After injection of local anesthetic on one side, repeat the above steps for the other side.

30.1.2.4 Local Anesthetic Application

- For children up to 7 years of age, 0.2 mL/kg 0.2 % ropivacaine is adequate.
- For older children, 0.2–0.3 mL/kg 0.5 % levobupivacaine should be used.

30.1.3 Ultrasound-Guided Technique

Subcutaneous structures of the rectus sheath at the level of L3–L4 are depicted in the MRI and corresponding ultrasound images in Fig. 30.2.

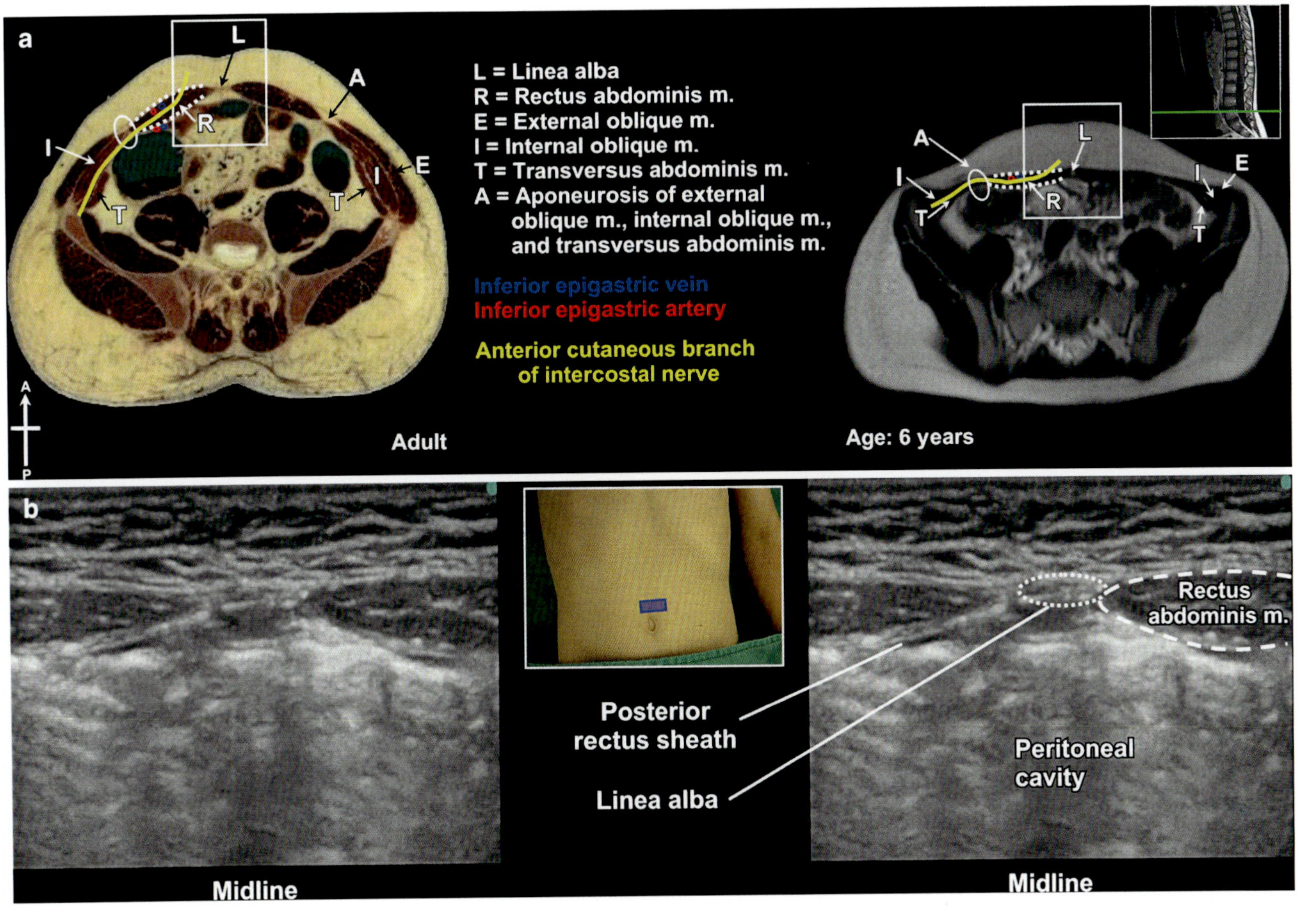

Fig. 30.2 (a) VHVS and MRI images of the abdominal wall, showing the rectus abdominal muscle and the rectus sheath. (b) Ultrasound image of the abdominal wall, showing the rectus abdominal muscle and the rectus sheath

30.1.3.1 Scanning Technique

- Multiple injections are required for a successful rectus sheath block. A typical approach is injection of local anesthetic on either side of the midline at the upper and lower ends of the excision for a total of four needle insertion points.
- A linear (6–15 MHz) transducer is placed in a transverse location on the anterior abdominal wall lateral to the proposed incision site.
- The required depth for penetration is usually 2–4 cm but varies with the depth of the subcutaneous layer.

30.1.3.2 Ultrasonographic Appearance (Fig. 30.2b)

- At the midline, the hyperechoic linea alba is seen between the belly of the rectus muscle on either side. The most superficial layer is subcutaneous fat.
- The peritoneum is seen behind the posterior rectus sheath.
- The muscles of the lateral abdominal wall (external oblique, internal oblique, and transversus abdominis, from superficial to deep) are seen lateral to the rectus muscle.
- The internal oblique muscle is on the same plane as the rectus muscle, and they are separated by the aponeurosis of the internal oblique.
- The target nerves are not visible. They course between internal oblique and transversus abdominis before piercing the posterior rectus sheath to traverse the belly of the rectus muscle.
- The target for injection is the lateral gutter between the posterior rectus sheath and the rectus muscle.
- The inferior epigastric vessels run through the rectus muscle. They may be seen if the Doppler function is utilized (Fig. 30.3). It is important to avoid puncturing or injecting local anesthetic into these vessels.

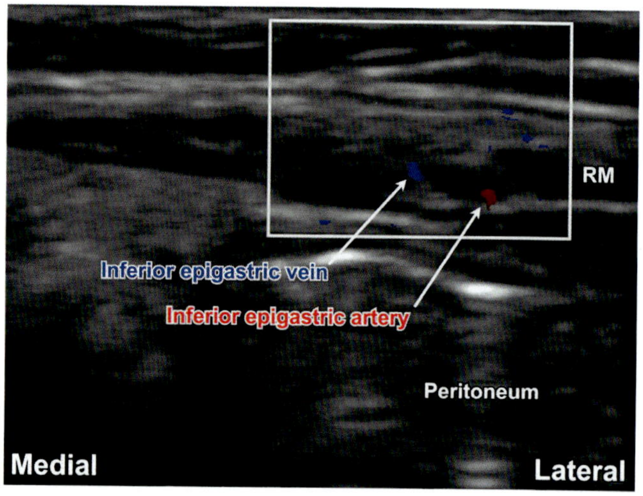

Fig. 30.3 Doppler ultrasound image showing location of inferior epigastric vessels in the rectus muscle (*RM*)

30.1.3.3 Needle Insertion

- Depending on subcutaneous fat depth, use a 4–10 cm, 22G needle.
- An in-plane (IP) approach is used (Fig. 30.4).
- Intermittent injection with D5W is recommended to confirm needle tip position.
- The needle is inserted from lateral to medial. To avoid puncturing the inferior epigastric vessels, a lateral needle insertion point is chosen. The needle is directed through the external and internal oblique muscles into the lateral gutter of the rectus muscle directly superficial to the posterior rectus sheath. Using this approach, the needle does not enter the belly of the rectus muscle and thereby avoids the inferior epigastric vessels.
- Needle tip position may be confirmed by injection of 1–2 mL D5W.

30.1.3.4 Local Anesthetic Application

- Performing a test dose with D5W is recommended prior to local anesthetic application to visualize the spread and confirm needle tip localization.
- Inject 0.2 mL/kg 0.2 % ropivacaine, 0.25 % bupivacaine, or 0.5 % bupivacaine on each side.
- The local anesthetic should be seen to spread between the posterior rectus sheath and the rectus muscle.

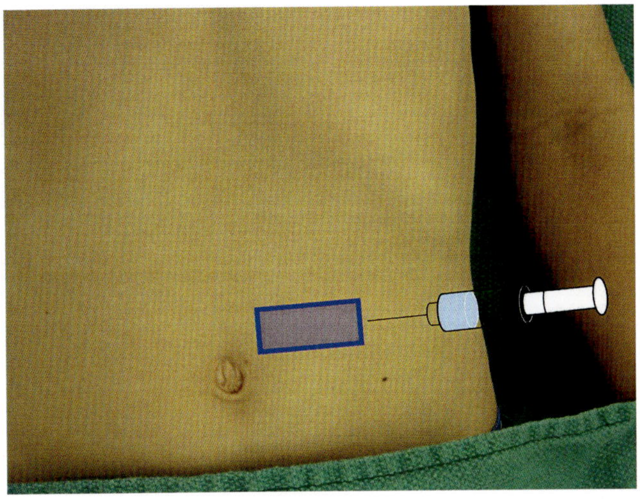

Fig. 30.4 In-plane needling technique for ultrasound-guided rectus sheath block. *Blue rectangle* indicates probe footprint

30.1.4 Current Literature in Ultrasound-Guided Approaches

For rectus sheath block, the probe is placed over the linea semilunaris (at the lateral aspect of the rectus abdominis muscle) at a level beneath the umbilicus, and the lateral edge of the rectus muscle is positioned at the edge of the screen. The posterior wall of the sheath may be poorly defined at locations caudad to the umbilicus (i.e., below the arcuate line) [1]. The peritoneum appears thick with a hyperechoic border beneath the muscles.

Willschke et al. described their approach for ultrasound-guided rectus sheath block in the clinical portion of their two-part study evaluating the sonoanatomy and clinical feasibility of this block [2]. They stated that their injection site was situated at the location where an optimal view of the posterior sheath was obtained. A short-beveled needle (e.g., 22G, 40 mm with facet tip) was inserted using an out-of-plane approach at the inferior edge of a linear hockey stick probe, using an angle most suitable for the depth of the sheath. The needle tip was placed just between the posterior rectus sheath and the posterior aspect of the rectus abdominis muscle. After negative aspiration (for epigastric vessel puncture), local anesthetic solution was injected; expansion of the space between the sheath and posterior aspect of the rectus muscle denoted proper placement of the needle.

The median depth of the posterior sheath in 30 children was 8.0 mm (range 5–13.8); moreover, there was poor correlation between the depth of the posterior rectus sheath and weight, height, or body surface area [3]. With the sheath's proximity to the peritoneum and without the possibility of reliable estimations or calculations of optimal needle depth, ultrasound imaging during the block is especially useful. It is also important to note that the posterior wall of the sheath is poorly defined below the arcuate line [1]. Placing the needle more lateral, and thus potentially avoiding puncture into the peritoneum, the umbilical nerve block targets the region lateral to the sheath where the nerves exit from their course between the transversus abdominis and internal oblique abdominal muscles.

Two recent studies compared ultrasound-guided rectus sheath block to the traditional method of local anesthetic infiltration for pain control during umbilical hernia repair. Both demonstrated a reduction in consumption of postoperative opioid and non-opioid analgesia in the rectus sheath block group [4, 5]. Gurnaney et al. [5] showed no difference in time to rescue analgesia between the groups, and Dingeman et al. [4] showed that postoperative pain scores were lower with the ultrasound-guided block. These studies' findings are supported by a case series of ultrasound-guided rectus sheath block for umbilical hernia repair which showed that patients receiving the block consumed less opioid analgesia in the post-op recovery unit [6]. These results also contrast those of a prior study [7] that did not use ultrasound to guide needle placement, suggesting that improved accuracy leads to more successful blocks.

30.1.4.1 Umbilical Nerve Block

For umbilical hernia repair, an umbilical nerve block can be performed. The scanning field of view should be increased to include the medial aspect of the lateral abdominal muscles and the region where their aponeuroses join to form the rectus sheath. Laterally, the lateral abdominal muscles may be delineated with oblique hyperechoic lines separating them. The external oblique abdominal muscle lies outermost, overlying the internal oblique abdominal and transversus abdominis muscles. The thick rectus abdominis muscle can be identified medially, as can the rectus sheath, formed by the aponeurosis of the transversus abdominis muscle and internal and external oblique abdominal muscles. The intercostal nerve(s) will likely not be visualized by ultrasound imaging. The nerves are small and run longitudinally, thus tangential, to the probe [1]. The hyperechoic and linear appearance of the nerves will closely resemble the aponeurosis of the musculature in this region.

De Jose Maria et al. [1] have described their approach to an ultrasound-guided umbilical nerve block. The probe (10 MHz frequency) was placed where a line between the tenth intercostal space and the umbilicus intersects the rectus abdominis muscle. They rotated the probe between transverse and longitudinal planes in order to obtain a good view clearly delineating the musculature and rectus sheath. The longitudinal plane was used during the block, and the ideal position of the probe was that which best captured the formation of the rectus sheath, by the aponeuroses of the transversus abdominis and internal oblique abdominal muscles. The needle was inserted using an in-plane approach to place the tip close to the lateral edge of the rectus muscle and between the aponeurosis of the abdominal muscles. The local anesthetic spread was observed behind the rectus abdominis muscle and under the internal oblique abdominal muscle.

30.1.4.2 Outcome Evaluation for Blocks at the Anterior Trunk

Earlier reports of the rectus sheath block, using "blind" techniques, describe successful blocks as performed in small numbers of patients [8, 9]. Using ultrasound guidance for rectus sheath blocks in 20 children, Willschke et al. reported a 100 % success rate for intra- and postoperative analgesia (until time to discharge at 4 h), using (predetermined volumes in their study) lower doses of local anesthetics (i.e., levobupivacaine 0.25 % 0.1 mL/kg versus bupivacaine 0.5 % 0.2 mL/kg) than previously described when using "blind" technique with the same injection protocol [3, 9]. Similar doses of local anesthetic have been used for the umbilical nerve block as those for the ultrasound-guided rectus sheath block (i.e., bupivacaine 0.25 % 0.1 mL/kg) [1].

30.1.5 Case Study

Rectus Sheath Block (*Provided By A. Spencer*)

A 4-year-old girl, 16 kg, presented for same-day repair of epigastric hernia. The patient underwent a general anesthetic combined with an ultrasound-guided periumbilical nerve block in line with the umbilicus (correlating with thoracic tenth dermatome level). A 22G 40 mm, B-beveled needle was inserted in-plane, and 3.5 mL ropivacaine 0.25 % with epinephrine was deposited bilaterally below the rectus abdominis muscle and posterior fascia (equivalent to 0.2 mL/kg per side) (Fig. 30.5). An additional 0.5 mL was injected into the aponeurosis adjoining the rectus abdominis muscle to the external and internal oblique and transversus abdominis muscles. Block duration was 6–12 h; time of surgery was 1 h 10 min.

Acetaminophen 15 mg/kg po liquid was administered preoperatively, and ketorolac 0.3 mg/kg was given perioperatively; no morphine was given during the case. The patient was comfortable in recovery 30 and 60 min post-op. No additional analgesia was required in the recovery room or on the day surgery ward prior to going home.

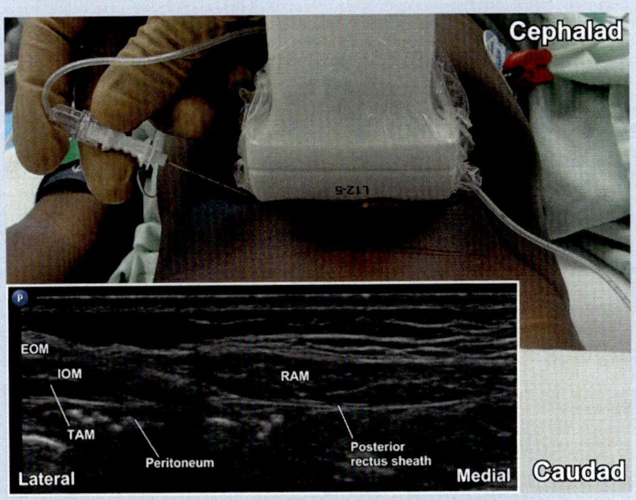

Fig. 30.5 Ultrasound-guided rectus sheath block. *EOM* external oblique muscle, *IOM* internal oblique muscle, *TAM* transversus abdominis muscle, *RAM* rectus abdominis muscle. See Case Study for details

30.2 Transversus Abdominis Plane (TAP) Block

30.2.1 Clinical Anatomy

- The sensory innervation of the abdominal wall is derived from anterior divisions of the thoracolumbar nerves (T6–L1).
- T6–T11 begin as intercostal nerves; T12 is the subcostal nerve; L1 is the ilioinguinal and iliohypogastric nerve.
- The thoracolumbar nerve roots exit the space that is bordered between the latissimus dorsi posteriorly and the transversus abdominis anteriorly, within the "lumbar triangle of Petit."
- There are often extensive anastomoses involving the segmental nerves that emerge from the costal margin, such that they rapidly lose their segmental origin [10].
- The intercostal nerves, subcostal nerves, and the first lumbar nerves run in a neurovascular plane known as the transversus abdominis plane (TAP) (Fig. 13.9).
- The TAP is situated between the internal oblique and transversus abdominis muscles; the plane allows adequate spread of local anesthetic.

30.2.2 Landmark-Based Technique

30.2.2.1 Patient Positioning

- The patient may be supine or lateral.
- When performing the block on an awake patient, it may be convenient to use a lateral position, which will increase exposure to the posterior axillary line and permit a more posterior approach.

30.2.2.2 Landmarks and Surface Anatomy

- Iliac crest
- Costal margin
- Triangle of Petit:
  - A weakness in the lateral abdominal wall that can be palpated when performing a landmark technique. Its base is the iliac crest, and it is bordered anteriorly by the external oblique muscle and posteriorly by latissimus dorsi (Fig. 30.6).

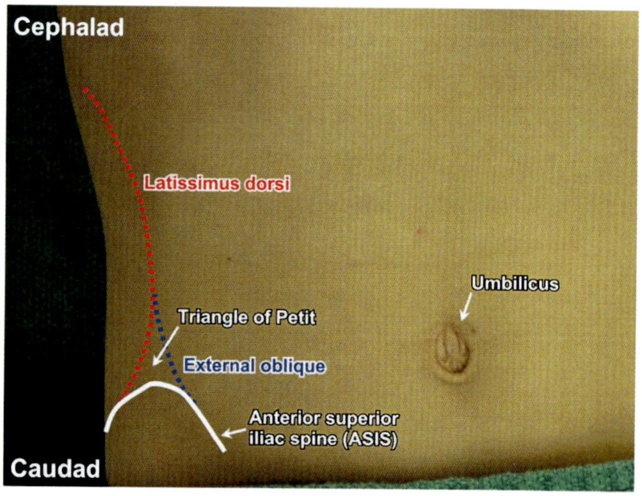

Fig. 30.6 Surface anatomy of transversus abdominis plane block showing the triangle of Petit landmark

30.2.2.3 Needle Insertion

- A blunt needle is recommended to facilitate easier detection of loss of resistance as the needle penetrates the external and internal oblique muscles.
- Insert the needle through the triangle of Petit, just anterior to the point at which the latissimus dorsi attaches to the external lip of the iliac crest, until the needle contacts the iliac crest. A "pop" may be felt as the needle passes through the external oblique muscle.
- The needle can then be "walked off" the iliac crest until an obvious "pop" is felt as the needle punctures the internal oblique muscle. The needle is now in the plane between the internal oblique and transversus abdominis muscles where the local anesthetic is to be injected.
- The above steps can be repeated for the other side of the abdomen.

30.2.2.4 Local Anesthetic Application

- For each side, 0.2–0.3 mL/kg of 0.25 % bupivacaine or 0.2 % ropivacaine can be used.
- Total dose of either drug should not exceed 3 mg/kg.

30.2.3 Ultrasound-Guided Technique

The abdominal wall with the associated musculature and rectus sheath is depicted in the MRI and corresponding ultrasound images in Fig. 30.7.

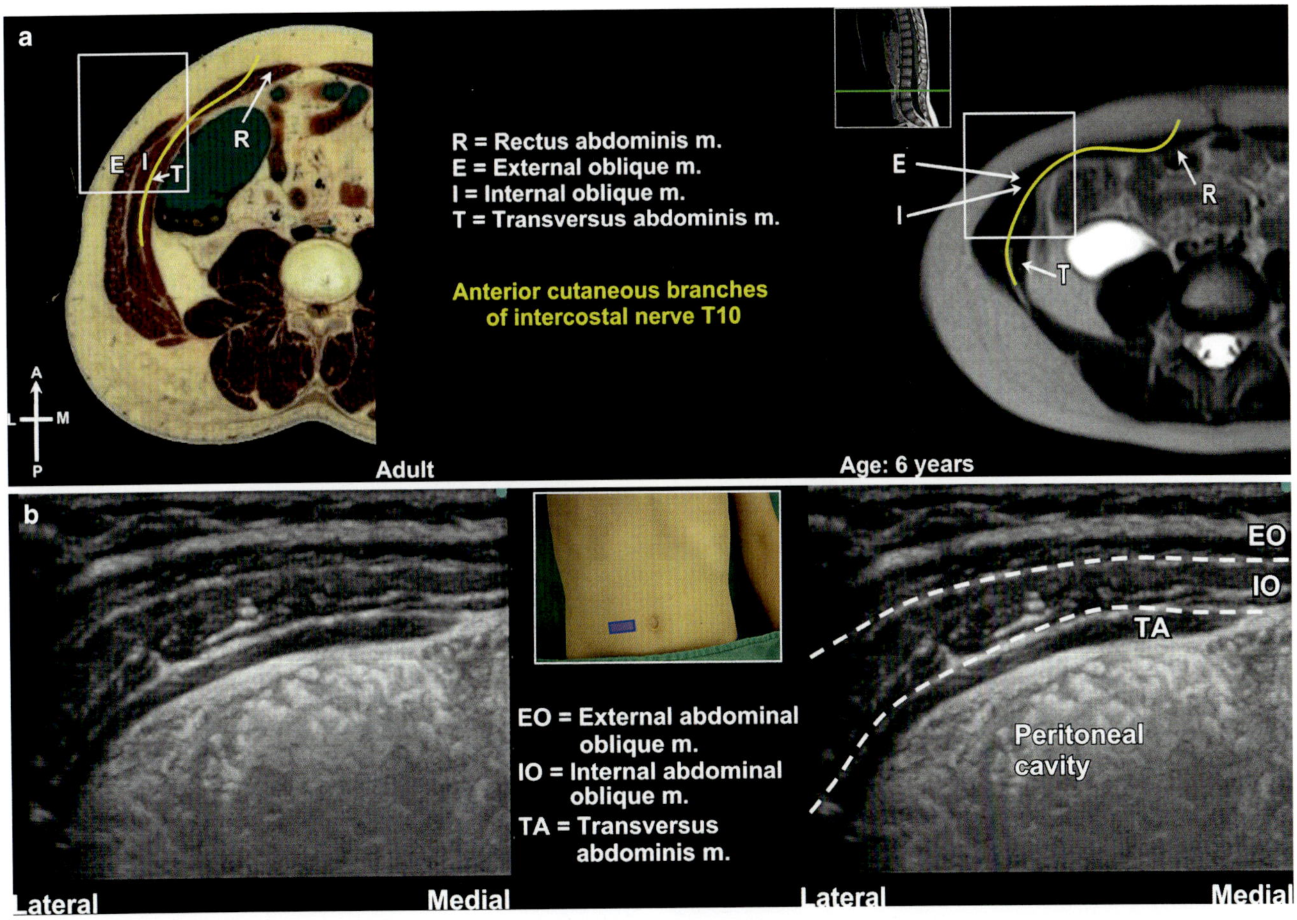

Fig. 30.7 (a) VHVS and MRI images showing the three layers of the lateral abdominal muscles. (b) Ultrasound image showing the three layers of the lateral abdominal muscles

30.2.3.1 Scanning Technique

- A linear (6–15 MHz) transducer is placed in a transverse location on the midaxillary line between the iliac crest and the costal margin.
- A curved probe may be used in obese patients, but the resultant image may be more challenging to interpret.
- The required depth for penetration is usually 2–4 cm but varies with the depth of the subcutaneous layer.
- The individual muscle layers may be difficult to identify; however, the internal oblique muscle is always the widest, and it is important to identify the superficial subcutaneous layer.

30.2.3.2 Ultrasonographic Appearance

- The nerves might not be visible; the target for injection is the fascial plane (TAP) which the nerves traverse.
- Three muscle layers can be seen, above which lies the subcutaneous fat (not to be mistaken for a muscle layer) and below which lies the peritoneum, peritoneal cavity, and loops of intestine (Fig. 30.7b).
- The most superficial layer is subcutaneous fat. This has a mostly hypoechoic appearance with occasional hyperechoic striations running through it.
- The muscle layers from superficial to deep are external oblique, internal oblique, and transversus abdominis muscles. They have a much greater hyperechogenic appearance than the superficial subcutaneous layer.
- The internal oblique muscle is the widest layer, and the transversus abdominis muscle is the thinnest.
- Each muscle layer is separated by a distinct hyperechoic fascial plane. The TAP separates the internal oblique from the transversus abdominis muscle.
- The transversalis fascia lies deep to the transversus abdominis muscle. The peritoneum is adherent to the transversalis fascia. The peritoneal cavity and intestines lie beneath this fascia.

30.2.3.3 Needle Insertion

- Depending on skin-to-TAP distance, use a 5- to 10 cm, 22G needle.
- Most commonly, an in-plane (IP) approach (Fig. 30.8) is used. The out-of-plane (OOP) approach (Fig. 30.9) is rarely used since it is difficult to visualize the needle tip due to the target depth. Intermittent injection with D5W is recommended to confirm needle tip position in this instance.
- For an IP approach, the needle is inserted 3–4 cm from the medial aspect of the probe and typically directed in a medial-to-lateral fashion at anterior axillary line, although some experts have also used a lateral-to-medial approach. This insertion point permits greater visibility as the needle is more parallel to the transducer. Because of the target depth, an insertion point close to the transducer surface would necessitate a steeper angle of approach and poor needle visibility.
  - A distinct "pop" may be felt as the needle penetrates the fascial planes. The needle tip position may be confirmed by injection of 1–2 mL of D5W.
- For the OOP approach, the ultrasound probe is placed in the same location as for the IP technique. The needle is then inserted in a cephalad-to-caudad direction. Due to the depth of the transverse abdominis plane, using a "walk-down" approach (see Chap. 4) is essential to avoid intraperitoneal needle insertion.

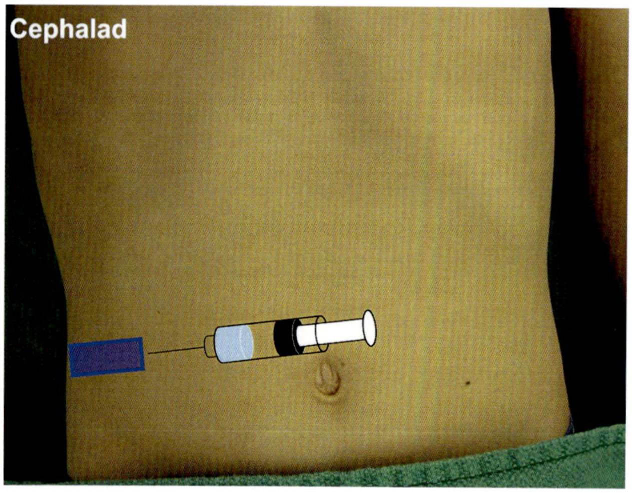

Fig. 30.8 In-plane needling technique for ultrasound-guided transversus abdominis plane block. *Blue rectangle* indicates probe footprint

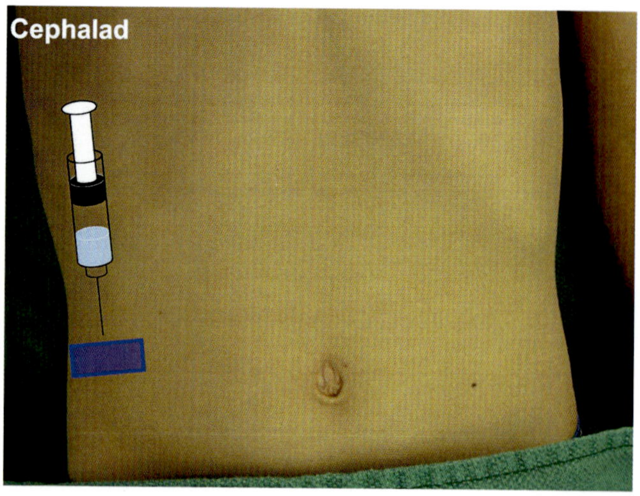

Fig. 30.9 Out-of-plane needling technique for ultrasound-guided transversus abdominis plane block. *Blue rectangle* indicates probe footprint

30.2.3.4 Local Anesthetic Application

- Performing a test dose with D5W is recommended prior to local anesthetic application to visualize the spread and confirm needle tip localization.
- 0.2–0.3 mL/kg of local anesthetic, (e.g., 0.2 % ropivacaine or 0.25 % bupivacaine) is injected per side.
- The correct response to injection is longitudinal spread of the hypoechoic-appearing local anesthetic within the TAP. Injection with the internal oblique or transversus abdominis muscles requires repositioning of the needle.

30.2.4 Catheter Placement Under Direct Visualization (Fig. 30.10)

An alternative to landmark- and ultrasound-guided placement of a TAP catheter(s) is placement under direct vision by the surgeon at the end of the procedure:

- Following closure of the transversus abdominis and rectus abdominis muscle layers, the catheter is inserted percutaneously through the abdominal wall cephalad to the incision at the lateral border of the transversus abdominis muscle.
- The catheter is inserted in a medial-to-lateral direction, and the catheter tip is positioned at the most lateral point of the incision.
- After full closure of the incision in three separate layers (transversus abdominis, internal oblique, external oblique), the catheter is affixed to the skin.
- Both unilateral and bilateral TAP catheters may be placed using this technique.
- The advantages of this approach include:
  - Familiarity of the surgeon with the anatomy of the abdominal wall musculature enables accuracy in catheter placement and positioning.
  - Removes the ambiguity of whether the fascial plane between the internal oblique and transversus abdominis muscles has been penetrated, [10] as is sometimes the case with landmark- and ultrasound-guided approaches.
  - Reduces significantly the risk of iatrogenic damage caused by advancement of the needle using blind or ultrasound-guided approaches.

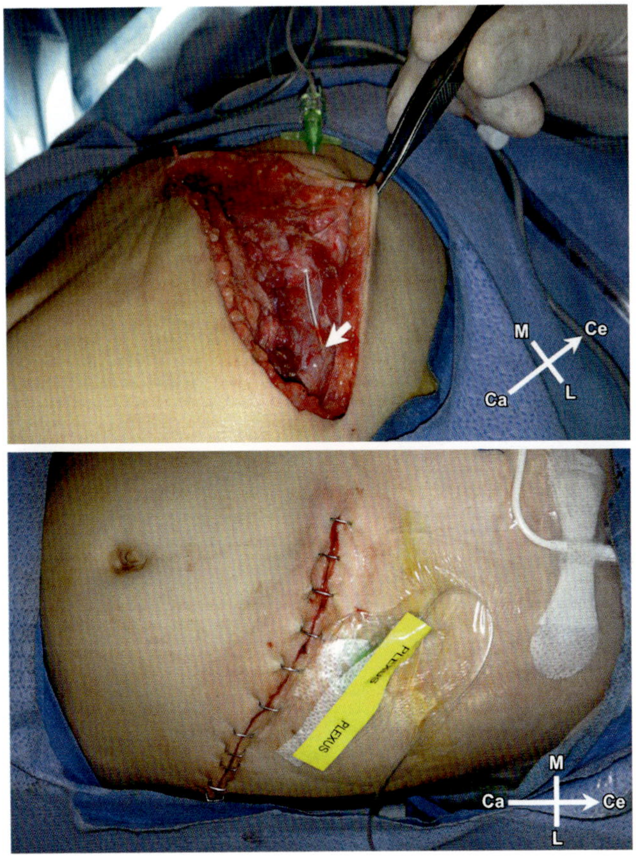

Fig. 30.10 Placement of a transversus abdominis plane catheter under direct visualization. The *top panel* shows placement of the catheter tip at the lateral point of the incision (*arrow*); *bottom panel* shows securement of the catheter following closure of the surgical site

30.2.5 Current Literature in Ultrasound-Guided Approaches

Mai et al. [11] recently published a comprehensive review of the use of TAP block in the pediatric population, including history, complications, and outcomes of published reports. Laghari et al. were first to describe an approach to performing an ultrasound-guided TAP block in children [12]. In a 9-year-old girl, these authors used an out-of-plane needle alignment to a linear probe placed in the flank above the iliac crest. The needle (21G, 50 mm insulated) was placed approximately 2 cm above the highest point of the iliac crest and directed cranially using a shallow angle. The needle was advanced until its tip was viewed in the TAP, thus between the transverse and internal oblique abdominal muscles. Local anesthetic was injected incrementally, and the spread was observed within the plane. No intraoperative analgesia was required, and excellent pain scores (0/10) were recorded soon after the open appendectomy. A simple technique for placement of the TAP block in infants and children has since been described with a step-by-step approach to performing this block in infants and children [13].

Fredrickson et al. [14] have described their early experience with TAP block under ultrasound guidance. They placed a linear probe in the axial plane above the iliac crest, or at a location where the three lateral abdominal muscle layers were most evident on the ultrasound screen. An in-plane needle alignment was used, with the needle (a short 22G spinal needle) directed from anterior to posterior to allow the needle to be viewed along its axis. Upon viewing the needle tip in the TAP, the local anesthetic was injected while observing the spread within the plane. The blocks were successful, with the exception of those patients who required intraoperative opioid supplementation due to spermatic cord manipulation (genitofemoral nerve). Following this report, the successful use of ultrasound-guided TAP blocks in neonates was demonstrated [15–17]. A recent audit of the use of ultrasound-guided TAP blocks, both unilateral and bilateral and for various surgeries, confirms the block's efficacy in controlling postoperative pain in neonates and infants [18].

Taylor et al. [19] published a report of two cases in which TAP catheters were installed under ultrasound guidance in children with a history of significant spina bifida. Both children underwent appendicovesicostomy and received bilateral TAP catheters through which a continuous infusion of bupivacaine was delivered. Pain control was excellent for both patients, and neither required supplementary analgesics during the postoperative period. A later case series described the use of TAP catheters installed under ultrasound guidance in low-weight (<15 kg) children in whom epidural anesthesia was contraindicated [20]. In these cases, all blocks were successful, with no adverse events reported.

Simpson et al. [21] described a case in which ultrasound-guided TAP block was administered for chronic pain associated with anterior cutaneous nerve entrapment syndrome (ANCES) in a 13-year-old patient. Bilateral TAP blocks were performed with a 22G needle inserted in-plane; 20 mL bupivacaine 0.25 % with 1:400,000 epinephrine was injected. Patient pain scores improved, and after 6 weeks, another set of TAP blocks was administered, extending pain relief for another month.

More recently, Sandeman et al. [22] showed that patients receiving ultrasound-guided TAP block for laparoscopic appendectomy reported reduced postoperative pain scores compared to patients not receiving a block. However, this study did not find a significant difference in time to first analgesia after surgery or opioid consumption. These results contrast those obtained by Elshaikh et al. and Sahin et al. [23, 24] which demonstrated significant reductions in pain scores and perioperative opioid consumption, as well as an increase in time to first analgesia, in patients receiving ultrasound-guided TAP blocks versus a control group which received systemic opioids for pain control. As an added benefit, the TAP group experienced less incidence of vomiting compared to the opioid group.

An observational study by Palmer et al. [25] studied the multilevel block properties of ultrasound-guided TAP block. Although pediatric guidelines have recommended TAP block for upper and lower abdominal surgeries [13], Palmer et al. found that only a quarter of patients experienced upper abdominal block extension. No significant correlation was found between dermatomal spread and local anesthetic dose, volume, or concentration.

Recently, the Pediatric Regional Anesthesia Network queried their database to provide information on complications, including puncture of vasculature/peritoneum/organs, pulmonary and/or neurological symptoms, hematoma, and infection, following TAP block [26]. A total of 1994 cases were assessed, of which, only two had complications. More concerning was the finding that a relatively wide range of doses (0.47–2.29 mg bupivacaine equivalents per kg) were used, with around 7 % of patients receiving potentially toxic doses. This survey reveals that, while TAP blocks have a relatively low incidence of complications in pediatric patients, care should be taken in determining dosing, with attention paid to avoiding delivery of a potentially toxic dose.

The TAP block provides analgesia to the abdominal wall, through blockade of the lower thoracic and first lumbar spinal nerves at the lateral aspect of the abdomen prior to their course between the transversus abdominis and internal oblique abdominal muscles. In adults, there may be reliance on palpating the "lumbar triangle of Petit" at the base of which lies the internal oblique muscle [27]. Because there is no distinctly palpable triangle of Petit in children (or one only enabling sensation of a tiny hole), ultrasound may be especially valuable for determining the point of needle puncture during this block. Indications for the TAP block include postoperative pain control following abdominal surgery including colostomy and laparotomy especially when a central neuraxial block is contraindicated as in children with spinal dysraphism (neural tube defect) or in children with coagulation abnormalities. Since this block includes blockade of the first lumbar nerve root, it may substitute the ilioinguinal/iliohypogastric block in cases when the region anterior and medial to the ASIS offers suboptimal imaging; the muscles in this region are apparently prone to anisotropy (i.e., artifactual images produced due to the beam penetration angle in relation to the muscles) [14].

30.2.6 Case Study

Transversus Abdominis Plane Block (*Provided By S. Suresh*)
A male toddler, 35 months old and weighing 13.5 kg, presented for laparoscopic gastrostomy tube insertion. The patient had a history of cystic fibrosis without mention of meconium ileus and failure to thrive and had previously undergone an X-ray of the upper gastrointestinal tract. An ultrasound-guided transversus abdominis plane block was performed using a 27G needle with an in-plane approach (see Fig. 30.11). Eight milliliters 0.25 % bupivacaine with 1:200,000 epinephrine was injected. Duration of surgery was 1 h, and block duration was 6 h. At 45 min post-op, the patient reported 5/10 for pain on the FLACC scale. A 7 mg injection of ketorolac (Toradol) was given 1 h post-op.

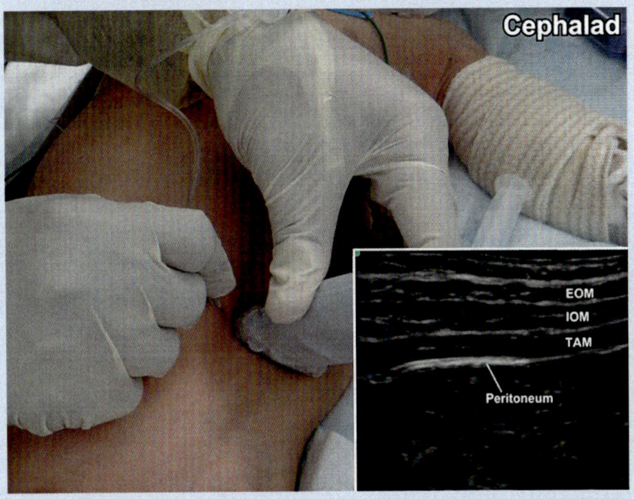

Fig. 30.11 Ultrasound-guided transversus abdominis plane block. *EOM* external oblique muscle, *IOM* internal oblique muscle, *TAM* transversus abdominis muscle (See Case Study for details)

References

1. de Jose MB, Gotzens V, Mabrok M. Ultrasound-guided umbilical nerve block in children: a brief description of a new approach. Pediatr Anesth. 2007;17:44–50.
2. Willschke H, Bosenberg A, Marhofer P, Johnston S, Kettner SC, Wanzel O, Kapral S. Ultrasonography-guided rectus sheath block in paediatric anaesthesia–a new approach to an old technique. Br J Anaesth. 2006;97:244–9.
3. Willschke H, Bosenberg A, Marhofer P, Johnston S, Kettner S, Eichenberger U, Wanzel O, Kapral S. Ultrasonographic-guided ilioinguinal/iliohypogastric nerve block in pediatric anesthesia: what is the optimal volume? Anesth Analg. 2006;102:1680–4.
4. Dingeman RS, Barus LM, Chung HK, Clendenin DJ, Lee CS, Tracy S, Johnson VM, Dennett KV, Zurakowski D, Chen C. Ultrasonography-guided bilateral rectus sheath block vs local anesthetic infiltration after pediatric umbilical hernia repair: a prospective randomized clinical trial. JAMA Surg. 2013;148:707–13.
5. Gurnaney HG, Maxwell LG, Kraemer FW, Goebel T, Nance ML, Ganesh A. Prospective randomized observer-blinded study comparing the analgesic efficacy of ultrasound-guided rectus sheath block and local anaesthetic infiltration for umbilical hernia repair. Br J Anaesth. 2011;107:790–5.
6. Alsaeed AH, Thallaj A, Khalil N, Almutaq N, Aljazaeri A. Ultrasound-guided rectus sheath block in children with umbilical hernia: case series. Saudi J Anaesth. 2013;7:432–5.
7. Isaac LA, McEwen J, Hayes JA, Crawford MW. A pilot study of the rectus sheath block for pain control after umbilical hernia repair. Pediatr Anesth. 2006;16:406–9.
8. Courreges P, Poddevin F, Lecoutre D. Para-umbilical block: a new concept for regional anaesthesia in children. Pediatr Anesth. 1997;7:211–4.
9. Ferguson S, Thomas V, Lewis I. The rectus sheath block in paediatric anaesthesia: new indications for an old technique? Pediatr Anesth. 1996;6:463–6.
10. Rozen WM, Tran TM, Ashton MW, Barrington MJ, Ivanusic JJ, Taylor GI. Refining the course of the thoracolumbar nerves: a new understanding of the innervation of the anterior abdominal wall. Clin Anat. 2008;21:325–33.
11. Mai CL, Young MJ, Quraishi SA. Clinical implications of the transversus abdominis plane block in pediatric anesthesia. Pediatr Anesth. 2012;22:831–40.
12. Laghari ZA, Harmon D. Ultrasound-guided transabdominus plane block. J Clin Anesth. 2008;20:156–8.
13. Suresh S, Chan VW. Ultrasound guided transversus abdominis plane block in infants, children and adolescents: a simple procedural guidance for their performance. Pediatr Anesth. 2009;19:296–9.
14. Fredrickson M, Seal P, Houghton J. Early experience with the transversus abdominis plane block in children. Pediatr Anesth. 2008;18:891–2.
15. Fredrickson MJ, Seal P. Ultrasound-guided transversus abdominis plane block for neonatal abdominal surgery. Anaesth Intensive Care. 2009;37:469–72.
16. Jacobs A, Thies KC. Ultrasound-guided transversus abdominis plane block for reversal of ileostomy in a 2-kg premature neonate. Pediatr Anesth. 2009;19:1237–8.
17. Tekin M, Gurkan Y, Solak M, Toker K. Ultrasound-guided bilateral transversus abdominis plane block in a 2-month-old infant. J Anesth. 2009;23:643–4.
18. Jacobs A, Bergmans E, Arul GS, Thies KC. The transversus abdominis plane (TAP) block in neonates and infants – results of an audit. Pediatr Anesth. 2011;21:1078–80.
19. Taylor LJ, Birmingham P, Yerkes E, Suresh S. Children with spinal dysraphism: transversus abdominis plane (TAP) catheters to the rescue! Pediatr Anesth. 2010;20:951–4.
20. Visoiu M, Boretsky KR, Goyal G, Cladis FP, Cassara A. Postoperative analgesia via transversus abdominis plane (TAP) catheter for small weight children-our initial experience. Pediatr Anesth. 2012;22:281–4.
21. Simpson DM, Tyrrell J, De RJ, Campbell FA. Use of ultrasound-guided subcostal transversus abdominis plane blocks in a pediatric patient with chronic abdominal wall pain. Pediatr Anesth. 2011;21:88–90.
22. Sandeman DJ, Bennett M, Dilley AV, Perczuk A, Lim S, Kelly KJ. Ultrasound-guided transversus abdominis plane blocks for laparoscopic appendicectomy in children: a prospective randomized trial. Br J Anaesth. 2011;106:882–6.
23. Elshaikh SM, Abdel Halim JMK, El-Awady GA, Saad A. Effects of preoperative ultrasonography-guided TAP block in pediatric patients undergoing major abdominal surgeries for intraabdominal malignancies on surgical outcome and postoperative analgesia. Egypt J Anaesth. 2009;25:335–43.
24. Sahin L, Sahin M, Gul R, Saricicek V, Isikay N. Ultrasound-guided transversus abdominis plane block in children: a randomised comparison with wound infiltration. Eur J Anaesthesiol. 2013;30:409–14.
25. Palmer GM, Luk VH, Smith KR, Prentice EK. Audit of initial use of the ultrasound-guided transversus abdominis plane block in children. Anaesth Intensive Care. 2011;39:279–86.
26. Long JB, Birmingham PK, De Oliveira GS Jr, Schaldenbrand KM, Suresh S. Transversus abdominis plane block in children: a multicenter safety analysis of 1994 cases from the PRAN (Pediatric Regional Anesthesia Network) database. Anesth Analg 2014;119:395–9.
27. Rafi AN. Abdominal field block: a new approach via the lumbar triangle. Anaesthesia. 2001;56:1024–6.

Suggested Reading

Bhalla T, Sawardekar A, Dewhirst E, Jagannathan N, Tobias JD. Ultrasound-guided trunk and core blocks in infants and children. J Anesth. 2013;27:109–23.

Karmakar MK, Kwok WH. Ultrasound-Guided Regional Anesthesia. In: Cote CJ, Lerman J, Anderson BJ, Eds. 5th ed. Philadelphia: WB Saunders; 2013. p. 880–908.

Ilioinguinal and Iliohypogastric Nerve Blocks

31

Ban C.H. Tsui

Contents

B.C.H. Tsui, Dip Eng, BSc (Math), B Pharm, MSc, MD, FRCPC
Department of Anesthesiology and Pain Medicine,
Stollery Children's Hospital/University of Alberta Hospital,
2-150 Clinical Sciences Building, Edmonton,
AB T6G 2G3, Canada
e-mail: btsui@ualberta.ca

B.C.H. Tsui, S. Suresh (eds.), *Pediatric Atlas of Ultrasound- and Nerve Stimulation-Guided Regional Anesthesia*,
DOI 10.1007/978-0-387-79964-3_31

31.1 Clinical Anatomy

- The ilioinguinal and iliohypogastric nerves are both extensions of the anterior rami of the L1 segmental nerve (Figs. 11.2 and 11.4).
- The nerves represent the most inferior spinal level of the segmental innervation of the body wall. Below L1, the anterior rami contribute to the lumbar and sacral plexuses to supply the lower limb, buttocks, and perianal region.
- Both nerves pass laterally on the quadratus lumborum muscle where they pierce the transversus abdominis to enter the transversus abdominis plane (TAP) between the transversus abdominis and internal oblique muscles.
- The iliohypogastric nerve continues within the TAP plane to segmentally supply the suprapubic skin, subcutaneous tissue, and muscles of the lower abdominal wall (Fig. 13.8). It also gives a lateral cutaneous branch which leaves the TAP at the iliac crest to supply the skin over the upper buttock behind where the T12 subcostal nerve provides cutaneous supply.
- The ilioinguinal nerve passes anteriorly in the TAP until it pierces the internal oblique at the superficial inguinal ring to lie on the spermatic cord or round ligament. It supplies the ipsilateral penile base, hemiscrotum, and a small area of medial thigh below the inguinal ligament.

31.2 Landmark-Based Technique (Fascial "Click" Method)

31.2.1 Patient Positioning

- The block is most easily performed with the patient supine.

31.2.2 Landmarks and Surface Anatomy

- Anterior superior iliac spine (ASIS): follow the iliac crest anteriorly to lateral abdomen and palpate the prominent spine.
- Umbilicus

31.2.3 Needle Insertion

There are several recommendations for determining the puncture point for needle insertion. Different sites may also necessitate variation in needle puncture angle. Low success rates may be attributed to anatomic variability or the needle puncture being too medial [1].

- The traditional puncture site places the needle above the ASIS at a point one-fourth, or sometimes one-third, of the way from the lateral aspect of a line between the ASIS and the umbilicus (Fig. 31.1); however, as Van Shoor et al. [1] suggested, this point may be too medial for most patients and instead recommend that the puncture point be just 2.5 mm from the ASIS on the above mentioned line (Fig. 31.1).
- Alternatively, the puncture site is considered at a point one fingerbreadth (of the patient) medial and inferior to the ASIS (the lower range for infants and young children) [2, 3].
- In a study of ultrasonographic imaging during ilioinguinal block, the ilioinguinal nerve was situated between 5 and 11.3 mm from the ASIS, depending on the weight of the child, although there was no significant correlation between weight and this distance [4].
- Any one of these points may be suitable, although in general, there is much variation in the nerves' locations, and ultrasound guidance is recommended for optimizing localization.
- A 3–4 cm, short-beveled or facet tipped, 22G–27G needle is inserted at a 45° angle to the midline at the puncture point (2.5 mm along the line between the ASIS and the umbilicus) until the characteristic "click" is detected after internal oblique muscle penetration.
- However, the author prefers to insert the needle perpendicularly at only one patient's fingerbreadth medial to the ASIS; this technique should reduce the risk of inadvertent bowel perforation.
- Although two "clicks" may be experienced upon crossing the external and internal oblique muscles, one "click" is often detected. In many patients, the external oblique muscle has already turned into an aponeurosis at this level.

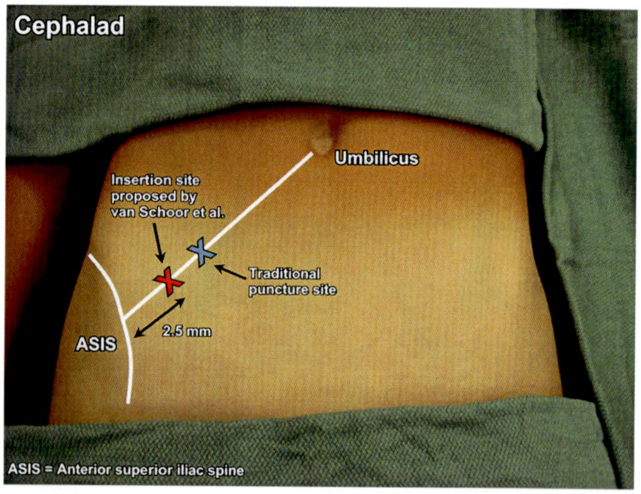

Fig. 31.1 Surface anatomy for ilioinguinal nerve block

31.2.4 Local Anesthetic Application

- Ensure negative aspiration prior to injecting local anesthetic.
- Inject local anesthetic (typically 0.3–0.5 mL/kg of 0.25 % levobupivacaine or 0.5 % bupivacaine when using "blind" technique) after detecting the fascial "click" upon penetration of the internal oblique muscle. A fanlike injection pattern, with both cephalad (toward the umbilicus) and caudad (toward the groin) directions, has been described.
- Alternatively, this author prefers to maintain the needle perpendicular to the skin while injecting one-third of the local anesthetic injection upon feeling the second "click" (internal oblique fascia), withdrawing the needle slightly and injecting another one-third above this layer, and then withdrawing slightly again and injecting the remaining one-third above the first "click" (external oblique fascia).
- An initial injection of some of the local anesthetic may be performed subcutaneously prior to advancing the needle to the intermuscular plane.
- Upon withdrawal of the needle, an additional 0.5–1 mL is deposited subcutaneously to ensure blockade of the iliohypogastric nerve.

31.3 Nerve Stimulation Technique

Nerve stimulation is not commonly performed for ilioinguinal nerve blocks.

31.4 Ultrasound-Guided Technique

The ilioinguinal nerve and surrounding musculature are depicted in the MRI and corresponding ultrasound images in Fig. 31.2. Prepare the needle insertion site and skin surface with antiseptic solution. Prepare the ultrasound probe surface by applying a sterile adhesive dressing to it prior to needling as discussed in Chap. 4.

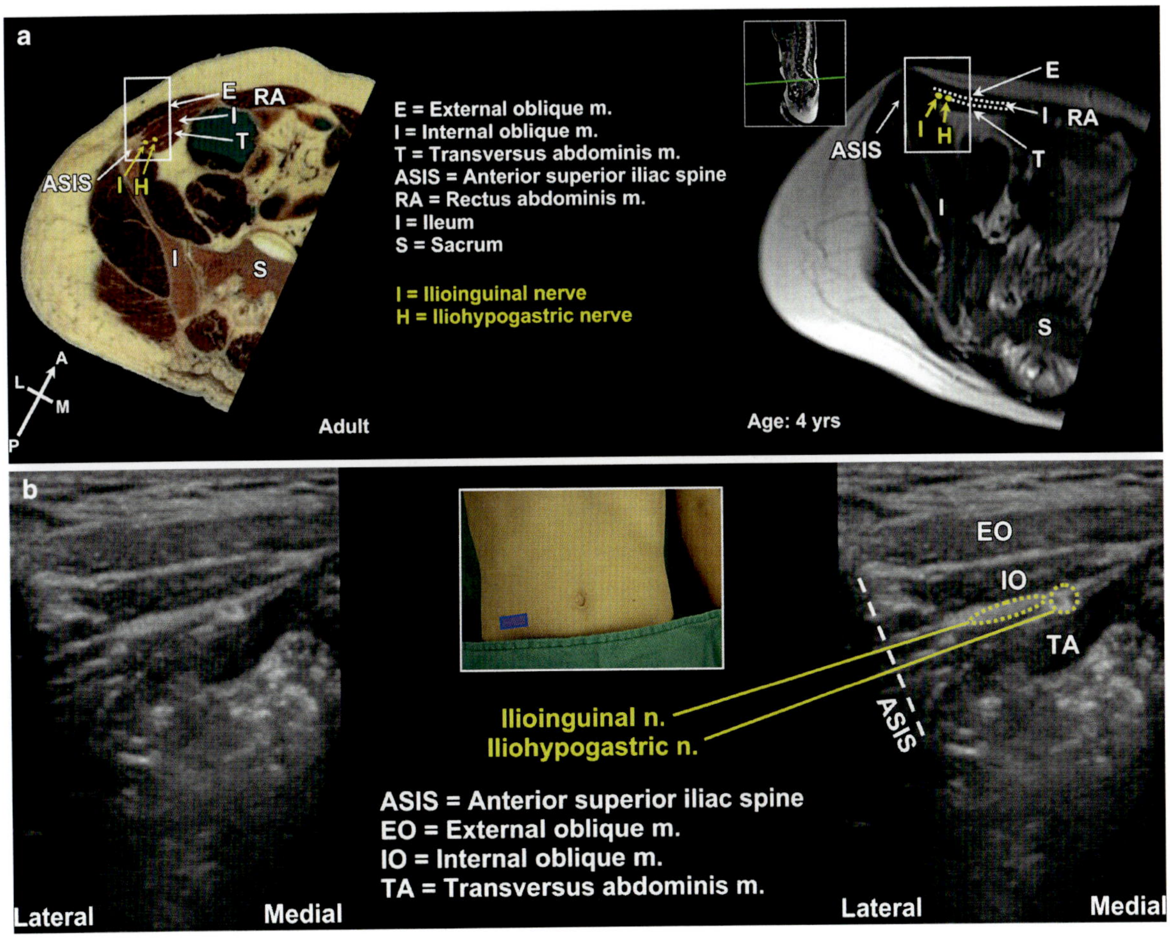

Fig. 31.2 (**a**) VHVS and MRI images showing the ilioinguinal nerve and surrounding musculature. (**b**) Ultrasound images showing the ilioinguinal nerve and surrounding musculature

31.4.1 Scanning Technique

- A linear (6–15 MHz) transducer is placed in an oblique location parallel to a line connecting the ASIS to the umbilicus.
- A curved probe may be used in obese patients, but the muscle and fascial layers will likely be more difficult to appreciate.
- The required depth for penetration is usually 1–4 cm but varies with the depth of the subcutaneous layer.
- The layers of the abdominal wall and underlying muscles, as well as bone and target nerves, should be able to be identified in children.

31.4.2 Ultrasonographic Appearance

- The layers of the abdominal wall should be visible, namely: skin, adipose tissue, external and internal oblique and transversus abdominis, peritoneum, and underlying bowel. The iliacus muscle and the ilium will be visible deeper to the working depth.
- The external oblique may in 50 % of patients be aponeurotic in this location [4].
- If the spermatic cord or round ligament is visible, then the probe is too medial and distal.
- The ilioinguinal and iliohypogastric nerves are usually in proximity to each other.
- The ilioinguinal and iliohypogastric nerves will be visible in children either between the external oblique and internal oblique or between the internal oblique and transversus abdominis muscle. The nerves are likely to much more difficult to appreciate in adults but may become more visible by using some fluid as contrast.
- Color flow Doppler may assist in identifying the neurovascular bundle; however, it is often too small to visualize.
- The endpoint for the block is to surround the identified ilioinguinal and iliohypogastric nerves with local anesthetic. Alternatively, if the nerves are not visible, for example, in adults or obese children, place local anesthetic in the TAP plane as well as the plane between the internal and external oblique muscles.

31.4.3 Needle Insertion

- Needle length will depend upon the adiposity of the patient. A 5–10 cm, short-beveled 22G needle or an 18G Tuohy needle should be utilized.
- Either an in-plane (IP) (Fig. 31.3) or out-of-plane (OOP) (Fig. 31.4) approach may be utilized. However, if the target is deep, the needle tip will be difficult visualize in an OOP approach. Intermittent injection with D5W is recommended to confirm needle tip position in this instance.
- For an IP approach, the needle is inserted at a shallow angle at the lateral end of the probe. The planes are often very shallow so that the needle is more parallel to the transducer.
- This angle of insertion has the advantage that if the needle inadvertently passes too deep, then either the iliacus muscle or ilium will likely be contacted and not the bowel.
- A distinct "pop" will usually be felt on passage through the fascial planes, as well as distinct "tenting" of the tissues on imaging. Needle tip position may be confirmed by injection of 1–2 mL of D5W.
- For the OOP approach, the ultrasound probe is placed in an oblique position along a line joining the ASIS and umbilicus. The needle should be inserted equidistant to the depth of the target nerve caudad or cephalad to the probe at a 45° angle, such that the needle tip can be visualized as it approaches the nerve.

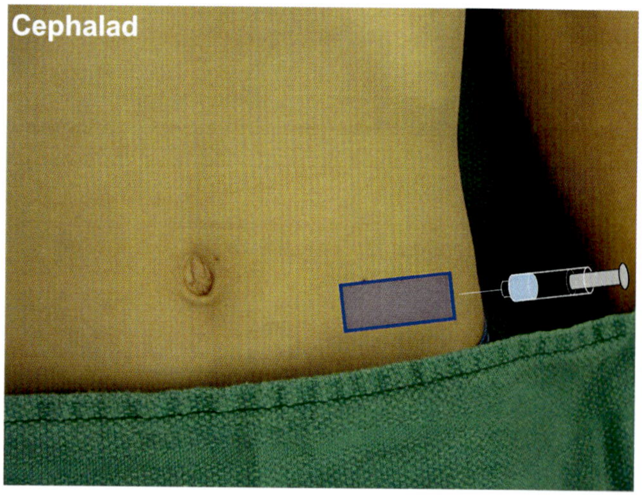

Fig. 31.3 In-plane needling technique for ultrasound-guided ilioinguinal/iliohypogastric nerve block. *Blue rectangle* indicates probe footprint

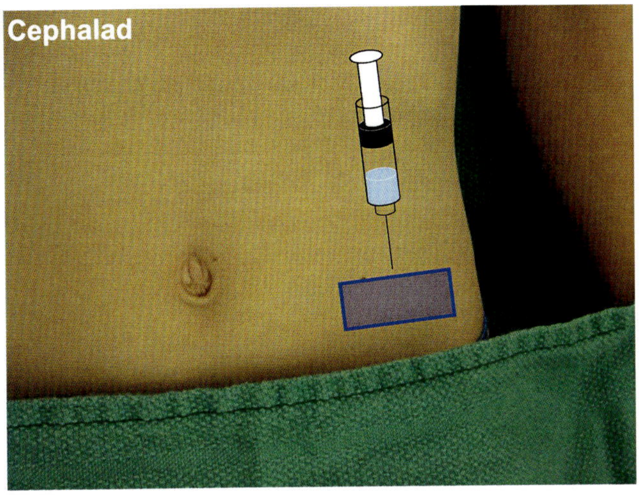

Fig. 31.4 Out-of-plane needling technique for ultrasound-guided ilioinguinal/iliohypogastric nerve block. *Blue rectangle* indicates probe footprint

31.4.4 Local Anesthetic Application

- Performing a test dose with D5W is recommended prior to local anesthetic application to visualize the spread and confirm needle tip localization.
- 10 mL of 0.25 % bupivacaine or 0.2 % ropivacaine surrounding the nerves (0.3–0.5 mL/kg in children) or 0.2 mL/kg in the TAP and 0.2 mL/kg between the external and internal oblique muscles if the nerves are not visible.
- The correct appearance is to have the hyperechoic nerves surrounded with hypoechoic local anesthetic. If intramuscular injection is evident, then the needle should be repositioned.

Clinical Pearls

- The probe may be positioned slightly obliquely toward the umbilicus for better visualization of the ilioinguinal and iliohypogastric nerves as they traverse down distally.
- When using an IP approach, a medial-to-lateral technique is preferred since the needle tip will be aiming toward the bony ASIS. Conversely, a lateral-to-medial technique will direct the needle toward the peritoneum.
- The authors have found it equally effective to use a landmark technique in which the needle is inserted perpendicularly at only one patient's fingerbreadth medial to the ASIS. While maintaining the needle perpendicular to skin, local anesthetic is injected as described in 31.2.4. Using this approach, the risk of inadvertent bowel perforation should be minimal.

31.5 Current Literature in Ultrasound-Guided Approaches

Willschke et al. [4] performed a prospective, randomized double-blinded study with 100 children scheduled for inguinal surgery to compare block efficacy between ultrasound-guided and conventional ilioinguinal/iliohypogastric nerve block. The endpoint in the ultrasound group was capturing a view of the local anesthetic solution surrounding the nerves. Detection of a fascial "click" was used to indicate injection in the traditional block group. Fewer children received intra- or postoperative (up to 4 h) analgesia in the ultrasound group (4 % and 6 %, respectively) than in the fascial click group (26 and 40 %). Furthermore, the volume of local anesthetic injected was lower in the ultrasound group (0.19 mL/kg versus 0.30 mL/kg).

Further evaluation of the optimal volume of local anesthetic required for ultrasound-guided ilioinguinal/iliohypogastric blocks was performed by this group in a subsequent study [5]. Using a modified step-up-step-down approach, with ten patients in each group starting at 0.2 mL/kg, a volume of 0.75 mL/kg was found to achieve 100 % block success for the first 4 h of postoperative care (longer analgesia may require higher volumes). These authors state that using lower volumes of local anesthetic could reduce the risk of local anesthetic toxicity and the incidence of adverse side effects, such as femoral nerve palsy.

Recent findings tend to support the use of lower volumes of local anesthetic when placing ilioinguinal blocks under ultrasound guidance, compared to the landmark-based technique [6]. In a pharmacokinetic study, plasma levels of ropivacaine were found to be higher using ultrasound guidance in comparison to a single "pop" technique (C_{max}: 1.78 [0.62] versus 1.23 [0.70] μg/mL). Although this finding is interesting and will likely encourage the planning of similar studies, the plasma levels reached in this study have never been associated with any clinical signs of toxicity.

Hong et al. [7] studied anatomical location of the ilioinguinal and iliohypogastric nerves in children of various age groups and attempted to examine whether a correlation exists between age and distance between the nerves and the ASIS. They found that ASIS-ilioinguinal distance correlated positively with age and ASIS-umbilicus distance, while ASIS-iliohypogastric distance correlated positively with age and ASIS-pubis distance. No correlations were made between distances and height or weight nor were any correlations detected between age and depth of nerves from the skin or distance from nerves to peritoneum.

Fredrickson et al. [8] recently tested the theory that ultrasound-guided TAP block could be used in place of the more common ultrasound-guided ilioinguinal block for pain control following pediatric inguinal surgery. The authors found that reporting of pain and oral analgesic intake was higher in the TAP group, suggesting that ilioinguinal blocks provide superior pain control for this procedure. However, ultrasound image quality was deemed better for the TAP blocks, and needle time under the skin was significantly greater for the ilioinguinal block group. Ultrasound-guided ilioinguinal blocks can also be given to enhance postoperative pain relief in children who receive caudal block for groin surgeries, particularly inguinal hernia repair.

31.6 Case Study

Ilioinguinal Nerve Block (*Provided by S. Suresh*)

A 7-year-old female, 20 kg, with no past medical history or relevant family history was presented for right inguinal hernia repair. An ilioinguinal block was performed under ultrasound guidance. Ten mL 0.125 % bupivacaine (epinephrine 1:200,000) was injected with a 22G needle (Fig. 31.5). Duration of the block was 6–12 h; surgery lasted 54 min. Pain control in recovery was reported at 0/10 (verbal) 1 h following the operation. Postoperative analgesia included acetaminophen (Tylenol), 240 mg orally (every 6 h as needed), and hydrocodone-acetaminophen 3–200 mg orally (every 6 h as needed).

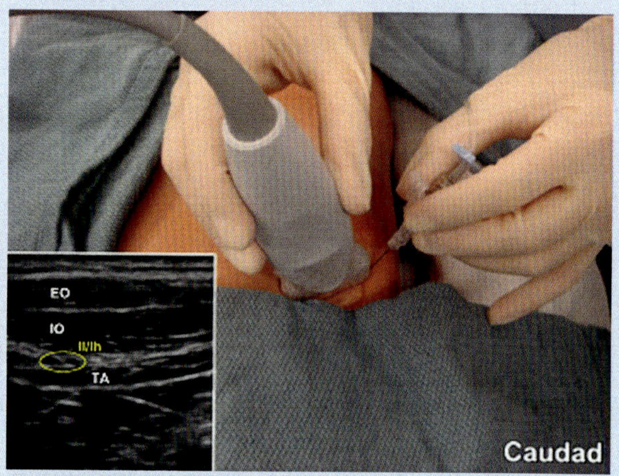

Fig. 31.5 Ultrasound-guided ilioinguinal/iliohypogastric nerve block. *EO* external oblique, *IO* internal oblique, *Il/Ih* ilioinguinal/iliohypogastric nerves, *TA* transversus abdominis muscle (See Case Study for details)

References

1. van Schoor AN, Boon JM, Bosenberg AT, et al. Anatomical considerations of the pediatric ilioinguinal/iliohypogastric nerve block. Pediatr Anesth. 2005;15:371–7.
2. Schulte-Steinberg O. Ilioinguinal and iliohypogastric nerve block. In: Saint-Maurice C, Schulte-Steinberg O, Armitage EN, editors. Regional anesthesia in children. Norwalk: Appleton & Lange; 1990. p. 156.
3. Sethna NF, Berde CB. Pediatric regional anesthesia. In: Gregory GA, editor. Pediatric anesthesia. New York: Churchill Livingston; 1989. p. 647–78.
4. Willschke H, Marhofer P, Bosenberg A, et al. Ultrasonography for ilioinguinal/iliohypogastric nerve blocks in children. Br J Anaesth. 2005;95:226–30.
5. Willschke H, Bosenberg A, Marhofer P, et al. Ultrasonographic-guided ilioinguinal/iliohypogastric nerve block in pediatric anesthesia: what is the optimal volume? Anesth Analg. 2006;102:1680–4.
6. Weintraud M, Lundblad M, Kettner SC, et al. Ultrasound versus landmark-based technique for ilioinguinal-iliohypogastric nerve blockade in children: the implications on plasma levels of ropivacaine. Anesth Analg. 2009;108:1488–92.
7. Hong JY, Kim WO, Koo BN, et al. The relative position of ilioinguinal and iliohypogastric nerves in different age groups of pediatric patients. Acta Anaesthesiol Scand. 2010;54:566–70.
8. Fredrickson MJ, Paine C, Hamill J. Improved analgesia with the ilioinguinal block compared to the transversus abdominis plane block after pediatric inguinal surgery: a prospective randomized trial. Pediatr Anesth. 2010;20:1022–7.

Suggested Reading

Dalens BJ. Blocks of nerves of the trunk. In: Dalens BJ, editor. Pediatric regional anesthesia. Boca Raton: CRC Press; 1990. p. 476–9.

Karmakar MK, Kwok WH. Ultrasound-Guided Regional Anesthesia. In: Cote CJ, Lerman J, Anderson BJ, Eds. 5th ed. Philadelphia: WB Saunders; 2013. p. 880–908.

Suresh S, Polaner DM, Cote CJ. Regional Anesthesia. In: Cote CJ, Lerman J, Anderson BJ, Eds. 5th ed. Philadelphia: WB Saunders; 2013. p. 835–79.

32 Penile Blocks

Heather Yizhen Z. Ting, Peter D. Metcalfe, and Ban C.H. Tsui

Contents

H.Y.Z. Ting, MD, FRCPC (✉)
Department of Anesthesiology and Pain Medicine,
University of Alberta Hospital, 8440-112 St NW, 2-150 Clinical Sciences Building, Edmonton, AB, Canada
e-mail: yizhenhe@ualberta.ca

P.D. Metcalfe, MD, MSc, FRCSC
Division of Pediatric Surgery, Division of Urology,
Department of Surgery, Stollery Children's Hospital,
University of Alberta Hospital, Edmonton, AB, Canada
e-mail: pmetcalf@ualberta.ca

B.C.H. Tsui, Dip Eng, BSc (Math), B Pharm, MSc, MD, FRCPC
Department of Anesthesiology and Pain Medicine,
Stollery Children's Hospital/University of Alberta Hospital,
2-150 Clinical Sciences Building, Edmonton,
AB T6G 2G3, Canada
e-mail: btsui@ualberta.ca

B.C.H. Tsui, S. Suresh (eds.), *Pediatric Atlas of Ultrasound- and Nerve Stimulation-Guided Regional Anesthesia*,
DOI 10.1007/978-0-387-79964-3_32

32.1 Clinical Anatomy

- The penis is supplied mainly by the two dorsal nerves of the penis, although there is some contribution to the base of the penis from the perineal, genitofemoral, and ilioinguinal nerves.
- The pudendal nerves (S2-S4) originate from the sacral plexus (Figure 12.1). At the distal pudendal canal where they run into ischial fossa, the pudendal nerves give off the inferior hemorrhoidal nerve and then divide into two terminal branches: (1) the perineal nerve which supplies the perineal muscles and scrotum, and (2) the dorsal nerve of the penis.
- The dorsal nerves (terminal branches of pudendal nerve; S2-S4) enter the subpubic space, pass under the pubic bone, and then lie deep in the suspensory ligament of the penis. The dorsal nerves then accompany the dorsal arteries of the penis bilaterally, in contact with the corpus cavernosum, encased by Buck's fascia (Figs. 32.1 and 32.2).
- From the base of the penis, the dorsal nerves divide several times and encircle the shaft of the penis before reaching the glans penis.
- The two dorsal nerves are usually blocked separately due to an often present anteroposterior septum (fundiform ligament) at the level of the suspensory ligament of the penis, which divides the subpubic space into two compartments.
- Two fascia envelop the penis; the superficial fascia of the penis, a continuation from the superficial fascia of the abdomen, and the deep layer (Buck's fascia), surrounding all three cavernous bodies, and which is continuous with Scarpa's fascia.
- The subpubic space is bordered anteriorly by the skin, subcutaneous tissue, the superficial fascia, and deep (Scarpa's) fascia of the abdomen. It is also bounded cranially by the pubis and caudally by the crura of corpora cavernosa.

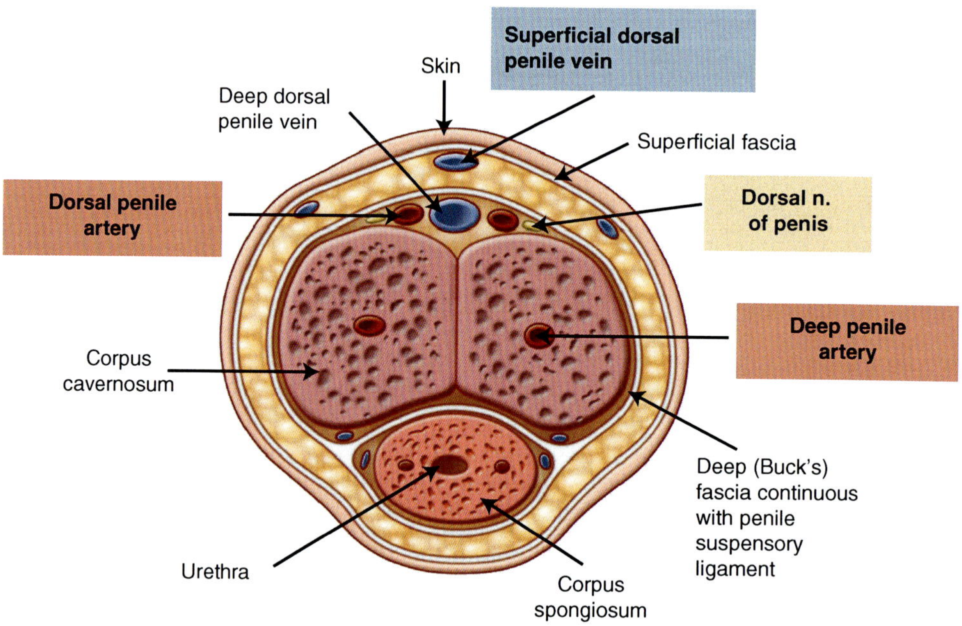

Fig. 32.1 Transverse section of penis

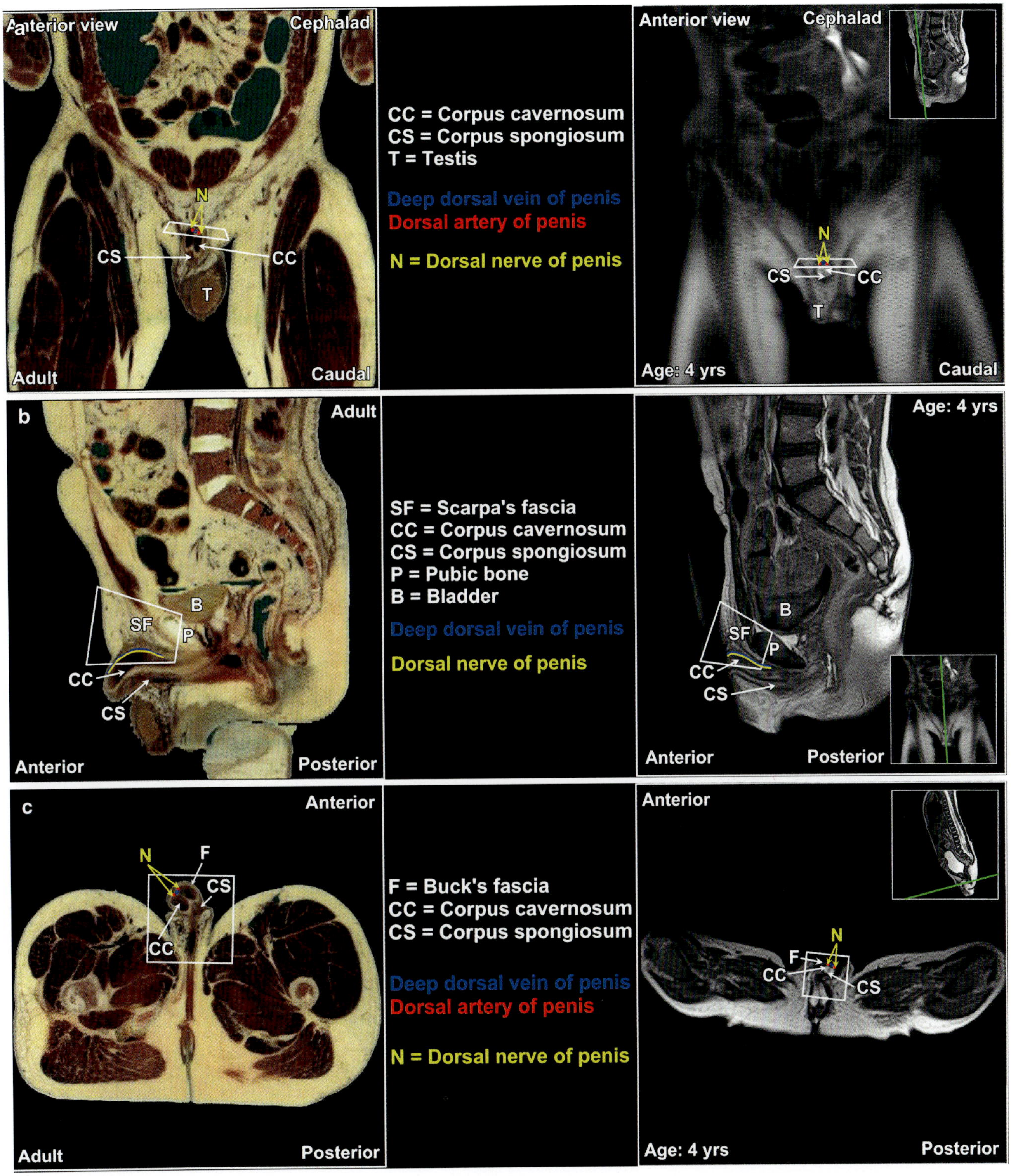

Fig. 32.2 VHVS and MRI images of anatomical structures surrounding the dorsal nerve of the penis; (**a**) anterior view, (**b**) sagittal view, (**c**) transverse view

32.2 Landmark-Based Technique (Subpubic Approach)

32.2.1 Patient Positioning

- The patient lies in the supine position.

32.2.2 Landmarks and Surface Anatomy

- Pubic symphysis
- Inferior border of the pubic rami

32.2.3 Needle Insertion

- Two marks are made on the lateral side of the pubic symphysis, just below each pubic ramus (0.5 cm for babies and 1 cm for older boys).
- With the penis held downward, the needle is inserted at the puncture site in a slight medial and caudal direction (10–15° to the vertical axis in both directions).
- A "pop" is felt as the needle penetrates Scarpa's fascia, approximately 8–30 mm below the skin (depth does not correlate with patient age or weight). A "pop" may also be felt as the needle passes through the superficial fascia (Fig. 32.3).
- Short-beveled 23G needles, 30 mm in length, are generally used for penile block.
- The dorsal penile block provides good analgesia, but may not block the ventral penis sufficiently, especially the frenulum. A ring block around the base of the penis [1] can ensure more effective coverage, especially when used in combination with the dorsal penile block. Ring block has been shown to be more effective than dorsal penile block or topical anesthetic for circumcision in neonates [2].
- The ring block can be performed with the same cutaneous puncture site as the dorsal block. The needle can be fanned out subcutaneously to the 3 and 9 o'clock position and then repositioned to these positions to administer subcutaneous local anesthetic through the 6 o'clock/scrotal area (see Fig. 32.4).
  - The ring block may interfere with hypospadias surgery or circumcision if done preoperatively; therefore, communication with the urologist is important to ensure that the tissue planes are not disrupted.

32.2.4 Local Anesthetic Application

- Bupivacaine 0.25–0.5 % is the local anesthetic of choice for penile block, although lidocaine is also effective. For each side, 0.1 mL/kg is injected up to a maximum of 5 mL per side. Blocks will last, on average, 5–12 h.
- Epinephrine is absolutely contraindicated since the dorsal arteries of the penis are terminal arteries.

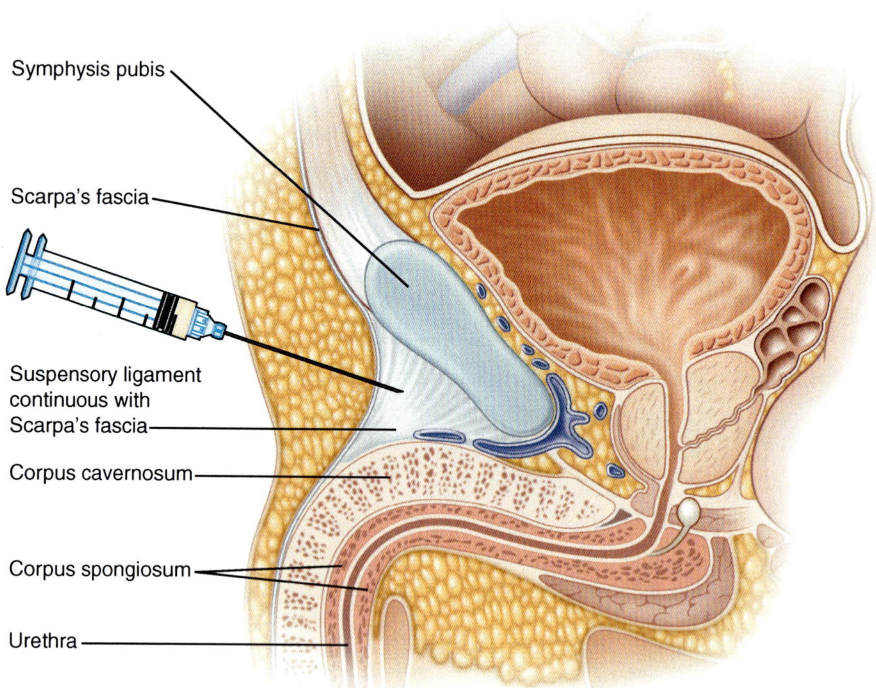

Fig. 32.3 Needle insertion through Scarpa's fascia into the subpubic space

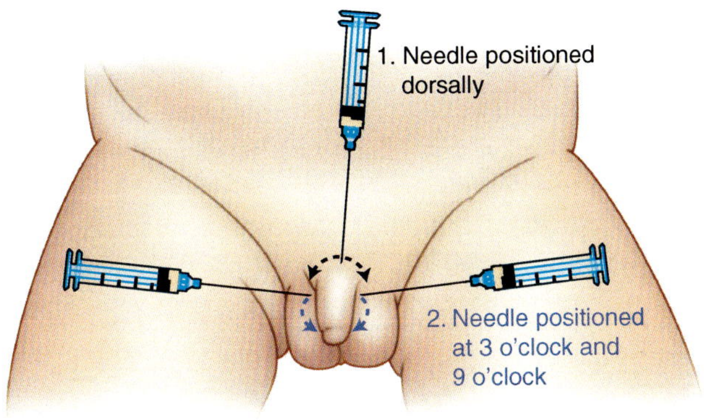

Fig. 32.4 Ring block of the penis. The needle is initially positioned dorsally and fanned out to the 3 o'clock and 9 o'clock positions while injecting local anesthetic. The needle is then repositioned to the 3 o'clock and 9 o'clock positions to ensure local anesthetic spread to the 6 o'clock/scrotal area

32.3 Ultrasound-Guided Technique

32.3.1 Scanning Technique

- A linear probe may be placed sagittally along the shaft of the penis, which will allow visualization of the subpubic space.

32.3.2 Ultrasonographic Appearance (Fig. 32.5)

- The subpubic space is identified as a triangle bordered by: Buck's fascia covering the corpora cavernosa and neurovascular bundle inferiorly; pubic symphysis superiorly; and by Scarpa's fascia anteriorly.
- The fundiform ligament, which forms a midline septum within the deep fascia of the penis, appears fan-shaped under ultrasound.
- Injection deep to Scarpa's fascia can be visualized with ultrasound; this will help to confirm the spread of local anesthetic.

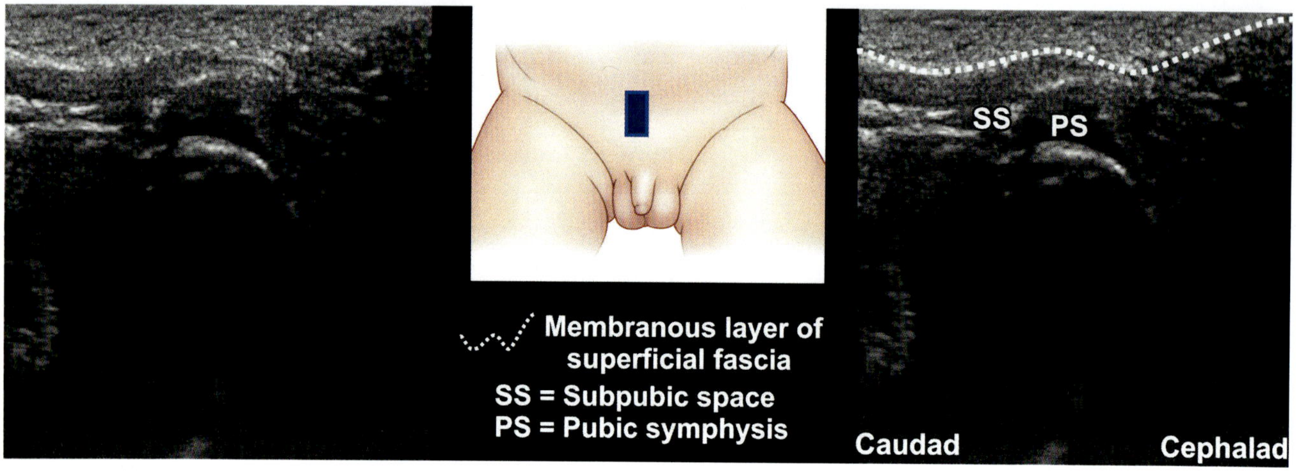

Fig. 32.5 Ultrasound image of the subpubic space for dorsal penile block

32.3.3 Needle Insertion

- As described above, the needle is inserted once on either side of the fundiform ligament (i.e., once on each side of the probe) to the depth of the subpubic space, deep to Scarpa's fascia. Ultrasound imaging will reveal the spread of local anesthetic in the subpubic space as a hypoechoic triangular area.

32.3.4 Local Anesthetic Application

- As described above, 0.1 mL/kg bupivacaine 0.25–0.5 % on each side is sufficient to provide adequate surgical anesthesia and postoperative analgesia.

32.4 Current Literature in Ultrasound-Guided Approaches

Sandeman and Dilley were the first to describe ultrasound-guided dorsal penile nerve block [3]. It was later shown that ultrasound-guided penile nerve block improved block efficacy compared to the traditional landmark-based technique with respect to postoperative pain during the first postoperative hour and the time to the first requirement for postoperative analgesia [4]. However, a later study by Sandeman et al. [5] demonstrated the advantages of ultrasound-guided dorsal penile nerve block compared to the landmark method and caudal epidural analgesia for circumcisions on boys aged 5 months to 15 years. The ultrasound and caudal epidural groups required significantly less morphine postoperatively and had shorter stays on the post-op ward compared to patients in the landmark-guided group. Furthermore, the ultrasound and landmark groups had significantly lower times to first analgesia administration compared to the caudal epidural group. Patients receiving ultrasound-guided blocks also required less intraoperative opiates than patients receiving landmark-guided blocks.

32.5 Case Study

Since the injection site for penile block is required to be close to the surgical field, many surgeons prefer to perform the block themselves during the procedure. An example is shown in Fig. 32.6. The patient received a landmark-guided dorsal penile nerve block for circumcision. After palpating the anterior edge of the symphysis pubis, a 23G pediatric needle was inserted slightly medially and cephalad until Buck's fascia was penetrated. Local anesthetic was injected at this location. Following caudal redirection of the needle, the remainder of the local anesthetic was injected in a subcutaneous wheal across the ventral surface of the midline of the penis. Pain control was excellent with no complications.

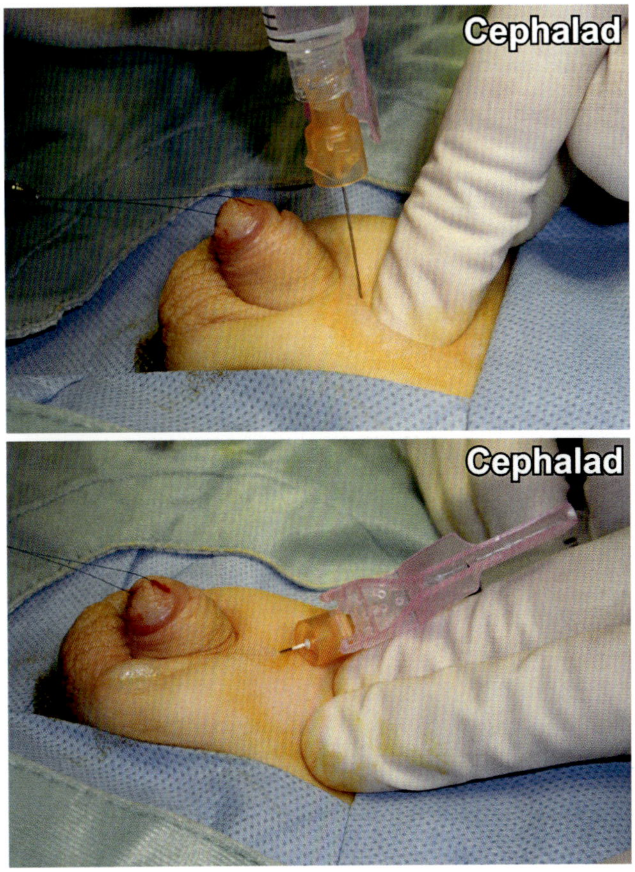

Fig. 32.6 Landmark-guided penile block performed by the surgeon, showing initial needle position (*top*) and needle position after redirection (*bottom*) (See Case Study for details)

References

1. Broadman LM, Hannallah RS, Belman AB, Elder PT, Ruttimann U, Epstein BS. Post-circumcision analgesia—a prospective evaluation of subcutaneous ring block of the penis. Anesthesiology. 1987;67: 399–402.
2. Lander J, Brady-Fryer B, Metcalfe JB, Nazarali S, Muttitt S. Comparison of ring block, dorsal penile nerve block, and topical anesthesia for neonatal circumcision: a randomized controlled trial. JAMA. 1997;278:2157–62.
3. Sandeman DJ, Dilley AV. Ultrasound guided dorsal penile nerve block in children. Anaesth Intensive Care. 2007;35:266–9.
4. Faraoni D, Gilbeau A, Lingier P, Barvais L, Engelman E, Hennart D. Does ultrasound guidance improve the efficacy of dorsal penile nerve block in children? Pediatr Anesth. 2010; 20:931–6.
5. Sandeman DJ, Reiner D, Dilley AV, Bennett MH, Kelly KJ. A retrospective audit of three different regional anaesthetic techniques for circumcision in children. Anaesth Intensive Care. 2010;38:519–24.

Suggested Reading

Dalens BJ. Blocks of nerves of the trunk. In: Dalens BJ, editor. Pediatric regional anesthesia. Boca Raton: CRC Press; 1990. p. 457–64.

Peutrell JM. Penile block. In: Peutrell JM, Mather SJ, editors. Regional anaesthesia for babies and children. Oxford: Oxford University Press; 1997. p. 130–40.

Suresh S, Polaner DM, Cote CJ. Regional Anesthesia. In: Cote CJ, Lerman J, Anderson BJ, Eds. 5th ed. Philadelphia: WB Saunders; 2013. p. 835–79.

Part XI

Neuraxial Blockade

Epidural and Caudal Anesthesia

33

Ban C.H. Tsui

Contents

B.C.H. Tsui, Dip Eng, BSc (Math), B Pharm, MSc, MD, FRCPC
Department of Anesthesiology and Pain Medicine,
Stollery Children's Hospital/University of Alberta Hospital,
2-150 Clinical Sciences Building, Edmonton,
AB T6G 2G3, Canada
e-mail: btsui@ualberta.ca

B.C.H. Tsui, S. Suresh (eds.), *Pediatric Atlas of Ultrasound- and Nerve Stimulation-Guided Regional Anesthesia*,
DOI 10.1007/978-0-387-79964-3_33

33.1 Epidural Anesthesia

33.1.1 Introduction

Epidural needle placement may fail for several reasons, including anatomical variability (e.g., limited interlaminar space, ossified or calcified ligamentum flavum, enlarged facet joints, or rotated vertebrae), faulty identification of the midline (e.g., obesity, scoliosis), and poor patient compliance or cooperation. In children, these issues may not be significant, but because the patients are usually under general anesthesia, the absence of any possible sensory warning of intrathecal or spinal cord placement adds inherent risks to the procedure.

Both epidural stimulation and ultrasound may be useful as adjuncts to other tests, such as loss of resistance to saline, for identifying needle entry into the epidural space. The epidural stimulation test may be especially beneficial to warn of a needle misplaced in the subdural or intrathecal spaces or if the needle is abutting a nerve root. The main benefit of ultrasound imaging is the ability to gauge the depth and direction to the epidural space prior to the procedure, which can help refine the point of needle puncture and angle of needle insertion. One may visualize the disruption caused by the injection of fluid into the epidural space when using the loss-of-resistance technique in the lumbar region in pediatric patients, but this observation is limited in the more compact thoracic spine (Fig. 33.1).

The distance of catheter threading will determine which technique to use for continuous blocks. The epidural stimulation test is useful when catheters are threaded at a distance into the epidural space but has only moderate application during direct placement of the catheter. In these cases, loss of resistance to saline will accurately determine epidural placement, and ultrasound guidance can be helpful. Nevertheless, the epidural stimulation test is useful in warning against unintentional intrathecal or intravascular local anesthetic injection.

Indications

Usually provides postoperative analgesia but occasionally provides surgical anesthesia for:

- Lower limb surgery
- Pelvic and urological surgery
- Abdominal surgery
- Thoracic surgery

33.1.2 Patient Positioning

Position an anesthetized patient in the lateral position; awake patients can be sitting up.

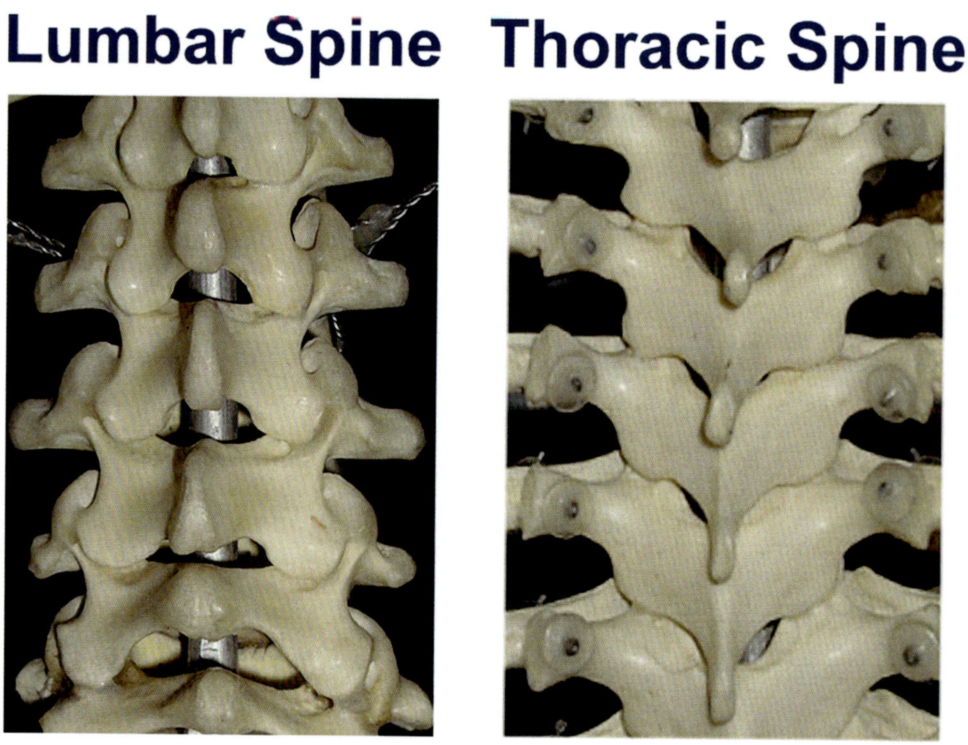

Fig. 33.1 Pediatric spine model showing spinal column in the thoracic and lumbar regions

33.1.3 Surface Anatomy

Lumbar (Fig. 33.2) and thoracic (Fig. 33.3) spine:

- Spinous Processes*
  - In the midline, palpate the spinous processes; a line drawn between the tips of the scapulae will run through the T7 vertebrae.
  - In the lumbar region, L4 is at level of the iliac crests, and S1 is on horizontal line drawn between the two posterior superior iliac spines.
- Transverse processes
  - These lie lateral to the midline in varying distances, depending on the age of the child.

  * The neural arches, forming the spinous processes, are not completely fused until the end of the first year (except at L5, where they fuse significantly later), so it is common to palpate two separate bony landmarks in infants.

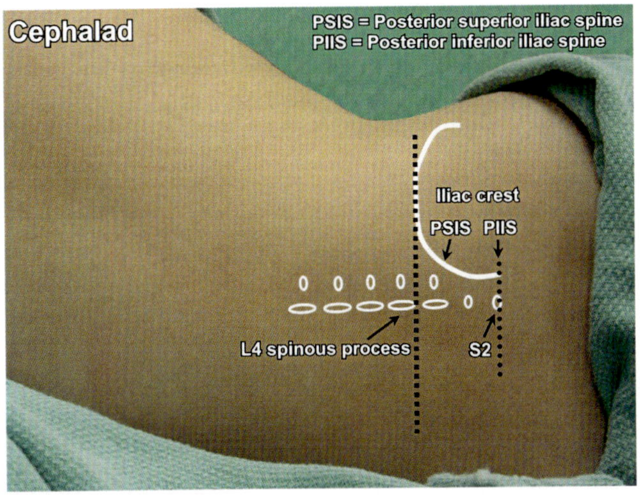

Fig. 33.2 Surface anatomy of the lumbar spine

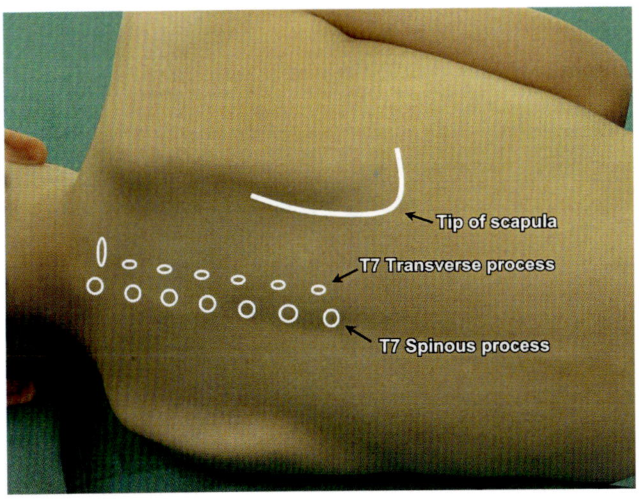

Fig. 33.3 Surface anatomy of the thoracic spine

33.1.4 Approaches

33.1.4.1 Direct Lumbar Approach

- Perform the lumbar epidural puncture with the patient in the lateral position.
- Locate iliac crests of pelvic and use this landmark to identify the spine of L4.
- Resistance to air or saline can be used to identify the lumbar epidural space, although both have their own advantages and disadvantages.
  - Air embolism (if needle accidently punctures a vein) and pneumoencephalocele are rare but potential risks when using loss of resistance (LOR) to air.
  - Occasionally, the loss of resistance to saline may be equivocal.
  - When using LOR to saline, use a small amount of saline to avoid diluting the local anesthetic.
  - The hanging drop technique can be used to identify the epidural space although this method is more suited to patients in the sitting position (i.e., not well suited for sedated pediatric patients).
- The skin to epidural space can be estimated as 1 mm/kg or [10 + (age in years ×2)] mm.
- Midline approach is typically used (Fig. 33.4), and paramedian approach is generally not needed or recommended unless abnormal anatomical landmarks are encountered or suspected in the lumbar region.
- When abnormal anatomical landmarks are encountered, a careful survey of the patient's spinal anatomy using ultrasound is strongly recommended to allow:
  - Identification of the midline
  - Measurement of epidural (ligamentum flavum) and dural space depth
  - Prediction of the best path (projection and angulation) that the needle should take to reach the epidural space

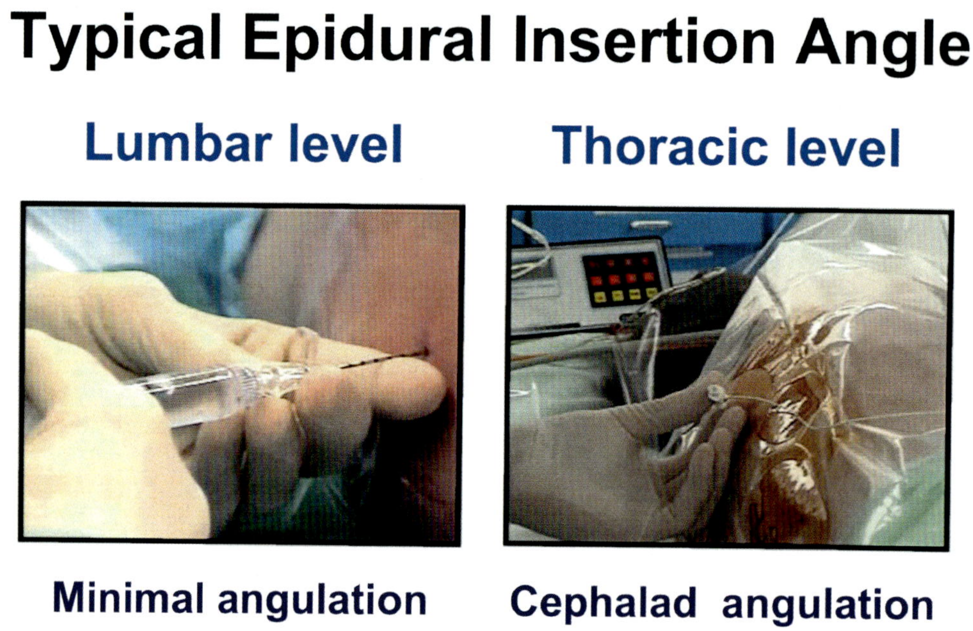

Fig. 33.4 Loss-of-resistance (LOR) technique. (*Left*) Midline approach. In the lumbar region, the needle is typically inserted with minimal angulation. (*Right*) Paramedian approach. In the thoracic region, cephalad angulation is often needed to reach the epidural space

33.1.4.2 Direct Thoracic Approach

In the pediatric population, continuous thoracic epidural anesthesia is used only for major surgery. Placement of a thoracic epidural requires a high skill level and can be a challenging procedure to perform. In children over the age of 6–12 months, the effectiveness of ultrasound guidance for thoracic epidural placement is limited since the bony anatomy of the region restricts and obstructs ultrasound visualization of the epidural space. Therefore, anesthesiologists continue to rely on a tactile approach with either a loss of resistance method or a hanging drop technique, both of which result in challenging needle insertion due to the angle required to access the thoracic epidural space. A median or paramedian approach can be used; however, each approach can be difficult and even dangerous if the patient is uncooperative. This procedure is therefore typically performed with the patient asleep. On rare occasions and for selective cases (i.e., mature teenager), it is occasionally possible to insert a thoracic epidural in an awake patient.

33.1.4.3 General Approaches

- Perform the thoracic epidural puncture with the patient in the lateral position; locate the prominent spine of the seventh cervical vertebra and use this landmark to calculate other vertebral levels. The lower extremity of the shoulder blade, which is at the level of the seventh thoracic vertebra, can also be used as a landmark.
- The paramedian approach allows one to choose the angle of insertion into the epidural space regardless of the space available between adjacent vertebral spines. However, the paramedian approach requires skill and experience to ensure that the needle tip is in the midline when it enters the epidural space.
- Compared to the lumbar region, the spinal canal at the level of T10–T12 is slightly superficial due to short spinous processes.
- Choose a needle that is appropriate for the size of the child; for children ≤12 kg, a 5 cm, 19G Tuohy needle is suitable, while an 18G version can be used for larger children. Also available is a thin-walled, 18G needle that allows a 20G catheter to be inserted through; an advantage of this needle is that when the needle is inserted with cephalad angulation, the bevel is parallel to the epidural space, reducing the risk of dural puncture by the needle tip.
- Similar to lumbar epidural, resistance to air or saline can be used to identify the thoracic epidural space. In children 1 year or older, the ligamentum flavum provides adequate resistance, and the negative pressure of the thoracic epidural space can be identified easily.
- For infants and young children, small 3 or 5 mL syringes can be used; for older patients, use a 5–10 mL syringe.

33.1.4.4 Median Approaches

A successful thoracic block will rely on an acute angle of insertion relative to the skin due to the angle of the spines. This is particularly noticeable when using the median approach in the midthoracic region compared to lumbar region, since the needle typically needs to be angulated more cephalad to reach the epidural space (Fig. 33.4). This technique may facilitate easier catheter movement in a cephalad direction within the epidural space.

33.1.4.5 Paramedian Approach

Most anesthesiologists find the paramedian approach to be the most effective technique for thoracic epidural placement. This technique involves the following steps (Fig. 33.5):

1. Insert the epidural needle 0.5–2 cm (e.g., one to two fingerbreadths distance) lateral to the spinous process of the vertebra. Note: Use the patient's finger as measurement of the distance lateral to the spinous process.
2. Advance the needle perpendicular to the skin until it contacts the lamina.
3. Redirect the needle approximately 15° medially to "walk off" the lamina.
4. Angle the needle cephalad, and continue the "walk off" technique to locate the epidural space.

Note: As shown in Fig. 33.6, steps 2 and 3 must be performed separately, as the epidural space may be missed if the needle is "walked off" diagonally (i.e., medial and cephalad angulation at the same time).

This procedure can be difficult to master. Accurate placement of the needle requires fine motor skills, which are best learned through hands-on practice. Training may be aided by a phantom model that reproduces the anatomy necessary to learn and practice the paramedian approach to thoracic epidurals.

33.1.5 Nerve Stimulation Technique

Electrical stimulation has been used in epidural anesthesia and for peripheral nerve blocks for many years. The epidural

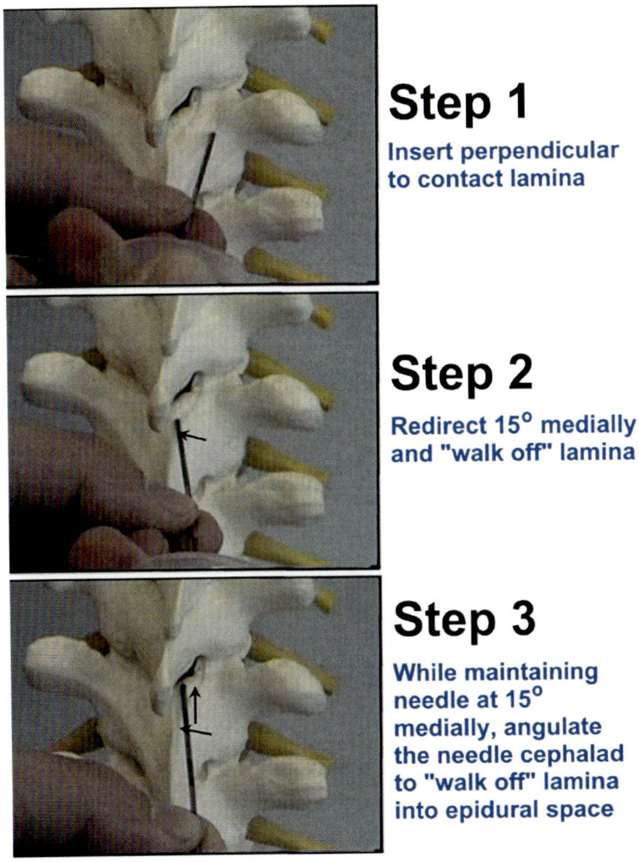

Fig. 33.5 Paramedian approach for thoracic epidural placement in a spine model. (*Top*) Insert needle lateral to spinous process and perpendicular to the skin to contact the lamina. (*Middle*) Redirect the needle approximately 15° medially to "walk off" the lamina. (*Bottom*) Angulate the needle cephalad while maintaining needle 15° medially, and continue to "walk off" to reach the epidural space

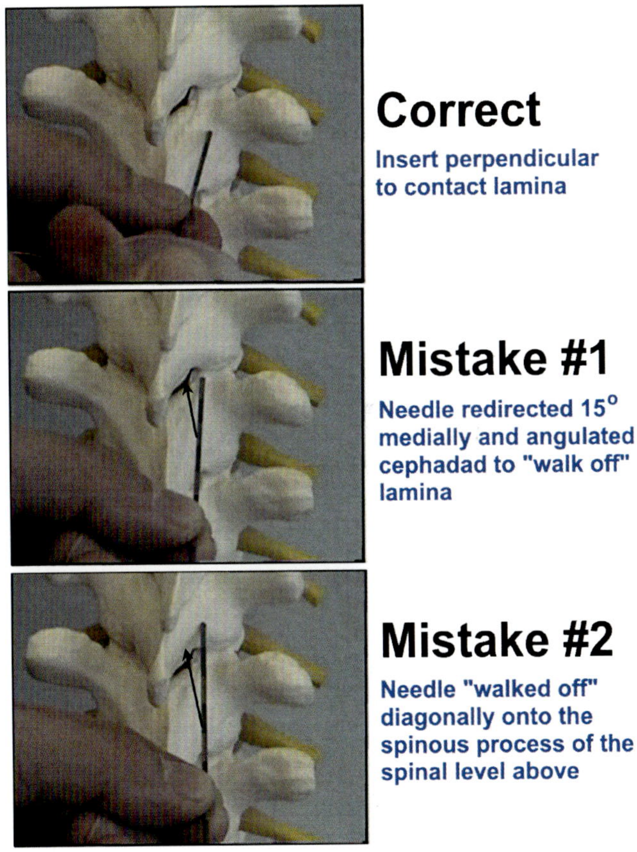

Fig. 33.6 Common mistakes: with simultaneous medial and cephalad angulation, the epidural space may be missed as the needle is "walked off" diagonally onto the spinous process or lamina of the spinal level above

Table 33.1 Catheter location determined by motor response and current threshold during the epidural stimulation test

Catheter location	Motor response	Current[a]
Subcutaneous	None	N/A
Subdural	Bilateral (many segments)	<1 mA
Subarachnoid	Unilateral or bilateral	<1 mA
Epidural space		
Against nerve root	Unilateral	<1 mA
Non-intravascular	Unilateral or bilateral	1–15 mA (threshold current increases after local anesthetic injection)
Intravascular	Unilateral or bilateral	1–15 mA (no change in threshold current after local anesthetic injected)

[a]Needle placement at the caudal and lumbar spine adheres well to these criteria, although placement at thoracic spinal levels may necessitate higher upper limits (up to 17 mA has been shown). The lower threshold applies to both catheter and needle placement

stimulation test (Tsui test) was developed to confirm epidural catheter placement, applying similar principles to those of peripheral nerve blockade (i.e., using electrical pulses and the current versus nerve-distance relationship). This test has demonstrated 80–100 % positive prediction for epidural catheter placement. It has also been shown to be effective to guide catheters to within two segmental levels (with radiologic confirmation), which can assist smooth placement to appropriate levels and allow adjustments in the event of catheter migration, kinking, or coiling. In addition to confirming and guiding epidural catheter placement, this test has been shown to be useful for detecting intrathecal, subdural, or intravascular catheter placement.

33.1.5.1 Needle Confirmation

The procedure is performed along with standard mechanical tests (e.g., loss of resistance to saline or air) for determining epidural needle placement:

- After sterile preparation, the nerve stimulator is attached to an 18G insulated Tuohy needle (see Fig. 1.3).
- The current is applied after skin puncture and during advancement; the epidural stimulation test is used together with detection of a "pop" or loss of resistance to saline.
- The threshold current range for determining correct needle placement is similar for the lumbar or caudal routes, but the higher limit of 10 mA may be extended for thoracic placement (mean of 11.1 mA and up to 17 mA) [1, 2].
- The test may provide further confirmation during direct epidurals, with the added benefit of warning that a needle is entering lumbar epidural space if the current is set above 6 mA [3]. However, this technique has not been applied widely in clinical practice except in the study environment.

33.1.5.2 Catheter Confirmation

- The same procedure as described above for an insulated needle applies, with the exception that the nerve stimulator is connected to an epidural stimulating catheter or a metal-containing epidural catheter using an electrode adaptor such as the Johans ECG adaptor (Fig. 2.9a).
- Prime the catheter and adaptor with sterile normal saline (0.2–1 mL).
- Attach the cathode lead of the nerve stimulator directly to the cable of the stimulating catheter or metal hub of the adaptor and the grounding anode lead to an electrode on the patient's body surface.
- Set the nerve stimulator to a low frequency and pulse width (2 Hz; 0.2 ms).
- Carefully and slowly increase the current intensity until motor activity begins.
- The characteristics of the various responses are compared in Table 33.1. Catheter location is identified, and the required adjustments are made depending to location indicated.

33.1.5.3 Mechanism of the Test

- Needle or catheter placement is confirmed by stimulating the spinal nerve roots (not spinal cord) with an electrically conducting catheter that conducts a low-amplitude electrical current through normal saline.
- An appropriate motor response (1–10 mA; Table 33.1) confirms accurate placement of the epidural catheter tip, defined as 1–2 cm from the nerve roots (see Fig. 2.8).
- Responses observed with a significantly lower threshold current (<1 mA), especially if substantially diffuse or bilateral, may warn of catheter placement in the intrathecal or subdural space (i.e., contacting highly conductive CSF) or in close proximity to a nerve root.
- The segmental level of the catheter tip may be predicted based on the progressive nature of the motor twitches as the catheter is advanced (i.e., lower limbs followed by intercostals and then upper limbs).
- A local anesthetic test dose helps confirm epidural versus intravascular location. If the catheter is localized in the epidural space, the motor threshold current should increase after injection of local anesthetic. Unintentional injection into the systemic circulation (i.e., removing local anesthetic from the vicinity of the nerve) will allow subsequent motor stimulation at the same current.

When Used for Needle Placement

- Insulated needles seem to provide lower electrical threshold current required for this test.
- The upper limit of the threshold current designating a positive test using needles is different depending on the level of needle placement (caudal = mean 3.7 mA; [4] lumbar = mean 3.84 mA; thoracic = mean 11.1 mA; intrathecal = mean 0.77 mA).
- The higher threshold currents that may be seen with direct thoracic level needle insertion may be related to the minimal depth of needle penetration that is inherently used for caution at this level.

33.1.5.4 Considerations for Test Performance and Interpretation

- Since local muscle contraction in the trunk region can be confused with epidural stimulation, it is recommended to place the anode lead on the upper extremity for lumbar epidurals and the lower extremity for thoracic epidurals.
- The 1–10 mA test criteria should be used as a guideline only. Epidural stimulation may occur outside this range. The reason we recommend this range is that it is easy to remember. In addition:
  - It is important to begin using the lowest current to allow detection of intrathecal placement or nerve root proximity; the lower limit of 1 mA applies to all situations.
  - Some cases will require stimulation upwards of 17 mA, particularly when using insulated needles in the thoracic region.
  - The best predictor of epidural placement is a combination of the threshold current level and the distribution of elicited motor responses (i.e., correlation with approximate segmental location) since subcutaneous placement would not elicit such predictive and segmental responses.

33.1.5.5 Detecting Intrathecal and Intravascular Catheter and Needle Placement (Table 33.1)

Aspiration should always be performed prior to local anesthetic injection. However, the inability to aspirate blood or CSF does not indicate that an epidural needle/catheter is not in the intrathecal or intravascular space. In pediatric patients, aspiration alone may fail to detect up to 86 % of intravascular entry of epidural needles or catheters [5]. The threshold current for a motor response during catheter and needle placement with the electrical stimulation test may help predict intrathecal placement. Intravascular placement may be detected with the electrical stimulation test in conjunction with a local anesthetic test dose.

Intrathecal

- When a needle/catheter is situated properly within the epidural space, a current greater than 1 mA should be required to elicit muscle twitches.
- Using insulated needles, currents to elicit a motor response in the epidural space (3.84 ± 0.99 mA and 5.2 ± 2.4 mA) are much higher than that for the intrathecal space (0.77 ± 0.32 mA and 0.6 ± 0.3 mA).
- If any motor response is detected with a current less than 1 mA, intrathecal catheter or needle placement should be suspected.

Intravascular

- Repeated injections of local anesthetic into a properly placed epidural catheter result in impairment of nerve conduction and require a gradual increase in the amplitude of electrical current to produce a positive motor response.
- If the local anesthetic is inadvertently injected into the intravascular space (i.e., systemic circulation, thereby reducing the concentration in the vicinity of the nerves), the threshold will remain the same instead of incrementally increasing with repeated application.
- Caution is required when extrapolating the intravascular information because this application has only been tested in a few adult obstetric patients and never in the pediatric population.
- An epinephrine test dose (0.5 μg/kg) should still be administered to identify inadvertent intravascular placement by observing specific ECG changes (i.e., >25 % increase in T-wave or ST segment changes irrespective of chosen lead).
- When using a the test dose in combination with the epidural stimulation test, one can confidently rule out the risk of accidental intravascular or intrathecal injection.

33.1.6 Electrocardiograph (ECG) Monitoring Technique (Fig. 33.7)

One limitation of the epidural stimulation technique is that it cannot be performed reliably if any significant clinical neuromuscular blockade is present or if local anesthetics have been administered in the epidural space. To overcome this limitation, an alternative monitoring technique using electrocardiograph (ECG) monitoring was developed [6]. Using epidural ECG, the anatomical position of the epidural catheter is determined by comparing the ECG signal from the tip of the catheter to a signal from a surface electrode positioned at the "target" segmental level. Thus, advancement of an epidural catheter from the lumbar or sacral region into the thoracic region can easily be monitored and placed within two vertebral spaces of the targeted level under ECG guidance.

Procedure

1. Place left-leg (red in figure) and left-arm (black in figure) electrodes at their standard positions.
2. Record a standard reference ECG (lead II) by connecting the right-arm electrode (white in figure) to a skin electrode on the patient's back at the target spinal level.
3. Connect the right-arm electrode (white in figure) to the metal hub of an electrode adaptor to record a tracing from the epidural catheter.

Interpreting the ECG Method

- When the epidural catheter tip is positioned in the lumbar and sacral regions, the amplitude of the QRS complex is relatively small since the recording electrode (epidural tip) is a considerable distance from the heart, and the vector of the cardiac electrical impulse is at approximately a 90° angle.

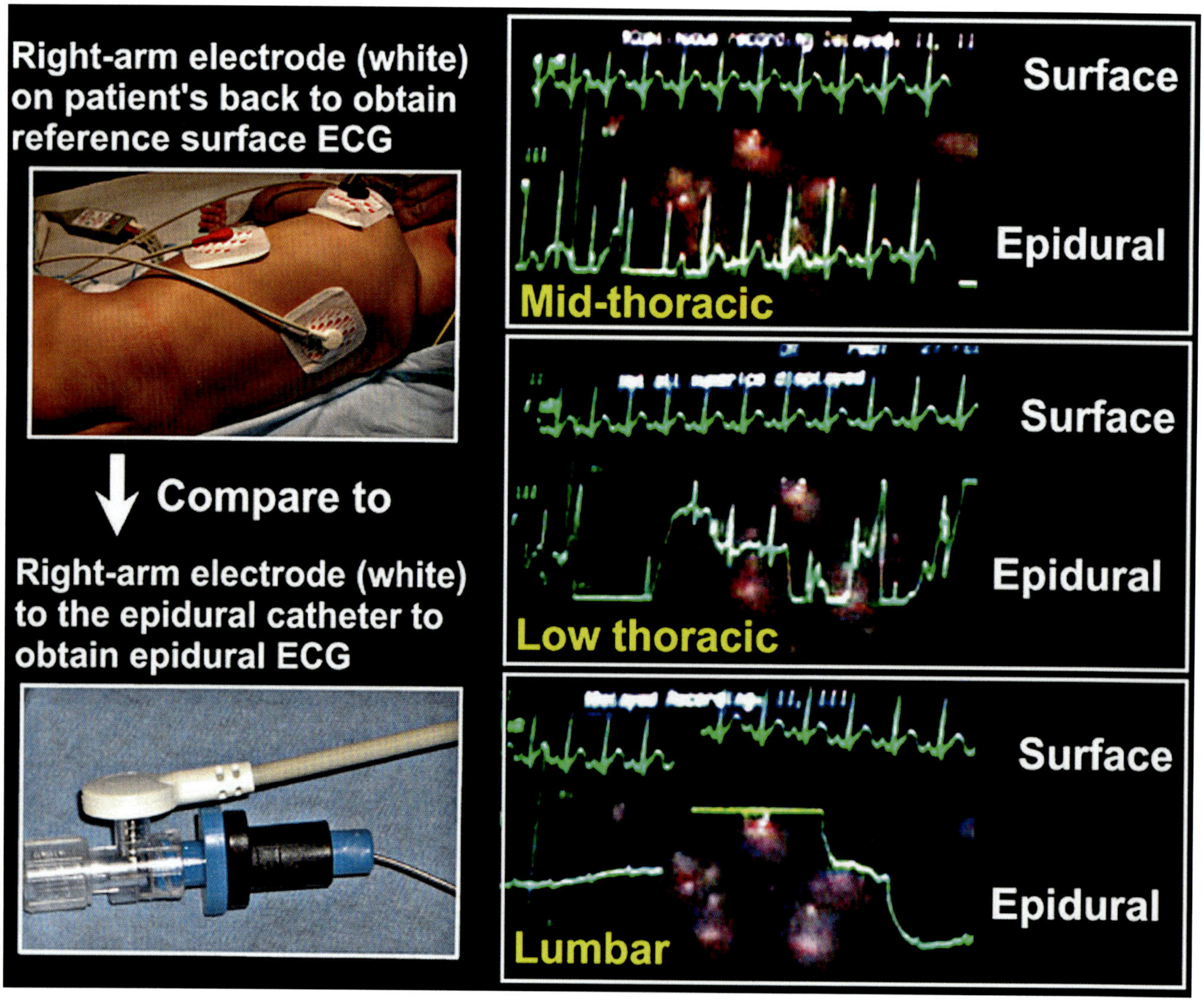

Fig. 33.7 ECG monitoring technique for thoracic epidural catheter placement via advancement from lumbar or caudal levels

- As the epidural tip advances toward the thoracic region, the amplitude of the QRS complex increases as the recording electrode comes closer to the heart and becomes more parallel to the cardiac electrical impulse.
- As the catheter tip passes the target level, the amplitude of QRS should match the amplitude of the reference surface electrode.

Limitations

The ECG technique cannot warn of a catheter placed in the intrathecal or intravascular space. In addition, this technique may not be suitable when threading catheters a short distance, as ECG changes may be too subtle to observe.

33.1.7 Ultrasound-Guided Technique

Generally, two approaches can be used for applying ultrasound imaging for epidural procedures. First, an "ultrasound-supported" approach employs a pre-procedural scan to identify the puncture site, depth of epidural space, and ideal needle trajectory. These procedures require multiple "still images" in different planes to capture accurate measurement with the ultrasound device. Second, real-time or "online" imaging can be used during epidural procedures to observe needle puncture, catheter placement, and local anesthetic application (each of these actions is improved through direct visualization of movement or by indirect means). There are some challenges with using ultrasound in neuraxial procedures, but it has demonstrable benefits for infants and neonates and may have some efficacy (e.g., reduced needle attempts and visibility of the sacral hiatus for caudal blocks) with older pediatric patients.

Generally, the lower lumbar region has the highest visibility (i.e., ultrasound "window"), as it is less compact than the more cephalad high-lumbar and thoracic levels. In pediatric patients, the ratio of visible to nonvisible segments to be 2:1 at the sacral, 1:1 at the lumbar, and 1:2 at the thoracic levels. Visibility of neuraxial structures in the lumbar and thoracic regions is best in patients 3 months of age and under, with age-dependent decreases in quality thereafter. As shown in Fig. 33.8, there will be variation in the structures that are visible in different planes of ultrasound scanning as illustrated in the skeleton model (i.e., paramedian longitudinal scanning will visualize the dura mater better than median longitudinal), and different techniques may require separate planes, although many approaches will require two or more planes for comprehensive assessment.

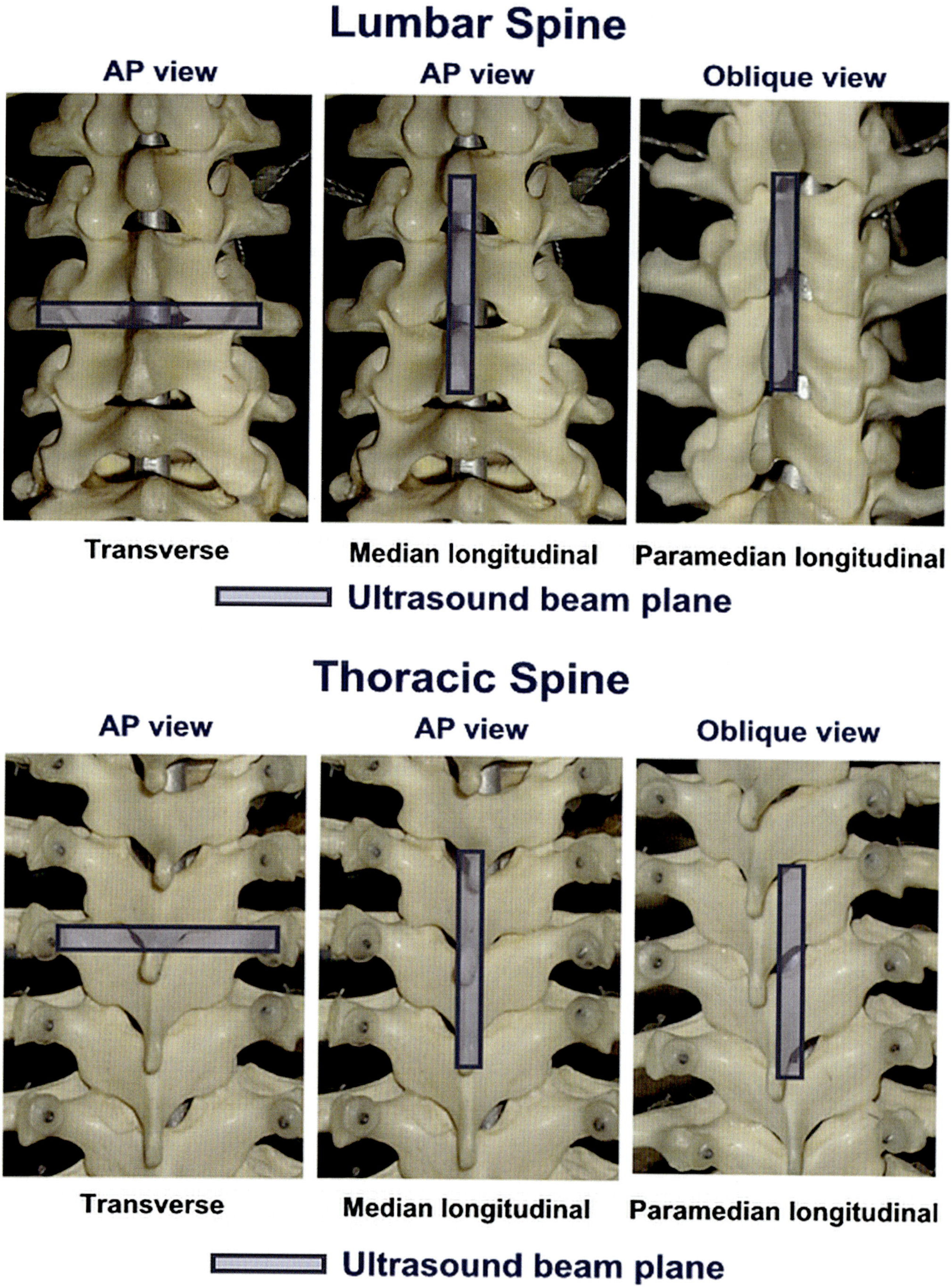

Fig. 33.8 Possible ultrasound views using a pediatric skeleton model. (*Top*) For the lumbar region, an ultrasound epidural window (i.e., no bone obstruction) can be obtained with both transverse and paramedian views. (*Bottom*) For the thoracic region, an epidural window cannot be seen easily and only with a paramedian view

33.1.7.1 Preparing the Needle Insertion Site

Sterile technique is critical during performance of neuraxial blocks due to the disastrous consequences of infection in the epidural space.

- Full aseptic technique should be undertaken, with the proceduralist gowned, gloved, and wearing a face mask and hat.
- The area should be prepped with a chlorhexidine and alcohol solution, which should be allowed to dry.
- Sterile draping of the area should be undertaken.
- The needle, catheter, and other equipment required should be assembled on a sterile tray and be easily accessible.

33.1.7.2 Scanning Technique

- Use a low-frequency (5–2 MHz) probe to scan the lumbar and thoracic spine in transverse and longitudinal planes.
- Figures 33.9 and 33.10 show the MRI anatomical structure and ultrasound appearance in the transverse plane at the lumbar and thoracic spine, respectively. Positioning the patient with a flexed spine will be advantageous for viewing in this plane since it will improve location of an ultrasound window between the vertebrae. If the spinous processes obstruct the view of dura, then the "expected position" of the dura can be estimated in most cases (see below for explanation).

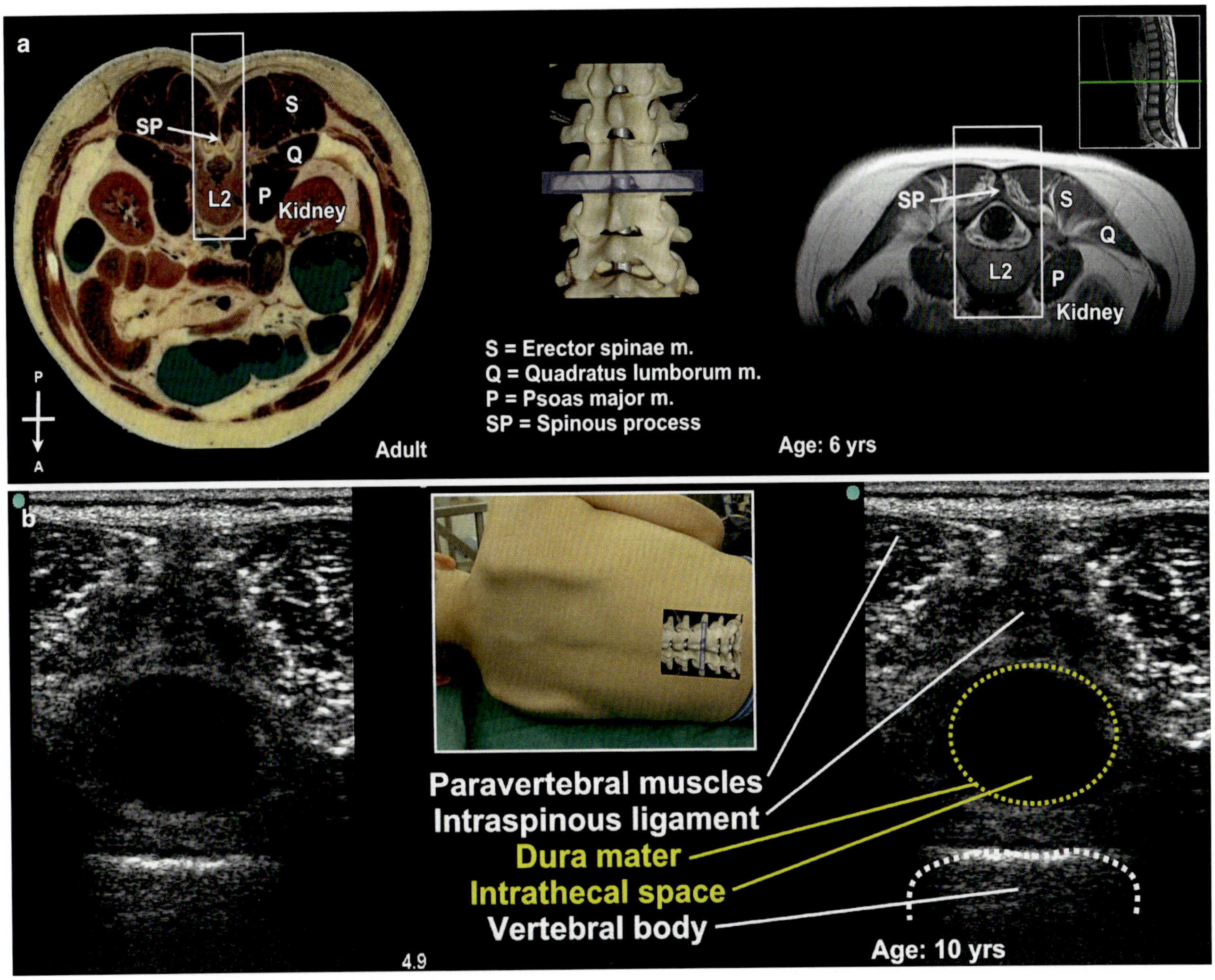

Fig. 33.9 (**a**) VHVS and MRI images of transverse plane at the lumbar spine. (**b**) Sonographic appearance of transverse plane at the lumbar spine

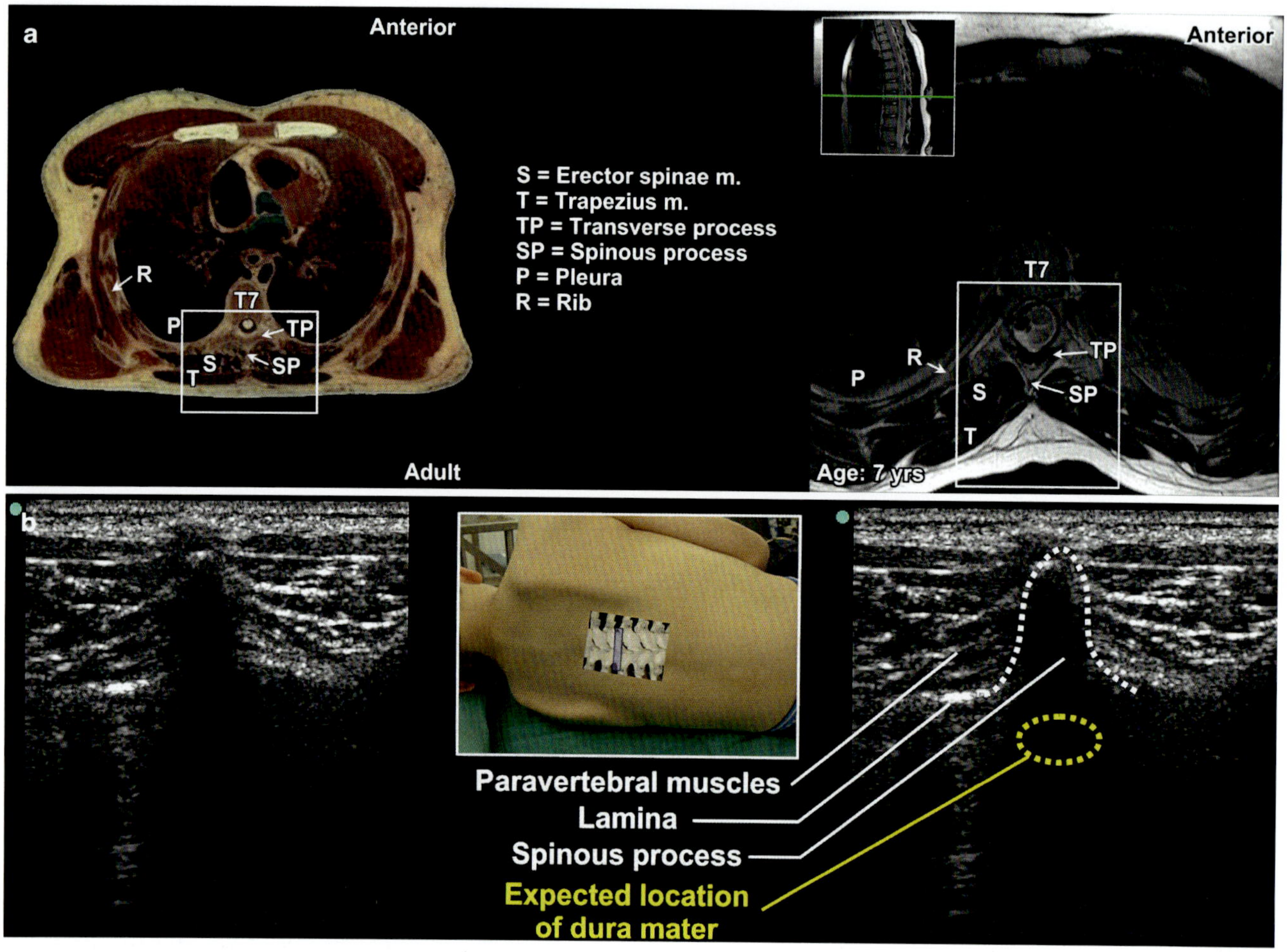

Fig. 33.10 (**a**) VHVS and MRI images of transverse plane at the thoracic spine. (**b**) Sonographic appearance of transverse plane at the thoracic spine

- Figures 33.11 and 33.12 show the MRI anatomical structure and ultrasound appearance in the midline and paramedian longitudinal plane at the lumbar and thoracic spine, respectively. The longitudinal paramedian plane will provide the best ultrasound window with reasonably good visibility of the dura mater for surrogate marking of the puncture site and loss of resistance depth (see below for explanation).

Fig. 33.11 (**a**) VHVS and MRI images of midline longitudinal plane at the lumbar spine. (**b**) Sonographic appearance of midline longitudinal plane at the lumbar spine. (**c**) VHVS and MRI images of paramedian longitudinal plane at the lumbar spine. (**d**) Sonographic appearance of paramedian longitudinal plane at the lumbar spine

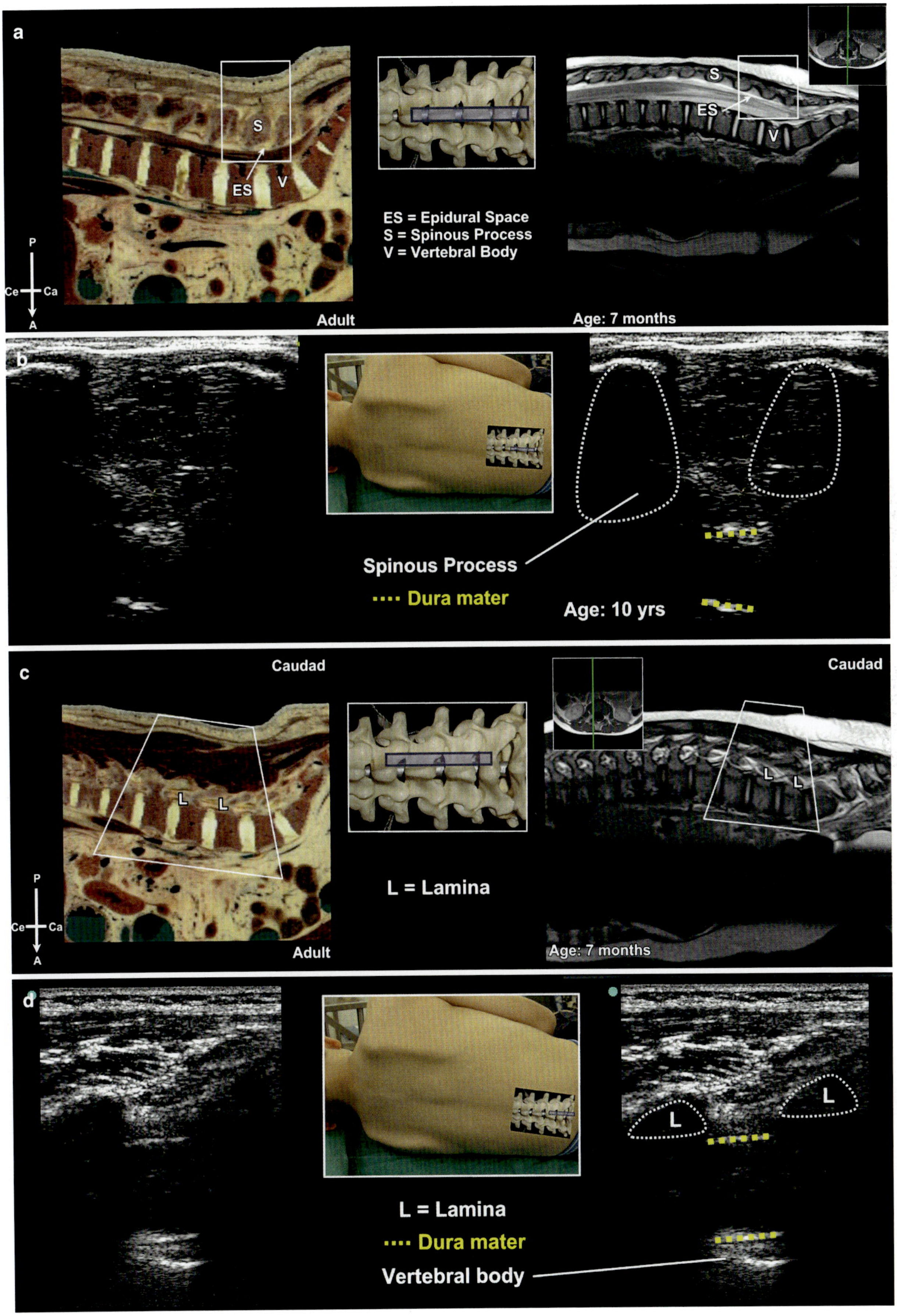
a
S
ES
V
P
Ce
Ca
A
ES = Epidural Space
S = Spinous Process
V = Vertebral Body
Adult
Age: 7 months
b
Spinous Process
···· Dura mater
Age: 10 yrs
c
Caudad
L
L = Lamina
Adult
Age: 7 months
d
L = Lamina
···· Dura mater
Vertebral body

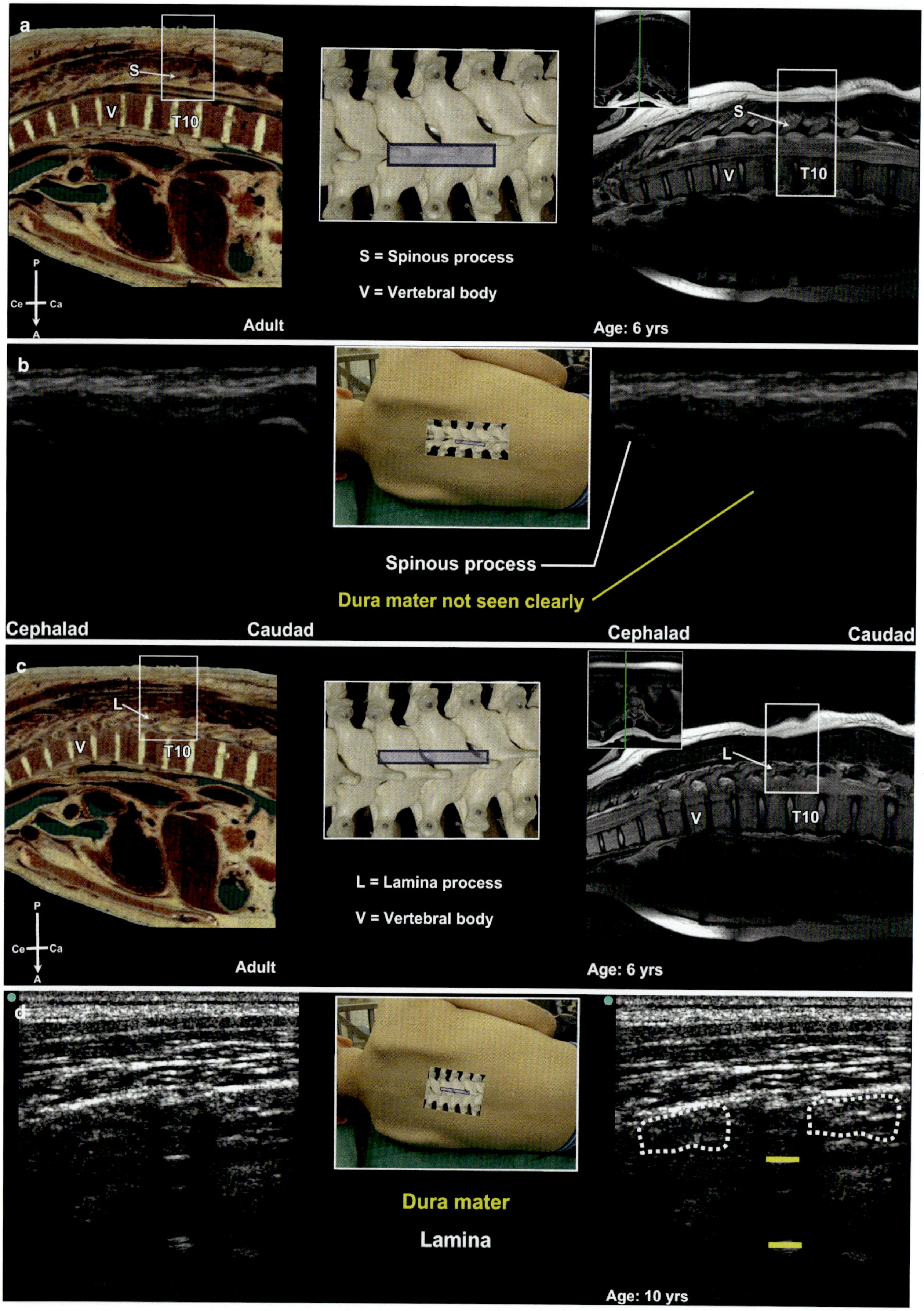

Fig. 33.12 (**a**) VHVS and MRI images of midline longitudinal plane at the thoracic spine. (**b**) Sonographic appearance of midline longitudinal plane at the thoracic spine. (**c**) VHVS and MRI images of paramedian longitudinal plane at the thoracic spine. (**d**) Sonographic appearance of paramedian longitudinal plane at the thoracic spine

33.1.7.3 Sonographic Appearance

As illustrated in Fig. 33.13, ultrasound imaging in neonates and infants (<12 months of age) results in a superior image.

Hyperechogenic Tissues (Bright)

- Dura mater: appears thin, linear, and bright, usually with a double-layered appearance in longitudinal view; it is best viewed in a longitudinal paramedian plane.
- Bony structures: highly reflective and bright on the surface, although they cast a dark shadow underneath.
- Conus medullaris and cauda equina: appear almost fibrillar with a nearly hyperechoic appearance.
- Catheter: appears as a double-linear structure in longitudinal view and as a single hyperechoic dot on short-axis view (see below).

Iso-/Hypoechoic Structures (Identical Density; Appear Grey)

- Epidural space: located beyond the relatively hyperechoic dura mater.
- Spinal cord: low echogenicity with a double line at the thoracic level.

Anechoic Structures/Substances (Black)

- Local anesthetic: upon injection, a hypoechogenic expansion is visible at the site of injection and often separates the neural and vascular structures.
- Intrathecal Space: filled with CSF

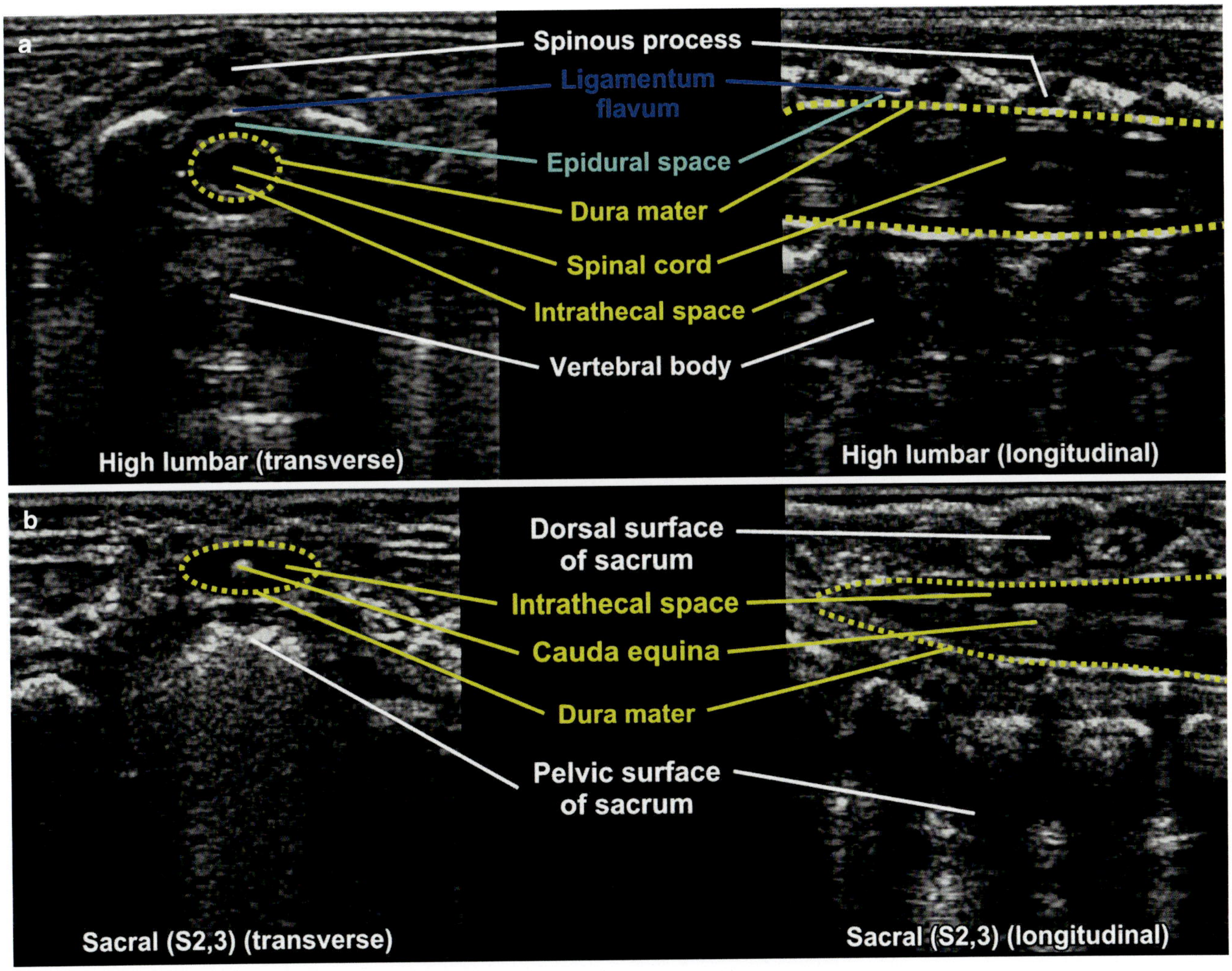

Fig. 33.13 Transverse and longitudinal ultrasound images at the high-lumbar (**a**) and sacral (**b**) levels in a 12-month-old infant. Note that there is more visibility in the infant spine due to the lack of calcification and fusion of the posterior elements of the canal

Lumbar spine of a 10-year-old:

Transverse axis (Fig. 33.9b):

- The center of the screen contains the circular subdural space within the vertebral (spinal) canal, with the internal anechoic CSF and hypoechoic intrathecal nerve roots (not viewed in Fig. 33.9) surrounded by a thin circular layer of hyperechoic dura.
- Superficially, it is possible to view the linear layer of hyperechoic subcutaneous tissue and inverted V-shape of the pedicles and spinous processes.

Paramedian longitudinal axis (Fig. 33.11d)

- The image contains an alternating dark (dorsal shadowing from bone) and bright (ultrasound "window") pattern (mainly intervertebral spaces).
- If seen, the conus medullaris and cauda equina have a hyperechoic and almost fibrillar appearance.
- Hypoechoic CSF lies adjacent to the spinal nerve roots and within the linear hyperechoic dura mater.
- The ligamentum flavum may be seen on the dorsal aspect of the dura and would also mark the epidural space.

Thoracic spine of a 10-year-old:

Transverse viewing (Fig. 33.10b):

- The "starry night" appearance of the paravertebral muscles is evident on either side of the hypoechoic matter (shadowing) from the long and thin spinous process.
- A wide scanning transverse view is often large enough to visualize the articular and transverse processes.
- In patients older than a few months, the central "window" of the spinal canal viewed in the lumbar and sacral spine is not nearly as well depicted in the thoracic region due to the compact nature of the bony elements.
- Generally, the hyperechoic meninges are not delineated, and the position of the dura is estimated at best.

Paramedian longitudinal viewing (Fig. 33.12d)

- Appears similar to that seen at the lumbar spine, except the spinal cord appears hypoechoic with the surrounding dura appearing as a thin hyperechoic line between shadows from the overlaying spinous processes.
- The ligamentum flavum may be seen and the epidural space determined to some extent.

Direct Imaging

- Transverse imaging shows the spinous processes with shadowing in the midline, the facet joints laterally, and the vertebral bodies being the deepest structure, with the potential for viewing intrathecal structures. Imaging of needle trajectory is limited except for indication of lateralization.
- Median longitudinal/sagittal imaging depicts the spinous processes and interspinous space quite clearly. Needle trajectory can be controlled through this approach
- In young patients, there is a good "soft tissue window," and the usually bilayered dura mater is clearly visualized, while the ligamentum flavum, intrathecal space, spinal cord, nerve roots, and fibers (including the cauda equina) all have intermediate but identifiable echogenicity.
- Paramedian longitudinal imaging can be used, allowing greatest visibility of the dura mater. There is less interference from ossification with this approach, allowing enhanced image quality and more visibility of the interspace.
- In the paramedian longitudinal view (Fig. 33.11d), the lamina and facet joints are visible, rather than the spinous processes (as seen more clearly with median longitudinal viewing).
- A remaining challenge with the paramedian longitudinal technique is the tangential (OOP; short-axis) relation of the needle (midline) and probe (paramedian), which only enables clear needle tip visibility and limits accurate angular positioning control of the shaft.

Indirect Imaging

- Continuous visualization of needle tip penetration and catheter advancement is sometimes difficult due to the ultrasound beam reflecting off bony structures.
- Needle punctures are often made visible by movements of the needle tip and displacement of the surrounding tissue.
- Occasionally, widening of the epidural space and ventral movement of the dura mater can be seen upon saline injection.
- Catheter advancement is generally visualized indirectly by the spread of injectate and movement of the dura in the vicinity of the catheter tip.
- This method limits the ability to reassess the catheter position post-procedure.
- It has been reported that the use of metal-coiled catheters, which appear bright with striated features, may help, but our experience shows that this effect is limited.

33.1.8 Needle Insertion Technique

Pre-procedural (ultrasound-supported) measurements:

- Use short- and long-axis scanning with a paramedian probe alignment.
- Ultrasound can be used to assess neuraxial anatomy and, depending on visibility, measure various distances in the vertebral (spinal) canal, including those from skin and bone to dural, epidural, and intrathecal spaces.
- Ultrasound-guided determination of epidural space depth and depth to loss of resistance may be beneficial with good correlation between ultrasound-measured and clinical loss of resistance depth.
  - This can be useful to assess the vertebral column (transverse and longitudinal views) and to estimate the epidural space (i.e., anticipated loss of resistance depths) (Fig. 33.14).
  - If the dura is seen:
    - Depth of the epidural space = slightly more shadow than skin-to-dural distance
  - If the lamina but not the dura is seen:
    - Depth of the epidural space = slightly deeper than skin-to-lamina distance
- Determination of the ideal puncture location and trajectory can be performed.
- Pre-procedural assessments can be performed prior to real-time ultrasound guidance or in isolation before proceeding with a standard loss-of-resistance technique.

Real-time guidance

- The value of dynamic ultrasound guidance in the thoracic region may be limited in patients older than a few months of age.
- The puncture is typically made with a midline approach at the required segment, and the probe is best aligned longitudinally along the paramedian plane.

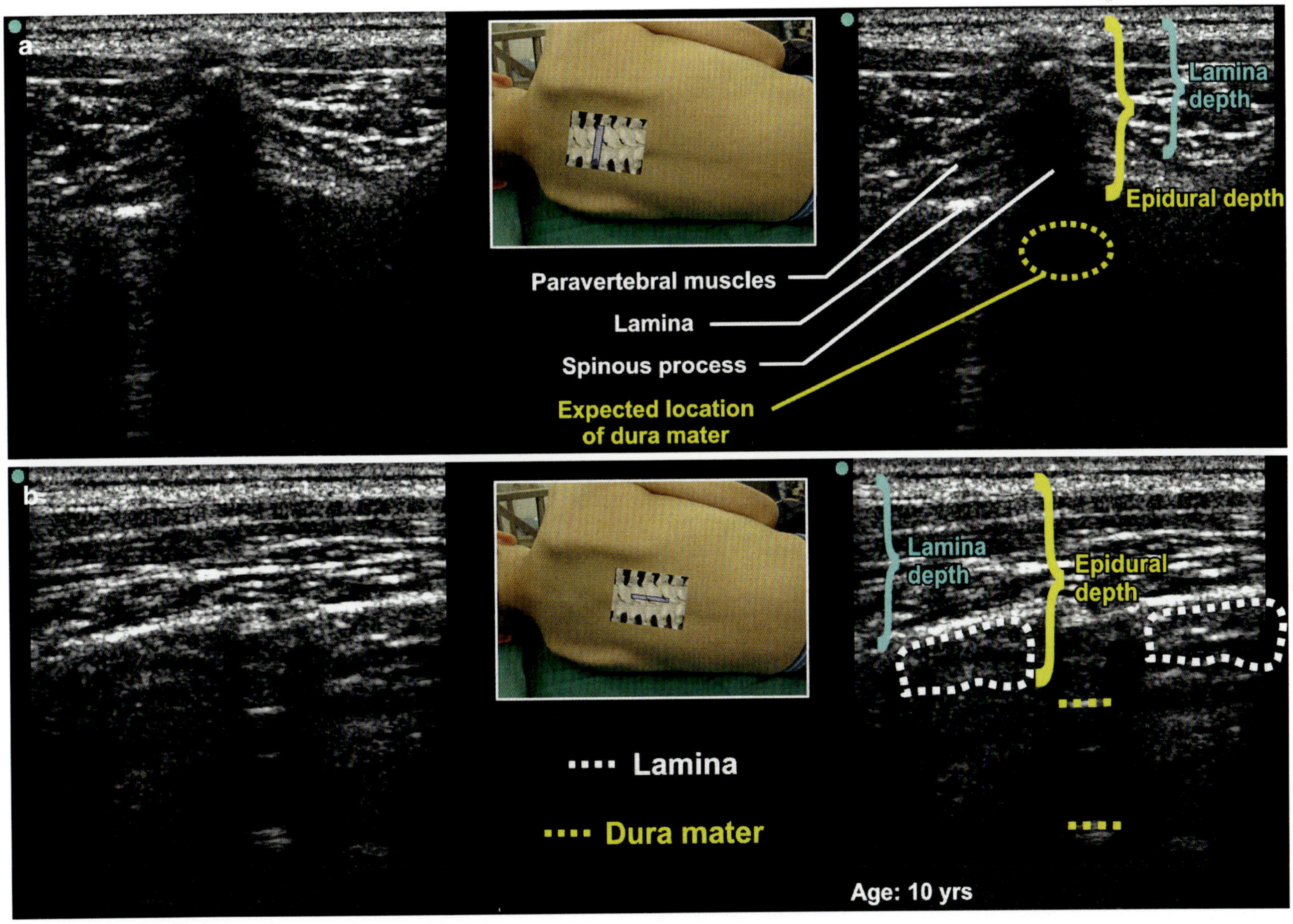

Fig. 33.14 (a) Estimation of epidural depth based on transverse plane images at the thoracic spine. (b) Estimation of epidural depth based on longitudinal plane images at the thoracic spine

- The needle shaft and probe beam are OOP, and only the needle tip may be seen.
- The loss-of-resistance technique is still required and may be aided by directly visualizing the needle penetrating the ligamentum flavum, particularly in the lumbar spine. However, confirmation of epidural space localization will generally occur by visualizing a test dose of local anesthetic and the subsequent dural movement it causes.
  - For ultrasound guidance during epidural anesthesia, an assistant will often be needed to perform the imaging, which allows the anesthesiologist to use both hands to perform the LOR (Fig. 33.15). Otherwise, the anesthesiologist will need to utilize an automotive device to detect LOR (e.g., Episure AutoDetect Syringe, Indigo Orb, CA, USA) to free a hand to manipulate the ultrasound probe.
- When performing ultrasound-guided epidural placements in infants (<10 kg), a 20G needle should be used.
- After epidural space confirmation, injection of the local anesthetic solution will be visualized with a caudal and cephalad spread.

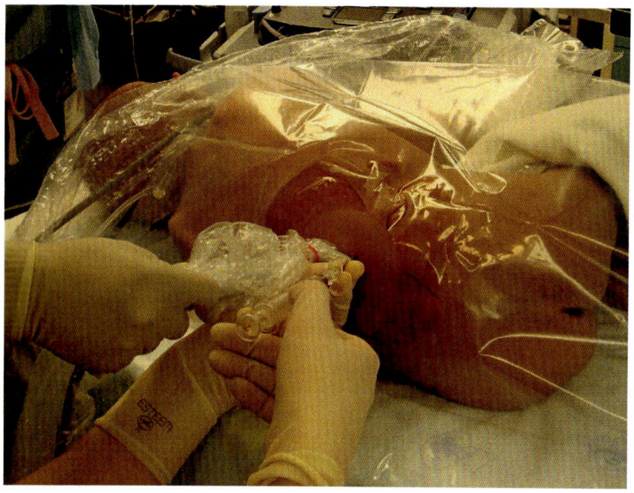

Fig. 33.15 Real-time (online) needling during a low-thoracic epidural showing out-of-plane alignment of the needle (median) and probe (paramedian). An assistant is needed to perform the ultrasound imaging

33.1.9 Catheter Insertion and Confirmation

- To confirm correct catheter insertion, we recommended using loss of resistance to saline technique despite the availability of ultrasound guidance or epidural stimulation testing.
- The catheter is introduced once the needle positioning in the epidural space has been confirmed by direct visualization of penetration and dural movement upon injection of a test dose of local anesthetic.
- The catheter tip may be visible upon entry and during advancement with local anesthetic injection.
- The epidural stimulation test may be used to confirm correct epidural needle entrance (i.e., to prevent intrathecal or intravascular placement), although its use in short-distance (2–5 cm) catheter advancement may be limited.
- Once correct catheter tip placement is confirmed, rule out intrathecal placement, and inject the local anesthetic. Epidural placement may be confirmed if the movement of dura is obvious and the catheter tip is visible. Catheter tip identification is possible in children under 3–6 years of age (see Fig. 33.16).

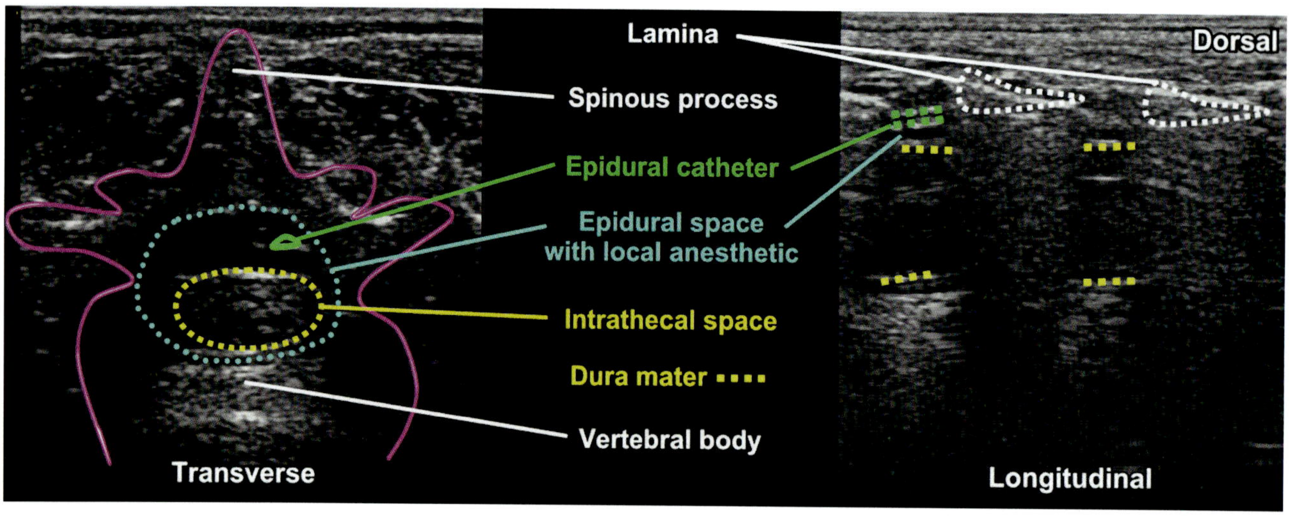

Fig. 33.16 Transverse and longitudinal views of an epidural catheter at the lumbar spine in a 14-month-old child

33.1.10 Case Study: Lumbar Epidural

Lumbar Epidural (*Provided by A. Spencer*)

A 2-month-old female, 3.3 kg, was scheduled to undergo a reversal of stoma and mucous fistula. The child had previously undergone a laparotomy due to meconium ileus; following this surgery, the patient remained intubated for 3 weeks due to difficulty with ventilation and sedation. The patient was also diagnosed with cystic fibrosis and pulmonary hypertension during this period. A lumbar epidural with insertion at the L2–L3 level was administered under ultrasound guidance. A pre-procedural ultrasound scan was performed to obtain a paramedian, longitudinal view of neuraxial structures, including the sacral, lumbar, and lower thoracic levels; the depth from skin to dura; and the location of the tip of the conus medullaris.

A 5 cm, 20G Tuohy needle was inserted, and a 24G multilumen epidural catheter was threaded into the epidural space (Fig. 33.17). An initial test dose of 0.3 mL lidocaine 1 % with epinephrine 1:200,000 was injected, followed by an initial bolus of 2.5 mL ropivacaine 0.25 %. Two 1 mL boluses of ropivacaine 0.25 % were given intraoperatively. Postoperatively, a continuous infusion of 1 mL/h ropivacaine 0.08 % (0.23 mg/kg/h) was ordered. Pain control was supplemented with acetaminophen 40 mg q6h per rectum for 2 days.

The patient was comfortable in recovery. Upon being moved to the surgical ward, a low-dose morphine infusion at 10 μg/kg/h was started since the patient seemed irritable and hungry but was NPO. Acute pain service followed the patient for 48 h, at which time the epidural was discontinued and removed.

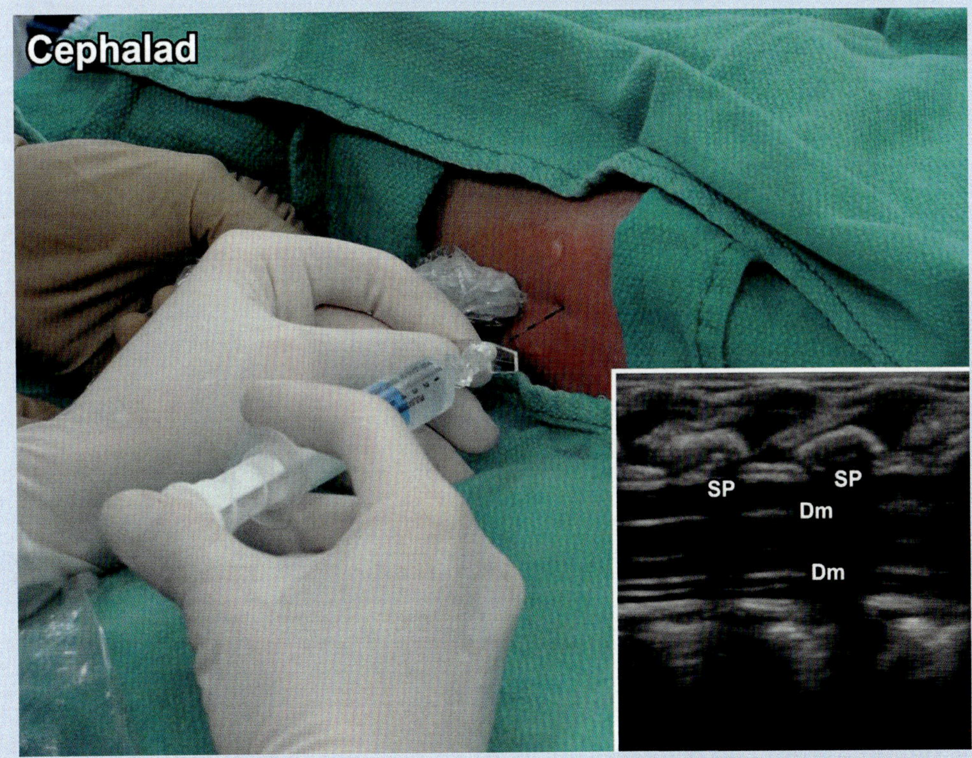

Fig. 33.17 Lumbar epidural block. *SP* spinous process, *Dm* dura mater (See Case Study for details)

33.2 Caudal Anesthesia

33.2.1 Introduction

Single-shot caudal epidural anesthesia is suitable for blockade of the lumbar and sacral dermatomes. Although needle puncture may be considerably safer at the sacral hiatus than at other regions in the spinal canal because it is below the spinal cord, there is still a high failure rate (up to 25 %) associated with needle placement into the caudal canal, and inadvertent vascular puncture occurs with some frequency (5–9 % of patients). Usually, a "pop" is detected as the needle enters the sacral canal through the sacral hiatus and posterior sacrococcygeal membrane, and this sign, together with ease of advancement of the angiocatheter and local anesthetic injection, is traditionally used to determine correct needle placement (Fig. 33.18).

The development of the epidural electrical stimulation test has enhanced the current repertoire of methods that assess correct needle placement in the caudal canal and is a more objective method than those currently available. Ultrasound may be useful to determine the best puncture site for caudal needle placement. As with other spinal levels, ultrasound imaging at the sacral spine may be most beneficial in young infants (<1 year old) since there is less ossification and therefore a good ultrasound "window" in this region. The main disadvantage with both ultrasound and nerve stimulation is that they do not provide immediate warning in cases of intravascular puncture.

Indications

Analgesia or surgical anesthesia for:

- Urogenital surgery
- Lower limb surgery

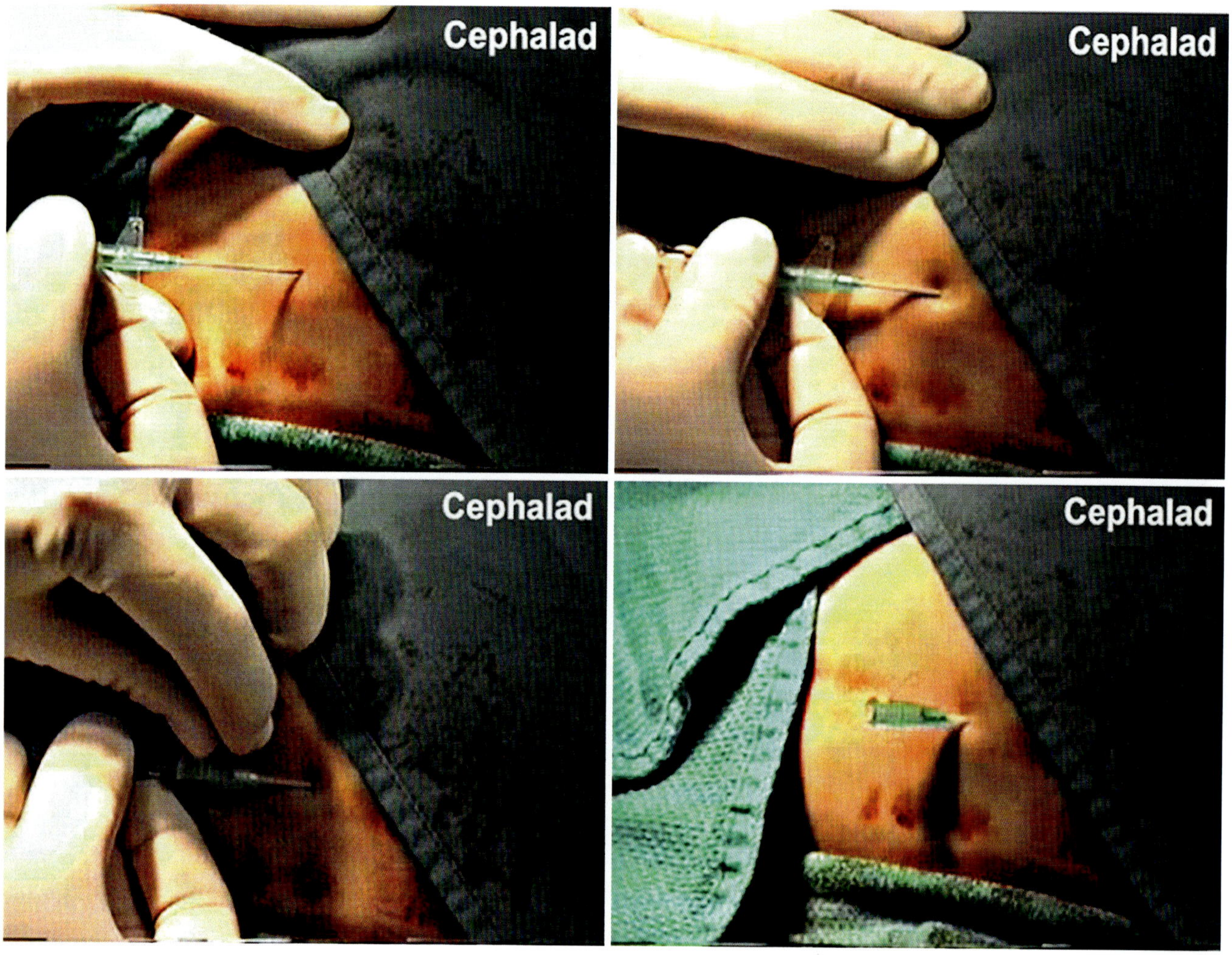

Fig. 33.18 Caudal blockade involves needle/catheter entry at the sacral hiatus and through the posterior sacrococcygeal ligament (*upper left*). As the needle enters the sacral canal and epidural space, a "pop" is usually felt (*upper right*). The ease of intravenous cannula advancement and local anesthetic injection is also used to confirm caudal epidural space localization

33.2.2 Patient Positioning

Position the patient in the lateral position.

33.2.3 Surface Anatomy (Fig. 33.19)

Iliac crests:
- Approximately at the level of the L4 spinous process
  Posterior superior iliac spines (PSIS):
- Approximately 4–5 cm lateral to S1/S2.

Median sacral crest:*
- Fused spinous processes of the sacrum (on dorsal surface)
- May be difficult to palpate in patients with excessive subcutaneous tissue

Sacral hiatus:*
- Sacral cornua (horns) can be palpated approximately 5 cm above the tip of the coccyx.
- The sacral hiatus lies at the midpoint between these cornua.

*These landmarks are suitable as reference points in older children only. Refer to Fig. 13.4 for more information.

Clinical Pearl

Using a landmark approach with an angiocatheter (Fig 33.18):
- The ease of intravenous cannula advancement is the most important sign to confirm caudal epidural location.
- Inadvertent intravascular placement can be detected easily by gentle aspiration once the needle is removed.

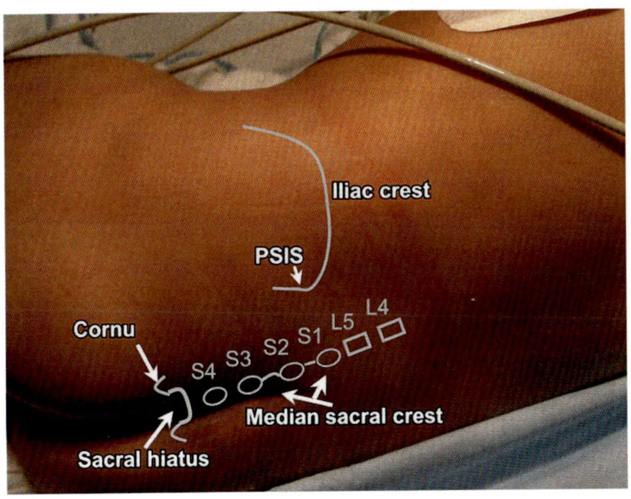

Fig. 33.19 Patient positioning and surface landmarks for caudal block

33.2.4 Nerve Stimulation Technique

- An insulated, sheathed 22G needle is required for the epidural stimulation test.
- After sterile preparation, connect a nerve stimulator to the needle.
- Attach the cathode (negative; black) lead of the nerve stimulator to the insulated needle, and attach the grounding anode (positive; red) lead to an electrode on the patient's body surface.
- Set the nerve stimulator to a low frequency and pulse width (1 or 2 Hz; 0.1 or 0.2 ms).
- Insert the needle perpendicular to the skin at the level of the sacral cornua (located by palpation).
- Advance the needle until the characteristic "give" or "pop" is felt, indicating entrance into the caudal epidural space.
- Carefully and slowly increase the current intensity until motor activity begins.
- The correct motor response is contraction of the anal sphincter (S2–S4) at a current threshold generally between 1 and 15 mA.
- Localized muscular twitches of the gluteal or back muscles are an incorrect response and indicate that the needle is likely in the subcutaneous space outside the sacrococcygeal ligament. Additionally, the current may be higher (>8 mA) in this case.
- Refer to Table 33.1 for information on the threshold current of motor response, particularly with respect to intrathecal placement.
- After negative aspiration for CSF, an epinephrine test dose (0.5 μg/kg) should be administered to identify inadvertent intravascular placement, as indicated by specific ECG changes (i.e., >25 % increase in T-wave or ST segment changes, irrespective of chosen lead).
- The presence of any physical signs of subcutaneous bulging or tissue resistance upon the injection of local anesthetic indicates improper needle placement and an unsuccessful caudal block.

33.2.5 Ultrasound-Guided Block

33.2.5.1 Preparing the Needle Insertion Site

The area should be prepared by cleaning with an alcohol-based chlorhexidine surgical wash and draping the area for sterility. Any catheter techniques should have the same meticulous attention to sterile technique as for epidural insertion.

33.2.5.2 Scanning Technique

- Begin with a short-axis transverse probe (5–12 MHz linear) orientation at the level of the fifth sacral vertebra to identify landmarks. The sacral cornua (bilateral horns of sacrum), dorsal surface of the sacrum and posterior sacrococcygeal ligament, and sacral hiatus may be visualized (Fig. 33.20).
- Upon skin puncture, rotate the probe 90° for long-axis (longitudinal) viewing between the two cornua (Fig. 33.21), which may allow IP imaging of the needle trajectory toward the entrance to the sacrococcygeal ligament; beyond this barrier, the characteristic "pop" can be used to confirm needle placement within the caudal epidural space.
- Linear probes are advantageous in most patients, although curvilinear array transducers with lower frequencies may be beneficial with older and/or obese patients. Smaller footprint (hockey stick) probes are more appropriate in smaller patients.
- After entry into the caudal epidural space, the probe can be rotated from a longitudinal to a transverse orientation to locate the needle in short axis (as a dot) between the sacrococcygeal ligament and the pelvic (ventral) surface of the sacrum (i.e., caudal epidural space).
- For young infants (best results in patients over 1 year old), the probe (7–12 MHz linear) can be placed over the midsacral level (S2–S3) due to the limited ossification of the sacral vertebrae (see Fig. 33.13). A long-axis view will allow clear visibility of the needle trajectory through the caudal entrance into the epidural space.

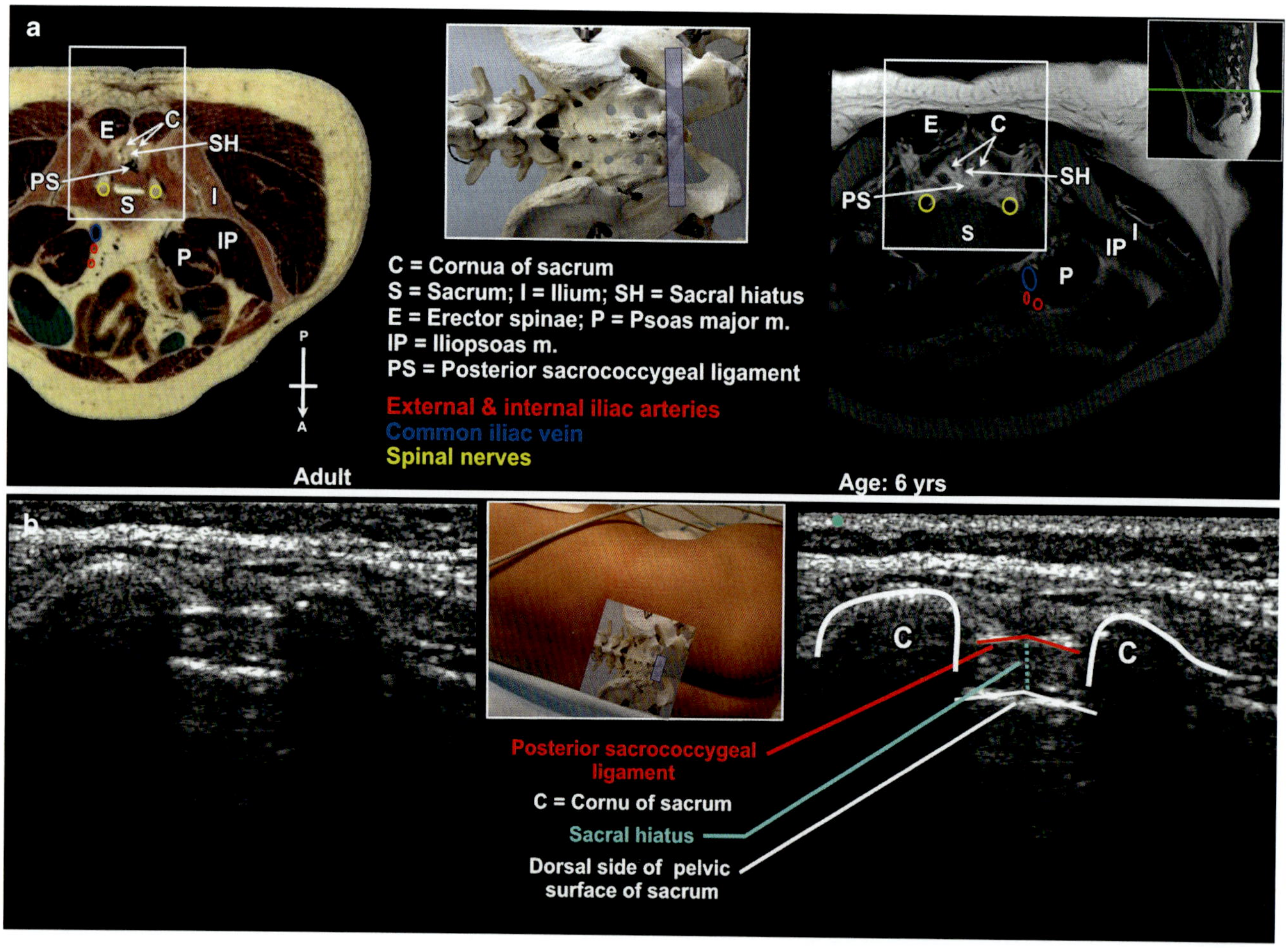

Fig. 33.20 (**a**) VHVS and MRI images of transverse plane of the caudal space. (**b**) Transverse/short-axis image captured by a linear probe at the level of the sacral hiatus in a 10-year-old patient

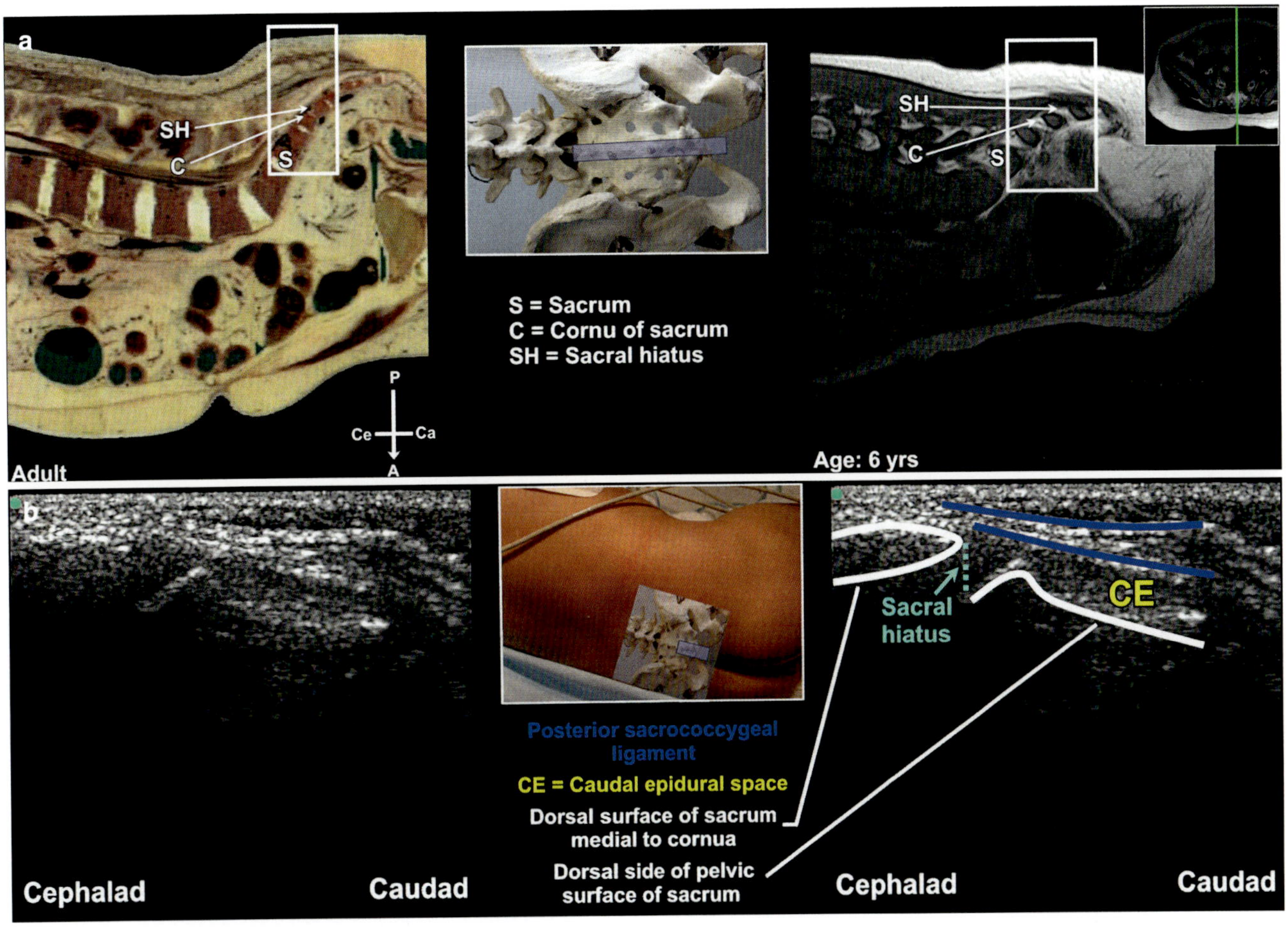

Fig. 33.21 (**a**) VHVS and MRI images of longitudinal plane of the caudal space. (**b**) Longitudinal/long-axis image captured by a linear probe placed between the sacral cornua of a 10-year-old patient

33.2.5.3 Sonographic Appearance

- Short-axis view at sacral hiatus (Fig. 33.20b):
  - Superficially, the two sacral cornua are seen as hyperechoic inverted U-shaped structures beneath the variably echogenic linear subcutaneous tissue.
  - Deep and between the cornua are two hyperechoic bands indicating the posterior sacrococcygeal membrane (first) and the dorsal side of the pelvic surface ("base") of the sacrum; the hypoechoic space between these is the sacral hiatus.
  - Deep to the cornua and bands, the image may show lateral darkening and a medial hypoechogenic epidural space; this will be variable.
  - The needle can be seen as a hyperechoic dot within the sacral hiatus following sacrococcygeal membrane puncture (not shown).
- Long-axis view at sacral hiatus (Fig. 33.21b):
  - The sacrococcygeal ligament appears broad, hyperechoic, and linear and is slanted at a caudal angle.
  - The dorsal surface of the sacrum appears hyperechoic deep and cephalad to the membrane.
  - The dorsal side of the ventral (pelvic) surface of the sacrum appears dark at the bottom of the image, with a moderately hypoechogenic space – the sacral hiatus – between the sacrococcygeal ligament and sacral bone (with the caudal epidural space cephalad and beneath the dorsal surface of the sacrum).
  - The needle may appear as a hyperechoic and linear structure outside the epidural space. The needle is not visible within the epidural space due to the beam reflection from the dorsum of the sacrum (not shown).

33.2.5.4 Caudal vs. Intrathecal Injection

- When performing caudal blocks, there is a risk of dural puncture leading to accidental intrathecal injection. Effects of intrathecal injection range from headache to total spinal blockade.
- Several methods, including the "whoosh" and "swoosh" tests, electrical stimulation, and imaging, have been used to guide needle placement and help ensure a caudal location.
- It was recently shown that color flow Doppler ultrasound can predict with high sensitivity and specificity whether injection is occurring in the caudal or intrathecal space; a clear signal is obtained with caudal injection, whereas intrathecal injection produces no detectable signal (Fig. 33.22).

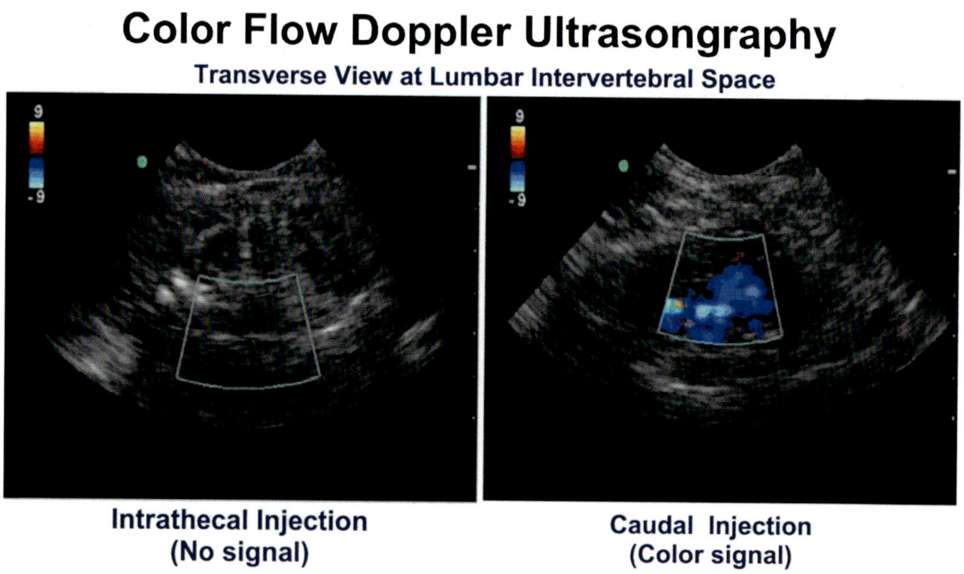

Fig. 33.22 Color Doppler ultrasound for confirming local anesthetic spread into the lumbar (L4) epidural space. Preinjection (*left*), no illumination and a central circular intrathecal space are seen; postinjection (*right*), local anesthetic appears as a medley of colors and expands the epidural space slightly

33.2.5.5 Needle Insertion and Local Anesthetic Application

In pediatric patients, caudal anesthesia follows general anesthesia in most cases.

For patients older than 1 year, position the probe at the sacral hiatus. For infants, place it at S2–S3.

- Insert a 22G needle perpendicular to the skin and in the midline at the sacral hiatus.
- With the probe placed longitudinally, the needle can be seen in long axis as it advances to and penetrates the sacrococcygeal ligament.
- Advance the needle until a "pop" is felt, signifying caudal epidural space entrance.
- The reduced fusion and calcification of the dorsal sacrum in infants may allow visibility of the needle tip beyond the ligament and within the epidural space.
- Rotate the probe to the short axis to confirm needle location (a bright dot in the epidural space) and inject the local anesthetic.
- Local anesthetic may be seen directly as an expansion of hypoechogenicity and indirectly through dural movement.

33.2.6 Case Study: Caudal Epidural

Caudal Epidural (*Provided by S. Suresh*)
A 9-month-old boy, 11 kg, was scheduled for a caudal block for hypospadias repair. The block was performed under ultrasound guidance with a 22G needle and 10 mL 0.25 % bupivacaine with epinephrine 1:200,000 (Fig. 33.23). Duration of surgery was 2 h; block duration was 4–6 h. No pain was reported in recovery (0 on FLACC scale). Postoperative analgesia consisted of a 6 mg injection of ketorolac (Toradol).

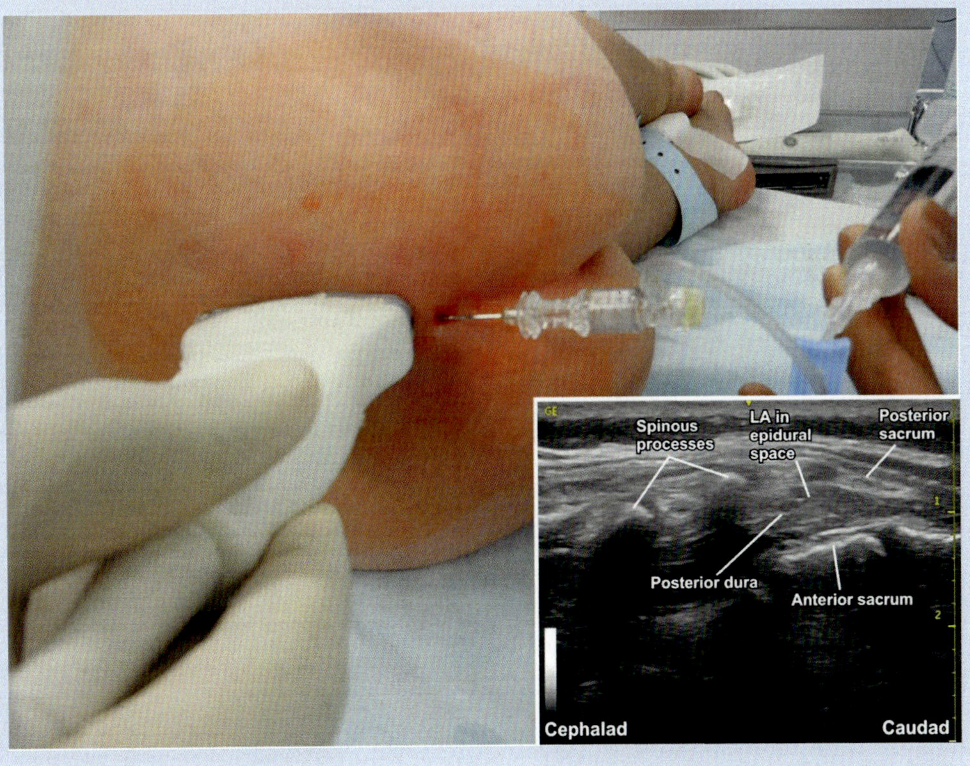

Fig. 33.23 Ultrasound-guided caudal epidural block (See Case Study for details)

33.3 Advancing a Catheter to the Lumbar or Thoracic Area from a Caudal Insertion Site

Advancing catheters from the sacral (or low lumbar) epidural space to lumbar or thoracic levels has the advantage of reducing the risk of direct spinal cord trauma (especially as there will be no sensory warning in anesthetized pediatric patients) and may be technically easier in patients with prior spinal surgery at higher levels. Confirmation of both proper catheter placement in the epidural space and monitoring the catheter's cephalad advancement is important, and both ultrasound and electrical epidural stimulations may be beneficial because of the dynamic nature of these techniques. The epidural stimulation test can provide a warning of intrathecal, and possibly intravascular, needle or catheter placement.

This is most successful in patients under 1 year of age since after this age, the lumbar curve becomes more pronounced, preventing easy advancement of epidural catheters from the caudal space. However, with specialized styletted catheters and using the epidural stimulation test to guide positioning, caudal catheter advancement is now possible in older children.

33.3.1 Epidural Stimulation Guidance Technique (Fig. 33.24)

Procedure

- Estimate the length necessary to thread a 20G styletted epidural stimulating catheter or metal-containing epidural catheter the required distance (Fig. 2.10).
- Adjust the stylet to a point within the distal end of the epidural catheter to obtain the desired stiffness.
- After sterile preparation, insert an 18G IV catheter, using similar technique to that of the single-shot approach into the caudal epidural space; correct placement will be characterized by the typical "give" or "pop" upon penetration of the sacrococcygeal ligament (Fig. 33.18).
- Use the electrode adaptor to connect a nerve stimulator to the epidural catheter.
- Prime the stimulating catheter and adaptor with sterile normal saline (1–2 mL).
- Attach the cathode lead of the nerve stimulator to the metal hub of the adaptor and the grounding anode lead to an electrode on the patient's body.

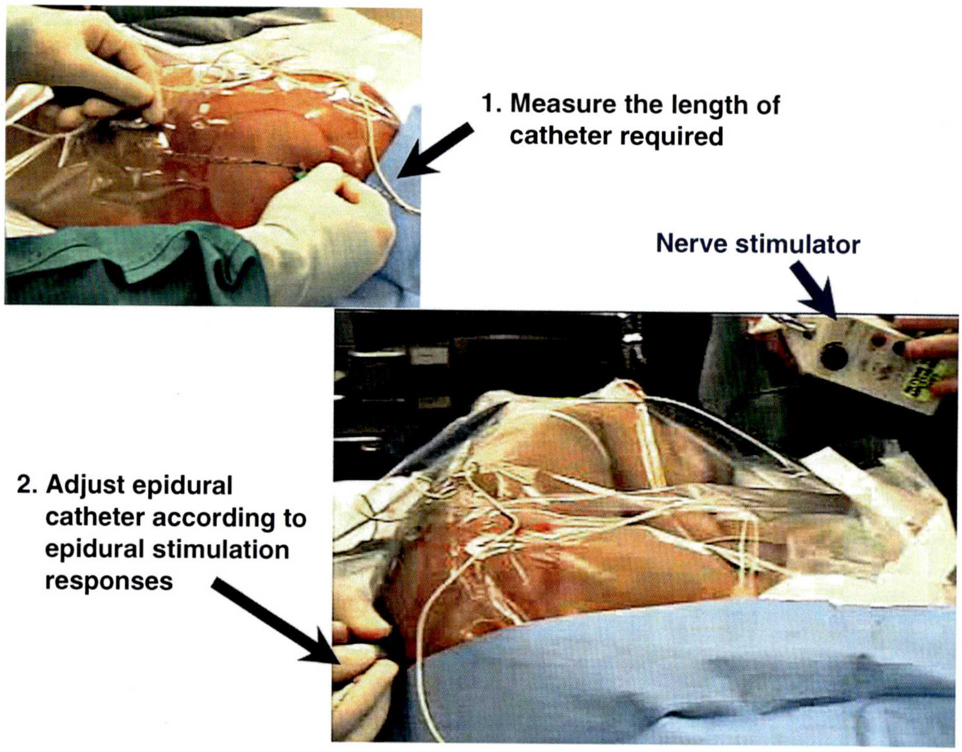

Fig. 33.24 Epidural catheter insertion using electrical epidural stimulation. First, estimate the length of a styletted metal-containing catheter. Secondly, insert the catheter into the caudal epidural space using traditional methods (i.e., loss of resistance), and advance the catheter. Observe responses to nerve stimulation to confirm epidural placement and the segmental level of catheter tip location

- Set the nerve stimulator to a low frequency and pulse width (2 Hz; 0.2 ms).
- For continuous caudal anesthesia, advance the catheter a few millimeters and gradually apply current to the catheter until motor activity or a twitch response of the anal sphincter (S2–S4) is visible.
- For threading to lumbar or thoracic levels, advance the catheter while gradually applying current.
- Follow progressive motor responses (from lower limbs and lumbar (back) to intercostals to thoracic and upper limbs) through cranial advancement until desired level is reached.
- Minor resistance encountered during catheter threading can be overcome by injecting normal saline through the catheter and/or simple flexion or extension of the patient's vertebral column.
- Inject a test dose of local anesthetic to rule out intravascular placement.
- Compare the total characteristics of the response to Table 33.1 to determine catheter placement and make any required adjustments.
- If the catheter does not reach the desired level, it can be pulled back and reinserted.
- Once optimally positioned, withdraw the 18G intravenous catheter and the stylet.
- Affix the catheter immediately cephalad to the site of insertion with several layers of occlusive dressing (Fig. 33.25).

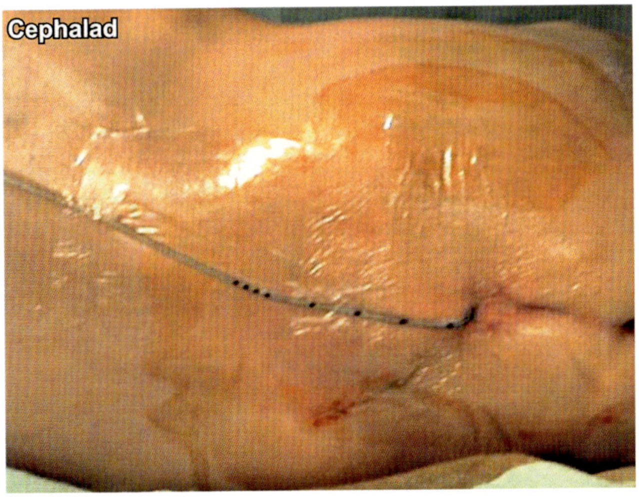

Fig. 33.25 Epidural catheter secured on an infant's back with sterile occlusive dressing to maintain sterility

33.3.2 Local Anesthetic Application ("Test") to Confirm Avoidance of Intravascular Placement

- After aspirating to rule out intrathecal placement, inject a test dose of local anesthetic (0.1 mL/kg lidocaine 1 % with 1:200,000 epinephrine) to confirm catheter placement and to ensure it is not intravascular.
- If catheter placement is correct, the current threshold should increase, and the motor response should cease upon local anesthetic injection.
- If the catheter tip is within the intravascular space, the local anesthetic will disperse systemically, and the motor response will remain the same with repeated injections of local anesthetic.
- Once intravascular placement is ruled out, the catheter can be affixed to the skin as described above.

33.3.3 Ultrasound-Guided Technique

This technique is most suitable for young infants (0–6 months) since, due to incomplete ossification of the vertebrae, the catheter tip and a greater number of anatomical structures are more easily visualized. The thoracic spine provides less of an "ultrasound window" due to its smaller size and overlapping spinous processes.

33.3.4 Scanning Technique

- An assistant must perform the ultrasound imaging during catheter placement.
- During caudal cannula placement and epidural catheter advancement, follow the scanning technique described earlier for caudal needle placement in young infants.
- For viewing the lumbar and thoracic regions of the spine, position the probe in a longitudinal median or paramedian plane (probe lateral to the spinous processes).
- Either alignment may be suitable for the lumbar spine, although paramedian may be superior, as it allows clear visibility of the dura, and dural movement upon catheter entrance has been shown to be a better indicator of ligamentum flavum penetration (as seen best through median alignment).
- The paramedian position (whether transverse or longitudinal axis) is the best choice for the thoracic spine as there is more ossification here, and the long, obliquely oriented spinous processes overlap each other significantly.

33.3.5 Sonographic Appearance

The appearance of the caudal epidural space will match that seen when performing single-shot anesthesia (see Figs. 33.20 and 33.21).

Catheter Visibility (14-Month-Old)

- At the lumbar spine, the tip of the catheter may be seen upon entry and during advancement (Fig. 33.16), although more than one imaging plane may be required. In children older than 3–6 years of age, the catheter tip may not be clearly identified following insertion.
- Generally, the catheter is viewed indirectly by observing movement of the dura upon fluid injection; the hypoechoic local anesthetic will appear to expand the epidural space and cause ventral movement of the dura.

Local Anesthetic Injection

- In general, local anesthetic cannot be seen directly, but occasionally, caudad and cephalad spread can be appreciated indirectly from displacement of the dura.

33.3.6 Catheter Insertion and Local Anesthetic Application

- On the exterior of the patient's body, measure the length of catheter required.
- Perform the block using an 18G IV cannula and a 20G epidural catheter (stimulating if using electrical epidural stimulation).
- If using epidural stimulation, follow the procedure in the previous section while viewing the catheter using ultrasound.
- If using ultrasound alone with the classic "pop" at the caudal epidural space, visualize catheter advancement either directly (in young infants) or with the aid of local anesthetic injection to cause movement of the dura.
- Once catheter tip placement is deemed correct, rule out inadvertent intrathecal placement (Table 33.1), and inject local anesthetic to check for inadvertent intravascular injection. Ultrasound may also be of use in this regard if the movement of dura is clear and if the catheter tip is visible in the epidural space.

33.3.7 Case Study: Thoracic Epidural

Thoracic Epidural (*Provided by B. Tsui*)

An 8-month-old child underwent open Nissen fundoplication surgery. After induction of general anesthesia without muscle relaxation, the child was placed in a lateral position. Under strict sterile conditions, an epidural catheter was introduced via the caudal space using similar technique to that shown in Figs. 33.18 and 33.24. Using nerve stimulation guidance, the catheter was advanced into the thoracic space. Once the catheter reached the desired location (with confirmation by nerve stimulation), it was secured as shown in Fig. 33.25. Real-time ultrasound imaging was performed during catheter advancement. A transverse view at L3/L4 (Fig. 33.26a) and paramedian longitudinal view (Fig. 33.26b) were obtained at the midthoracic level; the dura mater and epidural catheter can be easily appreciated in these images. The infant was wakened up without any signs of discomfort and was discharged to the ward postoperatively.

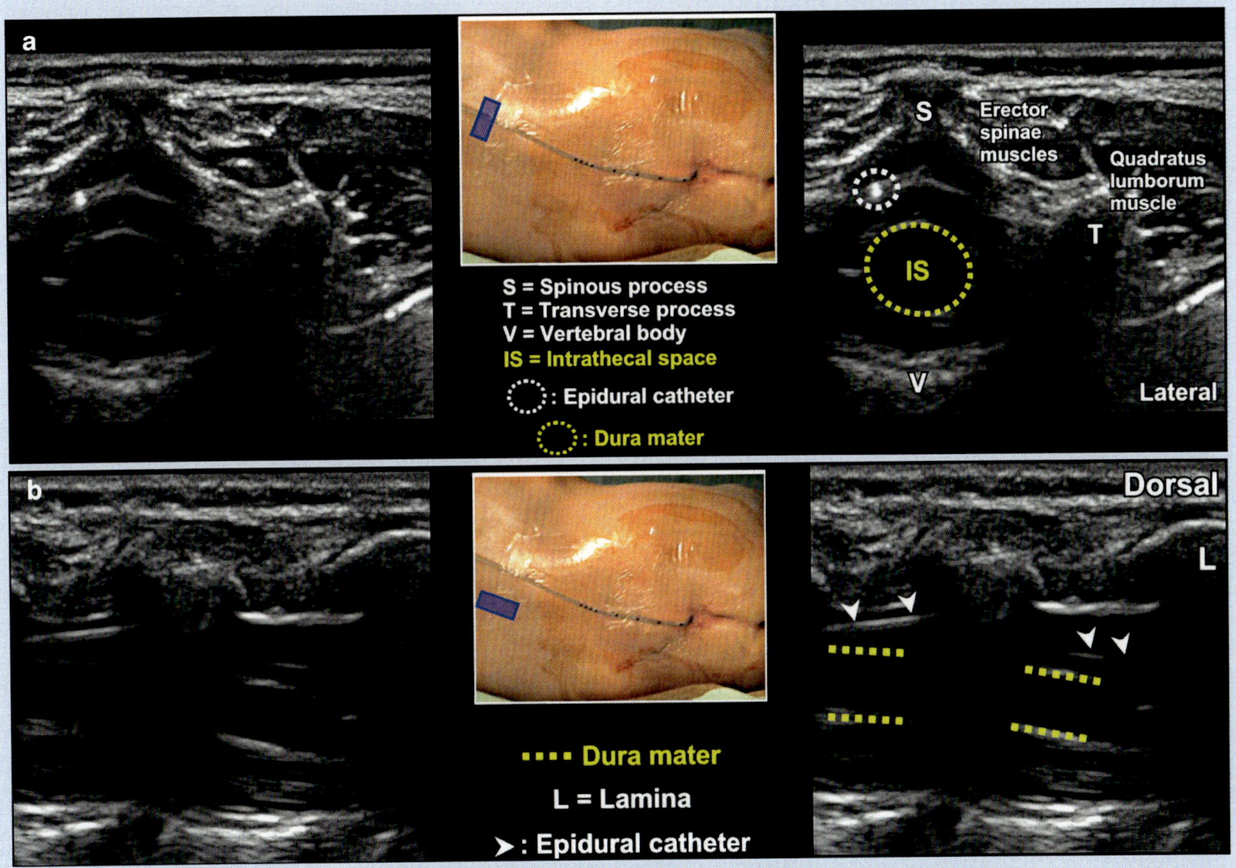

Fig. 33.26 Ultrasound-guided thoracic epidural catheter placement via caudal insertion. Transverse (**a**) and paramedian longitudinal (**b**) views are shown. *Blue rectangle* indicates probe footprint (See Case Study for details)

33.4 Current Literature in Ultrasound-Guided Approaches

There is a relative abundance of recent literature covering topics in ultrasound-guided techniques in pediatric practice. Most studies have compared ultrasound guidance to traditional non-ultrasound methods; an important outcome that this comparison addressed is needling time. For thoracic epidurals, Tachibana et al. [7] found a significantly shorter needling time in the ultrasound group compared to the control group (median 100 (77–116) vs. 165 (130–206) s) when ultrasound prescanning was used. Nevertheless, one consideration when ultrasound is used is the time taken to do the scan in the first place; in the Tachibana study, the scan to visualize neuraxial structure took, in most cases, over 2 min to perform. In certain circumstances, this may unnecessarily extend the overall needling time. In another study of block performance time, Wang et al. [8] compared ultrasound-guided caudal block by sacral hiatus injection to traditional sacral canal injection and reported a significantly shorter time for the ultrasound group (145 ± 23 vs. 164 ± 31 s), but did not comment on the time taken to perform the scan itself. Thus, ultrasound prescanning shortens actual needling time but will in all likelihood extend the overall block procedure time.

Success of neuraxial blocks under ultrasound guidance is another outcome that has been studied. Wang et al. [8] found that, although the overall success rate of caudal block was similar between groups whose blocks were performed under ultrasound guidance or using LOR (92.8 % vs. 95.7 %), success rates for the first puncture were significantly higher with ultrasound (92.8 % vs. 50 %). Similarly, Tachibana et al. [7] showed that the number of epidural puncture attempts was reduced when ultrasound prescanning was done, and those performing the blocks reported significantly more difficulty without a prescan. Shin et al. [9] compared two ultrasound-guided caudal block approaches – one involving the commonly used sacral hiatus and the other involving the S2–3 interspace. The first epidural puncture attempt success rate was significantly higher with the latter approach despite a similar overall success rate between the two approaches.

Several recent studies have assessed direct visualization of local anesthesia spread using ultrasound during neuraxial blockade. Lundblad et al. [10] used ultrasound imaging to show a significant inverse relationship with regard to age, weight, and height and maximum cranial spread after caudal blockade. Triffterer et al. [11] assessed local anesthetic injection speed (0.5 mL/s vs. 0.25 mL/s) during ultrasound-guided caudal block and found no significant difference in level of cranial spread or distance of spread relative to the conus medullaris in the epidural space. Ueda et al. [12] were able to demonstrate that transesophageal echocardiography could be used to visualize both catheter position and local anesthetic spread in three dimensions for thoracic epidural blocks. Finally, in a prospective observational study of children undergoing a surgical procedure or ongoing chemotherapy regime, Tsui et al. [13] found that color flow Doppler ultrasound could be used to successfully distinguish epidural injection from intrathecal injection.

Ultrasound has also been used to provide more information on subcutaneous neuraxial structures. Koo et al. [14] used ultrasound to examine movement of the dural sac depending on patient positioning; they observed significant cephalad shifts in dural sac position in the lateral flexed position versus a neutral position. The same group used ultrasound to determine the prevalence of spinal dysraphism in children with urogenital anomalies [15]. Children suspected of spinal cord tethering showed a lower level of conus medullaris and thicker filum terminale when compared to the normal group. Kim et al. [16] used information obtained from ultrasound scanning of the sacral hiatus to show that the traditional equiangular triangle method of identifying the sacral hiatus may not be reliable. Using ultrasound to estimate depth of structures, Tachibana et al. [7] showed a significant correlation between needle depth and ultrasound estimation of the skin-dura distance, while Shin et al. [9] revealed significant differences in depth of the sacral space at S2–3 when compared to the sacral hiatus.

With regard to block quality, Willschke et al. [17] retrospectively described the performance of ultrasound-guided thoracic epidural blocks for 20 infants with hypertrophic pylorus stenosis. Ultrasound-guided single-shot epidural blocks provided sufficient analgesia in all infants following surgery and were associated with stable heart rate and oxygen saturation intraoperatively.

References

1. Tsui BC, Wagner A, Cave D, Seal R. Threshold current for an insulated epidural needle in pediatric patients. Anesth Analg. 2004;99: 694–6.
2. Tsui BC, Wagner AM, Cunningham K, Perry S, Desai S, Seal R. Threshold current of an insulated needle in the intrathecal space in pediatric patients. Anesth Analg. 2005;100:662–5.
3. Tsui BC, Wagner AM, Cunningham K, Perry S, Desai S, Seal R. Can continuous low current electrical stimulation distinguish insulated needle position in the epidural and intrathecal spaces in pediatric patients? Pediatr Anesth. 2005;15:959–63.
4. Tsui BC, Tarkkila P, Gupta S, Kearney R. Confirmation of caudal needle placement using nerve stimulation. Anesthesiology. 1999; 91:374–8.
5. Fisher QA, Shaffner DH, Yaster M. Detection of intravascular injection of regional anaesthetics in children. Can J Anesth. 1997; 44:592–8.
6. Tsui BC. Thoracic epidural catheter placement in infants via the caudal approach under electrocardiographic guidance: simplification of the original technique. Anesth Analg. 2004;98:273.
7. Tachibana N, Yamauchi M, Sugino S, Watanabe A, Yamakage M. Utility of longitudinal paramedian view of ultrasound imaging for middle thoracic epidural anesthesia in children. J Anesth. 2012; 26:242–5.
8. Wang LZ, Hu XX, Zhang YF, Chang XY. A randomized comparison of caudal block by sacral hiatus injection under ultrasound guidance with traditional sacral canal injection in children. Pediatr Anesth. 2013;23:395–400.
9. Shin SK, Hong JY, Kim WO, Koo BN, Kim JE, Kil HK. Ultrasound evaluation of the sacral area and comparison of sacral interspinous and hiatal approach for caudal block in children. Anesthesiology. 2009;111:1135–40.
10. Lundblad M, Lonnqvist PA, Eksborg S, Marhofer P. Segmental distribution of high-volume caudal anesthesia in neonates, infants, and toddlers as assessed by ultrasonography. Pediatr Anesth. 2011;21:121–7.
11. Triffterer L, Machata AM, Latzke D, Willschke H, Rebhandl W, Kimberger O, Marhofer P. Ultrasound assessment of cranial spread during caudal blockade in children: effect of the speed of injection of local anaesthetics. Br J Anaesth. 2012;108:670–4.
12. Ueda K, Shields BE, Brennan TJ. Transesophageal echocardiography: a novel technique for guidance and placement of an epidural catheter in infants. Anesthesiology. 2013;118:219–22.
13. Tsui B, Leipoldt C, Desai S. Color flow Doppler ultrasonography can distinguish caudal epidural injection from intrathecal injection. Anesth Analg. 2013;116:1376–9.
14. Koo BN, Hong JY, Kim JE, Kil HK. The effect of flexion on the level of termination of the dural sac in paediatric patients. Anaesthesia. 2009;64:1072–6.
15. Koo BN, Hong JY, Song HT, Kim JM, Kil HK. Ultrasonography reveals a high prevalence of lower spinal dysraphism in children with urogenital anomalies. Acta Anaesthesiol Scand. 2012;56: 624–8.
16. Kim MS, Han KH, Kim EM, Jeong SH, Lee JR. The myth of the equiangular triangle for identification of sacral hiatus in children disproved by ultrasonography. Reg Anesth Pain Med. 2013;38: 243–7.
17. Willschke H, Machata AM, Rebhandl W, Benkoe T, Kettner SC, Brenner L, Marhofer P. Management of hypertrophic pylorus stenosis with ultrasound guided single shot epidural anaesthesia – a retrospective analysis of 20 cases. Pediatr Anesth. 2011;21:110–5.

Suggested Reading

Dalens B. Caudal anesthesia. In: Dalens B, editor. Regional anesthesia in infants, children, and adolescents. Philadelphia: Lippincott Williams & Wilkins; 1995. p. 171–94.

Dalens B. Lumbar epidural anesthesia. In: Dalens B, editor. Regional anesthesia in infants, children, and adolescents. Philadelphia: Lippincott Williams & Wilkins; 1995. p. 207–48.

Dalens B, Khandwala R. Thoracic and cervical epidural anesthesia. In: Dalens B, editor. Regional anesthesia in infants, children, and adolescents. Philadelphia: Lippincott Williams & Wilkins; 1995. p. 249–60.

Suresh S, Polaner DM, Cote CJ. Regional Anesthesia. In: Cote CJ, Lerman J, Anderson BJ, Eds. 5th ed. Philadelphia: WB Saunders; 2013. p. 835–79.

Tsui BC. Epidural anesthesia using electrical epidural stimulation and ultrasound guidance. In: Tsui BC, editor. Atlas of ultrasound and nerve stimulation-guided regional anesthesia. New York: Springer; 2007. p. 235–55.

Tsui BC. Caudal and epidural blockade. In: Tsui BC, editor. Atlas of ultrasound and nerve stimulation-guided regional anesthesia. New York: Springer; 2007. p. 271–93.

Spinal Anesthesia

34

Adam O. Spencer, Santhanam Suresh, and Ban C.H. Tsui

Contents

A.O. Spencer, MSc, MD, FRCPC
Vi Riddell Complex Pain and Rehabilitation Centre,
Alberta Children's Hospital, Calgary, AB, Canada
e-mail: adam.spencer@albertahealthservices.ca

S. Suresh, MD
Department of Pediatric Anesthesiology,
Ann & Robert Lurie Children's Hospital of Chicago,
Chicago, IL, USA

B.C.H. Tsui, Dip Eng, BSc (Math), B Pharm, MSc, MD, FRCPC (✉)
Department of Anesthesiology and Pain Medicine,
Stollery Children's Hospital/University of Alberta Hospital,
2-150 Clinical Sciences Building, Edmonton,
AB T6G 2G3, Canada
e-mail: btsui@ualberta.ca

B.C.H. Tsui, S. Suresh (eds.), *Pediatric Atlas of Ultrasound- and Nerve Stimulation-Guided Regional Anesthesia*,
DOI 10.1007/978-0-387-79964-3_34

34.1 Introduction

In 1885, James Leonard Corning administered the first spinal anesthetic published in a peer-reviewed medical journal [1]. It was not until 1901 that the use of spinal anesthesia in children was reported [2], and in 1909, Gray published the first pediatric case series [3]. Despite early pediatric successes and effective use of the technique in adults, it was not until the 1980s that the technique was resurrected for pediatric use by Abajian [4], who showed that spinal anesthesia could be used to mitigate the perioperative risks commonly associated with general anesthesia in the high-risk ex-premature neonate presenting for inguinal hernia repair. Today, spinal anesthesia continues to be most commonly used in neonates and infants when risk is increased with a general anesthetic.

It is important to be aware of some key age-dependent neuraxial anatomical differences between adult and pediatric patients with regard to spinal anesthesia, including:

- Conus medullaris: In early neonatal and infancy period, the spinal cord has been reported to extend to the L2–L3 level, whereas the conus ends at the L1–L2 level at 1 year of age and T12–L2 in adults [5] (Fig. 13.12).
- Dural sac: The dural sac of neonates and infants terminates more caudad at a level of S3 compared to adults at a level of S1.
- Subarachnoid space: The subarachnoid space is found at a much reduced depth in the pediatric patient. Compared to adults, there is a relationship between weight or body surface area and the depth to the subarachnoid space, especially in neonates and infants. Estimates of this depth increase from 10 to 15 mm at birth to 20 mm (3 years), 25 mm (5 years), and over 30 mm (10 years). In addition, the spinal canal space is also narrower, especially in the younger pediatric patient [6–8].
- Volume and distribution of cerebrospinal fluid (CSF): The total volume of CSF in infants has been estimated at 4 mL/kg vs. 2 mL/kg in adults, and there is a greater proportion of this volume in the spinal canal compared to adults. These are significant differences which may help explain the shorter duration of action of spinal anesthetics in infants despite a larger local anesthetic dose [9].

34.2 Indications

- Despite the use of spinal anesthesia for multiple procedures in pediatric anesthesia, it is usually restricted to infants, particularly premature infants with a history of apneas and bradycardias and chronic lung disease who would otherwise have received a general anesthetic or awake caudal block with high-dose local anesthetic [10].
- Some key advantages of a spinal anesthetic include:
  - Decreased use of sedatives and opioids and avoidance of airway manipulation
  - Quick onset
  - Favorable surgical conditions with complete sensory and motor block
  - Rapid postoperative recovery
- The technique is not limited to the premature population and has been used extensively in healthy and at-risk pediatric patients of all ages for a variety of surgical procedures including general, orthopedic, urological, spine, and cardiac surgery [11].

34.2.1 Clinical Use and Special Concerns

Spinal anesthesia is commonly used for lower abdominal, urological, and lower limb surgery. There are important considerations prior to proceeding with a spinal anesthetic:

- Coagulation status: Clinical history is insufficient to detect coagulation abnormalities in neonates and infants aged less than 1 year. Coagulation status in the ex-premature neonate is recommended prior to proceeding with a spinal anesthetic. Coagulation tests, including prothrombin time (PT/INR), activated partial thromboplastic time (APTT), and platelet counts, should be compared against age-specific reference ranges. See "Suggested Reading" for additional information [12, 13].
- Length of surgery: Although dependent on the local anesthetic and use of adjuvants, as a sole single-injection technique, a spinal will last up to a maximum of approximately 90 min. If surgery time is expected to take more

than 60–75 min, there is risk of needing additional sedation or general anesthetic. An alternate anesthetic plan should always be readily available.

- Patient position during surgery: Immediately following postspinal injection, it is necessary to avoid raising the legs or trunk above the level of the head as this can cause a high anesthetic block.

34.2.2 Contraindications

- Contraindications include patient or parent refusal, presence or suspicion of coagulopathy, infection (local or systemic), hypovolemia, and raised intracranial pressure.
- Relative contraindications specific to spinal anesthesia include anatomical abnormality of the spine, the presence of degeneration of or diseases affecting the central nervous system, and the presence of ventriculoperitoneal shunts or intrathecal catheters.

34.3 Technique

34.3.1 Preparation

- Due to the limited duration of the spinal anesthetic, it is necessary to have good communication with the surgical staff and for the team to be readied to begin surgery once the spinal is complete.
- Skin topicalization using 4% tetracaine (amethocaine; Ametop®, AnGel®) 30 min prior to the procedure or eutectic mixture of local anesthetic cream of lidocaine and prilocaine (EMLA) 1 h prior to the procedure can offer some local anesthesia for both intravenous access and spinal access. The topical gel or cream may be covered using a 3M Tegaderm® dressing. Depending on the anesthetic goal and age of the child, a premedication may be used in addition to skin topicalization.
- We recommend intravenous access prior to completing the spinal anesthetic. Several reasons include:
  1. The possibility of delaying the surgical start after spinal anesthesia due to unforeseen difficulties obtaining vascular access.
  2. Venous access allows premedication with atropine (10 μg/kg) prior to completing the spinal.
  3. Acute complications following the spinal without immediate vascular access (e.g., high spinal, profound apnea) may be more challenging to manage.

34.3.2 Patient Positioning

- Following intravenous access and premedication with atropine (10 μg/kg), the patient is placed in a lateral decubitus or sitting position based on the anesthesiologist's preference. The lateral position may help to create a more optimal flexed position in an awake infant or in an older child who has received sedation.
- In the lateral position (Fig. 34.1), a trained assistant flexes the patient's legs at the knees and hips while the neck and shoulders are gently flexed forward with careful attention to maintain a patent airway, especially in neonates and infants. The flexed fetal position facilitates palpation of bony landmarks and increases the accessible area between spinous processes.
- An alternative position for infants is to have an assistant hold the patient in a sitting position with the hips flexed and the head flexed forward. Cooperative adolescent patients can assume this sitting position themselves with a trained assistant facing them for support. The advantage of the sitting position is to increase the CSF pressure in the lumbar region and improve CSF flow through the spinal needle.

34.3.3 Surface Anatomy

Important surface anatomy landmarks that should be identified prior to sonographic assessment of the spine include:

- Spinous processes to ascertain midline and to assess for abnormal spine curvature: Due to delayed fusion in neonates and infants, these may be palpable as two adjacent bony landmarks.
- Iliac crests: An imaginary line between the anterior iliac crests, commonly known as the intercristal (or Truffier's) line, will cross the L5–S1 interspace in neonates and infants less than 1 year old and L4–L5 in older children (Fig. 34.2).
- Shoulders: Ensure that the left shoulder is not rotated forward and that both shoulders remain square to the bed. This will help ensure effective upper trunk flexion and alignment of the thoracic and lumbar spine, which may help with eventual dural puncture success.

Optimal positioning cannot be overemphasized and, once established, the Tegaderm® dressing should be removed and the residual gel wiped off. Prior to the spinal attempt, a sonographic assessment of the lumbar spine should be completed.

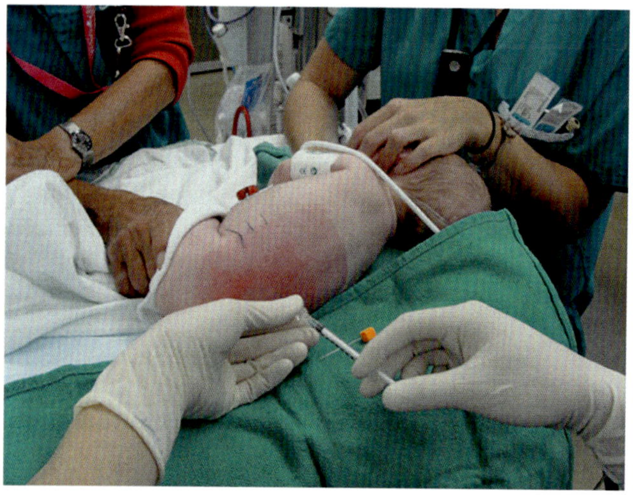

Fig. 34.1 Lateral positioning of patient for spinal anesthesia

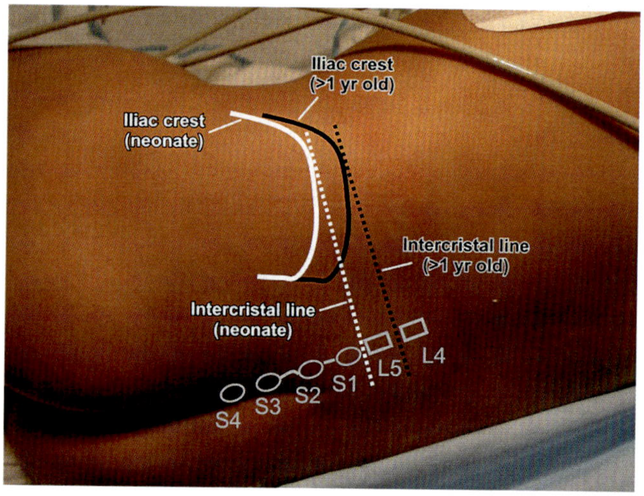

Fig. 34.2 Surface anatomy for pediatric spinal anesthesia. *White* and *black lines* indicate positions of iliac crests and intercristal line for neonates and children over 1 year old, respectively

34.3.4 Sonographic Assessment

- Sonographic assessment for spinal anesthesia is similar to that for lumbar epidural anesthesia (see Fig. 33.11). High-frequency (10–13 Hz) probes produce excellent resolution in small children and infants; however, in adolescents, the depth of neuraxial structures may necessitate a lower-frequency probe such as a curvilinear 2–6 MHz probe to gain adequate signal penetration.
- A wider footprint linear-array transducer (10–13 MHz) allows for an excellent median or paramedian longitudinal view. Occasionally, a paramedian longitudinal view provides better detail, but this usually adds little to a median view in neonates and infants that are less than 6 months of age.
- Expect the sonoanatomy to be excellent (>80 %) in children under 3 months of age, but it will gradually decline in quality to approximately 30–40 % by 9 months of age.
- There are significant benefits to completing a transverse and median or paramedian view of the lumbar spine prior to performing the spinal anesthetic. This allows one to:
  - Identify the lumbar and sacral levels prior to dural puncture.
  - Delineate the spinous processes and ideal needle trajectory.
  - Identify the conus medullaris to be confident that dural puncture is below the termination of the cord.
  - Estimate the depth to the subarachnoid space; the distance between skin and the dura can be estimated, which in neonates and infants can be narrow (6–8 mm) [6]. If significant pressure is used with the probe during the sonographic assessment, the estimated depth may be erroneous.
- Recently, it was demonstrated that real-time color flow Doppler ultrasound can be used to distinguish epidural injection from intrathecal injection (i.e., epidural injection produces a positive signal; intrathecal produces no signal) (see Fig. 33.22) [14].

Clinical Pearls

- Ultrasound may be useful for pre-scanning.
- Spinal anesthesia may be completed under real-time ultrasound guidance, but the merit of this approach is uncertain and may increase the risk of contamination due to the required extra equipment and personnel.

34.3.5 Nerve Stimulation Technique

The use of nerve stimulation to assist for spinal anesthesia in pediatric patients is not a common practice and therefore will not be described. However, the electrical epidural stimulation test can assist in distinguishing the epidural space (>1 mA) from the intrathecal space (<1 mA) when using an insulated needle (see Chap. 2) [15].

34.4 Equipment and Spinal Needle

- Similar to all regional anesthetic blocks, there should be strict adherence to aseptic technique.
- An absorbent pad should be placed between the warming blanket and the patient prior to the spinal anesthetic. Following the successful injection of the spinal anesthetic, the patient will occasionally have a bowel movement; an absorbent pad may be used to soak up these liquids that may otherwise inadvertently cool the patient over the course of the procedure.
- Once in position for the spinal, the skin should be prepped with a 2 % chlorhexidine gluconate and 70 % isopropyl alcohol solution and allowed to dry.
- A sterile clear plastic drape should be used, and a spinal needle and syringe containing the spinal anesthetic should be readily available.
- Ensure comfortable ergonomics for both the anesthesiologist and the assistant holding the patient. We suggest that the anesthesiologist sit for stability and improved dexterity when attempting a spinal on an awake younger pediatric patient in lateral decubitus position.
- If no topical gel or cream is used, infiltrate the skin with lidocaine 1 % using a 27G–30G needle prior to using the spinal needle.

34.4.1 Needles

- The lumbar puncture is performed using a midline approach, preferably with a short 25G–27G styletted spinal needle. The type of needle has not been shown to have an effect on success or postspinal complications in the pediatric population [16, 17]. However, a smaller needle size could reduce the risk of post-dural puncture headache which is difficult to assess in this population.
- Various types of spinal needles are available in pediatric sizes. Our approach is to use a 2.5 cm, 25G pencil-point needle (Pencan® Paed, B.Braun, Melsungen, Germany) and, if not successful, a 3.8 cm, 22G Quincke spinal needle. An introducer is not necessary in neonates and young infants.
- In children, the ligamentum flavum is soft, and a distinctive "pop" may not be appreciated when the dura is punctured.
- It is important to remove the stylet intermittently and examine for CSF flow. Initial CSF may be slightly blood tinged; ensure continued flow of clear fluid prior to injection of the anesthetic.
- In neonates and young infants, use a 1 mL syringe (tuberculin syringe with clear gradations) to inject the drug slowly. A good rule of thumb is to inject over a 15–20 s period while avoiding the barbotage method as it may result in unacceptably high levels of motor blockade.
- Once the subarachnoid block is performed, avoid elevating the legs or lower trunk. This will help to prevent cephalad spread of local anesthetic and is especially important during the application of the return pad which is typically fixed to the backs of neonates and young infants.

34.5 Local Anesthetics

- Many drugs have been used for pediatric spinal anesthesia in variable doses for various surgical procedures. These drugs have been used as sole agents and also in combination with sedation and general anesthesia. Intrathecal agents used in the pediatric population include bupivacaine, tetracaine, lidocaine, ropivacaine, and levobupivacaine; adjuvants include morphine, fentanyl, clonidine, epinephrine, neostigmine, and dextrose.
- The commonly used local anesthetics for pediatric spinal anesthesia include bupivacaine and tetracaine. Generally, a dose of 0.4–1 mg/kg of tetracaine or bupivacaine for spinal anesthesia will offer favorable surgical anesthesia. Higher doses per kg are preferred in the pediatric population, but the risk of a total spinal is rare as long as the procedure is carried out diligently. At our institution, the drug of choice is preservative-free plain bupivacaine 0.5 %. In neonates and infants weighing 5 kg or less, preservative-free plain bupivacaine 0.5 %, 1 mg/kg (0.2 mL/kg) is an effective dose that will provide 60 min of surgical anesthesia for inguinal hernia repair. Unfortunately, data for children outside the neonatal and infant stages are limited. As a general guide, the following suggested doses may be used:
  - 0.3–0.5 mg/kg bupivacaine 0.5 % for children 2 months to 12 years of age
  - 0.3–0.4 mg/kg hyperbaric tetracaine in children aged 12 weeks to 2 years
  - 0.2–0.3 mg/kg hyperbaric tetracaine in older children of >2 years

34.5.1 Adjuvants

- Clonidine (1 μg/kg) added to bupivacaine (1 mg/kg) has been used in spinal anesthesia in neonates and infants weighing 5 kg or less and provides almost twice the duration of spinal anesthesia when compared to local anesthetic alone [18]. Raising the intrathecal clonidine dose to 2 μg/kg provided no added benefit with propensity for transient drops in blood pressures intraoperatively and increased sedation in the postoperative period in this age group.
- The use of intravenous caffeine (5–10 mg/kg) has been shown to prevent potential apnea in the postoperative period, especially if clonidine is used in the spinal anesthetic solution [18, 19].
- An epinephrine washout of a tuberculin syringe may be preferred to a standard dose of intrathecal epinephrine (e.g., 0.01 mL/kg of 1:100,000 diluted epinephrine) for extending spinal block duration.
- When compared to a eubaric solution, hyperbaric solution with dextrose does not seem to alter the duration of the spinal block in children.

See Table 34.1 for a summary of suggested local anesthetics and adjuvants.

Table 34.1 Dosages of local anesthetics and additives for spinal anesthesia

Local anesthetic solution	
Bupivacaine	0.3–1 mg/kg
Tetracaine	0.4–1 mg/kg
Additives	
Epinephrine washout	
Clonidine	1 μg/kg
Morphine	5 μg/kg for postoperative analgesia in general pediatric procedures (e.g., scoliosis repair)
	10 μg/kg for cardiac surgical patients who will be ventilated postoperatively

34.6 Assessment of the Block Level

- Assessment of the sensory and motor block can be challenging, especially in neonates, small children, and sedated patients.
- In infants, response to cold stimuli (e.g., ice wrapped in a glove or an alcohol swab) can be used.
- A Bromage score (see Table 34.2) [20], which is the gold standard, can usually be obtained for children greater than 2 years of age.
- If a rapidly rising level of blockade is noted, the patient may be placed in reverse Trendelenburg position to prevent further cephalad spread of local anesthetic.

34.7 Complications

- The most common complications include multiple attempts, sensory and motor block failure requiring supplemental anesthetic, and surgical procedure outlasting the block.
- Other less common complications include bleeding and hematoma, infection, allergic reaction, local anesthetic toxicity, cardiovascular complications, and nerve injury. The risk of methemoglobinemia is present with the use of tetracaine.
- Although possible complications include post-dural puncture headache and transient radicular symptoms, these are less commonly reported in children.

Table 34.2 Bromage scale for spinal block assessment

Grade	Criteria	Degree of block
I	Free movement of legs and feet	Nil 0 %
II	Just able to flex knees with free movement of feet	Partial 33 %
III	Unable to flex knees but with free movement of feet	Almost complete 66 %
IV	Unable to move legs or feet	Complete 100 %

34.8 Current Literature in Ultrasound-Guided Approaches

There is limited literature regarding the use of ultrasound for spinal anesthesia in the pediatric population, as the landmark technique has traditionally been used with success in children. However, as discussed above, ultrasound has potential value in identifying neuraxial structures and verifying the presence of anatomic abnormalities if they are present. Koo et al. [21] demonstrated that ultrasound could be used on children with urogenital abnormalities to identify occult spinal dysraphism. Further discussion of the use of pre-procedural ultrasound scanning for neuraxial blocks is found in a review by Chin and Perlas [22].

34.9 Case Study

Case Study: Spinal Anesthetic (*Contributed by A. Spencer*)

A 56-day-old baby presented for repair of bilateral inguinal hernias. This triplet was born at 30 weeks gestational age and, at time of surgery, weighed 2.48 kg. After birth, the patient remained in the neonatal intensive care unit for 5 weeks due to apneic episodes associated with bradycardia and due to dietary issues and was ultimately discharged home at 36 weeks corrected age. She had no known drug allergies and was on no regular medications except for daily iron and multivitamins.

Thirty minutes prior to the spinal anesthetic, Ametop gel (tetracaine 4 %) was applied to the L3–L5 lumbar spinal level and covered with a Tegaderm® dressing. After induction with sevoflurane (up to 4 %), the patient was placed in left lateral decubitus position and held in fetal position by an operative nurse. The dressing was removed and the residual gel wiped off, and the skin was prepped with a 2 % chlorhexidine gluconate and 70 % isopropyl alcohol swab. A linear-array transducer (10–13 MHz) was used to image the patient's spine in a paramedian longitudinal view (Fig. 34.3). An assessment of the spinous processes, identification of lumbar levels, and assessment of the depth to the posterior dura and spinal cord and tip of the conus medullaris were completed. The sonogram of the lumbosacral region was then used to mark an entry level that would be below the conus. A 2.5 cm, 25G styletted spinal needle was used for dural puncture. Once cerebrospinal solution was found, 0.2 mL/kg (for a total volume of 0.5 mL) of preservative-free bupivacaine 0.5 % was slowly injected over 20 s. Block duration was 70 min; duration of surgery was 50 min.

Acetaminophen 15 mg/kg p.o. liquid was given preoperatively and q6h postoperatively for 48 h. The patient was comfortable 30 min post-op. The patient spent the next 24 h under observation in the pediatric intensive care unit due to her age and prematurity and history of apneas and bradycardia. This observation period was uneventful, and the patient was discharged home the next day.

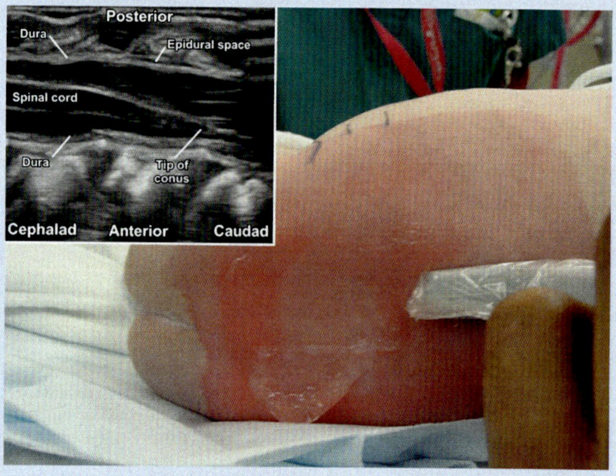

Fig. 34.3 Paramedian longitudinal ultrasound scan of neuraxial structures in an infant (see "Case Study" for details)

References

1. Frawley G, Ingelmo P. Spinal anaesthesia in the neonate. Best Pract Res Clin Anaesthesiol. 2010;24(3):337–51.
2. Bainbridge WS. A report of twelve operations on infants and young children using spinal analgesia. Arch Pediatr. 1901;18:570–4.
3. Gray HT. A study of spinal anaesthesia in children and infants. Lancet. 1909;2:913–7.
4. Abajian JC, Mellish RW, Browne AF, Perkins FM, Lambert DH, Mazuzan Jr JE. Spinal anesthesia for surgery in the high-risk infant. Anesth Analg. 1984;63:359–62.
5. Kesler H, Dias M, Kalapos P. Termination of the normal conus medullaris in children: a whole-spine magnetic resonance imaging study. Neruosurg Focus. 2007;23:E7.
6. Arthurs MM, Zubier M, Tooley J, Kelsall W. Ultrasonographic determination of neonatal spinal canal depth. Arch Dis Child Fetal Neonatal Ed. 2008;93:F451–4.
7. Bonadio W, Smith D, Metrou M, et al. Estimating lumbar-puncture depth in children. N Engl J Med. 1988;319:952–3.
8. Shenkman Z, Rathaus V, Jedeikin R, et al. The distance from the skin to the subarachnoid space can be predicted in premature and former-premature infants. Can J Anaesth. 2004;51:160–2.
9. Cote CJ, Lerman J, Todres ID. A practice of anesthesia for infants and children. Saunders, Elsevier: Philadelphia; 2009. Chapter 42 regional anesthesia, p. 877.
10. Cote CJ, Zaslavsky A, Downes JJ, Kurth CD, Welborn LG, Warner LO, Malviya SV. Postoperative apnea in former preterm infants after inguinal herniorrhaphy. A combined analysis. Anesthesiology. 1995;82:809–22.
11. Tobias JD. Spinal anaesthesia in infants and children. Pediatr Anesth. 2000;10:5–16.
12. Andrew M, Paes B, Milner R, Johnston M, Mitchell L, Tollefsen DM, Castle V, Powers P. Development of the human coagulation system in the healthy premature infant. Blood. 1988;72:1651–7.
13. De Saint Blanquat L, Simon L, Laplace C, Egu JF, Hamza J. Preoperative coagulation tests in former preterm infants undergoing spinal anaesthesia. Pediatr Anesth. 2002;12(4):304–7.
14. Tsui B, Leipoldt C, Desai S. Color flow Doppler ultrasonography can distinguish caudal epidural injection from intrathecal injection. Anesth Analg. 2013;116(6):1376–9.
15. Tsui BC, Wagner AM, Cunningham K, Perry S, Desai S, Seal R. Can continuous low current electrical stimulation distinguish insulated needle position in the epidural and intrathecal spaces in pediatric patients? Pediatr Anesth. 2005;15(11):959–63.
16. Kokki H, Heikkinen M, Turunen M, et al. Needle design does not affect the success rate of spinal anaesthesia or the incidence of postpuncture complications in children. Acta Anaesthesiol Scand. 2000;44:210–3.
17. Kokki H, Salonvaara M, Herrgard E, Onen P. Postdural puncture headache is not an age-related symptom in children: a prospective, open-randomized, parallel group study comparing a 22-gauge Quincke with a 22-gauge Whitacre needle. Pediatr Anesth. 1999;9:429–34.
18. Rochette A, Raux O, Troncin R, Dadure C, Verdier R, Capdevilla X. Clonidine prolongs spinal anesthesia in newborns: a prospective dose-ranging study. Anesth Analg. 2004;98(1):56–9.
19. Henderson-Smart DJ, Steer PA. Prophylactic caffeine to prevent postoperative apnoea following general anaesthesia in preterm infants. Cochrane Database Syst Rev. 2001;4:CD000048.
20. Bromage PR. A comparison of the hydrochloride and carbon dioxide salts of lidocaine and prilocaine in epidural analgesia. Acta Anaesthesiol Scand Suppl. 1965;16:55–69.
21. Koo BN, Hong JY, Song HT, Kim JM, Kil HK. Ultrasonography reveals a high prevalence of lower spinal dysraphism in children with urogenital anomalies. Acta Anaesthesiol Scand. 2012;56: 624–8.
22. Chin KJ, Perlas A. Ultrasonography of the lumbar spine for neuraxial and lumbar plexus blocks. Curr Opin Anaesthesiol. 2011;24: 567–72.

Suggested Reading

Dalens BJ. Spinal anesthesia. In: Dalens BJ, editor. Pediatric regional anesthesia. Boca Raton: CRC Press; 1990. p. 417–35.

Ganesh A, Kim A, Casale P, Cucchiaro G. Low-dose intrathecal morphine for postoperative analgesia in children. Anesth Analg. 2007;104:271–6.

López T, Sánchez FJ, Garzón JC, Muriel C. Spinal anesthesia in pediatric patients. Minerva Anestesiol. 2012;78:78–87.

Suresh S, Polaner DM, Cote CJ. Regional Anesthesia. In: Cote CJ, Lerman J, Anderson BJ, Eds. 5th ed. Philadelphia: WB Saunders; 2013. p. 835–79.

Puncuh F, Lampugnani E, Kokki H. Use of spinal anaesthesia in paediatric patients: a single centre experience with 1132 cases. Pediatr Anesth. 2004;14:564–7.

Rowney DA, Doyle E. Epidural and subarachnoid blockade in children. Anaesthesia. 1998;53:980–1001.

Saint-Maurice C. Spinal anesthesia. In: Dalens B, editor. Regional anesthesia in infants, children, and adolescents. Philadelphia: Lippincott Williams & Wilkins; 1995. p. 261–73.

Troncin R, Dadure C. Paediatric spinal anaesthesia. Update Anaesth. 2009;25:20–4.

Index

B.C.H. Tsui, S. Suresh (eds.), *Pediatric Atlas of Ultrasound- and Nerve Stimulation-Guided Regional Anesthesia*,
DOI 10.1007/978-0-387-79964-3

O

P

T

V

W

Y

Z